# From Acute to Chronic Back Pain

# From Acute to Chronic Back Pain

# Risk Factors, Mechanisms, and Clinical Implications

Edited by

## Monika I. Hasenbring
Department of Medical Psychology and Medical Sociology,
Faculty of Medicine,
Ruhr-University,
Bochum, Germany

## Adina C. Rusu
Department of Medical Psychology and Medical Sociology,
Faculty of Medicine,
Ruhr-University,
Bochum, Germany,
Department of Psychology, Royal Holloway,
University of London,
London, UK

## Dennis C. Turk
School of Medicine,
University of Washington,
Seattle, Washington, USA

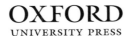

OXFORD
UNIVERSITY PRESS

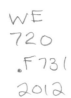

# OXFORD
UNIVERSITY PRESS

Great Clarendon Street, Oxford ox2 6DP

Oxford University Press is a department of the University of Oxford.
It furthers the University's objective of excellence in research, scholarship,
and education by publishing worldwide in

Oxford New York

Auckland Cape Town Dar es Salaam Hong Kong Karachi
Kuala Lumpur Madrid Melbourne Mexico City Nairobi
New Delhi Shanghai Taipei Toronto

With offices in

Argentina Austria Brazil Chile Czech Republic France Greece
Guatemala Hungary Italy Japan Poland Portugal Singapore
South Korea Switzerland Thailand Turkey Ukraine Vietnam

Oxford is a registered trade mark of Oxford University Press
in the UK and in certain other countries

Published in the United States
by Oxford University Press Inc., New York

British Library Cataloguing in Publication Data
Data available

Library of Congress Cataloging in Publication Data
Library of Congress Control Number: 2011943637

Typeset in Minion by Cenveo, Bangalore, India
Printed and bound by
CPI Group (UK) Ltd, Croydon, CR0 4YY

ISBN 978–0–19–955890–2

10 9 8 7 6 5 4 3 2 1

# Preface

Chronic back pain has been and continues to be a major cause of distress (both to people with persistent pain and their significant others), disability, work loss, and costs to society. Moreover, with the aging population, it is becoming even more prevalent and as a consequence is having an escalating impact upon the healthcare systems and society as a whole worldwide. A significant issue concerns understanding why, although the majority of people with acute back symptoms recover in a reasonable time, a significant minority evolve into patients with chronic pain and prolonged pain-related disability. Understanding the variables that contribute to chronicity could serve as a basis for early intervention to prevent the downward spiral. A growing number of studies have been conducted designed to discover predictors of chronicity and clinical trials have been initiated in an attempt to identify targets for intervention. To date there have been no volumes that have attempted to compile this research in a single source or that integrate the results of available studies in order to facilitate prevention and intervention in practice.

The identification of clinically relevant risk factors in low back pain has broad practical implications for the healthcare system globally. During the past 15 years, psychosocial risk factors and psychobiological mechanisms have been identified as important risk factors and have led to the development of early screening methods (e.g. 'yellow flag' diagnostics) and new psychosocial interventions by targeting treatment modalities to patients' particular characteristics and needs (risk factor-based interventions for pain and pain-related disability). Research is evolving from asking 'What treatments work?' to a set of inter-related questions: 'What treatments are most effective to people with what set of characteristics, provided when, on what outcome measures, compared to what alternatives, and at what costs?'. However, substantial aspects of the pathway from acute to chronic pain still remain unexplained. Recent neurobiological paradigms investigating genetic, neurophysiological, and biomechanical processes elucidate important mechanisms of chronic back pain, which represent important pathways from acute to chronic pain. We hope that these paradigms will lead to the development of new pharmacological and non-pharmacological treatment approaches, which might establish evidence that supports a comprehensive approach to assessment and treatment of back pain spanning the entire spectrum from acute through prevention and treatment of chronic pain and disability. Early and more appropriate interventions are needed to prevent long-term, disabling back pain with accompanying socioeconomic consequences.

This book was conceived following a series of discussions at international conferences and symposia about the future of evidence-based pain science and research between the three of us several years ago. We felt that there was an absence of a single volume that integrated the large but disparate body of knowledge of numerous specialties—medicine, psychology, and physiotherapy. The major aim of the symposia that preceded the development of the current publication was to present advances in basic pain research with a view to their relevance for the transition from acute to chronic pain. Thus, the meetings presented an opportunity for some of the most prominent pain scientists to present and critically discuss their current findings in an interdisciplinary setting. These conferences proved to be extremely stimulating to all parties and it revealed that much knowledge needs to be synthesized and transferred from research to the clinical practice. We hope that this book will fill a void by translating basic pain research to clinical practice in back pain.

The volume should be of equal interest to clinicians from multiple and diverse specialties who are involved in the treatment of back pain patients, as well as to pain researchers. Clinicians working with back pain patients and wanting to understand more about the basic mechanisms underlying back pain as well as novel developments in the clinical science will find a wealth of information in this book. To our knowledge, no other book has exactly this focus, and we hope that it may contribute to further increase the collaboration and the exchange of information between back pain experts and basic pain scientists.

We focused on three main themes in conceptualizing this text: (1) the mechanisms involved in the transition from acute to persistent pain; (2) the concept of treatment-relevant subgroups; and (3) how available research evidence can inform the prevention management of acute and chronic back pain. The volume brings together an internationally renowned group of contributors who are recognized as experts in their fields. It is organized in six inter-related sections. In Part 1, we introduced current developments in pain epidemiology. We also included chapters on recent neurobiological paradigms investigating genetic, neurophysiological (Part 2), biomechanical processes (Part 3), and psychosocial mechanisms including fear-avoidance, endurance, cognitive processing, and significant others/behavioral (Part 4) that may represent important pathways from acute to chronic pain. Part 5 delineates important advances in the practitioner's role in the process of care. Parts 6 to 9 summarize important advances to diagnostics and treatment of acute, subacute, and chronic back pain. In these final sections we extended the approach of treatment-relevant subgroups further and provide ideas on how to relate those findings to the prevention management of acute, sub-acute, and chronic back pain and disability.

Multi-author books take some years from initial conceptualization to publication. Hopefully, that wait will have been worthwhile, both for those readers who have been aware of impending completion of the text and for the authors themselves. When drafting the first outline of the current edited volume, we intended to develop a book that would stimulate discussion and offers avenues of future investigation and collaboration. Publication of this volume should be viewed as a status report and serve as a stimulus for additional research as there remains much that is not understood and much needs to be learned to prevent chronic pain and pain-related disability. Clinicians should find the materials as a useful guide for approach patients with acute, subacute, and chronic pain but they need to continue to follow research developments to enhance their approaches as evidence becomes available.

Monika I. Hasenbring
Adina C. Rusu
Dennis C. Turk
*Bochum, Germany* and *Seattle, Washington, USA March 2011*

# Contents

# List of Contributors

**A. Vania Apkarian**
Department of Physiology
Northwestern University
Feinberg School of Medicine
Chicago, IL, USA

**Gordon J.G. Asmundson**
Department of Psychology
University of Regina
Regina, SK, Canada

**Katja Boersma**
Örebro University
Center for Health and Medical
Psychology (CHAMP)
Örebro, Sweden

**Kay Brune**
Department of Experimental and Clinical
Pharmacology and Toxicology
FAU Erlangen-Nuremberg
Erlangen, Germany

**Kim Burton**
Spinal Research Unit
University of Huddersfield
Huddersfield, UK

**Annmarie Cano**
Department of Psychology
Wayne State University
Detroit, MI, USA

**R. Nicholas Carleton**
Department of Psychology
University of Regina
Regina, SK, Canada

**Peter R. Croft**
Arthritis Research Campaign
National Primary Care Centre
Keele University
Keele, UK

**Kate M. Dunn**
Arthritis Research Campaign
National Primary Care Centre
Keele University
Keele, UK

**Ida Flink**
Center for Health and Medical
Psychology
Örebro University
Örebro, Sweden

**Herta Flor**
Department of Cognitive and
Clinical Neuroscience
Central Institute of Mental Health
University of Heidelberg
Mannheim, Germany

**Sarah Gibson**
Meli Orhtopedics
Ft Lauderdale, FL, USA

**Richard H. Gracely**
Center for Neurosensory Disorders
University of North Carolina
Chapel Hill, NC, USA

**Dirk Hallner**
Department of Medical Psychology
and Medical Sociology
Faculty of Medicine
Ruhr-University of Bochum
Bochum, Germany

**Hermann O. Handwerker**
Department of Physiology &
Pathophysiology
Friedrich-Alexander Universität
Erlangen/Nürnberg
Erlangen, Germany

**Monika I. Hasenbring**
Department of Medical Psychology
and Medical Sociology
Faculty of Medicine
Ruhr-University of Bochum
Bochum, Germany

**Mark P. Jensen**
Department of Rehabilitation
Medicine
University of Washington
Seattle, WA, USA

**Sandra Kamping**
Department of Cognitive and
Clinical Neuroscience
Central Institute of Mental Health
University of Heidelberg
Mannheim, Germany

**Nicholas A.S. Kendall**
Health Services Consultant
Surbiton, Surrey, UK

**Robert D. Kerns**
Departments of Psychiatry, Neurology,
and Psychology
Yale University
West Haven, CT, USA; and
VA Central Office, and
Psychology Service
VA Connecticut Healthcare System
West Haven, CT, USA

**Bernhard W. Klasen**
Department of Medical Psychology
and Medical Sociology
Faculty of Medicine
Ruhr-University of Bochum
Bochum; and
Algesiologikum
Munich, Germany

**Bart Koes**
Department of General Practice
ErasmusMC-University Medical
Center Rotterdam
Rotterdam, The Netherlands

**Laura Leong**
Department of Psychology
Wayne State University
Detroit, MI, USA

**Steven J. Linton**
Center for Health and Medical Psychology
Örebro University
Örebro, Sweden

**John D. Loeser**
Departments of Neurological Surgery and
Anesthesiology and Pain Medicine,
University of Washington,
Seattle, WA, USA

**Gary J. Macfarlane**
Aberdeen Pain Research Collaboration
Epidemiology Group
University of Aberdeen
Aberdeen, UK

**Chris G. Maher**
The George Institute for
International Health
The University of Sydney
Sydney, Australia

**Chris J. Main**
Arthritis Research Campaign
National Primary Care Centre
Keele University
Keele, UK

**Anne F. Mannion**
Spine Center Division
Department of Research and Development
Schulthess Klinik
Zürich, Switzerland

**Marc O. Martel**
Department of Psychology
McGill University
Montreal, QC, Canada

**Arne May**
Department of Systems Neuroscience
University of Hamburg
Hamburg, Germany

**John McBeth**
Arthritis Research UK
Epidemiology Unit
University of Manchester
Manchester, UK

**Lance M. McCracken**
Health Psychology Section
Department of Psychology
Institute of Psychiatry
King's College London
London, UK

**Julia Metzner**
Institute of Pharmaceutical Chemistry
Goethe-University,
Frankfurt, Germany

**Michael K. Nicholas**
Pain Management Research Institute
University of Sydney at Royal North
Shore Hospital
St Leonards, NSW, Australia

**Warren R. Nielson**
Department of Medicine (Rheumatology)
University of Western Ontario and
St Joseph's Health Care
London, ON, Canada

**David O'Riordan**
Spine Center Division
Department of Research and Development
Schulthess Klinik
Zürich, Switzerland

**Tamar Pincus**
Department of Psychology
Royal Holloway
University of London
London, UK

**Andrea Power**
Human Pain Research Group
Hope Hospital
Salford, UK

**Glenn S. Pransky**
Liberty Mutual Research Institute for Safety
Hopkinton; and
University of Massachusetts Medical School
Worcester, MA, USA

**James Rainville**
Department of Physical Medicine and
Rehabilitation
Harvard Medical School, Boston;
New England Baptist Hospital
Boston, MA, USA

**Bertold Renner**
Department of Experimental and
Clinical Pharmacology and Toxicology
FAU Erlangen-Nuremberg
Erlangen, Germany

**James P. Robinson**
Department of Rehabilitation Medicine
University of Washington
Seattle, WA, USA

**Adina C. Rusu**
Department of Medical Psychology
and Medical Sociology
Faculty of Medicine
Ruhr-University
Bochum, Germany;
Department of Psychology,
Royal Holloway,
University of London,
London, UK

**Rita Santos**
Department of Psychology
Royal Holloway
University of London
London, UK

**William S. Shaw**
Liberty Mutual Research Institute
for Safety
Hopkinton; and
University of Massachusetts
Medical School
Worcester, MA, USA

**Rob J.E.M. Smeets**
Centre of Expertise in Rehabilitation and
Audiology
Adelante, Hoensbroek; and
Department of Rehabilitation Medicine
Caphri, Maastricht University,
Maastricht University Medical Centre
Maastricht, The Netherlands

**Blair H. Smith**
Medical Research Institute
University of Dundee
Dundee, UK

**J. Bart Staal**
Scientific Institute for Quality of Healthcare
Radboud University Medical Centre
Nijmegen, The Netherlands

**Michael J.L. Sullivan**
Departments of Psychology, Medicine
and Neurology
McGill University
Montreal, QC, Canada

**Pradeep Suri**
Department of Physical Medicine and
Rehabilitation
Harvard Medical School
Boston, MA USA; and
VA Boston Healthcare System
Boston, MA, USA

**Irmgard Tegeder**
Institute of Clinical Pharmacology
Goethe-University,
Frankfurt, Germany

**Kati Thieme**
Department of Medical Psychology
Philipps-University Marburg
Marburg, Germany

**Nicola Torrance**
Medical Research Institute
University of Dundee
Dundee, UK

**Dennis C. Turk**
Department of Anesthesiology
University of Washington
Seattle, WA, USA

**Linda Vancleef**
Department Clinical Psychological Science
Faculty of Psychology and Neuroscience
Maastricht University
Maastricht, The Netherlands

**Maurits van Tulder**
Department of Health Sciences and EMGO
Institute for Health and Care Research
Faculty of Earth & Life Sciences
VU University
Amsterdam, The Netherlands

**Jeanine Verbunt**
Adelante, Center of Expertise in
Rehabilitation and Audiology,
Adelante, Hoensbroek; and
Department of Rehabilitation Medicine,
Maastricht University and Maastricht
University Medical Center, Maastricht, the
Netherlands

**Johan Vlaeyen**
Pain and Disability Research Program
University of Leuven
Leuven, Belgium; and
Department Clinical Psychological Science
Faculty of Psychology and Neuroscience
Maastricht University
Maastricht, The Netherlands

**Steven Vogel**
British School of Osteopathy,
London, UK

**Michael Von Korff**
Group Health Research Institute
Seattle, WA, USA

**Harriet Wittink**
Research group Lifestyle and Health
Utrecht University of Applied Sciences
Utrecht, The Netherlands

# List of abbreviations

| | | | |
|---|---|---|---|
| ABPS-MP | Attitudes to Back Pain Scale for Musculoskeletal Practitioners | DTI | diffusion tensor imaging |
| | | EEG | electroencephalography |
| ACT | Acceptance and Commitment Therapy | EER | eustress-endurance response |
| | | EMG | electromyographic |
| ACC | anterior cingulate cortex | FABQ | Fear Avoidance Beliefs Questionnaire for Health Care Practitioners |
| ACTH | adrenocorticotropin hormone | | |
| ADL | activity of daily living | | |
| AEM | avoidance-endurance model | FAM | fear-avoidance model |
| AEQ | Avoidance-Endurance Questionnaire | FAR | fear-avoidance response |
| | | fMRI | functional magnetic resonance imaging |
| ALBP | acute low back pain | | |
| APAP | acetaminophen (paracetamol) | fMRI | fibromyalgia |
| AS | anxiety sensitivity | FNE | fear of negative evaluation |
| ASA | acetylicsalicylacid | FR | flexion-relaxation |
| BBQ | Back Beliefs Questionnaire | GI | gastrointestinal |
| BCI | brain–computer interface | GivE | graded in vivo exposure |
| BDI | Beck Depression Inventory | GnIH | gonadotropin inhibitory hormone |
| CA | central augmentation | GnRH | gonadotropin-releasing hormone |
| CBA | cognitive-behavioural approach | GP | general practitioner |
| CBP | chronic back pain | GWAS | genome-wide association studies |
| CBT | cognitive-behavioural therapy | HCP | healthcare professional |
| CCBT | contextual cognitive-behavioural therapy | HC-PAIRS | Health Care Providers Pain and Impairment Relationship Scale |
| CI | confidence interval | HPA | hypothalamic–pituitary–adrenal |
| CLBP | chronic low back pain | HPG | hypothalamic–pituitary–gonadal |
| COX | cyclo-oxygenase | HPGH | hypothalamic–pituitary–growth hormone |
| CPAQ | Chronic Pain Acceptance Questionnaire | | |
| | | IBCT | integrative behavioural couple therapy |
| CRH | corticotrophin releasing hormone | | |
| CSQ | Coping Strategies Questionnaire | IIS | illness/injury sensitivity |
| CST | coping skills training | IMF | initial median frequency |
| CT | computed tomography | IU | intolerance of uncertainty |
| CV | cardiovascular | IW | injured worker |
| CWP | chronic widespread pain | KPI | Kiel Pain Inventory |
| DER | distress-endurance response | LP | lumbopelvic |
| DHEA-s | dehydroepiandrosterone-sulphate | MAAS | Mindful Attention Awareness Scale |
| DLBP | disabling low back pain | MEG | magnetoencephalographic |
| DLPFC | dorsolateral prefrontal cortex | MET | metabolic equivalent |
| DNIC | diffuse noxious inhibitory control | MF | median frequency |
| DRAM | Distress Risk Assessment Method | MHPG | 3-methoxy-4-hydroxyphenylglycol |

| | |
|---|---|
| MMPI | Minnesota Multiphasic Personality Inventory |
| MPF | mean power frequency |
| mPFC | medial prefrontal cortex |
| MPI | Multidimensional Pain Inventory |
| MPRCQ | Multidimensional Pain Readiness to Change Questionnaire |
| MRI | magnetic resonance imaging |
| NPV | negative predictive value |
| NSAID | non-steroidal anti-inflammatory drug |
| NSAID | non-steroidal, antiphlogistic, inflammatory drugs |
| ÖMPSQ | Örebro Musculoskeletal Pain Screening Questionnaire |
| PAG | periaqueductal grey |
| PAIRS | Pain and Impairment Relationship Scale |
| PAL | physical activity in daily life |
| PAL | physical activity level |
| PARIS-CBA | pain risk screening-based cognitive-behavioural approaches |
| PASS | Pain Anxiety Symptoms Scale |
| PASS-20 | Pain Anxiety Symptoms Scale-20 |
| PCS | Pain Catastrophizing Scale |
| PDP | Pain-Disability Prevention [Programme] |
| PET | positron emission tomography |
| PFC | prefrontal cortex |
| PHODA | Photograph Series of Daily Activities |
| PMS | Positive Mood Scale |
| POMC | proopiomelanocortin |

| | |
|---|---|
| PPI | proton-pump inhibitors |
| PPV | positive predictive value |
| PSOCQ | Pain Stages of Change Questionnaire |
| RCBI | risk factor-based cognitive-behavioural interventions |
| RCT | randomized controlled trial |
| RER | respiratory exchange ratio |
| RISC-BP | RIsk SCreening of Back Pain |
| ROC | receiver operator curve |
| ROM | range of motion |
| RTW | return to work |
| SBDT | STarT Back Decision Tool |
| S-CST | spouse-assisted coping skills training |
| sEMG | surface electromyography |
| SEMP | Schema Enmeshment Model of Pain |
| SLC | sick leave certification |
| SNAP | Schedule for Nonadaptive and Adaptive Personality |
| SSRI | serotonin reuptake inhibitors |
| SST | Self-System Therapy |
| TMD | temporomandibular disorder |
| TSK | Tampa Scale for Kinesiophobia |
| TSS | Thought Suppression Scale |
| TTM | Transtheoretical Model of Behaviour Change |
| UDE | unwanted drug effects |
| $VO_2$ | maximum oxygen intake |
| WC | workers' compensation |
| WHO | World Health Organization |

# Part 1

## Current Developments in Epidemiology

# Chapter 1

# Epidemiology of Back Pain, from the Laboratory to the Bus Stop: Psychosocial Risk Factors, Biological Mechanisms, and Interventions in Population-Based Research

Blair H. Smith, Nicola Torrance, and
Gary J. Macfarlane

## 1.1 Introduction

### 1.1.1 Goals of epidemiology—improving health

Epidemiology is defined by MacMahon and Pugh (1970) as 'the study of the distribution and determinants of disease frequency in man'. It has its origins in the early days of modern medicine and continues to develop its science and expand its roles. In recognition of this, Porta et al.'s *Dictionary of Epidemiology* (2008) extends the definition to imply greater clinical relevance, and describes 'the study of the occurrence and distribution of health-related states or events in specific populations, including the study of the determinants influencing such states, and the application of this knowledge to control health problems' (Porta et al. 2008). It is the latter part of this definition that makes epidemiology an important clinical discipline, particularly for chronic low back pain (CLBP), an important purpose being to inform the provision of health services. Rothman and Greenland (1998) suggest that the ultimate goal of epidemiology is to identify the causes of disease, but good epidemiological data on chronic pain will also provide valuable information on a wide range of important areas (Box 1.1).

Epidemiological research should, therefore, have as one of its ultimate goals the development of effective healthcare interventions, through an understanding of the distribution and determinants of illnesses (Porta et al. 2008). The last 20 years has seen a large number of population-based epidemiological studies of chronic pain, including back pain, and these have provided important information for educational and clinical service resource requirements, and for prevention and management strategies (Verhaak et al. 1998; Manchikanti 2000; Harstall and Ospina 2003). These studies have consistently demonstrated that chronic back pain is a highly prevalent condition, with an important detrimental impact on individuals' health, the healthcare services and society, and for which successful treatment outcomes are difficult to achieve.

CLBP is a heterogeneous group of clinical conditions, a minority of which are associated with a specific, demonstrable structural disorder (such as lumbar disc degeneration or ankylosing spondylitis), and many of which coexist with chronic pain at other anatomical sites. (Smith et al. 2004a) The International Association for the Study of Pain classifies well over 100 different diagnostic categories of (low) back pain, though good evidence for the epidemiology of most of these

## Box 1.1 Beneficial outcomes of epidemiological study of chronic low back pain (CLBP)*

Good epidemiological data on CLBP will provide information on:

◆ Its *distribution*—this will allow an understanding of the profile of CLBP in the community.

◆ Its *aetiology* (determinants)—clinical or demographic factors that are associated with the presence of CLBP will be revealed by epidemiological study, as will the identification of factors which lead to or favour chronicity of pain.

◆ Possible *preventive measures*—having an awareness of aetiological factors or associations will allow consideration of interventions at an early stage of the development of CLBP, either to prevent chronicity or to minimize its impact.

◆ Improving *prognosis*—even if CLBP cannot be prevented, knowledge of the factors associated with the development of severe CLBP should inform the clinical management of the condition, thereby possibly limiting severity and minimizing disability. This would be best informed by longitudinal studies of CLBP to distinguish between determinants and effects.

◆ The *impact* on quality of life—this will provide an understanding of the importance of CLBP, as well as knowledge of the factors which are associated with high levels of physical, psychological or social adverse effects.

◆ *Definition* and *classification*—if CLBP can be classified in a clinically relevant way, management strategies can be targeted at subgroups in greatest need of treatment or with the greatest likelihood of improvement, while individuals with less severe CLBP can be identified with a view to prevention of exacerbation.

◆ The *evaluation* of treatment strategies—until the distribution, determinants, impact, and natural history of CLBP are understood, it is impossible to properly evaluate any intervention aimed at improving chronic pain.

◆ Allocation of *health service resources*—ideally this should be informed by robust epidemiological data. With a condition of the importance of CLBP, it is therefore crucial that research information is available for health service planning.

◆ Allocation of *educational resources*—as with financial and clinical resources, appropriate education of professionals and patients can be greatly assisted by epidemiological study.

* Smith et al. 1996.

remains elusive, and the great majority (90%) of back pain cases have no identifiable cause in any case (Manek and MacGregor 2005). Given that the majority of CLBP is managed in primary care, if anywhere (Croft et al. 1998), where neither the facilities nor expertise generally exist to render such specific diagnosis feasible or appropriate, it is often practically necessary to consider low back pain (LBP) as a single global entity (after excluding 'red flag' diagnoses such as fracture and malignancy (Royal College of General Practitioners 1999)). This is also true of population-based epidemiological research, which generally relies on questionnaires or interviews administered by non-specialists. A site-specific case definition, perhaps enhanced by a criterion referring to back pain-related disability (Dionne et al. 2008) is therefore the most frequently encountered classification of back pain, both clinically and epidemiologically. Despite this lack of specificity in case definition, there is remarkable consistency in studies across the world and in different population groups, on the risk factors (particularly mechanical, psychological, and social) and therefore prospective intervention targets for CLBP.

We therefore need generic treatment strategies, including pharmacological and non-pharmacological approaches that can address CLBP as a global entity. This should be reflected in the epidemiological approach to seeking aetiological and risk factors, while also seeking a deeper understanding of sub-groups of CLBP that might benefit from more specific, targeted therapeutic approaches. This chapter will review the outcomes of this approach to the chronic pain continuum, and consider the potential rewards of adding measurement of biological factors to the knowledge and methods developed to date.

### 1.1.2 Recent success of epidemiology in improving understanding of CLBP

In studies of chronic pain in the general population and in primary care, prevalence estimates of back pain vary, and it is generally acknowledged that the quality of the data is variable, based on the primary purpose of the investigation, the population sampled, and the definition of back pain.

From cross-sectional surveys, point prevalence estimates of LBP range from 12–35% in the general adult population, with lifetime incidence ranging from 49–70% (Andersson 1999). The majority of people who experience an episode of back pain recover quickly without residual functional loss, and most of these episodes, appropriately, are never brought to the consulting room (Papageorgiou et al. 1996). Overall it is estimated that 60–70% of patients recover by 6 weeks, and 80–90% by 12 weeks (Andersson 1999). However, recovery after 12 weeks is slow and uncertain, and fewer than half of those individuals disabled for longer than 12 months return to work, and after 2 years of absence from work, the return to work rate is close to zero (Andersson 1999). CLBP is not just 'the same as acute back pain lasting longer', but the result of a complex interplay of physical, psychological, and social factors in tandem with the onset of neck pain (Jayson 1997). Despite the above data on recovery, Croft et al. (1998) found that the great majority (75%) of those consulting with LBP in primary care remain disabled and in pain one year after consultation. Although an inception cohort in a more recent Australian study found a higher recovery rate, around one-third still had not recovered (Henschke et al. 2008) after one year, and therefore back pain for which healthcare is sought must be considered a serious condition, with epidemiological approaches that address this as CLBP.

### 1.1.3 Defining LBP in epidemiology studies

Standardized definitions of LBP, as distinct, global clinical conditions, have been proposed to allow comparisons of data derived from epidemiological prevalence studies (Dionne et al. 2008) (Box 1.2), recognizing the above argument that, although LBP encompasses a heterogeneous group of conditions, there is merit in grouping them together for epidemiological study. The main aim in reaching consensus on definitions is to improve the validity of future comparison of LBP prevalence figures for different countries, age groups, settings and occupational groups, among others. (Dionne et al. 2008).

## 1.2 Risk factors for LBP already established in population-based research

Large epidemiological studies have contributed considerably to our knowledge about potentially modifiable factors associated with the onset and outcome of developing a new episode of back

## Box 1.2 Proposed standardized definitions of low back pain (LBP)*

The 'minimal' definition for use in epidemiological prevalence studies, where there are likely to be many constraints, is ascertained by positive responses to two questions:

- 'In the past four weeks, have you had any pain in your lower back?'
- 'If yes, was this pain bad enough to limit your usual activities or change your daily routine for more than one day?'

The 'optimal' definition, for use in focused studies where the investigators have space or time for multiple questions, is derived from the minimal definition plus add-on questions covering:

- Frequency and duration of symptoms.
- Additional measures of severity, sciatica, and exclusions.

* Dionne et al. 2008.

pain, and our understanding of the influences on whether such an episode becomes chronic. At a population level, these known risk factors include physical, psychological, and social variables and some (though not all) are amenable to medical intervention. The presence of LBP is associated with demographic factors including female gender, older age, lower social class, as well as lifestyle factors, including lack of physical activity, obesity, and smoking (Elliott et al. 1999; Manchikanti 2000; Macfarlane 2006). Employment status and occupational factors have also identified the role of perceived workload (Linton 2005), mechanical load, posture and whole body vibration (Lis et al. 2007; see also Chapter 19). Factors that are not modifiable can nonetheless point to other productive lines of research. For example, the consistent finding of female preponderance in all chronic pain conditions has led to hypothesized endocrine (Macfarlane et al. 2002) and genetic (Mogil 2003, 2004) explanations that illuminate our understanding of pain pathways in general, and may inform interventions. The most important clinical risk factor for chronic pain at a specific site appears to be pain: either non-chronic pain (Croft et al. 1998; McBeth et al. 2001; Smith et al. 2004b) or chronic pain at other anatomical sites (Bergman et al. 2002; Papageorgiou et al. 2002; Smith et al. 2004b). The more severe the pain, and the greater the number of pain sites, the more likely is subsequent severe chronic pain (Bergman et al. 2002; Elliott et al. 2002). This highlights the need to intervene effectively with all presentations of pain. Poor general health (Elliott et al. 2002; Smith et al. 2004b), and a family or personal history of other related conditions ('functional somatic syndromes') (Clauw and Chrousos 1997; Wessely et al. 1999; Gran 2003; Bergman et al. 2002) are also risk factors for chronic pain. Known important psychosocial risk factors implicated in the transition to CLBP include psychological distress, pain catastrophizing, depressive mood, and more severe, persistent, or disabling symptoms at presentation, and to a lesser extent somatization (Pincus et al. 2002; Linton 2005; Henschke et al. 2008). Similarly, coping style, in particular passive coping, has been shown to be associated with increased risk of chronicity (Pincus et al. 2002; Jones et al. 2006). One of the strongest markers for developing chronic pain is illness behaviour, specifically people who have a history of frequent consultation and onward referral to specialist care. It could be hypothesized that this identifies individuals with a predisposition to somatization with high health anxiety. However, health anxiety has not been demonstrated to be a good predictor of the onset of chronic pain and the association with illness behaviour has been reported to be independent of markers of somatization (McBeth et al. 2003). It is likely that many of these risk factors or risk markers are caused by earlier experiences of chronic pain, (Jones et al. 2007) as well as causing future chronic pain, (Magni et al. 1993) and the concept of 'bi-directional aetiology' is important (Von Korff 1999), as is the possibility of a shared common aetiological mechanism

In summary, we now have considerable knowledge (albeit incomplete) about the aetiology of LBP—in particular the role of mechanical factors, psychological factors, and the role of the social environment as well as beliefs and behaviours. Accordingly, there have been efforts to address these with the development and testing of clinical interventions specifically targeting those we believe to be risk factors. We will now consider how this knowledge has been translated into management strategies in primary care.

## 1.3 **Evidence on management for LBP in primary care**

Community-based psychosocial interventions and physical therapies modelled on established risk factors have been found, at best, to be of marginal benefit in reducing LBP (UK BEAM Trial Team 2004; Hay et al. 2005; Heymans et al. 2005; Jellema et al. 2005b; Von Korff et al. 2005) though some have been effective in highly selected secondary care samples, and there are examples of interventions that have improved attitudes towards chronic back pain (Williams et al. 1996; Morley et al. 1999; van Tulder et al. 2000; Buchbinder and Jolley 2004).

For non-pharmaceutical interventions, the best evidence for effective management is that advice to remain active improves both short-term and long-term functions (Hagen et al. 2005). However, a systematic review found that strengthening and stabilizing exercises alone with other conservative interventions showed only small benefits in either short-term pain relief or functional outcomes (Hayden et al. 2005). Similarly, trials of spinal manipulation, (Assendelft et al. 2004) when compared to other traditionally advocated therapies, showed no differences in effectiveness of treatment (for more information see Chapter 25).

Research over the past decade which has emphasized the importance of psychosocial factors in the development of chronic or recurrent back pain (Pincus et al. 2002; Linton 2005; van der Windt et al. 2008) has led to recent interventions looking to test the effectiveness of either behavioural or multidisciplinary treatment programmes aimed at tackling these psychological and psychosocial factors. A number of trials have been conducted in primary care settings, in which primary healthcare professionals were trained to provide psychosocial interventions (Frost et al. 2004; Hay et al. 2005; Jellema et al. 2005b). All of these studies have included an active 'control' treatment arm to represent 'usual or best care' and include: a trial of a brief pain management programme in primary care compared with physical treatment (so called hands-on versus hands-off physiotherapy) (Hay et al. 2005); one session of assessment and advice versus routine physiotherapy (Frost et al. 2004); and another trial that compared a 20-minute consultation with general practitioners (GPs) who were trained to identify and discuss any potential psychosocial barriers to recovery with usual care (Jellema et al. 2005b). In a number of trials in primary care, providers (physiotherapists, nurses, or GPs) have been trained to deliver an intervention that uses a cognitive behavioural approach to the psychosocial management of back pain (Frost et al. 2004; UK BEAM Trial Team 2004; Hay et al. 2005; Jellema et al. 2005b; van der Windt et al 2008) with, at best, only marginal benefit.

Despite the considerable knowledge accrued from large population-based studies, the results from trials of management in the community/primary have proved disappointing, with no or only very modest improvements in patient outcome when compared with usual care/active control treatments. Before concluding that previously reported interventions did not work we have to understand better why current trials appear not to be working. A number of possible explanations for these 'negative' findings have been proposed. This could be because our information on psychosocial factors is still insufficient, because the interventions need better targeting, and/or because we need to consider other definitions and measures of successful outcomes of treatment (such as return to work, or patient-determined outcomes), and evaluations of the delivery of interventions (Macfarlane et al. 2006). For example, Jellema et al (2005a) showed some changes in GP behaviour and patient perceptions as a result of a psychosocial intervention, but that GPs rarely identified the psychosocial factors at which to target the intervention. In a systematic review of prospective studies, Hartvigsen et al. (2004) found relatively weak evidence for any single type of psychosocial factor being an important determinant of future onset of LBP. Research could look to identify which *clusters* of psychosocial factors, rather than picking out individual factors, influence LBP onset and outcome and their mechanism(s) of influence, in order to target intervention studies to population subgroups exhibiting these clusters.

Recent evidence suggests that it may be difficult to distinguish specific treatment effects in trials of complex interventions for chronic pain (i.e. the precise intervention under evaluation) from non-specific treatment effects (such as the duration of consultation, or the interest shown in the patient) (Newton-John and Geddes 2008). The latter may actually be more important than the former, with the result that any specific effect is overshadowed by the effects of treatment given to both the control arm and the treatment arm of a randomized controlled trial. Further research is beginning to suggest useful ways of identifying and harnessing these non-specific effects (Newton-John and Geddes 2008; van der Windt et al. 2008).

In interventions involving specific techniques, such as cognitive behavioural approaches, it is important that consistent messages are delivered by all care providers involved. Future trials should look to implement methods to measure skills and competencies of care providers, the actual content and delivery of the provided treatment/intervention, and adherence to protocols by patients and care providers. One way of tackling these issues may involve utilizing a 'mixed methods' approach, for example, combining a detailed qualitative content analysis of video-taped recordings of the intervention, together with conventional quantitative outcome measures (Lamb et al. 2007). Further investigation of what participants understood about the programme is also warranted (Lamb et al. 2007; Lambeek et al. 2007).

The outcome of an intervention is likely to be dependent upon several important, pre-existing patient factors, and it is important to consider the tailoring of interventions to individuals, or targeting subgroups of individuals with specific interventions, depending on either clinical factors, sociodemographic characteristics, or the type and extent of risk factors (Hay et al. 2008). A retrospective attempt to address this by secondary analysis of a large clinical trial of physical therapy, however, found the intervention still to be only marginally effective (Underwood et al. 2007). Patient preference for different interventions may also exert an effect on outcome and there is some evidence that patients' expectations and preferences may modify the outcome of treatment (Linde et al. 2007). New trial designs, such as 'enriched enrolment, randomised withdrawal' (McQuay et al. 2008) may be appropriate for addressing this in the future.

Further epidemiological, methodological, and clinical research would be valuable in each of these areas, as well as in refining and validating the measures we have for identifying high-risk groups, particularly psychosocial measures. Alternatively, or in addition, attention could focus on the identification and assessment of other risk factors for CLBP, or on approaches to assessing known variables that have been identified as potential risk factors. Taken along with our existing knowledge, this new work could inform the design or development of new interventions for application in the community, where most CLBP arises and is managed (Smith 2001).

## 1.4 **Potential biological risk factors hypothesized from existing research**

Epidemiological study has therefore been most successful in identifying the psycho-social components of the bio-psycho-social model of CLBP, though this has yet to be converted into effective interventions at a population level. We should turn our attention to the biological component, therefore, with a view to enhancing our aetiological understanding of CLBP in the community, and, potentially, the outcome of interventions. Studies in animals, and relatively small studies in humans, have proposed important biological mechanism in the development of CLBP that warrant further exploration in population-based research.

### 1.4.1 **Neurological**

Our understanding of the neurological mechanisms of acute and chronic (back) pain continues to advance, rapidly in recent years as a result of developing technology. Neurological imaging techniques, including functional magnetic resonance imaging (fMRI), now allow new views of the central processing of pain, and have demonstrated features specific to individuals who have chronic pain conditions (Gracely et al. 2002; Borsook and Becerra 2003; Cook et al. 2004). Perhaps most importantly for the current discussion, objective neurological evidence of lower pain thresholds and higher sensitivities has been found in individuals with chronic pain compared to those without (Sorensen et al. 1998; Banic et al. 2004). A detailed systematic review of studies of brain mechanisms in pain perception and regulation demonstrated the existence of a 'brain network' for acute pain perception, with many studies revealing the anatomical locations of network components, and postulated the nociceptive system as a separate sensory system (Apkarian et al. 2005, see also Chapters 7 and 8 for more detail). It also found consistent differences in the activation of this network, in response to acute pain stimuli, between those who had chronic pain and those who had not (Apkarian et al. 2005). Important similarities *and* differences were demonstrated in the parts of network involved in different chronic pain conditions, such as fibromyalgia, cardiac pain, neuropathic pain, and different types of headache. With reference to chronic back pain, imaging and neurochemistry studies have identified reduced activity and grey matter density in the prefrontal cortex and thalamus areas of the brain compared with those without chronic back pain (Apkarian et al. 2004; Apkarian et al. 2005; Baliki et al. 2006, 2008; Grachev et al. 2000). It is claimed that these variations account for up to 80% of the variance in duration and intensity of chronic pack pain (Baliki et al. 2008), whereas the social and demographic factors described above account for a much smaller proportion. The reduction in grey matter volume was equivalent to between 10 and 20 years of normal ageing, with the amount of loss correlating positively with the duration of back pain (Apkarian et al. 2004). Different patterns of brain involvement were found between neuropathic and non-neuropathic back pain (Apkarian et al. 2004) and between back pain and other causes of chronic pain (Apkarian et al. 2005; Baliki et al. 2008). Extending this further, some of these activity patterns were reversed with analgesic treatment (Baliki et al. 2008), corresponding with symptomatic relief of chronic back pain. These findings provide some clues as to mechanisms of CLBP, and to its comorbidities, and may be helpful in the design of targeted treatment strategies. The prefrontal cortex areas involved are also those associated with certain emotional experiences, such as anxiety and depression, in whose presence the patterns of activation differ (Grachev et al. 2001, 2002, 2003). They are also co-located with regions concerned with the emotional view of the self, where a persistently negative response to suffering, and consequent maladaptive behaviour can be initiated (Melzack and Casey 1968; Baliki et al. 2006). These findings support the hypothesis (above) of shared aetiological mechanisms between these clinical conditions. The neurological findings also raise the possibility of biomarkers for chronic back pain or objective markers of response to treatment. These could be in the form of imaging (Baliki et al. 2008) or neurochemistry (Grachev et al. 2000).

It is important to note that the studies contributing to our understanding of neural mechanisms of CLBP have, for excellent practical reasons, been cross-sectional, on small sample sizes. As such, they need confirmation in other populations and in larger samples, where their importance at a population level can also be assessed. Furthermore, they cannot distinguish between cause and effect, and we cannot tell whether altered brain activity patterns precede the onset of back pain, whether they arise as a result of chronic back pain, or whether other factor(s), such as lifestyle are the cause of both. This understanding can only come from well-designed longitudinal studies.

### 1.4.2 **Endocrine and immunological**

Disorders of the hypothalamic–pituitary–adrenal (HPA) axis have been implicated in both regional musculoskeletal and chronic widespread pain (CWP) (Vaeroy 1989; Griep et al. 1998; Haddad et al. 2002) although the precise aspects of function associated with symptoms vary between studies. Other research has demonstrated that, amongst people free of CWP but at high risk of its development (based on known risk markers), aspects of HPA axis function, such as loss of diurnal rhythm and failure to suppress cortisol secretion after an overnight dexamethasone test, increased the risk of future onset of CWP (McBeth et al. 2005). It is not clear how this may relate to back pain, but patients with CLBP and an abnormal dexamethasone suppression test responded better to a high-intensity aerobic exercise programme in a recent randomized controlled trial (Chatzitheodorou et al. 2008). Abnormalities of HPA axis function have also been found in conditions such as depression and fatigue, (Gaab et al. 2005; Jerjes et al. 2005, 2006; Smith et al. 2006) both common comorbidities among people with chronic (back) pain. An intriguing hypothesis linking these data with previous observations of the possible role of early life factors (Jones et al. 2007) is that such adverse or traumatic life events may alter the stress response, which then makes individuals vulnerable to future adverse events. Testing such a hypothesis requires large long-term studies.

Cytokines and neuropeptides have been implicated in chronic pain conditions including back pain (MacGregor et al. 2004; Manek and MacGregor 2005) neuropathic pain (Abbadie et al. 2003), polymyalgia rheumatica and rheumatoid arthritis (Pountain et al. 1998), and fibromyalgia (Staud 2004). These generally reflect inflammatory processes, and show certain consistency in the biochemical profile elicited between these pain conditions, including important roles for substance P and the interleukins (Omoigui 2007). Although, in theory, this information could lead to the development of biomarkers to promote an understanding and diagnosis of conditions such as disc degeneration, results have so far been disappointing, with a comprehensive search for candidate markers in spinal fluid lavage yielding no measurable cytokines (Scuderi et al. 2006).

Noradrenaline, dopamine, and serotonin metabolites have also been found to have important roles in chronic widespread pain and fibromyalgia, as have neuropeptides such as substance P, nerve growth factor, and dynorphin A (Russell et al. 1992, 1998). In a prospective study of 67 adults with acute back pain, Hasselhorn et al. (2001) found that low serum levels of 3-methoxy-4-hydroxyphenylglycol (MHPG), dehydroepiandrosterone-sulphate (DHEA-s), and beta-endorphin each predicted persistent disability after 6 months. They postulated that these links with stress response, anabolism, and the opioid system could help to explain the known associations with some of psychological variables described above. However, as with studies of neurological mechanisms of back pain, these findings need to be confirmed and assessed in large, population-based studies, which would ideally be prospective in order to distinguish the cause/effect relationship. The precise nature of the role, and the overall importance of these endocrine factors in the development of chronic back pain therefore remain poorly understood, but initial results suggest that this could be an important area for further research (Staud 2004), for understanding the biology of pain, for developing biomarkers and treatment biomarkers, and measuring the response to these treatments (see also Chapter 5).

### 1.4.3 **Genetic**

There are three questions to address, and therefore areas of research in the consideration of genetic risk factors for CLBP: (1) is CLBP a heritable condition? (2) Is there a genetic basis to pain mechanisms generally? (3) Is there a genetic basis to specific causes of CLBP? Despite many recent advances in both genetics and pain research, approaches to these questions are still in their relative infancy. When addressing the last of these, and despite the comments above, this is one area when the consideration of CLBP as a single global entity may be less helpful than its consideration as a group of specific disorders, each of which has distinct pathophysiology, a distinct molecular origin, and therefore distinct genetic associations. However, there is likely to be an important interaction between the molecular origins of any back pain condition, and the perception of this as an individually important and disabling condition. The latter perception may be more vulnerable to generic factors, including genetic and environmental factors, and the picture is likely to be complex (see also Chapter 3 in this volume).

There is some evidence that chronic pain (Edwards et al. 1985) and back pain (Matsui et al. 1997; Postacchini et al. 1998) cluster in families, suggesting a heritable component. While much of this may be due to social, psychological, and behavioural factors within families (a 'maternal effect'), (Lau et al. 1990; Terre and Ghiselli 1997; Hotopf et al. 1998; MacGregor et al. 2004), studies comparing monozygotic and dizygotic twins have identified a specific genetic contribution to back pain (Sambrook et al. 1999). Depending on the definition of back pain applied, heritability estimates were found in more recent twin studies to range from 30–46% (Battié et al. 2007), with perhaps as much as 57% of the variance in population liability to severe disabling back pain attributable to genetic factors (MacGregor et al. 2004). Heritability was found to be greater in more severe back pain (Battié et al. 2007), but the genetic contribution to decrease with increasing age (Hartvigsen et al. 2004). MacGregor et al. (2004) found considerable overlap between the genetic predictors of back pain and of psychological well-being, suggesting a partially common genetic aetiology that requires further exploration. In contrast to these studies, however, an earlier twin study (MacGregor et al. 1997) found no evidence of a genetic component to pain threshold, ascribing the variability to shared environmental influences. Other research has found no evidence of familial aggregation of recurrent pain complaints (Koutantji et al. 1998; Borge and Nordhagen 2000), or of back pain (Hartvigsen et al. 2004).

Biologically, there is evidence in mice of genetic transmission of nociception (Mogil et al. 1999), and there is growing evidence of specific genetic contributions to some pain conditions in humans (Mogil 2004; Diatchenko et al. 2006; Limer et al. 2008; Max and Stewart 2008). This suggests that at least some components of the pain pathway are subject to the effects of measurable genetic variation, irrespective of the cause of the pain. This makes sense given the central role for molecular mechanisms, either as originators of pain sensations or as their modulators in interaction with external, environmental factors (Diatchenko et al. 2006). In addition to providing valuable insights into mechanisms of pain processing, specific polymorphisms in some of these genes may be associated with the development or perception of chronic pain. These include the genes coding for μ-opioid receptors (Yu 2004), serotonin receptors 1A and 1B (Bondy et al. 1999; Pata et al. 2004), and transporter (5-HTT) (Herken et al. 2001; Szilagyi et al. 2006), and val-158-met catecholamine-o-methyltransferase (COMT) (Gursoy et al. 2003; Zubieta et al. 2003). The list of genes whose variants are purported to be involved in human pain conditions, either as single nucleotide polymorphisms or with haplotype variants, is constantly growing, but includes those listed in Box 1.3. In addition, genetic polymorphisms of the cytochrome P450 enzyme system (Wolf et al. 2000; Fishbain et al. 2004) and of opioid receptors (Mogil 2004) are likely to be important in determining responses to pharmacological pain treatment, and warrant epidemiological study. The latter are examples of how genetic research might directly influence the treatment of chronic pain conditions, for example, by targeting drug treatment on an individual basis, optimizing its effectiveness on the basis of a known genetically-tested profile relating to the relevant cell receptors and metabolic pathways ('personalized medicine'). This is an important aim of research in this area (Max and Stewart 2008), though its transfer to clinical practice is still some way off.

With respect to the genetics of conditions that cause CLBP, most evidence relates to causes of lumbar disc degeneration. Inherited lumbar disc degeneration was recently confirmed to be an important cause of CLBP (Battié et al. 2007), with up to one-quarter of the genetic effect on back pain explicable by genetic causes of disc degeneration. The mode of inheritance is likely to be complex, involving multiple factors including multiple genes (Kalichman and Hunter 2008).

---

## Box 1.3  Genes implicated in human pain conditions*

- 5-HTR2A
- ABCB1 or MDR1
- ACE
- ADRA2A, ADRA2C
- ADRB2
- ATP1A2
- CACNA1A
- COMT
- CYP2D6
- DRD2
- DRD4
- GCH1
- HSN2
- HTR2A
- HTR3A
- HTR3B
- IFNB2
- IKBKAP or IKAP

- IL10
- IL1A, IL1B, and IL1RN
- IL4
- IL6
- LTA
- MAOA
- MC1R
- MTHFR
- NGFB
- NOS3
- NTRK1 or TRKA
- OPRM1 or MOR
- SCN1A
- SCN9A
- SERPINA1
- SLC6A3 or DAT1
- SLC6A4, or 5-HTT, or SERT
- SPTLC1 or SPT1
- TNF

* Diatchenko et al. 2007; Limer et al. 2008.

Polymorphisms of the genes coding for interleukin 1 (IL-1) (Solovieva et al. 2004a, 2004b), vitamin D receptor (Jones et al. 1998; Videman et al. 1998; Kawaguchi et al. 2002), IX collagen (Annunen et al. 1999; Paassilta et al. 2001), and aggrecan (Kawaguchi et al. 1999) have been found, among other polymorphisms, to be associated with lumbar disc degeneration and chronic back pain (Ala-Kokko 2002). The association between ankylosing spondylitis and the *HLA B27* gene has been long established, and links between back pain and other genes coding for inflammatory markers are also apparent (Valdes et al. 2005), but the biological mechanisms behind these associations remain unclear.

Most of the evidence associating (back) pain conditions with genetic polymorphisms is based on small twin or case–control studies, and further confirmatory evidence is called for (Max 2004), ideally on large population samples. A range of epidemiological approaches is required to determine the prevalence of candidate polymorphisms, and their interaction with other, environmental factors. In addition, a continuing search for polymorphisms at other sites that may be associated with chronic pain is important (Solovieva et al. 2004b, Eisenach 2004). The *COMT* gene was the first, and perhaps the most researched gene in pain, with single nucleotide and haplotype variants being found in small studies to be associated with pain perception or development, yet with conflicting evidence found in confirmatory studies (Max and Stewart 2008). Larger sample sizes still are required for definitive evidence. The increasing use and falling costs of genome-wide association studies (GWAS), perhaps using collaborative consortia of samples derived from different studies offer further exciting opportunity for identifying multiple candidate genes and testing them in large samples (http://www.wtccc.org.uk/).

If any of these genetic factors are found to be important at a population level, rather than just in the small samples so far tested, developing work in the field of proteomics could potentially provide the basis for identifying measurable markers of risk for future chronic pain, with the prospect of early intervention or prevention.

## 1.5 The need and potential benefit of population-based studies of hypothesized biological risk factors

These biological factors may be important as variables on the path to development of chronic pain (as in possible HPA dysfunction), as effect modifiers (as in some of the fMRI changes, or genetic polymorphisms) and/or as risk markers (as in cerebral spinal fluid substance P levels, or proteomic measurement based on genetic polymorphisms). The proposed factors do not operate in isolation, and many will interact with each other, as well as with existing known factors (Diatchenko et al. 2006). For example, brain imaging studies demonstrate that psychological modulation of pain processing contributes to chronic pain, completing a hypothetically demonstrable pathway from genes to prefrontal cortex in CLBP (Apkarian et al. 2005). The task is not, therefore, to isolate new risk factors so much as to identify important ones, and assess their interaction with each other. Studying the biology of CLBP will both extend our knowledge of risk factors and potential intervention points, and improve our understanding of the biological mechanisms by which other risk factors exert their effects on the pain pathways.

The importance of the proposed biological factors in the community, particularly of those that may inform interventions, needs now to be tested. This will require population-based studies to determine: (1) whether any observed associations between proposed risk factors and CLBP extrapolate to larger, representative samples; (2) the strength of these associations in CLBP as it occurs in the community; and (3) the prevalence of the proposed factors. The technology and opportunity now exist to conduct such studies, addressing a number of potential risk factors that have been demonstrated. Studies should include and compare distinct diagnostic or structural disorders, as well as the global entity of CLBP, including unexplained causes; these will present different challenges in terms of sample size requirements, recruitment, and interpretation, but will all contribute to the developing picture. Evidence from research on psychosocial factors suggests that there will be some biological markers found for specific back conditions (such as the genes associated with degenerative back pain), but that others will relate to several chronic pain conditions (such as the *COMT* gene), or to chronic pain as a single entity (such as altered neuronal pathways).

Epidemiologists will need a new set of tools in their box for this. In addition to continuing to measure demographic and psychosocial risk factors in population-based studies, they will need to take biological samples for DNA testing and storage and biochemical measurements, and to consider, where appropriate, the use of brain imaging techniques such as fMRI (Borsook and Becerra 2003). Ideally, in order to assess the predictive importance of clusters of risk factors, prospective cohort studies are required. These may either be established *de novo*, or, with additional funding represent added value to existing or planned cohorts such as the UK Biobank (www.ukbiobank.ac.uk) or Generation Scotland (Smith et al. 2006). These studies are expensive, however and will not produce useful data for several years. Other study designs (such as cross-sectional and case–control studies) will also be valuable though will lack the ability to distinguish cause from effect with dynamic (non-genetic) markers, and will therefore be less helpful in informing interventions. In all cases, close collaborations will be required between epidemiologists, pain and generalist clinicians, radiologists, laboratory scientists, and geneticists, as well as with the psychologists and sociologists with whom pain epidemiologists have more traditionally consorted. Importantly, these collaborations should be bi-directional, with the epidemiology research informing the focus of laboratory and imaging research, as well as vice versa.

### 1.5.1 **Beyond the bedside**

The results of this new effort will include new understandings of the development and persistence of chronic back pain, informing the development of new prevention and treatment strategies for the population. These can either be applied on a large scale, if important, prevalent risk factors can be addressed, or targeted accurately for maximum benefit using the knowledge of distribution that the research will provide. In the UK, the Medical Research Council aims to translate research 'from the laboratory to the bedside and back again' (www.mrc.ac.uk/index/current-research/current-clinical_research.htm). Similarly the National Institutes of Health in the USA promote and reward 'bench-to-bedside' research (www.nih.gov/news/pr/jun2006/cc-07.htm). However, in the case of CLBP, where only a small proportion of sufferers are treated in hospital and many do not even attend a family practitioner, this translation must reach beyond the bedside, into community-based consulting rooms, and beyond—from the laboratory to the bus stop, and back again (Smith et al. 2007).

### References

Abbadie, C., Lindia, J.A., Cumiskey, A.M., *et al.* (2003). Impaired neuropathic pain responses in mice lacking the chemokine receptor CCR2. *Proceedings of the National Academy of Sciences of the United States of America,* **100**, 7947–52.

Ala-kokko, L. (2002). Genetic risk factors for lumbar disc disease. *Annals of Medicine,* **34**, 42–7.

Andersson, G.B. (1999). Epidemiological features of chronic low-back pain. *Lancet,* **354**, 581–85.

Annunen, S., Passilta, P., Lohiniva, J., *et al.*(1999). An allele of COL9A2 associated with intervertebral disc disease. *Science,* **285**, 409–12.

Apkarian, A.V., Sosa, Y., Sonty, S., *et al.* (2004). Chronic back pain is associated with decreased prefrontal and thalamic gray matter density. *The Journal of Neuroscience,* **24**, 10410–15.

Apkarian, A.V., Bushnell, M.C., Treede, R.D. and Zubieta, J.K. (2005). Human brain mechanisms of pain perception and regulation in health and disease. *European Journal of Pain*, **9**, 463–84.

Assendelft, W.J., Morton, S.C., Yu, E.I., Suttorp, M.J. and Shekelle, P.G. (2004). Spinal manipulative therapy for low back pain. *Cochrane Database of Systematic Reviews*, **1**, CD000447.

Baliki, M.N., Chialvo, D.R., Geha, P.Y., *et al.* (2006). Chronic pain and the emotional brain: specific brain activity associated with spontaneous fluctuations of intensity of chronic back pain. *The Journal of Neuroscience*, **26**, 12165–73.

Baliki, M.N., Geha, P.Y., Jabakhanji., Harden, N., Schnitzer, T.J. and Apkarian, A.V. (2008). A preliminary fMRI study of analgesic treatment in chronic back pain and knee osteoarthritis. *Molecular pain*, **4**, 47.

Banic, B., Petersen-Felix, S., Andersen, O.K., *et al.* (2004). Evidence for spinal cord hypersensitivity in chronic pain after whiplash injury and in fibromyalgia. *Pain*, **107**, 7–15.

Battie, M.C., Videman, T., Levalahti, E., Gill, K., and Kaprio, J. (2007). Heritability of low back pain and the role of disc degeneration. *Pain*, **131**, 272–80.

Bergman, S., Herrstrom, P., Jacobsson, L.T., and Petersson, I.F. (2002). Chronic widespread pain: a three year followup of pain distribution and risk factors. *The Journal of Rheumatology*, **29**, 818–25.

Bondy, B., Spaeth, M., Offenbaecher, M., *et al.* (1999). The T102C polymorphism of the 5-HT2A-receptor gene in fibromyalgia. *Neurobiology of Disease*, **6**, 433–39.

Borge, A.I. and Nordhagen, R. (2000). Recurrent pain symptoms in children and parents. *Acta Paediatrica*, **89**, 1479–83.

Borsook, D. and Becerra, L. (2003). Pain imaging: future applications to integrative clinical and basic neurobiology. *Advanced Drug Delivery Reviews*, **55**, 967–86.

Buchbinder, R. and Jolley, D. (2004). Population based intervention to change back pain beliefs: three year follow up population survey. *British Medical Journal*, **28**, 321.

Chatzitheodorou, D., Mavromoustakos, S. and Milioti, S. (2008). The effect of exercise on adrenocortical responsiveness of patients with chronic low back pain, controlled for psychological strain. *Clinical Rehabilitation*, **22**, 319–28.

Clauw, D.J. and Chrousos, G.P. (1997). Chronic pain and fatigue syndromes: overlapping clinical and neuroendocrine features and potential pathogenic mechanisms. *Neuroimmunomodulation*, **4**, 134–53.

Cook, D.B., Lange, G., Ciccone, D.S., Liu, W.C., Steffner, J., and Natelson, B.H. (2004). Functional imaging of pain in patients with primary fibromyalgia. *The Journal of Rheumatology*, **31**, 364–78.

Croft, P.R., Macfarlane, G.J., Papageorgiou, A.C., Thomas, E., and Silman, A.J. (1998). Outcome of low back pain in general practice: a prospective study. *British Medical Journal*, **316**, 1356–59.

Diatchenko, L., Nackley, A.G., Slade, G.D., Fillingim, R.B., and Maixner, W. (2006). Idiopathic pain disorders—pathways of vulnerability. *Pain*, **123**, 226–30.

Diatchenko, L., Nackley, A.G., Tchivileva, I.E., Shabalina, S.A., and Maixner, W. (2007). Genetic architecture of human pain perception. *Trends in Genetics*, **23**, 605–13.

Dionne, C.E., Dunn, K.M., Croft, P.R., *et al.* (2008). A consensus approach toward the standardization of back pain definitions for use in prevalence studies. *Spine*, **33**, 95–103.

Edwards, P.W., Zeichner, A., Kuczmierczyk, A.R., and Boczkowski, J. (1985). Familial pain models: the relationship between family history of pain and current pain experience. *Pain*, **21**, 379–84.

Eisenach, J.C. (2004). Fishing for genes: practical ways to study genetic polymorphisms for pain. *Anesthesiology*, **100**, 1343–4.

Elliott, A.M., Smith, B.H., Penny, K.I., Smith, W.C., and Chambers, W.A. (1999). The epidemiology of chronic pain in the community. *Lancet*, **354**, 1248–52.

Elliott, A.M., Smith, B.H., Hannaford, P.C., Smith, W.C. and Chambers, W.A. (2002). The course of chronic pain in the community: results of a 4-year follow-up study. *Pain*, **99**, 299–307.

Fishbain, D.A., Fishbain, D., Lewis, J., *et al.* (2004). Genetic testing for enzymes of drug metabolism: does it have clinical utility for pain medicine at the present time? A structured review. *Pain Medicine*, **5**, 81–93.

Frost, H., Lamb, S.E., Doll, H.A., Carver, P.T., and Stewart-Brown, S. (2004). Randomised controlled trial of physiotherapy compared with advice for low back pain. *British Medical Journal,* **329**, 708.

Gaab, J., Baumann, S., Budnoik, A., Gmunder, H., Hottinger, N., and Ehlert, U. (2005). Reduced reactivity and enhanced negative feedback sensitivity of the hypothalamus-pituitary-adrenal axis in chronic whiplash-associated disorder. *Pain,* **119**, 219–24.

Gracely, R.H., Petzke, F., Wolf, J.M., and Clauw, D.J. (2002). Functional magnetic resonance imaging evidence of augmented pain processing in fibromyalgia. *Arthritis and Rheumatism,* **46**, 1333–43.

Grachev, I.D., Frerickson, B.E., and Apkarian, A.V. (2000). Abnormal brain chemistry in chronic back pain: an in vivo proton magnetic resonance spectroscopy study. *Pain,* **89**, 7–18.

Grachev, I.D., Fredickson, B.E., and Apkarian, A.V. (2001). Dissociating anxiety from pain: mapping the neuronal marker N-acetyl aspartate to perception distinguishes closely interrelated characteristics of chronic pain. *Molecular Psychiatry,* **6**, 256–8.

Grachev, I.D., Fredrickson, B.E., and Apkarian, A.V. (2002). Brain chemistry reflects dual states of pain and anxiety in chronic low back pain. *Journal of Neural Transmission,* **109**, 1309–34.

Grachev, I.D., Ramachandran, T.S., Thomas, P.S., Szeverenyi, N.M. and Fredrickson, B.E. (2003). Association between dorsolateral prefrontal N-acetyl aspartate and depression in chronic back pain: an in vivo proton magnetic resonance spectroscopy study. *Journal of Neural Transmission,* **110**, 287–312.

Gran, J.T. (2003). The epidemiology of chronic generalized musculoskeletal pain. *Best Practice & Research. Clinical Rheumatology,* **17**, 547–61.

Griep, E.N., Boersma, J.W., Lentjes, E.G., Prins, A.P., Van Der Korst, J.K., and De Kloet, E.R. (1998). Function of the hypothalamic-pituitary-adrenal axis in patients with fibromyalgia and low back pain. *The Journal of Rheumatology,* **25**, 1374–81.

Gursoy, S., Erdal, E., Herken, H., Madenci, E., Alaeshirli, B., and Erdal, N. (2003). Significance of catechol-O-methyltransferase gene polymorphism in fibromyalgia syndrome. *Rheumatology International,* **23**, 104–7.

Haddad, J.J., Saade, N.E., and Safieh-Garabedian, B. (2002). Cytokines and neuro-immune-endocrine interactions: a role for the hypothalamic-pituitary-adrenal revolving axis. *Journal of Neuroimmunology,* **133**, 1–19.

Hagen, K.B., Jamtvedt, G., Hilde, G., and Winnem, M.F. (2005). The updated cochrane review of bed rest for low back pain and sciatica. *Spine,* **30**, 542–6.

Harstall, C. and Ospina, M. (2003). How prevalent is chronic pain? *Pain Clinical Updates,* **11**, 1–4.

Hartvigsen, J., Christensen, K., Frederiksen, H., and Petersen, H.C. (2004). Genetic and environmental contributions to back pain in old age: a study of 2,108 Danish twins aged 70 and older. *Spine,* **29**, 897–901.

Hasselhorn, H.M., Theorell, T., Vingard, E., and Musculoskeletal Intervention Center (MUSIC)-NORRTALJE Study Group (2001). Endocrine and immunologic parameters indicative of 6-month prognosis after the onset of low back pain or neck/shoulder pain. *Spine,* **26**, E24–9.

Hay, E.M., Mullis, R., Lewis, M., *et al.* (2005). Comparison of physical treatments versus a brief pain-management programme for back pain in primary care: a randomised clinical trial in physiotherapy practice. *Lancet,* **365**, 2024–30.

Hay, E.M., Dunn, K.M., Hill, J.C., *et al.* (2008). A randomised clinical trial of subgrouping and targeted treatment for low back pain compared with best current care. The STarT Back Trial Study Protocol. *BMC Musculoskeletal Disorders,* **9**, 58.

Hayden, J.A., Van Tulder, M.W., Malmivaara, A. and Koes, B.W. (2005). Exercise therapy for treatment of non-specific low back pain. *Cochrane Database of Systematic Reviews,* **3**(3), CD000335.

Henschke, N., Maher, C.G., Regshauge, K.M., *et al.* (2008). Prognosis in patients with recent onset low back pain in Australian primary care: inception cohort study. *British Medical Journal,* **337**, 171.

Herken, H., Erdal, E., Mutlu, N., *et al.* (2001). Possible association of temporomandibular joint pain and dysfunction with a polymorphism in the serotonin transporter gene. *American Journal of Orthodontics and Dentofacial Orthopedics,* **120**, 308–13.

Heymans, M.W., Van Tulder, M.W., Esmail, R., Bombardier, C., and Koes, B.W. (2005). Back schools for non-specific low-back pain: a systematic review within the framework for the Cochrane Collaboration Back Review Group. *Spine,* **30**, 2153–63.

Hotopf, M., Carr, S., Mayou, R., Wadsworth, M., and Wessely, S. (1998). Why do children have chronic abdominal pain, and what happens to them when they grow up? Population based cohort study. *British Medical Journal,* **316**, 1196–200.

Jayson, M.I. (1997). Why does acute back pain become chronic? *British Medical Journal,* **314**, 1639–40.

Jellema, P., Van Der Windt, D.A., Van Der Horst, H.E., Blankenstein, A.H., Bouter, L.M., and Stalman, W.A. (2005a). Why is a treatment aimed at psychosocial factors not effective in patients with (sub) acute low back pain? *Pain,* **118**, 350–9.

Jellema, P., Van Der Windt, D.A., Van Der Horst, H.E., Twisk, J.W., Stalman, W.A., and Bouter, L.M. (2005b). Should treatment of (sub)acute low back pain be aimed at psychosocial prognostic factors? Cluster randomised clinical trial in general practice. *British Medical Journal,* **331**, 84–8.

Jerjes, W.K., Cleare, A.J., Wessley, S., Wood, P.J. and Taylor, N.F. (2005). Diurnal patterns of salivary cortisol and cortisone output in chronic fatigue syndrome. *Journal of Affective Disorders,* **87**, 299–304.

Jerjes, W.K., Peters, T.J., Taylor, N.F., Wood, P.J., Wessley, S., and Cleare, A.J. (2006). Diurnal excretion of urinary cortisol, cortisone, and cortisol metabolites in chronic fatigue syndrome. *Journal of Psychosomatic Research,* **60**, 145–53.

Jones, G., White, C., Sambrook, P., and Eisman, J. (1998). Allelic variation in the vitamin D receptor, lifestyle factors and lumbar spinal degenerative disease. *Annals of Rheumatic Diseases,* **57**, 94–9.

Jones, G.T., Johnson, R.E., Wiles, N.J., *et al.* (2006). Predicting persistent disabling low back pain in general practice: a prospective cohort study. *The British Journal of General Practice,* **56**, 334–41.

Jones, G.T., Silman, A.J., Power, C., and Macfarlane, G.J. (2007). Are common symptoms in childhood associated with chronic widespread body pain in adulthood? Results from the 1958 British Birth Cohort Study. *Arthritis and Rheumatism,* **56**, 1669–75.

Kalichman, L. and Hunter, D.J. (2008). The genetics of intervertebral disc degeneration. Familial predisposition and heritability estimation. *Joint Bone Spine,* **75**, 383–7.

Kawaguchi, Y., Osada, R., Kanamori, M., *et al.* (1999). Association between an aggrecan gene polymorphism and lumbar disc degeneration. *Spine,* **24**, 2456–60.

Kawaguchi, Y., Kanamori, M., Ishihara, H., Ohmori, K., Matsui, H., and Kimura, T. (2002). The association of lumbar disc disease with vitamin-D receptor gene polymorphism. *The Journal of bone and Joint Surgery,* **84-A**(11), 2022–8.

Koutantji, M., Pearce, S.A., and OakelyY, D.A. (1998). The relationship between gender and family history of pain with current pain experience and awareness of pain in others. *Pain,* **77**, 25–31.

Lamb, S.E., Lall, R., Hansen, Z. and the Back Skills Training Trial (BeST) Team (2007). Design considerations in a clinical trial of a cognitive behavioural intervention for the management of low back pain in primary care: Back Skills Training Trial. *BMC Musculoskeletal Disorders,* **8**, 14.

Lambeek, L.C., Anema, J.R., Van Royen, B.J., *et al.* (2007). Multidisciplinary outpatient care program for patients with chronic low back pain: design of a randomized controlled trial and cost-effectiveness study. *BMC Public Health,* **7**, 254.

Lau, R.R., Quadrel, M.J., and Hartman, K.A. (1990). Development and change of young adults' preventive health beliefs and behavior: influence from parents and peers. *Journal of Health and Social Behavior,* **31**, 240–59.

Limer, K.L., Nicholl, B.I., Thomson, W., and McBeth, J. (2008). Exploring the genetic susceptibility of chronic widespread pain: the tender points in genetic association studies. *Rheumatology,* **47**, 572–7.

Linde, K., Witt, C.M., Streng, A., *et al.* (2007). The impact of patient expectations on outcomes in four randomized controlled trials of acupuncture in patients with chronic pain. *Pain,* **128**, 264–71.

Linton, S.J. (2005). Do psychological factors increase the risk for back pain in the general population in both a cross-sectional and prospective analysis? *European Journal of Pain,* **9**, 355–61.

Lis, A.M., Black, K.M., Korn, H., and Nordin, M. (2007). Association between sitting and occupational LBP. *European Spine Journal*, **16**, 283–98.

Macfarlane, G.J. (2006). Who will develop chronic pain and why? In: H. Flor, E. Kalso, and J.O. Dostrovsky (eds) *The Epidemiological Evidence Proceedings of the 11th World Congress on Pain*. Seattle, WA: International Association for the Study of Pain (IASP) Press.

Macfarlane, G.J., Jones, G.T., and Hannaford, P.C. (2006). Managing low back pain presenting to primary care: where do we go from here? *Pain*, **122**, 219–22.

Macfarlane, T.V., Blinkhorn, A., Worthington, H.V., Davies, R.M., and Macfarlane, G.J. (2002). Sex hormonal factors and chronic widespread pain: a population study among women. *Rheumatology*, **41**, 454–7.

MacGregor, A.J., Griffiths, G.O., Baker, J., and Spector, T.D. (1997). Determinants of pressure pain threshold in adult twins: evidence that shared environmental influences predominate. *Pain*, **73**, 253–7.

MacGregor, A.J., Andrew, T., Sambrook, P.N., and Spector, T.D. (2004). Structural, psychological, and genetic influences on low back and neck pain: a study of adult female twins. *Arthritis and Rheumatism*, **51**, 160–7.

MacMahon, B. and Pugh, T.F. (1970). *Epidemiology: Principles and Methods*. Boston, MA: Little Brown.

Magni, G., Marchetti, M., Moreschi, C., Merskey, H. and Luchini, S.R. (1993). Chronic musculoskeletal pain and depressive symptoms in the National Health and Nutrition Examination. I. Epidemiologic follow-up study. *Pain*, **53**, 163–8.

Manchikanti, L. (2000). Epidemiology of low back pain. *Pain physician*, **3**, 167–92.

Manek, N.J. and MacGregor, A.J. (2005). Epidemiology of back disorders: prevalence, risk factors, and prognosis. *Current Opinion in Rheumatology*, **17**, 134–40.

Matsui, H., Maeda, A., Tsuji, H., and Naruse, Y. (1997). Risk indicators of low back pain among workers in Japan. Association of familial and physical factors with low back pain. *Spine*, **22**, 1242–7.

Max, M.B. (2004). Assessing pain candidate gene studies. *Pain*, **109**, 1–3.

Max, M.B. and Stewart, W.F. (2008). The molecular epidemiology of pain: a new discipline for drug discovery. *Nature Reviews. Drug Discovery*, **7**, 647–58.

McBeth, J., Macfarlane, G.J., Hunt, I.M., and Silman, A.J. (2001). Risk factors for persistent chronic widespread pain: a community-based study. *Rheumatology*, **40**, 95–101.

McBeth, J., Harkness, E.F., Silman, A.J., and Macfarlane, G.J. (2003). The role of workplace low-level mechanical trauma, posture and environment in the onset of chronic widespread pain. *Rheumatology*, **42**, 1486–94.

McBeth, J., Chui, Y.H., Silman, A.J., *et al.* (2005). Hypothalamic-pituitary-adrenal stress axis function and the relationship with chronic widespread pain and its antecedents. *Arthritis Research & Therapy*, **7**, R992–R1000.

McQuay, H.J., Derry, S., Moore, R.A., Poulain, P., and Legout, V. (2008). Enriched enrolment with randomised withdrawal (EERW): Time for a new look at clinical trial design in chronic pain. *Pain*, **135**, 217–20.

Melzack, R. and Casey, K. (1968). Sensory, motivational, and central control determinants of pain. In: D.R. Kenshalo (ed.) *The skin senses*, 2nd edn., pp. 423–43. Springfield, IL: Charles C. Thomas.

Mogil, J.S., Wilson, S.G., Bon, K., et al. (1999). Heritability of nociception I: responses of 11 inbred mouse strains on 12 measures of nociception. *Pain*, **80**, 67–82.

Mogil, J.S., Wilson, S.G., Chesler, E.J., *et al.* (2003). The melanocortin-1 receptor gene mediates female-specific mechanisms of analgesia in mice and humans. *Proceedings of the National Academy of Sciences of the United States of America*, **100**, 4867–72.

Mogil, J.S. (ed) (2004). *The Genetics of Pain (Progress in Pain Research and Management)*. Seattle, WA: IASP Press.

Morley, S., Eccleston, C., and Williams, A. (1999). Systematic review and meta-analysis of randomized controlled trials of cognitive behaviour therapy and behaviour therapy for chronic pain in adults, excluding headache. *Pain*, **80**, 1–13.

Newton-John, T.R. and Geddes, J. (2008). The non-specific effects of group-based cognitive—behavioural treatment of chronic pain. *Chronic illness*, **4**, 199–208.

Omoigui, S. (2007). The biochemical origin of pain: the origin of all pain is inflammation and the inflammatory response. Part 2 of 3 - inflammatory profile of pain syndromes. *Medical hypotheses*, **69**, 1169–78.

Paassilta, P., Lohiniva, J., Goring, H.H., *et al.* (2001). Identification of a novel common genetic risk factor for lumbar disk disease. *Journal of the American Medical Association*, **285**, 1843–9.

Papageorgiou, A.C., Croft, P.R., Thomas, E., Ferry, S., Jayson, M.I., and Silman, A.J. (1996). Influence of previous pain experience on the episode incidence of low back pain: results from the South Manchester Back Pain Study. *Pain*, **66**, 181–5.

Papageorgiou, A.C., Silman, A.J., and Macfarlane, G.J. (2002). Chronic widespread pain in the population: a seven year follow up study. *Annals of the Rheumatic Diseases*, **61**, 1071–4.

Pata, C., Erdal, E., Yazc, K., Camdeviren, H., Ozkaya, M., and Ulu, O. (2004). Association of the -1438 G/A and 102 T/C polymorphism of the 5-Ht2A receptor gene with irritable bowel syndrome 5-Ht2A gene polymorphism in irritable bowel syndrome. *Journal of Clinical Gastroenterology*, **38**, 561–6.

Pincus, T., Burton A.K., Vogel, S., and Field, A.P. (2002). A systematic review of psychological factors as predictors of chronicity/disability in prospective cohorts of low back pain. *Spine*, **27**, E109–20.

Porta, M., Greenland, S., and Last, J.M. (eds). (2008). *A Dictionary of Epidemiology*, 5th edn. New York: Oxford University Press.

Postacchini, F., Lami, R., and Pugliese, O. (1988). Familial predisposition to discogenic low-back pain. An epidemiologic and immunogenetic study. *Spine*, **13**, 1403–6.

Pountain, G., Hazelman, B., and Cawston, T.E. (1998). Circulating levels of IL-1beta, IL-6 and soluble IL-2 receptor in polymyalgia rheumatica and giant cell arteritis and rheumatoid arthritis. *British Journal of Rheumatology*, **37**, 797–8.

Rothman, K.J. and Greenland, S. (1998). *Modern Epidemiology*, 2nd edn. Oxford: Oxford University Press.

Royal College of General Practitioners (1999). *Clinical Guidelines for the Management of Acute Low Back Pain*. London: Royal College of General Practitioners.

Russell, I.J. (1998). Advances in fibromyalgia: possible role for central neurochemicals. *The American Journal of the Medical Sciences*, **315**, 377–84.

Russell, I.J., Vaeroy, H., Javors, M. and Nyberg, F. (1992). Cerebrospinal fluid biogenic amine metabolites in fibromyalgia/fibrositis syndrome and rheumatoid arthritis. *Arthritis and Rheumatism*, **35**, 550–6.

Sambrook, P.N., Macgregor, A.J., and Spector, T.D. (1999). Genetic influences on cervical and lumbar disc degeneration: a magnetic resonance imaging study in twins. *Arthritis and Rheumatism*, **42**, 366–72.

Scuderi, G.J., Brusovanik, G.V., Anderson, D.G., *et al.* (2006). Cytokine assay of the epidural space lavage in patients with lumbar intervertebral disk herniation and radiculopathy. *Journal of Spinal Disorders & Techniques*, **19**, 266–9.

Smith, A.K., White, P.D., Aslakson, E., Vollmer-Conna, U., and Rajeevan, M.S. (2006). Polymorphisms in genes regulating the HPA axis associated with empirically delineated classes of unexplained chronic fatigue. *Pharmacogenomics*, **7**, 387–94.

Smith, B.H. (2001). Chronic pain: a challenge for primary care. *British Journal of General Practice*, **51**, 524–6.

Smith, B.H., Chambers, W.A., and Smith, W.C. (1996). Chronic pain: time for epidemiology. *Journal of the Royal Society of Medicine*, **89**, 181–3.

Smith, B.H., Elliott, A.M. and Hannaford, P.C. (2004a). Is chronic pain a distinct diagnosis in primary care? Evidence arising from the Royal College of General Practitioners' Oral Contraception study. *Family practice*, **21**, 66–74.

Smith, B.H., Elliott, A.M., Hannaford, P.C., Chambers, W.A., and Smith, W.C. (2004b). Factors related to the onset and persistence of chronic back pain in the community: results from a general population follow-up study. *Spine*, **29**, 1032–40.

Smith, B.H., Campbell, H., Blackwood, D., *et al.* (2006). Generation Scotland: the Scottish Family Health Study; a new resource for researching genes and heritability. *BMC Medical Genetics,* **7**, 74.

Smith, B.H., Macfarlane, G.J., and Torrance, N. (2007). Epidemiology of chronic pain, from the laboratory to the bus stop: time to add understanding of biological mechanisms to the study of risk factors in population-based research? *Pain,* **127**, 5–10.

Solovieva, S., Kouhia, S., Leino-Arjas, P., *et al.* (2004a). Interleukin 1 polymorphisms and intervertebral disc degeneration. *Epidemiology,* **15**, 626–33.

Solovieva, S., Leino-Arjas, P., Saarela, J., Luoma, K., Raininko, R., and Riihimaki, H. (2004b). Possible association of interleukin 1 gene locus polymorphisms with low back pain. *Pain,* **109**, 8–19.

Sorensen, J., Graven-Nielsen, T., Henriksson, K.G., Bengtsson, M., and Arendt-Nielsen, L. (1998). Hyperexcitability in fibromyalgia. *The Journal of Rheumatology,* **25**, 152–5.

Staud, R. (2004). Fibromyalgia pain: do we know the source? *Current Opinion in Rheumatology,* **16**, 157–63.

Szilagyi, A., Boor, K., Orosz, I., Szantai, E., *et al.* (2006). Contribution of serotonin transporter gene polymorphisms to pediatric migraine. *Headache,* **46**, 478–85.

Terre, L. and Ghiselli, W. (1997). A developmental perspective on family risk factors in somatization. *Journal of Psychosomatic Research,* **42**, 197–208.

UK BEAM Trial Team (2004). United Kingdom back pain exercise and manipulation (UK BEAM) randomised trial: effectiveness of physical treatments for back pain in primary care. *British Medical Journal,* **329**, 1377.

Underwood, M.R., Morton, V., Farrin, A. and UK BEAM Trial Team (2007). Do baseline characteristics predict response to treatment for low back pain? Secondary analysis of the UK BEAM dataset. *Rheumatology,* **46**, 1297–302.

Vaeroy, H. (1989). Impaired neuroendocrine axis and FMS. *The Journal of Rheumatology,* **16**, 1460–5.

Valdes, A.M., Hassett, G., Hart, D.J., and Spector, T.D. (2005). Radiographic progression of lumbar spine disc degeneration is influenced by variation at inflammatory genes: a candidate SNP association study in the Chingford cohort. *Spine,* **30**, 2445–51.

Van Der Windt, D., Hay, E., Jellema, P., and Main, C. (2008). Psychosocial interventions for low back pain in primary care: lessons learned from recent trials. *Spine,* **33**, 81–9.

Van Tulder, M.W., Ostelo, R., Vlaeyen, J.W., Linton, S.J., Morley, S.J., and Assendelft, W.J. (2000). Behavioral treatment for chronic low back pain: a systematic review within the framework of the Cochrane Back Review Group. *Spine,* **25**, 2688–99.

Verhaak, P.F., Kerssens, J.J., Dekker, J., Sorbi, M.J., and Bensing, J.M. (1998). Prevalence of chronic benign pain disorder among adults: a review of the literature. *Pain,* **77**, 231–9.

Videman, T., Leppavuori, J., Kaprio, J., *et al.* (1998). Intragenic polymorphisms of the vitamin D receptor gene associated with intervertebral disc degeneration. *Spine,* **23**, 2477–85.

Von Korff, M. (1999). Epidemiological methods In: I.K. Crombie, P.R. Croft, S.J. Linton, L. Leresche, and M. Von Korff (eds.) *Epidemiology of Pain,* pp. 7–15. Seattle, WA: IASP Press.

Von Korff, M., Balderson, B.H., Saunders, K., *et al.* (2005). A trial of an activating intervention for chronic back pain in primary care and physical therapy settings. *Pain,* **113**, 323–30.

Wessely, S., Nimnuan, C., and Sharpe, M. (1999). Functional somatic syndromes: one or many? *Lancet,* **354**, 936–9.

Williams, A.C., Richardson, P.H., Nicholas, M.K., *et al.* (1996). Inpatient vs. outpatient pain management: results of a randomised controlled trial. *Pain,* **66**, 13–22.

Wolf, C.R., Smith, G., and Smith, R.L. (2000). Science, medicine, and the future: Pharmacogenetics. *British Medical Journal,* **320**, 987–90.

Yu, L. (2004). Pharmacogentics: the OPRM (mu-opioid-receptor) gene. In: J.S. Mogil (ed.) *The Genetics of Pain (Progress in Pain research and Management),* pp. 239–56. Seattle, WA: IASP Press.

Zubieta J.K., Heitzeg, M.M., Smith, Y.R., *et al.* (2003). COMT val158met genotype affects mu-opioid neurotransmitter responses to a pain stressor. *Science,* **299**, 1240–3.

Chapter 2

# Defining Chronic Pain by Prognosis

Kate M. Dunn, Michael Von Korff, and Peter R. Croft

This book addresses the transition 'from acute to chronic back pain', but do we really know what 'chronic' means? The International Association for the Study of Pain (IASP) defines chronic pain as pain lasting beyond the normal healing time, which is usually defined as 3 months or 6 months (International Association for the Study of Pain 1986). Is this retrospective approach to defining chronic pain sufficient, or are there better ways to characterize patients with chronic pain? In this chapter we reconsider the duration-based, retrospective approach to defining chronic pain, consider reasons why it might be inadequate, and develop an alternative approach to assessing and defining chronic pain, based on its prognosis and multiple prognostic indicators grounded in the biopsychosocial model of pain.

The prognostic approach to defining chronic pain developed in this chapter rests upon three propositions that can be tested empirically. The first proposition is that chronic pain is better characterized by a failure of pain and associated dysfunction to resolve than by progression to a qualitatively distinct chronic pain state. That is, severe pain, pain-related activity limitations, psychological distress, and other features used to characterize chronic pain patients are observable soon after pain onset. What typically differentiates 'chronic pain' from 'acute pain' is that severe pain and associated dysfunction does not show meaningful improvement. While progressive worsening of pain and pain dysfunction may be observed in some patients, this clinical course is less common. The second proposition is that the seeds of chronic pain (prognostic indicators) are observable early in the course of a pain condition, providing a basis for early identification of patients at risk of an unfavourable outcome. The third proposition is that varied and multi-faceted prognostic indicators can be summarized in a single measure—a prognostic risk score. This prognostic risk score measures how likely it is that clinically significant pain will continue to be present at a future point in time, providing a simple and clinically relevant metric for quantifying chronic pain in terms of its future prognosis rather than its past duration considered in isolation.

## 2.1 Duration-based definitions of chronic pain

In 1953, Bonica described chronic pain as pain persisting beyond normal healing time (Bonica 1953). The Classification of Chronic Pain of the IASP (International Association for the Study of Pain 1986) defined chronic pain as pain that persists for at least 3 or 6 months for non-malignant pain, corresponding to the time required for inflammation to subside or acute injuries to repair. Similar definitions exist for specific pain conditions. Nachemson and Andersson (1982) defined chronic back pain as back pain lasting 3 months or longer based on a study showing that 90% of patients recovered within that time. The International Classification of Headache Disorders defined chronic secondary headache disorders as headache persisting over a period longer than 3 months, and chronic primary headache disorders as attacks of headache occurring on most days for over 3 months (International Headache Society 2004).

These definitions are each based on the assumption that duration or persistence of pain is the critical defining feature of chronic pain. Duration-based definitions of chronic pain differentiate persons with chronic pain empirically, as the passage of time sorts out those with chronic pain from those with acute pain. However, as Loeser and Melzack pointed out (1999), 'it is not the duration of pain that distinguishes acute from chronic pain'. This statement reflects the implicit understanding, shared by clinicians and patients alike, that the term 'chronic pain' carries greater significance than a simple descriptive statement about how long pain has lasted. Defining chronic pain by duration alone neglects other features of pain that have equal or greater prognostic value (e.g. pain intensity, pain-related interference with activities, the diffuseness of pain, emotional distress), and that have greater import for patient functioning and quality of life than pain duration considered in isolation.

The conceptual underpinnings of duration-based definitions of chronic pain are problematic. There are four significant limitations of defining chronic pain by duration alone:

◆ *Multidimensionality*—it is widely recognized that pain is a multidimensional phenomenon (Waddell 1998; Loeser and Melzack 1999). Raspe et al. (2003) observed that 'back pain is more than pain in the back'. The traditional definition of chronic pain implies that acute and chronic pain can be differentiated by pain duration alone, whereas physical and emotional suffering, behavioural deactivation, and social role disability are important clinical features of chronic pain.

◆ *Early identification*—duration-based definitions do not provide a basis for identifying patients at risk of a poor outcome *early* in the clinical course of a pain condition, when prevention might be most effective. This is illustrated by Patient A (Box 2.1). According to a duration

## Box 2.1 Examples of typical back pain patients

### Patient A

This person presents to his primary care physician having had back pain for 1 month. His pain is severe and he is clinically depressed. He reports pain in many other anatomical locations as well. He is off work and has no plans to return to work, and is spending most of his time resting and watching television. He has significant sleep disturbance.

### Patient B

This person visits his doctor during an unusually severe flare-up of back pain. He has had back pain almost every day for many years. The pain typically fluctuates during the day, but is not too bothersome once he is up and about. He sometimes finds it difficult to make certain movements due to his back pain, but he generally regards it as a minor nuisance that does not substantially limit his activities. He does not experience significant psychological distress, and his pain is limited to the lower back. The patient has had these flare-ups before, and they always improve to his usual low level, typically within 3–5 days.

### Patient C

This person comes to see her doctor because her back pain has gotten worse again. She has had pain in the lower back for over a year, and this appears to be an exacerbation. She also says that she is having headaches and cannot sleep because of the pain. Over the last 6 months, the patient has taken time off work several times, which is worrying her, and she is no longer getting much satisfaction out of her job. She is also having trouble doing the shopping as it hurts her back to carry shopping bags.

based definition, this patient has acute back pain, and would not be classified as having chronic back pain until his pain had lasted another 2 months. A primary care physician who focused on pain duration to evaluate prognosis would manage this patient according to acute low back pain guidelines, and might even advise the patient that he could expect to be 'pain-free' in a matter of days or weeks. However, the other factors reported by this patient are established indicators of significant psychosocial dysfunction linked to poor prognosis, and these might not be detected, or might be regarded as understandable manifestations of severe (but time-limited) back pain, that could be expected to resolve as the patient's back pain improved with the tincture of time.

◆ *Timescale of neurophysiological and somatosensory mechanisms*—as noted above, chronic pain is traditionally distinguished from acute pain on a timescale measured in months. This does not correspond to the timescale of neurophysiological changes hypothesized to contribute to chronic pain.[1] For example, long-term potentiation of nociceptive synaptic transmission can be induced over a time scale measured in milliseconds to seconds (Klein et al., 2004). Wind-up, or central pain sensitization, has been observed to take place over a timescale measured in seconds to minutes (Staud et al. 2001). Burn sensitization occurs over a timescale of minutes to hours (Woolf and McMahon 1985). And, inflammation has been observed to produce central changes in pain pathways over a timescale measured in hours to days (Pitcher et al. 2007). Thus, neurophysiological changes that may contribute to induction of chronic pain can occur early in the development of a pain condition, rather than unfolding gradually over a period of months. At the same time, individual differences in susceptibility to induction of chronic pain may be associated with premorbid somatosensory characteristics, such as somatization or hypochondriasis, that are relatively stable over long periods of time (Barsky et al. 1998; De Gucht 2003; Fishbain et al. 2009). These more stable prognostic indicators may be identifiable early in the course of a pain condition, or prior to onset. This raises the question of the extent to which there is a transition from acute pain to a qualitatively distinct chronic pain state that takes months to unfold or whether essential features of chronic pain are observable early on. Duration-based definitions of chronic pain imply that there is a transition from acute to chronic pain that takes months to unfold.

◆ *Convergent validity*—there is not a clear association between pain duration and the extent of pain dysfunction. In addition, manifestations often referred to as identifying features of 'chronic' pain (e.g. severe pain, depression, pain-related activity limitations) are often present in the acute phase of pain. If 'chronic' pain implies only that pain has lasted for 3 months or more, the weak association of pain duration and pain dysfunction would be of limited import. However, it is sometimes assumed that people with long-standing pain problems almost always have greater dysfunction and require different treatment than persons with pain of more recent origin. In fact, there is no clear cut-off for pain duration that alone is a strong predictor of the severity of pain dysfunction (Von Korff et al. 1992; Dunn and Croft 2006). Moreover, among people with long pain duration and significant pain dysfunction, some go on to improve significantly even through they continue to experience pain. For such persons, is their pain more chronic due to increased duration, or less chronic due to reduced pain dysfunction? In the population-at-large, there are many individuals with persistent or recurrent pain who do not experience substantial activity limitations and suffering. For example,

---

[1] We gratefully acknowledge Gregory Terman for pointing out the difference between the traditional timescale used to differentiate chronic from acute pain (3 to 6 months) and the much briefer time intervals over which neuroplastic changes hypothesized to induce chronic pain have been observed.

although a substantial proportion of people with 'chronic' pain have a poor prognosis, up to 40% completely recover within a year (Costa et al. 2009). Among persons with comparably long pain duration, those with less intense pain, lower levels of activity limitation, lower levels of emotional distress, and less diffuse pain are more likely to recover (that is, their pain is less likely to run a chronic course). This is illustrated by Patient B in Box 2.1, who has had long-standing back pain, but whose pain is likely to improve to a manageable level as there are no indicators of poor back pain prognosis other than pain of long duration.

In light of these conceptual difficulties with defining chronic pain by duration alone, there is a need to consider approaches to defining chronic pain that address shortcomings of traditional, duration-based definitions of chronic pain.

## 2.2 **Conceptual bases for defining chronic pain[2]**

Defining chronic pain by duration is based on the view that acute pain signals potential tissue damage, whereas chronic pain results from central and peripheral sensitization in which pain is sustained after nociceptive inputs have diminished (Bonica 1990). From this perspective, chronic pain is a progressive condition characterized by changes in central and peripheral nerves facilitating transmission of pain signals at lower thresholds (e.g. allodynia and hyperalgesia) (Staud and Spaeth 2008). Such changes in pain transmission may be accompanied by psychological changes (e.g. onset of depressed mood, disturbed sleep), by behavioural changes (e.g. reduced activity levels), and, in severe cases, by disruption of social role function (e.g. unemployment). The transition from acute to chronic pain is hypothesized to take place over a 3–6-month period in which a qualitatively different chronic pain state emerges.

A contrasting perspective is that chronic pain reflects deficiencies in endogenous pain inhibition systems, individual differences in somatosensory processing, and differences in abilities to cope with pain that are observable soon after pain onset or even prior to pain onset. Edwards has hypothesized that individual differences in pain sensitivity and pain inhibition, differences which reflect variability in central nervous system pain processing, influence chronic pain risk across anatomic sites (Edwards 2005). Individuals with inadequate endogenous pain inhibition are at increased risk that pain conditions will not spontaneously resolve. Individual differences in somatosensory processing, indicated by diffuse somatic symptoms and/or hypochondriasis, may also be related to unfavourable prognostic risk (Celestin et al. 2009; Fishbain et al. 2009). The biopsychosocial perspective holds that psychological and behavioural domains are also integral determinants of risks of pain dysfunction being sustained over time. Catastrophizing, emotional distress, and helplessness reflect deficiencies in abilities to adapt to pain (Keefe et al. 2004). Individuals with these characteristics may be less able to restore normal functioning. This perspective focuses on factors present early in a pain episode (and prior to onset) that differentiate persons likely to have favourable pain outcomes from those less likely to recover. Chronic pain represents a failure of homeostatic systems (neurophysiological, psychological, behavioural) to control pain expression and restore normal functioning, rather than as a transition to a qualitatively different chronic pain state. Manifestations of chronic pain (e.g. severe pain, depression, activity limitations) are present early on, while chronic pain is usually characterized by a failure

----

2  The authors are indebted to Judith Turner, Gregory Terman, Mark Sullivan, Ruth Landau, Alex Cahana, and Gary Franklin for discussions that contributed to ideas discussed in the section of this chapter on 'Conceptual bases for defining chronic pain'.

of these manifestations to resolve, rather than progressive worsening over time being a typical clinical course. However, this perspective leaves room for a cumulative effect of the experience of pain over time to interact with the psychological and behavioural characteristics mentioned above. Thus, pain persistence (or duration) is a significant prognostic indicator for two reasons: (1) pain persistence is an indicator of deficiencies in pain inhibitory systems; and (2) pain persistence also reflects increased opportunity for interaction between the experience of pain and psychological and behavioural processes which may influence the subsequent course of pain and associated dysfunction.

A critical question addressed by this chapter is the extent to which outcomes can be predicted early in an episode of a painful condition. If chronic pain is predominantly a progressive condition, marked by a transition from acute to chronic pain, then it may be necessary to rely on the passage of time to empirically sort out patients who develop chronic pain, which would justify relying on pain duration as the critical defining feature of chronic pain. However, if indicators of deficient endogenous pain inhibition, somatosensory amplification and inadequate pain coping can be identified in the early stages of pain episodes, then it may be possible to identify patients at high risk of unfavourable pain outcomes for early intervention. This chapter considers the extent to which patients at high risk of clinically significant persistent pain, and associated dysfunction, can be empirically identified without relying primarily on the passage of time to distinguish those for whom clinically significant pain does not resolve spontaneously. The prognostic variables considered in this chapter include self-report measures of pain (intensity, persistence, diffuseness), depression, and pain-related dysfunction. However, the prognostic approach developed in this chapter could, and should, be extended to incorporate psychophysical measures of deficiencies in pain modulation such as tests of diffuse noxious inhibitory control (DNIC) and mechanical temporal summation (Granot et al. 2006, 2008). DNIC is a measure of endogenous pain inhibition capacity, specifically, the degree to which exposure to an ongoing painful 'conditioning' stimulus inhibits the pain caused by a brief, repeated painful 'test' stimulus. Mechanical temporal summation is an indicator of the excitatory mechanism of pain processing. Other measures of somatosensory processing (e.g. somatization, hypochondriasis) and pain coping (e.g. catastrophizing, fear-avoidance) should be considered as prognostic indicators as well.

## 2.3 **Duration-based and prognostic approaches**

Duration-based definitions of chronic pain have been commonly used for research purposes. For example, traditionally designed prognostic studies rely on an inception cohort (of acute patients), determined by episode duration (Henschke et al. 2008) or healthcare use (Croft et al. 1998). Similarly, patients recruited to randomized controlled trials of chronic pain are often identified based on the duration of their symptoms, e.g. low back pain for at least 6 months (Spinhoven et al. 2004) or a minimum of 3 months (Katz et al. 2003). However, it is often unclear exactly how this duration is determined, for example does the pain have to be present every day, or most days? It is rare that the exact question used to define duration is presented with information supporting its reliability and validity. Research comparing different questions used to determine back pain episode duration has shown poor reliability between different definitions. For example, 38% of people who said their back pain had been present for less than 3 months also reported they had not had a whole month without back pain for over a year (Dunn et al. 2006a). Such difficulties likely result from the nature of pain, which commonly runs a recurrent or episodic course (Von Korff et al. 1993a). A definition of chronic pain based purely on duration implies a linear course of pain (Cedraschi et al. 1998), making it difficult to accurately classify persons with recurrent pain as either acute or chronic. In a clinical consultation, it may be possible to clarify the duration of pain by requesting further information from the patient, but in a research setting where data collection is standardized, this is a difficult task.

Researchers have recognized these difficulties, and proposed alternate definitions of chronic pain. Definitions can take the episodic nature of some pain conditions into account, e.g. defining chronic back pain as pain present on at least half the days in a 12-month or a 6-month period (Von Korff 1994). Consensus definitions about how an episode should be defined more specifically have been proposed. De Vet et al. (2002) defined episodes of low back pain, care for low back pain, and work absence due to low back pain, summarized in Box 2.2. The definition of low back pain episodes has been examined among primary care back pain patients and found to have good reliability and validity (Dunn et al. 2006a). However, there are still many problems in defining duration. In a recent Delphi study, back pain researchers had substantial difficulty in reaching consensus on how to operationalize back pain duration (Dionne et al. 2008). In the end, the participants agreed to recommend using time since the last pain-free month to assess duration, but with an additional category to identify patients with less than 3 months duration.

Apart from conceptual difficulties, the empirical bases for the cutpoints used to define chronicity are not well supported. The justification that 90% of patients recover within 3 months (Nachemson and Andersson 1982) has since been refuted. Hestbaek et al. carried out a systematic review including 36 articles, and reported that an average of 62% of patients consulting with low back pain still experienced pain after 12 months (Hestbaek et al. 2003). Furthermore, research comparing primary care back pain patients with different episode durations did not support a cut-off at 3 months' duration, and offered only limited support for a cut-off at 6 months' duration (Dunn and Croft 2006).

Prior episodes of pain have been found to be one of the main predictors of outcome (Papageorgiou et al. 1996; Hestbaek et al. 2003). This suggests that defining chronicity purely on the basis of the duration of the current episode, and ignoring prior history, might not be the most appropriate approach. So-called 'inception cohorts' may not actually identify people at a

---

## Box 2.2 Definitions of low back pain episodes

### Episode of low back pain

Definition: a period of pain in the lower back lasting over 24 hours, preceded and followed by 1 month or more without low back pain (de Vet et al. 2002).

Question for current pain sufferers: 'How long is it since you had a whole month without any back pain?' (Dunn and Croft 2006).

Question for general population samples: 'If you had low back pain in the past 4 weeks, how long was it since you had a whole month without any low back pain?' (Dionne et al. 2008).

### Episode of care for low back pain

Definition: a consultation or a series of consultations for low back pain, preceded and followed by at least 3 months without consultation for low back pain (de Vet et al. 2002).

### Episode of work absence due to low back pain

Definition: a period of work absence due to low back pain, preceded and followed by a period of at least 1 day at work in the normal job (de Vet et al. 2002).

common point in the course of their condition, if measured by duration of the current episode, when prior back pain episodes are taken into account.

## 2.4 **Chronic pain as a multidimensional phenomenon**

Risk factors for chronic pain come from a range of domains. Biological mechanisms can include factors such as genetics (Hartvigsen et al. 2004; Hestbaek et al. 2004) or abnormalities in the hypothalamic–pituitary–adrenal (HPA) stress-response system (McBeth et al. 2007), and biomechanical factors may incorporate components such as muscle strength (Smeets and Wittink 2007) or central sensitization (Werneke and Hart 2001). Psychological factors can involve factors such as distress or depressive mood (Pincus et al. 2002). Social factors may include job stress (Turner et al. 2008) or social isolation (Steenstra et al. 2005). These factors are all known prognostic indicators, but also characterize people with chronic pain. For example, 20% of people with chronic pain also have major depression (Currie and Wang 2004), and chronic pain patients are much more likely to have fear avoidance beliefs than acute pain patients (Grotle et al. 2004). Studies including factors from several domains have confirmed the multidimensional nature of chronic pain for a range of conditions including hand and wrist problems, back pain, shoulder pain, and neck pain (Smith et al. 2004; Carragee et al. 2005; Kamper et al. 2008; Reilingh et al. 2008; Spies-Dorgelo et al. 2008).

The recommendations for management of chronic pain also highlight the multidimensional nature of the problem. For example, the European guidelines for the management of chronic non-specific low back pain recommend assessment of domains including work-related factors, psychological distress and depressive mood, and point out that no single intervention is likely to be effective due to the multidimensional nature of chronic low back pain (Airaksinen et al. 2006; see also Chapter 24). The guidelines for persistent pain from the American Geriatrics Society recommend assessment of pain characteristics and impairments in physical and social function, as well as factors such as attitudes and beliefs about pain (American Geriatrics Society Panel on Persistent Pain in Older Persons 2002). The basis for such assessment stems from systems such as Turk and Rudy's Multiaxial Assessment of Pain, which integrated physical, psychosocial, and behavioural information (Turk and Rudy 1987). The assessment of psychological factors has been significantly advanced by the 'yellow flags' approach to assessment of back pain (ACC and the National Health Committee 1997; Kendall et al. 2009; Nicholas et al. 2011), complementing the 'red flag' indicators of serious underlying conditions (Croft 1999; Henschke et al. 2009), and 'blue flags' addressing individual-level occupational factors (Shaw et al. 2009). These 'flags' are now commonly recommended for use in conditions such as low back pain (Samanta et al. 2003; Main and Spanswick 2003; see also Chapter 13). This approach to back pain assessment is consistent with the prognostic approach to defining chronic pain developed in this chapter.

Despite the acceptance of prognostic factors for chronic pain from multiple domains, and the integration of the multidimensional approach into back pain assessment and treatment guidelines, the definition of chronic pain by duration is widely employed. For example, 'chronic' pain patients are still identified for randomized controlled trials (e.g. Smeets et al. 2006; Critchley et al. 2007) and cohort studies (e.g. Keeley et al. 2008; Reilingh et al. 2008) using duration-based definitions of chronicity. As stated by Cedraschi et al. over 10 years ago, there is a 'necessity to include not only clinical findings but also elements in relation to a biopsychosocial model of low back pain in the definition of chronicity' (Cedraschi et al. 1998). Limiting ourselves to studying chronic pain in terms of duration restricts the investigation of genetic, neurophysiological and biomechanical processes, and psychosocial mechanisms that may represent important influences on the development and course of chronic pain.

## 2.5 **Chronic pain—static or dynamic?**

The term 'chronic' can be interpreted as meaning unlikely to change (Von Korff and Dunn 2008), but chronic pain is *not* a static phenomenon. Descriptions of the course of low back pain, for example, describe pain episodes with exacerbations and pain-free intervals (Deyo 1993). Chronic pain is most commonly characterized by recurrences or repeated episodes (Von Korff et al. 1993a). Population studies appear to give a slightly more stable picture of chronic pain, with a study in Scotland showing that almost 80% of people with chronic pain still had reported pain 4 years later (Elliott et al. 2002), but this apparent stability in the presence of pain masks large variability in pain severity. Recent in-depth analysis of pain trajectories over time has found highly variable patterns of pain over time. Among primary care back pain consulters, groups could be characterized as having recovering, persistent mild, fluctuating or severe chronic pain trajectories (Dunn et al. 2006b).

Labelling patients as having 'chronic pain' has negative connotations in clinical practice, implying a problem patient (Cedraschi et al. 1999), or someone with long-standing psychiatric problems for whom treatment is likely to be ineffective (American Geriatrics Society Panel on Persistent Pain in Older Persons 2002). From a patient's perspective, defining chronic pain based on the duration of symptoms only gives information on their pain experience up to that point, and gives no indication of likely pain outcomes (Richardson et al. 2006). This lack of knowledge about the future course of pain compounds the overall uncertainty of many pain conditions, prevents planning, and may be a barrier to accepting and coping with pain (Richardson et al. 2006).

Interestingly, research from clinical practice has shown that clinicians (rheumatologists and chiropractors) actually do not simply use pain duration to define chronicity. Rather, they incorporate a broader psychosocial context including symptoms and signs, psychological difficulties, and working conditions (Cedraschi et al. 1999). And individuals with chronic pain themselves may be expressing different things when they are reporting chronicity, for example they may take the wider experience of their symptoms or the severity of the effects of pain on their daily lives into account, rather than simply referring to the duration of their pain.

Despite problems with purely duration-based approaches, episode duration as reported and perceived by patients does have some prognostic value and should not be discarded. Patients with different episode durations have different characteristics and different prognoses, even after adjustment for other factors (Bot et al. 2005; Dunn and Croft 2006; Demmelmaier et al. 2008). Episode duration may also influence treatment outcomes, for example back pain patients in a disability rehabilitation programme with 3–6 months' duration of sick leave did better than those with over 6 months' duration (Sullivan et al. 2008). Classification systems, such as that produced by the Quebec Task Force (Spitzer et al. 1987), do include duration alongside other prognostic indicators.

Alternative approaches to defining chronic pain that are consistent with the prognostic approach developed in this chapter have been proposed and evaluated. As mentioned earlier, the Multiaxial Assessment of Pain (Turk and Rudy's Dysfunctional Chronic Pain taxonomy) assesses chronic pain status in terms of dimensions including activity interference, emotional distress, pain intensity, and perceived support (Turk and Rudy 1987). The Chronic Pain Grade (Von Korff et al. 1992) is a widely used method of classifying dysfunctional chronic pain. It was developed on samples of patients with headache, back pain, and temporomandibular pain, and has since been used in other conditions such as neck pain (Côté et al. 1998), hand pain (Dziedzic et al. 2007), and hip pain (Dasch et al. 2008), and in population-based samples (Cassidy et al. 1998; Elliott et al. 1999; Thomas et al. 2004). It incorporates information on pain intensity and pain interference to classify individuals into one of five severity grades and persistent versus non-persistent pain.

While it considers pain intensity and pain-related interference with activities, it is not multi-dimensional, as factors now recognized to be important, such as yellow flag psychosocial indicators, are not included.

Overall, chronic pain is characterized by its uncertainty (Richardson et al. 2006), and should not be seen as an inherently fixed or stable trait, but as being mutable over time (Von Korff and Dunn 2008). In the following section, we describe an approach to integrating multidimensional prognostic variables relevant to chronic pain, using this information to predict probabilities of unfavourable pain outcomes.

## 2.6 **Defining chronic pain by outcome probability**

A prognostic approach to defining chronic pain combines information on past and current pain status, with information on other prognostic variables, into a definition based on outcome probabilities. This approach was initially developed by Von Korff and Miglioretti using data from a cohort of primary care back pain consulters in Washington State, USA (Von Korff and Miglioretti 2005, 2006), and was subsequently replicated across several pain conditions in independent studies (Dunn et al. 2008; Thomas et al. 2008; Von Korff and Dunn 2008).

## 2.7 **Development of the approach**

The definition of chronic pain used in the development of the approach was clinically significant pain likely to be present 1 or more years in the future. This outcome (clinically significant pain) was operationalized using Chronic Pain Grades II to IV (Von Korff et al. 1992) at the follow-up time points. This identifies people with moderate to severe pain intensity and mild to severe dysfunction 1, 2, or 5 years after the baseline evaluation, which typically occurred about 2–4 weeks after an index pain visit in a primary care setting.

In the initial work, latent transition regression analysis was used to identify categories of latent pain severity: no pain, mild pain, moderate pain/limitation, and severe limiting pain. The observed probabilities of severe pain at the subsequent observation demonstrated the utility of pain severity measures in predicting risk of future clinically significant pain, as people with severe pain tended to continue to have severe pain, and people with mild or moderate pain were very unlikely to develop severe pain. This observation suggested that chronicity could be measured by the probability of clinically significant pain continuing at a future point in time.

The next step was to consider prognostic variables other than pain severity, to further differentiate people with lower or higher risk of future clinically significant pain. The variables considered were: depression, measured using the SCL-90-R (Derogatis et al. 1974), the number of days with pain in the previous 6 months, and the number of other pain sites (headache, abdominal pain, chest pain, and facial pain). These variables were then combined with ratings of pain intensity and interference with activities to produce a risk score. Table 2.1 shows the scoring rules used to calculate the risk score for each patient. The items were scored using a limited number of categories established by examining distributional properties of individual items, with 0 scores assigned to low values. It was subsequently assessed whether the predictive accuracy of scoring could be improved by optimizing the scoring weights for each of the items. It was found that predictive validity was not materially improved by using regression-based scoring weights.

The ability of the risk score to predict chronic pain at follow-up was then assessed using a smoothed plot of the baseline risk score against the probability of clinically significant pain 1 year after the index consultation. Probable chronic pain was defined by an 80% or greater probability of future clinically significant pain, possible chronic pain as a 50% or greater probability, and

**Table 2.1** Scoring rules for estimating prognostic risk score

| Item | Item value | Risk score value |
|---|---|---|
| Average pain intensity | 0–3 | 0 |
| | 4–6 | 1 |
| | 7–10 | 2 |
| Worst pain intensity | 0–4 | 0 |
| | 5–7 | 1 |
| | 8–10 | 2 |
| Current pain intensity | 0–2 | 0 |
| | 3–4 | 1 |
| | 5–10 | 2 |
| Interference with usual activities | 0–2 | 0 |
| | 3–4 | 1 |
| | 5–10 | 2 |
| Interference with work/household activities | 0–2 | 0 |
| | 3–4 | 1 |
| | 5–10 | 2 |
| Interference with family/social activities | 0–2 | 0 |
| | 3–4 | 1 |
| | 5–10 | 2 |
| Days of activity limitation due to pain in prior 3 months | 0–2 | 0 |
| | 3–6 | 1 |
| | 7–15 | 2 |
| | 16–24 | 3 |
| | 25–90 | 4 |
| SCL-90-R[†] Depression score | <0.50 | 0 |
| | 0.50–<1.0 | 1 |
| | 1.0–<1.5 | 2 |
| | 1.5–<2.0 | 3 |
| | 2.0–4.0 | 4 |
| Number of other pain sites | 0 | 0 |
| | 1 | 1 |
| | 2 | 2 |
| | 3 | 3 |
| | 4 | 4 |

**Table 2.1** (continued) Scoring rules for estimating prognostic risk score (*Continued*)

| Item | Item value | Risk score value |
|---|---|---|
| Number of days with index pain in prior 6 months | 0–30 | 0 |
| | 31–89 | 1 |
| | 90–120 | 2 |
| | 121–160 | 3 |
| | 161–180 | 4 |
| Total risk score | | 0–28 |

* Risk score values are summed across items.

‡ Measured on 0–10 numerical rating scale.

† Symptom Checklist-90-R (Derogatis et al. 1974).

intermediate risk as a 20% or greater probability of future clinically significant pain, with low risk below 20%. Cut-points on the risk score were then determined from the probability plot to define chronic pain status in terms of the probability of having clinically significant pain at a future time point. Low risk was determined as risk scores of 0–7 (31% of the sample), intermediate risk from 8–15 (43%), possible chronic pain as a score of 16–21 (20%) and probable chronic pain as a risk score of 22 or more (6% of the sample). These categories strongly predicted clinically significant pain at 1 year, as would be expected (see Table 2.2), but they also strongly predicted clinically significant pain at the 2-year and 5-year follow-ups.

These findings provided initial support for the predictive validity of a prognostic approach to defining chronic pain, and supported a multivariable approach to defining chronic pain in terms of outcome probabilities.

## 2.8 Generalizability of the prognostic approach to other samples

Since the initial development of the prognostic approach, it has been tested in a number of other situations. Dunn et al. (2008) investigated the generalizability of the prognostic approach among another low back pain sample, this time in UK primary care consulters. The researchers used the same definitions of chronic pain as the original study, and had the same pain severity variables. They also measured the same prognostic domains, although the measurement instruments used

**Table 2.2** Probability of clinically significant pain at follow-up (percent of each risk score group with chronic pain grade II–IV at follow-up)

| Sample | Baseline risk score group | | | |
| | Low risk (0–7) | Intermediate risk (8–15) | Possible chronic pain (16–21) | Probable chronic pain (22+) |
|---|---|---|---|---|
| US LBP 1 year[1] | 10.9 | 32.1 | 58.7 | 82.1 |
| UK LBP 1 year[2] | 22.9 | 29.9 | 51.1 | 90.3 |
| UK knee 18 months[3] | 20.3 | 51.1 | 84.3 | 88.6 |

LBP, low back pain.
[1] Von Korff and Miglioretti (2005).
[2] Dunn et al. (2008).
[3] Thomas et al. (2008).

to assess these domains were different, e.g. the Hospital Anxiety and Depression Scale (Zigmond and Snaith 1983) was used to measure depression, rather than the SCL-90-R (Derogatis et al. 1974), and time since the last pain-free month (Dunn and Croft 2006) was used to measure pain duration, rather than days with pain in the prior 6 months. The results showed that the prognostic approach was applicable to UK primary care patients. For example, over 90% of people defined with probable chronic back pain actually had clinically significant pain a year later (see Table 2.2). These results also supported the feasibility of substituting different measures of the prognostic indicators when the originally tested prognostic indicators are not available, suggesting that these results are robust across alternative measures of the same prognostic indicator.

Von Korff and Dunn (2008) investigated the use of the prognostic approach in another primary care low back pain sample in the USA. Again, the results showed predictive validity of the approach for predicting chronic pain. They also showed that the prognostic risk scores significantly predicted unemployment and long-term opioid use, as well as the pain itself, with 'probable' chronic back pain sufferers having 15 times the odds of being unemployed, and three times the odds of being on long-term opioid therapy compared to people in the low-risk score group.

The prognostic approach has also been evaluated in conditions other than back pain. In samples of primary care patients with headache and orofacial pain, it was shown to have good predictive validity with similar cut-points to those initially proposed (Von Korff and Dunn 2008). Thomas et al. (2008) have explored the use of the prognostic Risk Score in a general population sample of older adults with knee pain in the UK. They showed that the approach had good prognostic ability in this population as well. For example, 89% of people defined with probable chronic knee pain at baseline had clinically significant pain a year later (see Table 2.2). The findings were consistent when considered across different time-frames. This sample was population-based, and therefore contained a mixture of people seeking healthcare for their knee pain, and those who had not sought care. This work suggested that risk score cut-points may need to be modified for use in general population samples, with lower cut-points being employed in general population samples than in primary care samples.

These studies have shown that using a multifactorial prognostic approach to defining chronic pain is applicable to individuals with back pain, headache, orofacial pain, and knee pain, in both US and UK settings, and in primary care and population settings. While the approach appears to be generalizable, the absolute risk score cut-points did differ between primary care and general population samples when the likelihood of clinically significant pain at follow-up was considered. Thus, while the general approach is reproducible and useful, it may be that cut-points (e.g. for probable or possible chronic pain) need to be determined for particular situations. Specifically, primary care samples assessed in proximity to an initial visit are assessed in a period of pain exacerbation, whereas general population samples are assessed at an arbitrary point in time in the course of their pain condition. For this reason, lower cut-points for possible and probable chronic pain may be appropriate in a general population sample than in patients seeking treatment for a pain condition. Additional research on this issue is needed before a prognostic risk score is used to estimate the prevalence of chronic pain in a general population sample. With that caveat, research to date suggests that the risk score approach not only predicts clinically significant pain, but also behavioural outcomes such as unemployment and medication use, supporting its utility for predicting a range of outcomes that are associated with chronic pain.

Application to the general population is useful for estimating the prevalence of chronic pain in the population-at-large. Applying the original cut-points to a previous general population study (Von Korff et al. 1988, 1993b), the prevalence of probable chronic back pain, headache, or facial pain was approximately 1%. An additional 8% of people had possible chronic pain using this definition. When risk score cut-points defined for general population samples were employed

(18 for probable chronic pain and 12 for possible chronic pain), the prevalence of prognostically defined chronic pain was 5% for probable chronic pain and 19% for possible chronic pain (or 24% of the population having possible or probable chronic pain considering back pain, headache and orofacial pain in combination).

## 2.9 **Comparison of prognostic and duration approaches**

One important part of the assessment of the prognostic approach to defining chronic pain was to compare it to more traditional duration-based approaches. In the UK back pain sample, classifying the sample by duration showed that 52% of people with over 3 months of pain had a poor outcome, whereas classification using the risk score approach indicated that 67% of people with possible or probable chronic pain had a poor outcome (Dunn et al. 2008). Extending this to the US back pain, headache, and orofacial pain samples, the risk score was consistently a better predictor of future clinically significant pain than pain days in the previous year (Von Korff and Dunn 2008). In the population-based knee pain sample, Risk score again proved to have improved prognostic ability when compared to pain duration alone, with the area under the receiver-operating characteristic curve being 0.82 (95% confidence interval [CI]: 0.78, 0.85) for the prognostic approach compared to 0.56 (CI: 0.51, 0.61) for pain duration alone (Thomas et al. 2008), where area under of the curve of 0.50 represents no better than chance prediction.

The evidence shows that the prognostic approach to defining chronic pain shows improved predictive abilities when compared to using measures of pain duration alone, but it has a number of conceptual advantages as well. Traditional duration-based approaches group people into acute and chronic categories. Research into episode duration has shown that the reality is more of a continuum, with little support for the traditional cut-points (Dunn and Croft 2006). Evaluation of the risk score approach has shown that it provides a continuum, where increasing scores indicate increasing risk of future clinically significant pain. The use of cut-points can provide a useful categorization of these scores, and the labels of probable and possible chronic pain are appropriate for a condition where uncertainty about clinical course is inherent. Labelling patients as 'chronic' without indicating the potential for change can have potentially stigmatizing effects. Of greatest importance, the risk score integrates information on pain severity, pain duration, and other prognostic indicators (e.g. depression, number of pain sites), summarizing the results of a multidimensional assessment of chronic pain status, consistent with the biopsychosocial model, in terms of a single risk score that quantifies long-term outcome probabilities.

## 2.10 **Clinical implications**

This chapter challenges the notion that acute and chronic pain, defined by the length of time the pain has been present, should be a predominant basis for prognostic classification of pain patients. For all patients, whether pain duration is brief or long, more accurate prediction of likely outcome than that based on pain duration alone is possible. Persons with recent onset pain who have multiple risk indicators may have a less favourable prognosis than persons with long-lasting pain who have few other unfavourable prognostic indicators. With a more accurate prognostic evaluation, Patient A (see Box 2.1) would be found to be at high risk of chronic dysfunction and steps could be taken to manage his pain, increase his activity levels, and get the patient back to work as soon as possible. Similarly, people who have had their pain for a long time may still have a high likelihood of a favourable outcome if they have few unfavourable prognostic characteristics (see Patient B in Box 2.1). With an accurate prognostic evaluation, the lack of risk factors would be clarified, and the clinician could recognize that the patient is likely to recover to his normal manageable pain levels soon. The patient could be reassured to expect improvement, and offered short-term palliative remedies if desired by the patient. If Patient B's physician focused on pain duration alone, the patient might be offered more aggressive or longer-term medical treatments than warranted. The prognostic approach provides a useful basis for assessing patients, while acknowledging the inherent uncertainty of pain and its variability over time.

For clinicians, using a prognostic approach to defining chronic pain could help to identify targets for intervention early in the clinical course of a pain condition, before social role dysfunction has become entrenched. The prognostic approach focuses attention on what can be done to improve the likelihood of a favourable outcome rather than labelling patients as intractable and unlikely to change. For patients with a short-term problem and no other risk factors, the approach may give a clinician more confidence in offering reassurance and short-term pain relief. The prognostic approach can also provide information to facilitate better management of back pain patients with long term problems. For Patient C (Box 2.1), a clinician using a duration-based definition of chronic might simply tell the person that she is not likely to get better. But using a prognostic approach, prognostic indicators might provide a basis for discussion of how to increase the likelihood of a more favourable outcome, by increasing activity levels in work and family life. This multidimensional approach provides a basis for communicating with patients about what can be done to reduce risks of an unfavourable pain outcome rather than an exclusive focus on medical treatments to 'cure' the underlying condition.

The prognostic approach is consistent with current pain management guidelines, which take a biopsychosocial approach and encourage assessment of a wide range of factors. Using a probabilistic definition incorporates the assumption that the future course of symptoms and prognosis is inherently uncertain, while at the same time identifying possible targets for intervention. This is in contrast to labelling patients as 'chronic', which provides little information to the patient or clinician, and can have connotations of an intractable and enduring problem about which little can be done. Of course, a probabilistic statement about pain prognosis could also be used to label patients as unlikely to improve, or hopeless, but that is contrary to our intent. The term chronic pain is qualified to reflect a possible or probable outcome, not a certainty. And, each patient's risk score is quantified in terms of prognostic factors that can be modified even if pain cannot be eliminated. For these reasons, we believe a prognostic approach to chronic pain is less likely to be used to label and inadvertently stigmatize patients, and more likely to be used to focus attention on a broader set of prognostic factors that can be influenced to improve patient outcomes than pain alone.

Research on a prognostic approach to defining chronic pain has used a range of measurement instruments to assess prognostic factors. It is entirely appropriate to substitute different measures of pain intensity, interference, number of pain sites, pain duration, and psychological distress for those used in prior research. In fact, results have been generally comparable when different measures have been employed. Given the time and cost constraints usually present in clinical practice, briefer instruments may provide the necessary information without taking up too much time. However, the use of risk scores is increasingly feasible in settings that use electronic medical records, and various risk scores are being evaluated for clinical use in many different areas of clinical management of chronic disease and prevention (Ferrer et al. 2005). There is a need for additional research which tests the prognostic ability of alternative self-report measures for predicting long-term pain outcomes to improve the predictive power of this approach. It would also be entirely consistent with a prognostic approach to defining chronic pain to employ psychophysical measures (e.g. diffuse noxious inhibitory control) or genetic markers, if these variables were found to improve prediction of long-term pain outcomes. Research assessing the prognostic value of measures of pain coping and somatosensory functioning could also be evaluated to assess their contribution of prediction of future clinically significant pain. Such research could not only enhance the accuracy of a prognostic classification of chronic pain, it could also shed light on the nature and underlying mechanisms of chronic pain.

To some, viewing a patient in a broader context than the duration of their pain alone may seem obvious. Many clinicians intuitively incorporate indicators of prognosis into their assessment and management of back pain patients already. The adoption of a more structured approach to defining chronic pain by multiple prognostic indicators could result in these approaches being used more consistently across settings and healthcare professionals, providing an evidence-based foundation for patient care. Thus, a prognostic approach to defining chronic pain has the potential to provide a theory-based and evidence-based approach to classification of diverse chronic pain conditions for epidemiological, clinical, and basic research. It could also provide a useful classification for clinical practice, but further research is needed to examine applicability to clinical care.

## 2.11 **Conclusions**

In this chapter, traditional duration-based approaches to defining chronic pain have been contrasted with multifactorial models of pain based in the biopsychosocial model. A new approach to defining chronic pain based on outcome probabilities that are a function of multiple prognostic indicators is proposed. We believe that this approach offers improved predictive validity, as well as better conceptual links to the biopsychosocial model, than approaches based on pain duration alone. It is consistent with current guidelines for managing chronic pain, and is likely to provide more useful information to patients and clinicians.

As an alternative to the IASP definition of chronic pain, we propose that chronic pain be defined by the risk that clinically significant pain and associated dysfunction will be present at a future time point, where the likelihood of future pain and dysfunction is predicted by multiple prognostic factors. The prognostic indicators currently investigated for this purpose include pain severity, pain duration, number of anatomical pain sites, the severity of pain-related activity limitations, and psychological distress. However, these should not be considered as a restrictive or exhaustive list. Other prognostic indicators should be evaluated as they are identified or as the purpose fits, including psychological, psychophysical, and genetic variables. Such factors should be investigated and incorporated while keeping in mind that any assessment has to be acceptable and practical in the setting where it will be applied. The current approach, and any future extensions of the approach, will require testing in clinical practice to establish validity and utility outside the research setting. This definition of chronic pain based on risk of future clinically significant pain defines chronic pain status in probabilistic terms (possible and probable chronic pain), indicating to patients and providers alike that change in pain status over time, both improvement and deterioration, is common. This may help patients and clinicians to view chronic pain as a dynamic process, with potential for change, rather than a label applied to patients deemed unlikely to improve or hopeless. The fact that outcomes are a function of multiple factors calls attention to the possibility that chronic pain outcomes can be improved in ways other than reducing pain alone.

The proposed prognostic approach should not be seen as representing a linear progression over time, although changes in any of the variables included in the risk score may indicate a transition between pain status categories. For example, an increase in the level of depression reported could move someone from having possible to probable chronic pain. Equally, a reduction in pain intensity could move someone from probable to possible chronic pain. Changes in the number of anatomical sites with pain or pain interference could also trigger shifts between categories of pain status. There is no underlying implication in the prognostic approach that pain sufferers progress from low risk through to probable chronic pain over time. This contrasts with a purely duration-based approach which, by its definition, implies deterioration in status or worsening prognosis over time, but is not based on strong empirical evidence and does not give further information on what should be done to improve outcomes other than eliminating pain.

Using a definition of chronic pain based on pain duration alone seems inappropriate when biomedical, psychological and social factors are all accepted contributors to the experience, assessment, mechanisms and management of chronic pain. A definition based on prognosis, quantified in terms of outcome probabilities, encompasses both the complexity and the variability of pain, and appears to be more consistent with the biopsychosocial model of pain.

## References

ACC and the National Health Committee. (1997). *New Zealand Acute Low Back Pain Guide.* Wellington: Accident Rehabilitation & Compensation Insurance Corporation of New Zealand and the National Health Committee.

Airaksinen, O., Brox, J.I., Cedraschi, C., *et al.* (2006). European guidelines for the management of chronic nonspecific low back pain. *Eur Spine J,* **15,** S192–S300.

American Geriatrics Society Panel on Persistent Pain in Older Persons. (2002). The management of persistent pain in older persons. *J Am Geriatr Soc,* **50,** S205–24.

Barsky, A.J., Fama, J.M., Bailey, E.D., Ahern, D.K. (1998). A prospective 4- to 5-year study of DSM-III-R hypochondriasis. *Arch Gen Psychiatry,* **55,** 737–44.

Bonica, J.J. (1953). *The Management of Pain.* Philadelphia, PA: Lea & Febiger.

Bonica, J.J. (1990). General considerations of chronic pain. In Bonica J.J. (ed.) *The Management of Pain,* pp. 159–79. Philadelphia, PA: Lea and Febiger.

Bot, S.D., van der Waal, J.M., Terwee, C.B., *et al.* (2005). Predictors of outcome in neck and shoulder symptoms: a cohort study in general practice. *Spine,* **30,** E459–70.

Carragee, E.J., Alamin, T.F., Miller, J.L., Carragee, J.M. (2005). Discographic, MRI and psychosocial determinants of low back pain disability and remission: a prospective study in subjects with benign persistent back pain. *Spine J,* **5,** 24–35.

Cassidy, J.D., Carroll, L.J., Côté, P. (1998). The Saskatchewan health and back pain survey. The prevalence of low back pain and related disability in Saskatchewan adults. *Spine,* **23,** 1860–6.

Cedraschi, C., Nordin, M., Nachemson, A.L., Vischer, T.L. (1998). Health care providers should use a common language in relation to low back pain patients. *Baillière's Clin Rheumatol,* **12,** 1–15.

Cedraschi, C., Robert, J., Goerg, D., Perrin, E., Fischer, W., Vischer, T.L. (1999). Is chronic non-specific low back pain chronic? Definitions of a problem and problems of a definition. *Br J Gen Pract,* **49,** 358–62.

Celestin, J., Edwards, R.R., Jamison, R.N. (2009). Pretreatment psychosocial variables as predictors of outcomes following lumbar surgery and spinal cord stimulation: a systematic review and literature synthesis. *Pain Med,* **10,** 639–53.

Costa, L.C., Maher, C.G., McAuley, J.H., *et al.* (2009). Prognosis for patients with chronic low back pain: inception cohort study. *BMJ,* **339,** b3829.

Côté, P., Cassidy, J.D., Carroll, L. (1998). The Saskatchewan Health and Back Pain Survey. The prevalence of neck pain and related disability in Saskatchewan adults. *Spine,* **23,** 1689–98.

Critchley, D.J., Ratcliffe, J., Noonan, S., Jones, R.H., Hurley, M.V. (2007). Effectiveness and cost-effectiveness of three types of physiotherapy used to reduce chronic low back pain disability: a pragmatic randomized trial with economic evaluation. *Spine,* **32,** 1474–81.

Croft, P.R. (1999). Diagnosing regional pain: the view from primary care. *Baillière's Best Pract Res Clin Rheumatol,* **13,** 231–42.

Croft, P.R., Macfarlane, G.J., Papageorgiou, A.C., Thomas, E., Silman, A.J. (1998). Outcome of low back pain in general practice: a prospective study. *BMJ,* **316,** 1356–9.

Currie, S.R. and Wang, J. (2004). Chronic back pain and major depression in the general Canadian population. *Pain,* **107,** 54–60.

Dasch, B., Endres, H.G., Maier, C., *et al.* (2008). Fracture-related hip pain in elderly patients with proximal femoral fracture after discharge from stationary treatment. *Eur J Pain,* **12,** 149–56.

De Gucht, V. (2003). Stability of neuroticism and alexithymia in somatization. *Compr Psychiatry,* **44,** 466–71.

de Vet, H.C., Heymans, M.W., Dunn, K.M., *et al.* (2002). Episodes of low back pain: a proposal for uniform definitions to be used in research. *Spine,* **27,** 2409–16.

Demmelmaier, I., Lindberg, P., Asenlof, P., Denison, E. (2008). The associations between pain intensity, psychosocial variables, and pain duration/recurrence in a large sample of persons with nonspecific spinal pain. *Clin J Pain,* **24,** 611–19.

Derogatis, L.R., Lipman, R.S., Rickels, K., Uhlenhuth, E.H., Covi, L. (1974). The Hopkins Symptom Checklist (HSCL): a self-report symptom inventory. *Behav Sci,* **19,** 1–15.

Deyo, R.A. (1993). Practice variations, treatment fads, rising disability. Do we need a new clinical research paradigm? *Spine,* **18,** 2153–62.

Dionne, C.E., Dunn, K.M., Croft, P.R., *et al.* (2008). A consensus approach toward the standardization of back pain definitions for use in prevalence studies. *Spine,* **33,** 95–103.

Dunn, K.M., and Croft, P.R. (2006). The importance of symptom duration in determining prognosis. *Pain,* **121,** 126–32.

Dunn, K.M., de Vet, H.C., Hooper, H., Ong, B.N., Croft, P.R. (2006a). Measurement of back pain episode inception in questionnaires: a study combining quantitative and qualitative methods. *J Musculoskeletal Pain,* **14,** 29–37.

Dunn, K.M., Jordan, K., Croft, P.R. (2006b). Characterising the course of low back pain: a latent class analysis. *Am J Epidemiol,* **163,** 754–61.

Dunn, K.M., Croft, P.R., Main, C.J., Von Korff, M. (2008). A prognostic approach to defining chronic pain: replication in a UK primary care low back pain population. *Pain,* **135,** 48–54.

Dziedzic, K., Thomas, E., Hill, S., Wilkie, R., Peat, G., Croft, P.R. (2007). The impact of musculoskeletal hand problems in older adults: findings from the North Staffordshire Osteoarthritis Project (NorStOP). *Rheumatology (Oxford),* **46,** 963–7.

Edwards, R.R. (2005). Individual differences in endogenous pain modulation as a risk factor for chronic pain. *Neurology,* **65,** 437–43.

Elliott, A.M., Smith, B.H., Penny, K.I., Smith, W.C., Chambers, W.A. (1999). The epidemiology of chronic pain in the community. *Lancet,* **354,** 1248–52.

Elliott, A.M., Smith, B.H., Hannaford, P.C., Smith, W.C., Chambers, W.A. (2002). Assessing change in chronic pain severity: the chronic pain grade compared with retrospective perceptions. *Br J Gen Pract,* **52,** 269–74.

Ferrer, J., Neyro, J.L., Estevez, A. (2005). Identification of risk factors for prevention and early diagnosis of a-symptomatic post-menopausal women. *Maturitas,* **52**(Suppl 1), S7–22.

Fishbain, D.A., Lewis, J.E., Gao, J., Cole, B., Steele, R.R. (2009). Is chronic pain associated with somatization/hypochondriasis? An evidence-based structured review. *Pain Pract,* **9,** 449–67.

Granot, M., Granovsky, Y., Sprecher, E., Nir, R.R., Yarnitsky, D. (2006). Contact heat-evoked temporal summation: tonic versus repetitive-phasic stimulation. *Pain,* **122,** 295–305.

Granot, M., Weissman-Fogel, I., Crispel, Y., *et al.* (2008). Determinants of endogenous analgesia magnitude in a diffuse noxious inhibitory control (DNIC) paradigm: do conditioning stimulus painfulness, gender and personality variables matter? *Pain,* **136,** 142–9.

Grotle, M., Vøllestad, N.K., Veierød, M.B., Brox, J.I. (2004). Fear-avoidance beliefs and distress in relation to disability in acute and chronic low back pain. *Pain,* **112,** 343–52.

Hartvigsen, J., Christensen, K., Frederiksen, H., Pedersen, H.C. (2004). Genetic and environmental contributions to back pain in old age: a study of 2,108 Danish twins aged 70 and older. *Spine,* **29,** 897–901.

Henschke, N., Maher, C.G., Refshauge, K.M., *et al.* (2008). Prognosis in patients with recent onset low back pain in Australian primary care: inception cohort study. *BMJ,* **337,** a171.

Henschke, N., Maher, C.G., Refshauge, K.M., *et al.* (2009). Prevalence of and screening for serious spinal pathology in patients presenting to primary care settings with acute low back pain. *Arthritis Rheum,* **60,** 3072–80.

Hestbaek, L., Leboeuf-Yde, C., Manniche, C. (2003). Low back pain: what is the long-term course? A review of studies of general patient populations. *Eur Spine J,* **12,** 149–65.

Hestbaek, L., Iachine, I.A., Leboeuf-Yde, C., Kyvik, K.O., Manniche, C. (2004). Heredity of low back pain in a young population: a classical twin study. *Twin Res,* **7,** 16–26.

International Association for the Study of Pain Subcommittee on Taxonomy (1986). Classification of chronic pain. Descriptions of chronic pain syndromes and definitions of pain terms. *Pain Suppl,* **3,** S1–226.

International Headache Society H.C.S. (2004). Definition of terms. *Cephalalgia,* **24,** 150–51.

Kamper, S.J., Rebbeck, T.J., Maher, C.G., McAuley, J.H., Sterling, M. (2008). Course and prognostic factors of whiplash: A systematic review and meta-analysis. *Pain,* **138,** 617–29.

Katz, N.P., Ju, W.D., Krupa, D.A., *et al.* (2003). Efficacy and safety of rofecoxib in patients with chronic low back pain: results from two 4-week, randomized, placebo-controlled, parallel-group, double-blind trials. *Spine,* **28,** 851–59.

Keefe, F.J., Rumble, M.E., Scipio, C.D., Giordano, L.A., Perri, L.M. (2004). Psychological aspects of persistent pain: current state of the science. *J Pain,* **5,** 195–211.

Keeley, P., Creed, F., Tomenson, B., Todd, C., Borglin, G., Dickens, C. (2008). Psychosocial predictors of health-related quality of life and health service utilisation in people with chronic low back pain. *Pain,* **135,** 142–50.

Kendall, N.A.S., Burton, A.K., Main, C.J., Watson, P.J. (2009). *Tackling musculoskeletal problems, a guide for the clinic and workplace: Identifying obstacles using the psychosocial flags framework.* London: The Stationery Office.

Klein, T., Magerl, W., Hopf, H-C., Sandkühler, J., Treede, R-D. (2004). Perceptual Correlates of Nociceptive Long-Term Potentiation and Long-Term Depression in Humans. *J Neurosci,* **24,** 964–71.

Loeser, J.D. and Melzack, R. (1999). Pain: an overview. *Lancet,* **353,** 1607–9.

Main, C.J. and Spanswick, C. (2003). *Pain management: an interdisciplinary approach.* Edinburgh: Churchill Livingstone.

McBeth, J., Silman, A.J., Gupta, A., *et al.* (2007). Moderation of psychosocial risk factors through dysfunction of the hypothalamic-pituitary-adrenal stress axis in the onset of chronic widespread musculoskeletal pain: findings of a population-based prospective cohort study. *Arthritis Rheum,* **56,** 360–71.

Nachemson, A.L. and Andersson, G.B. (1982). Classification of low-back pain. *Scand J Work Environ Health,* **8,** 134–6.

Nicholas, M.K., Linton, S.J., Watson, P.J., Main, C.J., "Decade of the Flag" Working Group (2011). Early identification and management of psychological risk factors ("yellow flags") in patients with low back pain: a reappraisal. *Phys Therapy,* **91,** 737–53.

Papageorgiou, A.C., Croft, P.R., Thomas, E., Ferry, S., Jayson, M.I., Silman, A.J. (1996). Influence of previous pain experience on the episode incidence of low back pain: results from the South Manchester Back Pain Study. *Pain,* **66,** 181–5.

Pincus, T., Burton, A.K., Vogel, S., Field, A.P. (2002). A systematic review of psychological factors as predictors of chronicity/disability in prospective cohorts of low back pain. *Spine,* **27,** E109–20.

Pitcher, M.H., Ribeiro-da-Silva, A., Coderre, T.J. (2007). Effects of inflammation on the ultrastructural localization of spinal cord dorsal horn group I metabotropic glutamate receptors. *J Comp Neurol,* **505,** 412–23.

Raspe, H., Huppe, A., Matthis, C. (2003). Theories and models of chronicity: on the way to a broader definition of chronic back pain. *Schmerz,* **17,** 359–66.

Reilingh, M.L., Kuijpers, T., Tanja-Harfterkamp, A.M., van der Windt, D.A. (2008). Course and prognosis of shoulder symptoms in general practice. *Rheumatology,* **47,** 724–30.

Richardson, J.C., Ong, B.N., Sim, J. (2006). Remaking the future: contemplating a life with chronic widespread pain. *Chronic Illness,* **2,** 209–18.

Samanta, J., Kendall, J., Samanta, A. (2003). 10-minute consultation. Chronic low back pain. *BMJ,* **326,** 535.

Shaw, W.S., van der Windt, D.A., Main, C.J., Loisel, P., Linton S.J. (2009). Early patient screening and intervention to address individual-level occupational factors ('blue flags') in back disability. *J Occup Rehabil,* **19,** 64–80.

Smeets, R.J. and Wittink, H. (2007). The deconditioning paradigm for chronic low back pain unmasked? *Pain,* **130,** 201–202.

Smeets, R.J., Vlaeyen, J.W., Hidding, A., *et al.* (2006). Active rehabilitation for chronic low back pain: Cognitive-behavioral, physical, or both? First direct post-treatment results from a randomized controlled trial [ISRCTN22714229]. *BMC Musculoskelet Disord,* **7,** 5.

Smith, B.H., Elliott, A.M., Hannaford, P.C., Chambers, W.A., Smith, W.C. (2004). Factors Related to the Onset and Persistence of Chronic Back Pain in the Community: Results From a General Population Follow-up Study. *Spine,* **29,** 1032–40.

Spies-Dorgelo, M.N., van der Windt, D.A., Prins, A.P., Dziedzic, K.S., van der Horst, H.E. (2008). Clinical course and prognosis of hand and wrist problems in primary care. *Arthritis Rheum,* **59,** 1349–57.

Spinhoven, P., Ter Kuile, M., Kole-Snijders, A.M., Hutten, M.M., Den Ouden, D.J., Vlaeyen, J.W. (2004). Catastrophizing and internal pain control as mediators of outcome in the multidisciplinary treatment of chronic low back pain. *Eur J Pain,* **8,** 211–19.

Spitzer, W.O., LeBlanc, F.E., Dupuis, M., *et al.* (1987). Scientific approach to the assessment and management of activity-related spinal disorders: A monograph for clinicians. Report of the Quebec Task Force on Spinal Disorders. *Spine* **12**(7 Supp ), S1–S59.

Staud, R. and Spaeth, M. (2008). Psychophysical and neurochemical abnormalities of pain processing in fibromyalgia. *CNS Spectr,* **13,** 12–17.

Staud, R., Vierck, C.J., Cannon, R.L., Mauderli, A.P., Price, D.D. (2001). Abnormal sensitization and temporal summation of second pain (wind-up) in patients with fibromyalgia syndrome. *Pain,* **91,** 165–75.

Steenstra, I.A., Verbeek, J.H., Heymans, M.W., Bongers, P.M. (2005). Prognostic factors for duration of sick leave in patients sick listed with acute low back pain: a systematic review of the literature. *Occupational and Environmental Medicine,* **62,** 851–60.

Sullivan, M.J., Adams, H., Tripp, D., Stanish, W.D. (2008). Stage of chronicity and treatment response in patients with musculoskeletal injuries and concurrent symptoms of depression. *Pain,* **135,** 151–9.

Thomas, E., Peat, G., Harris, L., Wilkie, R., Croft, P.R. (2004). The prevalence of pain and pain interference in a general population of older adults: cross-sectional findings from the North Staffordshire Osteoarthritis Project (NorStOP). *Pain,* **110,** 361–68.

Thomas, E., Dunn, K.M., Mallen, C.D., Peat, G. (2008). A prognostic approach to chronic pain: application to knee pain in older adults. *Pain,* **139,** 389–97.

Turk, D.C. and Rudy, T.E. (1987). Towards a comprehensive assessment of chronic pain patients. *Behav Res Ther,* **25,** 237–49.

Turner, J.A., Franklin, G., Fulton-Kehoe, D., *et al.* (2008). ISSLS prize winner: Early predictors of chronic work disability: a prospective, population-based study of workers with back injuries. *Spine,* **33,** 2809–18.

Von Korff, M. (1994). Studying the natural history of back pain. *Spine,* **19,** 2041S–2046S.

Von Korff, M. and Dunn, K.M. (2008). Chronic pain reconsidered. *Pain,* **138,** 267–76.

Von Korff, M. and Miglioretti, D.L. (2005). A prognostic approach to defining chronic pain. *Pain,* **117,** 304–13.

Von Korff, M. and Miglioretti, D.L. (2006). A prospective approach to defining chronic pain. In Flor H., Kalso E., Dostrovsky J.O. (eds.) *Proceedings of the 11th World Congress on Pain.* pp. 761–9. Seattle, WA: IASP Press.

Von Korff, M., Dworkin, S.F., Le Resche, L., Kruger, A. (1988). An epidemiologic comparison of pain complaints. *Pain,* **32,** 173–83.

Von Korff, M., Ormel, J., Keefe, F.J., Dworkin, S.F. (1992). Grading the severity of chronic pain. *Pain,* **50,** 133–49.

Von Korff, M., Deyo, R.A., Cherkin, D.C., Barlow, W. (1993a). Back pain in primary care. Outcomes at 1 year. *Spine,* **18,** 855–62.

Von Korff, M., Le Resche, L., Dworkin, S.F. (1993b). First onset of common pain symptoms: a prospective study of depression as a risk factor. *Pain,* **55,** 251–8.

Waddell, G. (1998). *The Back Pain Revolution.* Edinburgh: Churchill Livingstone.

Werneke, M. and Hart, D.L. (2001). Centralization phenomenon as a prognostic factor for chronic low back pain and disability. *Spine,* **26,** 758–64.

Woolf, C.J. and McMahon, S.B. (1985). Injury-induced plasticity of the flexor reflex in chronic decerebrate rats. *Neuroscience,* **16,** 395–404.

Zigmond, A.S. and Snaith, R.P. (1983). The Hospital Anxiety and Depression Scale. *Acta Psychiatr Scand,* **67,** 361–70.

Part 2

## Risk Factors of Chronic Back Pain and Disability: Biological Mechanisms

# Chapter 3

# Genetic Factors Modulating Chronic Back Pain

Julia Metzner and Irmgard Tegeder

## 3.1 Introduction

The manifestation of back pain is contributed by structural, psychosocial, and occupational influences (Hartvigsen et al. 2004). Biochemical and inflammatory factors modulate the transition of acute towards chronic pain and genetic factors may impact on any of these factors. Research has been mainly focused on genes that determine bone and cartilage structure and are accompanied by morphological signs in magnetic resonance imaging (MRI). Genetic associations were found for disc height narrowing, disc herniation, and different definitions of back pain, such as duration of the worst back pain episode and hospitalization for back problems (Battie et al. 2007). The heritability estimates for these back pain variables ranged from 30–45% (Battie et al. 2007).

However, only a minority of the genetic influences was caused by genes affecting disc degeneration suggesting that genes involved in pain perception, signalling, and psychological processing (Foulkes and Wood 2008), and genetic variants of immune genes (Solovieva et al. 2004b) contribute to the proportion of heritability of chronic back pain. The genetic variability in pain signalling pathways contributes to the variance in pain sensitivity and the individual response to treatment strategies. In this chapter we will summarize genetic factors that specifically modify intervertebral disc stability and pain signalling that may independently impact on the risk of developing chronic back pain.

## 3.2 Polymorphisms associated with subtle modulations of pain sensitivity

MRI signs of bone and cartilage structure are weakly predictive for chronic back pain suggesting that interindividual differences in pain sensation and processing contribute to the individual risk of chronic back pain. Genetic variants in genes modifying pain sensation and signalling are likely to explain a certain proportion of the high heritability estimates for chronic back pain. Only recently it has been increasingly recognized that some frequent genetic polymorphisms are associated with modulations of pain sensitivity or the development of hyperalgesia. These frequent polymorphisms are not the cause of serious diseases but may change the risk for chronic pain including chronic back pain. Associations between candidate genes and chronic back pain with lumbar root pain were evaluated in patients following lumbar disc surgery (Tegeder et al. 2006). The patients suffered from serious long-lasting radicular sciatic pain before surgery. In the first 2 years after surgery, pain scores for frequency and intensity at rest and during walking were recorded. The statistical analysis revealed that patients with a defined set of single nucleotide polymorphisms (SNPs) in the gene of the GTP cyclohydrolase 1 (*GCH1*) had consistently less pain than non-carriers and a significantly better outcome after surgery (Tegeder et al. 2006). The polymorphisms in *GCH1* that were associated with reduced pain constitute a certain haplotype, referred to as 'pain-protective' haplotype of *GCH1*, with a frequency of about 16% in the Caucasian population. The GTP cyclohydrolase is the rate-limiting enzyme in the synthesis of the enzyme cofactor, tetrahydrobiopterin which is essential for the production of biogenic amines (Blau and Niederwieser 1985) and nitric oxide (Gross and Levi 1992). It has been confirmed in further studies that the 'pain-protective' haplotype is associated with a reduction of the sensitivity to mechanical and heat stimulation and particularly the development of hyperalgesia (Tegeder et al. 2008). Functionally, this haplotype prevents the up-regulation of *GCH1* and overproduction of tetrahydrobiopterin that normally occurs upon pro-inflammatory stimulation or peripheral nerve injury (Tegeder et al. 2006, 2008).

Other genetic polymorphisms have been associated with reduced pain sensitivity (Oertel and Lötsch 2008) but most studies did not specifically address chronic back pain. However, it appears reasonable to hypothesize that polymorphisms that modulate other types of chronic pain may also impact on the liability to develop chronic back pain. Such pain-modulating gene variants were found for catechol-O-methyltransferase (*COMT*), transient receptor potential channel A1 (*TRPA1*), melanocortin-1 receptor (*MC1R*), fatty acid amide hydrolase (*FAAH*), and the μ-opioid receptor (*OPRM1*). *COMT* modulates specific aspects of human pain perception and the risk for developing complex pain conditions including migraine (Diatchenko et al. 2006). *COMT* metabolizes catecholamines and modifies thereby the transmission of dopaminergic, adrenergic and noradrenergic pathways in the brain. A single nucleotide exchange in the coding region of *COMT* leads to an amino acid substitution of valine to methionine at position 158 (V158M), with impaired translation of *COMT*-mRNA, reduction of its enzyme activity and reduced thermostability (Diatchenko et al. 2006). The V158M genotype was primarily associated with the rate of temporal summation of heat pain (Diatchenko et al. 2006). Other SNPs of *COMT* exert a greater influence on baseline nociceptive sensitivity and are inversely correlated with enzyme activity and the risk of developing the myogenous temporomandibular joint disorder (TMD) (Slade et al. 2007). TMD is a common pain syndrome with a prevalence of about 10% and 3:1 female to male ratio with high heritability estimates (Oakley and Vieira 2008; Stohler 2006) and is often associated with chronic back pain (Oakley and Vieira 2008; Stohler 2006).

Variants of the melanocortin 1 receptor gene (*MC1R*) were reported to reduce pain sensitivity (Mogil et al. 2005) although this finding was not reproduced in another human cohort (Liem et al. 2005). Nevertheless, in humans with red-hair and fair skin, which is the visible phenotype associated with non-function variants in the *MC1R* gene, the analgesic efficacy of μ-opioid agonists was increased in both women and men, whereas κ-agonists reduced pain only in females (Mogil et al. 2005). Interestingly, female but not male carriers of a genetic variant of the cold receptor, *TRPA1* had increased sensitivity to cold-induced pain compared to carriers of the wild-type allele (Kim et al. 2006a).

The sensitivity to pain and to opioid analgesia and side effects is known to be modulated by variants in opioid receptors (Lötsch and Geisslinger 2005). The μ-opioid receptor, encoded by the *OPRM1* gene (*OPRM1*), is the primary site of action of endogenous and of the most potent exogenous common clinical opioid analgesics such as morphine, fentanyl, or methadone. A large number of polymorphisms have been identified in the promoter region, in exons and introns of *OPRM1* (Ikeda et al. 2005; Lötsch and Geisslinger 2005). So far, most information has been accumulated about the *OPRM1* 118A>G SNP in exon 1 leading to an amino acid substitution from asparagine to aspartate at position 40 of the protein thereby deleting a putative extracellular glycosylation site. This SNP is highly prevalent in the population with an allele frequency of approximately 16% in Caucasians. At the molecular level, it is thought to either decrease μ-opioid receptor expression (Zhang et al. 2005) or, in a brain-region dependent manner, agonist-stimulated receptor signalling (Oertel et al. 2008). With respect to pain sensitivity, carriers of this variant displayed higher pain thresholds (Fillingim et al. 2005) or lower cortical responses to experimental pain stimuli (Lötsch et al. 2006b). With respect to pain treatment with exogenous opioids, the 118A>G SNP significantly reduced the potency of morphine-6-glucuronide (Lötsch et al. 2002; Skarke et al. 2003), morphine (Skarke et al. 2003), or levomethadone (Lötsch et al. 2006a) in experimental studies in healthy volunteers that evaluated pupil constrictory effects of the opioids (Lötsch et al. 2002). The *OPRM1* 118A>G polymorphism reduced both analgesic (Oertel and Lötsch 2008; Oertel et al. 2006) and respiratory depressive (Oertel et al. 2006) effects of alfentanil suggesting that the efficacy of various μ-opioid receptor agonists is affected by this variant. In the clinical setting, carriers of the *OPRM1* 118A>G polymorphism required significantly higher doses of morphine in the early postoperative period following knee surgery (Chou et al. 2006b), abdominal hysterectomy (Chou et al. 2006a), or other major abdominal surgical interventions (Hayashida et al. 2008). Cancer patients homozygous for the 118 G allele also needed higher morphine doses to achieve pain control (Klepstad et al. 2004), further modulated when these patients had the wild type *COMT* Val/Val genotype (Reyes-Gibby et al. 2007).

Endogenous cannabinoids, cannabis, and its congeners reduce pain and modify emotional components of pain through agonistic action at peripheral and central cannabinoid-1 CB1 receptors (Agarwal et al. 2007; Manning et al. 2001). Cannabinoids additionally modify the immune response through cannabinoid CB2 receptors. Tetrahydrocannabinol, one of the constituents of marihuana has the potential to reduce serious neuropathic pain in patients with multiple sclerosis or other neuropathic pain syndromes (Svendsen et al. 2004). However, polymorphisms in the CB1 gene *CNR1* have not been associated with specific pain phenotypes, but were associated with obesity (Aberle et al. 2008; Russo et al. 2007), schizophrenia or efficacy of neuroleptic treatment (Hamdani et al. 2008; Ujike et al. 2002) and drug and alcohol dependence (Agrawal et al. 2008; Zhang et al. 2004; Zuo et al. 2007). Polymorphisms in the CB2 gene *CNR2* play a role in osteoporosis (Karsak et al. 2005) and thereby possibly chronic back pain that is often caused by osteoporosis of the spine with and without vertebral fractures. Genetic variances in *CNR2* might also modulate the susceptibility to autoimmune disorders (Sipe et al. 2005) such as rheumatic diseases. The endocannabinoid anandamide is rapidly metabolized by fatty acid amide hydrolase (FAAH) (Thomas et al. 1997) and FAAH inhibitors reduce pain due to a prolonged half life of anandamide (Lichtman et al. 2004). Polymorphisms in the *FAAH* gene (Doehring et al. 2007) result in decreased FAAH enzyme catalytic activity (Kim et al. 2006a) and slightly reduced sensitivity to cold pain in experimental settings in healthy volunteers (Kim et al. 2006a). The potential modulation of the susceptibility to chronic back pain has not been addressed. However, considering the functions of endocannabinoids on bone formation and density and pain signalling (Ofek et al. 2006; Tam et al. 2008) it is likely that alterations in their metabolism affect the susceptibility to chronic back pain.

## 3.3 Genetic polymorphisms associated with intervertebral disc disease

Intervertebral disc disease (IDD) is characterized by disc degeneration and herniation and is often associated with low back pain and lumbar radicular pain due to nerve root compression or inflammation. Sensory neurons and afferent fibres from multiple spinal cord levels innervate intervertebral discs (Zhang et al. 2006) explaining the often widespread back pain. An increased risk of low back pain was found in relation to all signs of disc degeneration (Luoma et al. 2000;

Sakai et al. 2007). However, structural aspects alone are of limited predictive value for chronic back pain.

Collagen is a major component of the extracellular matrix and regulates cartilage fibril formation within intervertebral discs. It is a heterotrimeric protein consisting of three α-chains. Polymorphisms in the genes coding for the α2 and α3 chains of collagen IX, *COL9A2*, and *COL9A3* were associated with alterations in the mechanical properties of human intervertebral discs and contribute to the susceptibility for lumbar disc herniation and back pain (Annunen et al. 1999; Paassilta et al. 2001; Seki et al. 2006). Several IDD associated *COL9A2* alleles were identified. The so called Trp2 allele representing a Gln326Trp amino acid exchange in the α2 chain was associated with premature disc degeneration and back pain in Finnish, Japanese and Chinese populations (Annunen et al. 1999; Higashino et al. 2007; Jim et al. 2005). The Trp2 variant however was not detected in Germans (Knoeringer et al. 2008) but a high relapse rate of lumbar disc disease after surgery was detected in carriers of the Gln326Arg variant of *COL9A2* (Knoeringer et al. 2008). A Trp3 variant of the α3 chain was also associated with an increased risk of disc degeneration (Paassilta et al. 2001). Presumably, the collagen IX variants reduce the stability of the intervertebral cartilage and thereby increase the risk of disc degeneration and herniation.

Type X1 collagen in the annulus fibrosus and nucleus pulposus also plays a major role in the stability of the intervertebral disc. It is also composed of three α-chains, α1(XI), α2(XI), and α3(II), which are encoded by *COL11A1*, *COL11A2*, and *COL2A1*, respectively. Type XI collagen regulates the diameter of cartilage collagen fibrils. Genetic variants in *COL11A1* were associated with an increased risk of lumbar disc herniation in a Japanese cohort (Mio et al. 2007). A single nucleotide polymorphism in the coding region of *COL11A1* showed the strongest association with disc herniation. The stability of the transcript of the disease-associated allele was reduced and the expression level inversely correlated with the severity of disc degeneration (Mio et al. 2007). In a Finnish population, carriers of a deletion splice site variant of *COL11A2* encoding the α2(XI) chain had a lower risk for degenerative spinal stenosis with radicular pain than carriers of the more abundant 'wild-type' allele (Noponen-Hietala et al. 2003).

Carriers of the so called Sp1 promoter variant of type I collagen (*COL1A1*) were at risk to develop intervertebral disc degeneration (Pluijm et al. 2004), reduced bone mineral density and osteoporotic bone fractures particularly in postmenopausal women (Ashford et al. 2001; MacDonald et al. 2001; Pluijm et al. 2004). The Sp1 variant interferes with the binding of the transcription factor Sp1 resulting in reduced expression of *COL1A1* (Grant et al. 1996). Osteoporosis represents a major cause of chronic low back pain (Schneider et al. 2007) and polymorphisms of various other genes such as transforming growth factor beta (Dick et al. 2003; Langdahl et al. 2003), oestrogen receptor (Kung et al. 2006), the vitamin D receptor (Hustmyer et al. 1994; Morrison et al. 1994) and the low density lipoprotein genes *LRP5* and *LRP6* (Richards et al. 2008; van Meurs et al. 2008) contribute to the pathogenesis of osteoporosis and may therefore contribute to the development of back pain.

Intervertebral disc disease was also associated with 'variable number of tandem repeats' (VNTR) in the coding region of the human aggrecan gene (*AGAN)* (Solovieva et al. 2007). Thirteen different alleles have been identified, with repeat numbers ranging from 13 to 33. The polymorphism results in individuals with differing length aggrecan core proteins, bearing different numbers of potential attachment sites for chondroitin sulfate. Magnetic resonance imaging in healthy volunteers revealed the association of *ACAN* polymorphisms with MRI-signs of intervertebral disc disease (Solovieva et al. 2007). Particularly, multilevel and severe disc degeneration was present in the patients with shorter VNTR length of the aggrecan gene whereas a higher number of repeats (>25) had protective effects (Kawaguchi et al. 1999).

Variants of the gene coding for the cartilage intermediate layer protein (CILP) (Kalichman and Hunter 2008; Seki et al. 2005) were recently reported to be associated with intervertebral disc degeneration (Seki et al. 2005). CILP was expressed abundantly in intervertebral discs, and its expression increased during progression of disc degeneration. CILP colocalized with transforming growth factor TGF-β1 and directly inhibited TGF-1 mediated induction of cartilage matrix genes and TGF-β1 mediated inhibition of metalloproteinase transcription. The aberrantly increased inhibitory effects of CILP attributed to the variant allele probably perturb the balance of TGF-β control over chondrocyte metabolism and intervertebral disc tissue maintenance.

A single adenine insertion/deletion polymorphism (6A/5A) in the metalloproteinase-3 (*MMP3*) promoter region was associated with MRI so-called modic changes in endplates of lumbar vertebral bodies in Finnish male workers, particularly if carriers of the *MMP3* variant had additional polymorphisms in interleukin-1 locus genes (Karppinen et al. 2008). In a cohort of Japanese middle-aged women *MMP3* genotypes with the shorter allele (5 adenine nucleotides) were associated with degenerative changes in lumbar intervertebral discs (Takahashi et al. 2001). The 5A promoter has higher activity compared to that of the 6A allele. Thus, subjects without the variant 5A allele would be predicted to have higher expression and activity of MMP3. As MMP3 plays a major role in the neuroimmune responses following nerve injury and contributes to the development of neuropathic pain in rodents (Kawasaki et al. 2008) this variant may additionally increase the susceptibility to radicular sciatic pain in degenerative disc disease.

In addition to *MMP3*, a single missense polymorphism in metallaoproteinase-9 (*MMP9*) was strongly associated with lumbar disc herniation in two independent Japanese cohorts (Hirose et al. 2008). This polymorphism showed a combinatorial effect with a non-coding variant of the thrombospondin-2 gene. The *THBS2*-SNP caused differences on exon 11 skipping rates, with decreased thrombospondin-2 interaction with MMP2 and MMP9 (Hirose et al. 2008). MMP9 also plays a major role in the manifestation of neuropathic pain following nerve injury (Kawasaki et al. 2008) suggesting that variants in thrombospondin and *MMP9* may also increase the risk of pain hypersensitivity in carriers of these variants.

Carriers of some variants of the vitamin D receptor gene may also be at a higher risk for intervertebral disc disease and osteoporosis. A common polymorphism in exon 2 of the vitamin D receptor gene (*VDR*) introduces a new translation start site and produces a protein that differs in length by three amino acids. Some studies suggest that the longer variant is correlated with lower bone mineral density in some populations (Morrison et al. 1994) and lumbar disc degeneration (Videman et al. 1998).

As extracellular matrix protein polymorphisms increase the susceptibility to degeneration of discs and/or bone of the spine they may increase the risk for chronic back pain. However, these genetic variants presumably do not directly affect pain sensation or signalling or adaptations of peripheral and central pain circuits, with exception of the metalloproteinase polymorphisms. The risk conferred by genetic variants of ECM-genes is further contributed by the risk conferred by inflammatory genes.

## 3.4 Polymorphisms in pro-inflammatory genes

Inflammation plays a major role in the development of intervertebral disc disease (Battie et al. 1995). The extent and resolution of inflammation is modified by genetic variants in cytokine genes. Particularly, polymorphisms in the interleukin-1 gene (IL-1) locus contribute to the development of low back pain. Variants in the genes of IL-1α, IL-1β and the IL-1 receptor antagonist (*IL1RN*) modify bone mineral density (Kim et al. 2006b) and promote intervertebral disc disease with low back pain (Solovieva et al. 2004a; Solovieva et al. 2006). Herniated discs produce several inflammatory mediators such as IL-1, IL-6 and tumour necrosis factor alpha (TNFα) which maintain the inflammatory process and sensitize nociceptors that innervate the affected discs or the surrounding tissue. In a Finnish study in middle-aged men carriers of the IL-1 receptor antagonist G1821>A allele had an increased risk of low back pain (Solovieva et al. 2004b). In addition, carriers of this allele in combination with variants of IL-1α or IL-1β had a higher risk to develop low back pain than non-carriers, and reported more days with pain and higher intensities of low back pain (Solovieva et al. 2004b). The results suggest that IL-1 gene locus polymorphisms promote or prolong low back pain, supported by a recent study that revealed MRI changes in endplates of lumbar vertebral bodies in carriers of combined polymorphisms in *IL1a* and the 5-adenine promoter polymorphism of metalloproteinase-3 (Karppinen et al. 2008). In addition to IL-1, polymorphisms in the IL-6 gene were associated with intervertebral disc disease in patients with discogenic lumbar radicular pain (Noponen-Hietala et al. 2005). Several other pro-inflammatory gene polymorphisms including variants of IL-2, TNF-α, IL-4 and INFγ were analysed but had almost identical allele frequencies in low back pain patients and controls.

## 3.5 Polymorphisms contributing to chronic widespread musculoskeletal pain

Chronic back pain is often associated with widespread pain in complex musculoskeletal pain syndromes such as fibromyalgia (Arnold et al. 2008), temporomandibular joint disorder (Wiesinger et al. 2007), and chronic fatigue syndrome (Meeus et al. 2007). Fibromyalgia is a generalized widespread chronic pain disorder characterized by diffuse muscle pain throughout the body, most often including chronic back and neck pain, muscle weakness, fatigue, increased negative mood, sleep disturbance (Arnold et al. 2008) and comorbidity with anxiety and depression (Thieme et al. 2004). The precise role of genetic factors in the aetiopathology is still unclear but polymorphisms in genes of the serotoninergic and catecholaminergic systems have been associated with an increased risk of fibromyalgia and chronic fatigue syndrome. *COMT* polymorphisms may contribute to the pathogenesis because approximately 74% of fibromyalgia patients had low or intermediate *COMT* activity resulting in low catecholamine degradation (Gursoy et al. 2003; Tander et al. 2008).

Polyarthropathic diseases such as ankylosing spondylitis, rheumatoid arthritis, psoriatic arthritis, or systemic lupus erythematosus cause inflammatory back pain due to arthritis of the small intervertebral or sacroiliacal joints and myositis. Polymorphisms in the major histocompatibility complex (MHC) molecules contribute to the development of these diseases (Brown et al. 1998a; Brown et al. 1998b). However, several other immune genes such as immunoglobulin receptors, TNF receptor, transcription factors such as Stat4, various cytokines and chemokines were shown to be associated with the risk to develop these chronic inflammatory autoimmune diseases and to modify the response to pharmacologic treatments with e.g. anti-TNF monoclonal antibodies or immunosuppressive agents.

## 3.6 Polymorphisms causing complex syndromes with a loss of pain perception

Several hereditary maladies with complete loss of pain sensitivity have been genetically defined. Although the molecular mechanisms differ among them, all syndromes are characterized by an interruption of transmission or processing at key points of the nociceptive system (for full details, see the 'Online Mendelian Inheritance in Man' database (OMIM): http://www.ncbi.nlm.nih.gov/sites/entrez?db=omim) (Oertel and Lötsch 2008). This includes (1) the channelopathy associated insensitivity to pain, which is based on loss-of-function mutations of the alpha-subunit of the voltage-gated sodium channel, Na(v)1.7 (Cox et al. 2006; Goldberg et al. 2007), (2) the Hereditary sensory and autonomic neuropathy type I (HSAN-I), caused by mutations in the serine palmitoyltransferase, long chain base subunit 1 gene (Bejaoui et al. 2001; Dawkins et al. 2001; Verhoeven et al. 2006), (3) the HSAN-II, based on mutations in the hereditary sensory neuropathy, type II (Lafreniere et al. 2004; Riviere et al. 2004; Cho et al. 2006; Roddier et al. 2005), (4) the HSAN-III due to mutations in the inhibitor of kappa light polypeptide gene enhancer in B-cells, kinase complex-associated protein gene (Slaugenhaupt and Gusella 2002; Anderson et al. 2001; Leyne et al. 2003), (5) the HSAN-IV, also called congenital insensitivity to pain with anhidrosis (CIPA) and based on mutations in the neurotrophic tyrosine kinase, receptor, type 1 gene (Indo et al. 1996; Miura et al. 2000), and (6) the HSAN-V caused by mutations in the nerve growth factor, beta polypeptide gene (Einarsdottir et al. 2004). All these syndromes are very rare affecting a few families. Therefore, their specific association with back pain has not been shown but it is reasonable to assume that patients with these syndromes will not develop back pain.

## 3.7 **Summary**

Several genetic factors contribute to the risk for chronic back pain and widespread pain syndromes. The experience of pain results from a complex interaction between several genetic variants involved in different steps of neuronal processing of nociceptive information with additional contribution of other genetic, structural, environmental and psychosocial factors. The investigation of interactions between genetic variants that modify pain signalling and the variants affecting the bone and intervertebral cartilage and the identification of the molecular consequences of functional variants are further required to understand the genetics of pain and specially to identify genetic predictors of chronic back pain.

## References

Aberle, J., Flitsch, J., Beck, N.A., *et al.* (2008). Genetic variation may influence obesity only under conditions of diet: analysis of three candidate genes. *Mol Genet Metab* **95**, 188–91.

Agarwal, N., Pacher, P., Tegeder, I., *et al.* (2007). Cannabinoids mediate analgesia largely via peripheral type 1 cannabinoid receptors in nociceptors. *Nat Neurosci* **10**, 870–9.

Agrawal, A., Wetherill, L., Dick, D.M., *et al.* (2008). Evidence for association between polymorphisms in the cannabinoid receptor 1 (CNR1) gene and cannabis dependence. *Am J Med Genet B Neuropsychiatr Genet* **150B**(5), 736–40.

Anderson, S.L., Coli, R., Daly, I.W., *et al.* (2001). Familial dysautonomia is caused by mutations of the IKAP gene. *Am J Hum Genet* **68**, 753–8.

Annunen, S., Paassilta, P., Lohiniva, J., *et al.* (1999). An allele of COL9A2 associated with intervertebral disc disease. *Science* **285**, 409–12.

Arnold, B.S., Alpers, G.W., Suss, H., *et al.* (2008). Affective pain modulation in fibromyalgia, somatoform pain disorder, back pain, and healthy controls. *Eur J Pain* **12**, 329–38.

Ashford, R.U., Luchetti, M., McCloskey, E.V., *et al.* (2001). Studies of bone density, quantitative ultrasound, and vertebral fractures in relation to collagen type I alpha 1 alleles in elderly women. *Calcif Tissue Int* **68**, 348–51.

Battie, M.C., Videman, T., Gibbons, L.E., Fisher, L.D., Manninen, H., and Gill, K. (1995). 1995 Volvo Award in clinical sciences. Determinants of lumbar disc degeneration. A study relating lifetime exposures and magnetic resonance imaging findings in identical twins. *Spine* **20**, 2601–12.

Battie, M.C., Videman, T., Levalahti, E., Gill, K., and Kaprio, J. (2007). Heritability of low back pain and the role of disc degeneration. *Pain* **131**, 272–80.

Bejaoui, K., Wu, C., Scheffler, M.D., *et al.* (2001). SPTLC1 is mutated in hereditary sensory neuropathy, type 1. *Nat Genet* **27**, 261–2.

Blau, N., and Niederwieser, A. (1985). GTP-cyclohydrolases: a review. *J Clin Chem Clin Biochem* **23**, 169–76.

Brown, M.A., Kennedy, L.G., Darke, C., *et al.* (1998a). The effect of HLA-DR genes on susceptibility to and severity of ankylosing spondylitis. *Arthritis Rheum* **41**, 460–5.

Brown, M.A., Pile, K.D., Kennedy, L.G., *et al.* (1998b). A genome-wide screen for susceptibility loci in ankylosing spondylitis. *Arthritis Rheum* **41**, 588–95.

Cho, H.J., Kim, B.J., Suh, Y.L., An, J.Y., and Ki, C.S. (2006). Novel mutation in the HSN2 gene in a Korean patient with hereditary sensory and autonomic neuropathy type 2. *J Hum Genet* **51**, 905–8.

Chou, W.Y., Wang, C.H., Liu, P.H., Liu, C.C., Tseng, C.C., and Jawan, B. (2006a). Human opioid receptor A118G polymorphism affects intravenous patient-controlled analgesia morphine consumption after total abdominal hysterectomy. *Anesthesiology* **105**, 334–7.

Chou, W.Y., Yang, L.C., Lu, H.F., *et al.* (2006b). Association of mu-opioid receptor gene polymorphism (A118G) with variations in morphine consumption for analgesia after total knee arthroplasty. *Acta Anaesthesiol Scand* **50**, 787–92.

Cox, J.J., Reimann, F., Nicholas, A.K., *et al.* (2006). An SCN9A channelopathy causes congenital inability to experience pain. *Nature* **444**, 894–8.

Dawkins, J.L., Hulme, D.J., Brahmbhatt, S.B., Auer-Grumbach, M., and Nicholson, G.A. (2001). Mutations in SPTLC1, encoding serine palmitoyltransferase, long chain base subunit-1, cause hereditary sensory neuropathy type I. *Nat Genet* **27**, 309–12.

Diatchenko, L., Nackley, A.G., Slade, G.D., *et al.* (2006). Catechol-O-methyltransferase gene polymorphisms are associated with multiple pain-evoking stimuli. *Pain* **125**, 216–24.

Dick, I.M., Devine, A., Li, S., Dhaliwal, S.S., and Prince, R.L. (2003). The T869C TGF beta polymorphism is associated with fracture, bone mineral density, and calcaneal quantitative ultrasound in elderly women. *Bone* **33**, 335–41.

Doehring, A., Geisslinger, G., and Lötsch, J. (2007). Rapid screening for potentially relevant polymorphisms in the human fatty acid amide hydrolase gene using Pyrosequencing. *Prostaglandins Other Lipid Mediat* **84**, 128–37.

Einarsdottir, E., Carlsson, A., Minde, J., *et al.* (2004). A mutation in the nerve growth factor beta gene (NGFB) causes loss of pain perception. *Hum Mol Genet* **13**, 799–805.

Fillingim, R.B., Kaplan, L., Staud, R., *et al.* (2005). The A118G single nucleotide polymorphism of the mu-opioid receptor gene (OPRM1) is associated with pressure pain sensitivity in humans. *J Pain* **6**, 159–67.

Foulkes, T., and Wood, J.N. (2008). Pain genes. *PLoS Genet* **4**, e1000086.

Goldberg, Y.P., MacFarlane, J., MacDonald, M.L., *et al.* (2007). Loss-of-function mutations in the Nav1.7 gene underlie congenital indifference to pain in multiple human populations. *Clin Genet* **71**, 311–19.

Grant, S.F., Reid, D.M., Blake, G., Herd, R., Fogelman, I., and Ralston, S.H. (1996). Reduced bone density and osteoporosis associated with a polymorphic Sp1 binding site in the collagen type I alpha 1 gene. *Nat Genet* **14**, 203–5.

Gross, S.S., and Levi, R. (1992). Tetrahydrobiopterin synthesis. An absolute requirement for cytokine-induced nitric oxide generation by vascular smooth muscle. *J Biol Chem* **267**, 25722–9.

Gursoy, S., Erdal, E., Herken, H., Madenci, E., Alasehirli, B., and Erdal, N. (2003). Significance of catechol-O-methyltransferase gene polymorphism in fibromyalgia syndrome. *Rheumatol Int* **23**, 104–7.

Hamdani, N., Tabeze, J.P., Ramoz, N., *et al.* (2008). The CNR1 gene as a pharmacogenetic factor for antipsychotics rather than a susceptibility gene for schizophrenia. *Eur Neuropsychopharmacol* **18**, 34–40.

Hartvigsen, J., Christensen, K., Frederiksen, H., and Pedersen, H.C. (2004). Genetic and environmental contributions to back pain in old age: a study of 2,108 danish twins aged 70 and older. *Spine* **29**, 897–901; discussion 902.

Hayashida, M., Nagashima, M., Satoh, Y., *et al.* (2008). Analgesic requirements after major abdominal surgery are associated with OPRM1 gene polymorphism genotype and haplotype. *Pharmacogenomics* **9**, 1605–16.

Higashino, K., Matsui, Y., Yagi, S., *et al.* (2007). The alpha2 type IX collagen tryptophan polymorphism is associated with the severity of disc degeneration in younger patients with herniated nucleus pulposus of the lumbar spine. *Int Orthop* **31**, 107–11.

Hirose, Y., Chiba, K., Karasugi, T., *et al.* (2008). A functional polymorphism in THBS2 that affects alternative splicing and MMP binding is associated with lumbar-disc herniation. *Am J Hum Genet* **82**, 1122–9.

Hustmyer, F.G., Peacock, M., Hui, S., Johnston, C.C., and Christian, J. (1994). Bone mineral density in relation to polymorphism at the vitamin D receptor gene locus. *J Clin Invest* **94**, 2130–4.

Ikeda, K., Ide, S., Han, W., Hayashida, M., Uhl, G.R., and Sora, I. (2005). How individual sensitivity to opiates can be predicted by gene analyses. *Trends Pharmacol Sci* **26**, 311–17.

Indo, Y., Tsuruta, M., Hayashida, Y., *et al.* (1996). Mutations in the TRKA/NGF receptor gene in patients with congenital insensitivity to pain with anhidrosis. *Nat Genet* **13**, 485–88.

Jim, J.J., Noponen-Hietala, N., Cheung, K.M., *et al.* (2005). The TRP2 allele of COL9A2 is an age-dependent risk factor for the development and severity of intervertebral disc degeneration. *Spine* **30**, 2735–42.

Kalichman, L., and Hunter, D.J. (2008). The genetics of intervertebral disc degeneration. Associated genes. *Joint Bone Spine* **75**, 388–96.

Karppinen, J., Daavittila, I., Solovieva, S., *et al.* (2008). Genetic factors are associated with modic changes in endplates of lumbar vertebral bodies. *Spine* **33**, 1236–41.

Karsak, M., Cohen-Solal, M., Freudenberg, J., *et al.* (2005). Cannabinoid receptor type 2 gene is associated with human osteoporosis. *Hum Mol Genet* **14**, 3389–96.

Kawaguchi, Y., Osada, R., Kanamori, M., *et al.* (1999). Association between an aggrecan gene polymorphism and lumbar disc degeneration. *Spine* **24**, 2456–60.

Kawasaki, Y., Xu, Z.Z., Wang, X., *et al.* (2008). Distinct roles of matrix metalloproteases in the early- and late-phase development of neuropathic pain. *Nat Med* **14**, 331–6.

Kim, H., Mittal, D.P., Iadarola, M.J., and Dionne, R.A. (2006a). Genetic predictors for acute experimental cold and heat pain sensitivity in humans. *J Med Genet* **43**, e40.

Kim, J.G., Lim, K.S., Ku, S.Y., Kim, S.H., Choi, Y.M., and Moon, S.Y. (2006b). Relations between interleukin-1, its receptor antagonist gene polymorphism, and bone mineral density in postmenopausal Korean women. *J Bone Miner Metab* **24**, 53–7.

Klepstad, P., Rakvag, T.T., Kaasa, S., *et al.* (2004). The 118 A > G polymorphism in the human mu-opioid receptor gene may increase morphine requirements in patients with pain caused by malignant disease. *Acta Anaesthesiol Scand* **48**, 1232–9.

Knoeringer, M., Reinke, A., Trappe, A.E., and Schlegel, J. (2008). Absence of the mutated Trp2 allele but a common polymorphism of the COL9A2 collagen gene is associated with early recurrence after lumbar discectomy in a German population. *Eur Spine J* **17**, 463–67.

Kung, A.W., Lai, B.M., Ng, M.Y., Chan, V., and Sham, P.C. (2006). T-1213C polymorphism of estrogen receptor beta is associated with low bone mineral density and osteoporotic fractures. *Bone* **39**, 1097–106.

Lafreniere, R.G., MacDonald, M.L., Dube, M.P., *et al.* (2004). Identification of a novel gene (HSN2) causing hereditary sensory and autonomic neuropathy type II through the Study of Canadian Genetic Isolates. *Am J Hum Genet* **74**, 1064–73.

Langdahl, B.L., Carstens, M., Stenkjaer, L., and Eriksen, E.F. (2003). Polymorphisms in the transforming growth factor beta 1 gene and osteoporosis. *Bone* **32**, 297–310.

Leyne, M., Mull, J., Gill, S.P., *et al.* (2003). Identification of the first non-Jewish mutation in familial Dysautonomia. *Am J Med Genet A* **118A**, 305–8.

Lichtman, A.H., Leung, D., Shelton, C.C., *et al.* (2004). Reversible inhibitors of fatty acid amide hydrolase that promote analgesia: evidence for an unprecedented combination of potency and selectivity. *J Pharmacol Exp Ther* **311**, 441–8.

Liem, E.B., Joiner, T.V., Tsueda, K., and Sessler, D.I. (2005). Increased sensitivity to thermal pain and reduced subcutaneous lidocaine efficacy in redheads. *Anesthesiology* **102**, 509–14.

Lötsch, J., and Geisslinger, G. (2005). Are mu-opioid receptor polymorphisms important for clinical opioid therapy? *Trends Mol Med* **11**, 82–89.

Lötsch, J., Skarke, C., Grosch, S., Darimont, J., Schmidt, H., and Geisslinger, G. (2002). The polymorphism A118G of the human mu-opioid receptor gene decreases the pupil constrictory effect of morphine-6-glucuronide but not that of morphine. *Pharmacogenetics* **12**, 3–9.

Lötsch, J., Skarke, C., Wieting, J., *et al.* (2006a). Modulation of the central nervous effects of levomethadone by genetic polymorphisms potentially affecting its metabolism, distribution, and drug action. *Clin Pharmacol Ther* **79**, 72–89.

Lötsch, J., Stuck, B., and Hummel, T. (2006b). The human mu-opioid receptor gene polymorphism 118A > G decreases cortical activation in response to specific nociceptive stimulation. *Behav Neurosci* **120**, 1218–24.

Luoma, K., Riihimaki, H., Luukkonen, R., Raininko, R., Viikari-Juntura, E., and Lamminen, A. (2000). Low back pain in relation to lumbar disc degeneration. *Spine* **25**, 487–92.

MacDonald, H.M., McGuigan, F.A., New, S.A., *et al.* (2001). COL1A1 Sp1 polymorphism predicts perimenopausal and early postmenopausal spinal bone loss. *J Bone Miner Res* **16**, 1634–41.

Manning, B.H., Merin, N.M., Meng, I.D., and Amaral, D.G. (2001). Reduction in opioid- and cannabinoid-induced antinociception in rhesus monkeys after bilateral lesions of the amygdaloid complex. *J Neurosci* **21**, 8238–46.

Meeus, M., Nijs, J., and Meirleir, K.D. (2007). Chronic musculoskeletal pain in patients with the chronic fatigue syndrome: a systematic review. *Eur J Pain* **11**, 377–86.

Mio, F., Chiba, K., Hirose, Y., *et al.* (2007). A functional polymorphism in COL11A1, which encodes the alpha 1 chain of type XI collagen, is associated with susceptibility to lumbar disc herniation. *Am J Hum Genet* **81**, 1271–7.

Miura, Y., Mardy, S., Awaya, Y., *et al.* (2000). Mutation and polymorphism analysis of the TRKA (NTRK1) gene encoding a high-affinity receptor for nerve growth factor in congenital insensitivity to pain with anhidrosis (CIPA) families. *Hum Genet* **106**, 116–24.

Mogil, J.S., Ritchie, J., Smith, S.B., *et al.* (2005). Melanocortin-1 receptor gene variants affect pain and mu-opioid analgesia in mice and humans. *J Med Genet* **42**, 583–7.

Morrison, N.A., Qi, J.C., Tokita, A., *et al.* (1994). Prediction of bone density from vitamin D receptor alleles. *Nature* **367**, 284–7.

Noponen-Hietala, N., Kyllonen, E., Mannikko, M., *et al.* (2003). Sequence variations in the collagen IX and XI genes are associated with degenerative lumbar spinal stenosis. *Ann Rheum Dis* **62**, 1208–14.

Noponen-Hietala, N., Virtanen, I., Karttunen, R., *et al.* (2005). Genetic variations in IL6 associate with intervertebral disc disease characterized by sciatica. *Pain* **114**, 186–94.

Oakley, M., and Vieira, A.R. (2008). The many faces of the genetics contribution to temporomandibular joint disorder. *Orthod Craniofac Res* **11**, 125–35.

Oertel, B., and Lötsch, J. (2008). Genetic mutations that prevent pain: implications for future pain medication. *Pharmacogenomics* **9**, 179–94.

Oertel, B.G., Preibisch, C., Wallenhorst, T., *et al.* (2008). Differential opioid action on sensory and affective cerebral pain processing. *Clin Pharmacol Ther* **83**, 577–88.

Oertel, B.G., Schmidt, R., Schneider, A., Geisslinger, G., and Lötsch, J. (2006). The mu-opioid receptor gene polymorphism 118A>G depletes alfentanil-induced analgesia and protects against respiratory depression in homozygous carriers. *Pharmacogenet Genomics* **16**, 625–36.

Ofek, O., Karsak, M., Leclerc, N., *et al.* (2006). Peripheral cannabinoid receptor, CB2, regulates bone mass. *Proc Natl Acad Sci U S A* **103**, 696–701.

Paassilta, P., Lohiniva, J., Goring, H.H., *et al.* (2001). Identification of a novel common genetic risk factor for lumbar disk disease. *Jama* **285**, 1843–9.

Pluijm, S.M., van Essen, H.W., Bravenboer, N., *et al.* (2004). Collagen type I alpha1 Sp1 polymorphism, osteoporosis, and intervertebral disc degeneration in older men and women. *Ann Rheum Dis* **63**, 71–7.

Reyes-Gibby, C.C., Shete, S., Rakvag, T., *et al.* (2007). Exploring joint effects of genes and the clinical efficacy of morphine for cancer pain: OPRM1 and COMT gene. *Pain* **130**, 25–30.

Richards, J.B., Rivadeneira, F., Inouye, M., *et al.* (2008). Bone mineral density, osteoporosis, and osteoporotic fractures: a genome-wide association study. *Lancet* **371**, 1505–12.

Riviere, J.B., Verlaan, D.J., Shekarabi, M., *et al.* (2004). A mutation in the HSN2 gene causes sensory neuropathy type II in a Lebanese family. *Ann Neurol* **56**, 572–5.

Roddier, K., Thomas, T., Marleau, G., *et al.* (2005). Two mutations in the HSN2 gene explain the high prevalence of HSAN2 in French Canadians. *Neurology* **64**, 1762–7.

Russo, P., Strazzullo, P., Cappuccio, F.P., *et al.* (2007). Genetic variations at the endocannabinoid type 1 receptor gene (CNR1) are associated with obesity phenotypes in men. *J Clin Endocrinol Metab* **92**, 2382–6.

Sakai, Y., Matsuyama, Y., Hasegawa, Y., *et al.* (2007). Association of gene polymorphisms with intervertebral disc degeneration and vertebral osteophyte formation. *Spine* **32**, 1279–86.

Schneider, S., Mohnen, S.M., Schiltenwolf, M., and Rau, C. (2007). Comorbidity of low back pain: representative outcomes of a national health study in the Federal Republic of Germany. *Eur J Pain* **11**, 387–97.

Seki, S., Kawaguchi, Y., Chiba, K., *et al.* (2005). A functional SNP in CILP, encoding cartilage intermediate layer protein, is associated with susceptibility to lumbar disc disease. *Nat Genet* **37**, 607–12.

Seki, S., Kawaguchi, Y., Mori, M., *et al.* (2006). Association study of COL9A2 with lumbar disc disease in the Japanese population. *J Hum Genet* **51**, 1063–7.

Sipe, J.C., Arbour, N., Gerber, A., and Beutler, E. (2005). Reduced endocannabinoid immune modulation by a common cannabinoid 2 (CB2) receptor gene polymorphism: possible risk for autoimmune disorders. *J Leukoc Biol* **78**, 231–38.

Skarke, C., Darimont, J., Schmidt, H., Geisslinger, G., and Lötsch, J. (2003). Analgesic effects of morphine and morphine-6-glucuronide in a transcutaneous electrical pain model in healthy volunteers. *Clin Pharmacol Ther* **73**, 107–21.

Slade, G.D., Diatchenko, L., Bhalang, K., *et al.* (2007). Influence of psychological factors on risk of temporomandibular disorders. *J Dent Res* **86**, 1120–25.

Slaugenhaupt, S.A., and Gusella, J.F. (2002). Familial dysautonomia. *Curr Opin Genet Dev* **12**, 307–11.

Solovieva, S., Kouhia, S., Leino-Arjas, P., *et al.* (2004a). Interleukin 1 polymorphisms and intervertebral disc degeneration. *Epidemiology* **15**, 626–33.

Solovieva, S., Leino-Arjas, P., Saarela, J., Luoma, K., Raininko, R., and Riihimaki, H. (2004b). Possible association of interleukin 1 gene locus polymorphisms with low back pain. *Pain* **109**, 8–19.

Solovieva, S., Lohiniva, J., Leino-Arjas, P., *et al.* (2006). Intervertebral disc degeneration in relation to the COL9A3 and the IL-1ss gene polymorphisms. *Eur Spine J* **15**, 613–19.

Solovieva, S., Noponen, N., Mannikko, M., *et al.* (2007). Association between the aggrecan gene variable number of tandem repeats polymorphism and intervertebral disc degeneration. *Spine* **32**, 1700–5.

Stohler, C.S. (2006). TMJD 3: a genetic vulnerability disorder with strong CNS involvement. *J Evid Based Dent Pract* **6**, 53–57.

Svendsen, K.B., Jensen, T.S., and Bach, F.W. (2004). Does the cannabinoid dronabinol reduce central pain in multiple sclerosis? Randomised double blind placebo controlled crossover trial. *Bmj* **329**, 253.

Takahashi, M., Haro, H., Wakabayashi, Y., Kawa-uchi, T., Komori, H., and Shinomiya, K. (2001). The association of degeneration of the intervertebral disc with 5a/6a polymorphism in the promoter of the human matrix metalloproteinase-3 gene. *J Bone Joint Surg Br* **83**, 491–95.

Tam, J., Trembovler, V., Di Marzo, V., *et al.* (2008). The cannabinoid CB1 receptor regulates bone formation by modulating adrenergic signaling. *Faseb J* **22**, 285–94.

Tander, B., Gunes, S., Boke, O., *et al.* (2008). Polymorphisms of the serotonin-2A receptor and catechol-O-methyltransferase genes: a study on fibromyalgia susceptibility. *Rheumatol Int* **28**, 685–91.

Tegeder, I., Adolph, J., Schmidt, H., Woolf, C.J., Geisslinger, G., and Lötsch, J. (2008). Reduced hyperalgesia in homozygous carriers of a GTP cyclohydrolase 1 haplotype. *Eur J Pain* **12**, 1069–77.

Tegeder, I., Costigan, M., Griffin, R.S., *et al.* (2006). GTP cyclohydrolase and tetrahydrobiopterin regulate pain sensitivity and persistence. *Nat Med* **12**, 1269–77.

Thieme, K., Turk, D.C., and Flor, H. (2004). Comorbid depression and anxiety in fibromyalgia syndrome: relationship to somatic and psychosocial variables. *Psychosom Med* **66**, 837–44.

Thomas, E.A., Cravatt, B.F., Danielson, P.E., Gilula, N.B., and Sutcliffe, J.G. (1997). Fatty acid amide hydrolase, the degradative enzyme for anandamide and oleamide, has selective distribution in neurons within the rat central nervous system. *J Neurosci Res* **50**, 1047–52.

Ujike, H., Takaki, M., Nakata, K., *et al.* (2002). CNR1, central cannabinoid receptor gene, associated with susceptibility to hebephrenic schizophrenia. *Mol Psychiatry* **7**, 515–18.

van Meurs, J.B., Trikalinos, T.A., Ralston, S.H., *et al.* (2008). Large-scale analysis of association between LRP5 and LRP6 variants and osteoporosis. *Jama* **299**, 1277–90.

Verhoeven, K., Timmerman, V., Mauko, B., Pieber, T.R., De Jonghe, P., and Auer-Grumbach, M. (2006). Recent advances in hereditary sensory and autonomic neuropathies. *Curr Opin Neurol* **19**, 474–80.

Videman, T., Leppavuori, J., Kaprio, J., *et al.* (1998). Intragenic polymorphisms of the vitamin D receptor gene associated with intervertebral disc degeneration. *Spine* **23**, 2477–85.

Wiesinger, B., Malker, H., Englund, E., and Wanman, A. (2007). Back pain in relation to musculoskeletal disorders in the jaw-face: a matched case-control study. *Pain* **131**, 311–19.

Zhang, P.W., Ishiguro, H., Ohtsuki, T., *et al.* (2004). Human cannabinoid receptor 1: 5' exons, candidate regulatory regions, polymorphisms, haplotypes and association with polysubstance abuse. *Mol Psychiatry* **9**, 916–31.

Zhang, Y., Kerns, J.M., Anderson, D.G., *et al.* (2006). Sensory neurons and fibers from multiple spinal cord levels innervate the rabbit lumbar disc. *Am J Phys Med Rehabil* **85**, 865–71.

Zhang, Y., Wang, D., Johnson, A.D., Papp, A.C., and Sadee, W. (2005). Allelic expression imbalance of human mu opioid receptor (OPRM1) caused by variant A118G. *J Biol Chem* **280**, 32618–24.

Zuo, L., Kranzler, H.R., Luo, X., Covault, J., and Gelernter, J. (2007). CNR1 variation modulates risk for drug and alcohol dependence. *Biol Psychiatry* **62**, 616–26.

# Chapter 4

# Peripheral and Central Sensitization as Risk Factors of Low Back Pain

Hermann O. Handwerker

## 4.1 Introduction

Acute low back pain is one of the most common complaints of adult humans, probably due to degenerative and/or use-dependent damages of the vertebral column and surrounding structures. When low back pain becomes chronic, it is a disabling disease. Chronic low back pain (CLBP), probably the most common chronic pain disease, is very difficult to treat (see Chapter 25). Though pathological processes at and around the vertebral column are the source of the pain, there is surprisingly little correlation between the magnitude e.g. of degenerative alterations of the spine and the pain intensity.

Chronic pain states are generally due to a complex interplay between peripheral and central nociceptive mechanisms. In CLBP this interplay is particularly complex, since it includes not only sensitized nociceptors from vertebrae, muscles, tendons, and small joints, but very often also has neuropathic components from damaged vertebral nerve roots. Sensitized nociceptors, or damaged axons, may bombard the central nervous system and this may lead to a disordered matrix of central nociceptive neuronal populations. In this respect, marked differences exist between muscle and skin nociceptors. Muscle pain has a much stronger tendency to be referred and to become chronic and this tendency is particularly strong in low back muscles (Taguchi et al. 1985, 1986). In addition, nocifensive reflexes may induce inadequate contractions of the spinal musculature which again create a changed micro-environment of the nociceptor terminals and hence lead to further nociceptor sensitization.

This short review of the pathophysiology of CLBP concentrates on three sources of chronic pain:

1) Nociceptor sensitization and damage.
2) Altered processing at central synapses.
3) Changes of the reactivity and structure of the brain in chronic pain states.

Indirect influences, e.g. the role of hormonal processes are covered by another chapter of this book (see Chapter 5) and only marginally implemented in this review. Details about the interaction of muscle activation and CLBP are discussed in two other chapters of this book (see Chapters 8 and 9).

## 4.2 Nociceptor functions

The term 'nociceptor' denominates a large subpopulation of primary afferent neurons. Each nociceptor consists of a cell body in a dorsal root ganglion (DRG), an axon running in a nerve which terminally diverts in branches and sprouts into the target tissue. The nociceptor terminals in the periphery are equipped with a mosaic of membrane proteins functioning as receptors and membrane channels. The central branches of the nociceptor axons project into the spinal cord dorsal horn. A review of nociceptor functions has been recently published by Woolf (2007). The author of this chapter has published an audio-seminar on nociceptor functions (Handwerker 2009).

It has long been known that nociceptors constitute a heterogeneous population of primary afferent neurons with respect to functions of their terminals, conduction velocity of axons, and central projections. According to their neurogenesis two major classes can be distinguished: a peptidergic population defined by the presence of calcitonin-gene related peptide (CGRP) and often also substance P. These neurons express the membrane receptor trkA (a receptor tyrosine kinase of the Trk family) and are dependent on the nerve growth factor (NGF). By contrast, non-peptidergic nociceptors express Ret, the receptor for the glial cell line-derived neuro-trophic factor. These neurons are histochemically characterized by binding isolectin B4 (IB4). However, the two cell populations are not entirely exclusive (Snider and McMahon 1998; Gold and Gebhart 2010).

Part of the peptidergic primary afferents release CGRP (and in some species also substance P) from their peripheral terminals and these neuropeptides may have a function in safeguarding the integrity of the innervated tissues (Kruger 1988). In the course of sensitization this release of afferent transmitters can be markedly increased leading to neurogenic inflammation (Richardson and Vasko 2002). Apart of the important distinction in peptidergic and non-peptidergic units various classes of nociceptors have been distinguished according to the function of their peripheral terminals (Handwerker 2010). The most common type has been named 'polymodal nociceptor' some decades ago (Bessou and Perl 1969). These units are characterized by unmyelinated axons and sensitivity to heating and strong mechanical stimulation. Though this characterization was originally made for cutaneous nociceptors, the term has been transferred to nociceptor populations in other tissues. Nociceptors with thin myelinated axons may have similar properties, or serve exclusively as high threshold mechanoreceptors (Adriaensen et al. 1983). 'Polymodal nociceptors' can probably be found in the peptidergic and in the non-peptidergic neuronal population. It is not always clear which units belong to this group in different tissues, species and preparations (Handwerker 2009).

During the last decade another group of nociceptors emerged which are insensitive to mechanical stimulation—as long as the tissue surrounding their terminals is intact. Afferents of this kind were first described in the knee joint of the cat. They become activated, however, in the time course of the development of joint inflammation. (Schaible and Schmidt 1983). The authors called these fibres 'sleeping nociceptors'. From these early findings it became immediately clear that this group of nociceptors must play a salient role in the development of inflammatory pain and hyperalgesia. Later on similar types of nociceptors responding to electrical stimulation of their axons, but not to mechanical stimulation of their terminals were found in the monkey skin. They were termed MIAs (mechanically insensitive afferents) (Meyer et al. 1991). Finally, mechanically insensitive nociceptors were encountered in microneurography experiments in human skin nerves and named CMi (for mechanically insensitive C-fibres) (Schmidt et al. 1995). This latter group of units is peptidergic and responsible for the axon reflex flare provoked by the CGRP release from the terminals (Schmelz et al. 2000). CMi units are characterized by very slow conduction velocities of their axons and very large receptive fields indicating extensive arborization of their terminals in the skin. It has been shown that CMi units become mechanically responsive, when their receptive field is treated with irritants, such as capsaicin (ligand of the TRPV1-receptor, see below), or mustard oil (ligand of the TRPA1-receptor). CMi units play a decisive role in the development of mechanical hyperalgesia of inflamed tissues (Torebjörk et al. 1996; Schmidt et al. 2000).

Unfortunately detailed analyses of the nociceptive afferents from the vertebral column and surrounding tissues are not available and their properties have to be deduced from comparisons with those of larger muscles and joints, in some cases even from skin (see below).

### 4.2.1 Transduction and transformation processes in nociceptor terminals.

It has long been known that plasticity of the nociceptor function and nociceptor sensitization is a major source of hyperalgesia (which has been termed 'primary' hyperalgesia when due to sensitized nociceptor terminals). Two steps are involved in the excitation of nociceptor (and other) receptor terminals: at first, in a transduction process stimuli generate depolarizations of the terminals (generator potentials). In a second step these local depolarizations are transformed into sequences of action potentials. In nociceptors these two processes are not easy to distinguish, since they occur in parallel at the same sites of the terminal membrane (Carr et al. 2009). Several types of trans-membrane proteins play a role in the transduction: ion channels, G-protein coupled receptors (GPCRs), receptors for cytokines and for neurotrophins. The different composition of these protein populations are a major source of the diversity of nociceptors. Several comprehensive reviews on transduction processes in nociceptors have been published (Woolf and Ma 2007; Gold and Gebhart 2010), and only a non-comprehensive summary of the processes most important for CLBP can be given in this chapter.

- ◆ *Membrane channels* are the prototypic transducing molecules. *Transient receptor potential* (TRP) channels seem to play a key role in nociception, most importantly TRPV1 and TRPA1. The former is gated by heating, low pH and by an exogenous irritant, capsaicin. Endogenous gating substances have been hypothesized (e.g. anandamide). TRPA1 is gated by various chemical irritants. Other channels found in nociceptors are gated by ATP, belonging to the P2X channel family. In addition channels that influence passive membrane properties, the two-pore $K^+$ channels TREK 1 (Patel and Honore 2001) and TRAAK (Maingret et al. 1999) contribute to the terminal membrane potential. Though TREK and TRAAK channels are gated by mechanical forces (Chemin et al. 2007), they probably do not contribute to the mechanical activation of nociceptors, and neither does one of the above channels. This is an important gap in our knowledge in particular in the context of low back pain which is in part initiated by mechanical forces. Important in muscle nociception and the development of hyperalgesia are channels gated by the low PH of inflamed tissue, the ASIC channels and TRPV1. Also purinergic membrane receptors (P2X3) gated by ATP seem to play a greater role than in skin nociceptors (Sluka et al. 2001; Ellrich and Makowska 2007; Heinricher et al. 2009; Walder et al. 2010).

- ◆ **G protein-coupled receptors** do not directly change the membrane potential, but are important for the sensitization of nociceptors. Many of them bind to inflammatory substances, e.g. EP-receptors for prostaglandines, BK-receptors for bradykinin, but also receptors binding to histamine (H1), serotonin (5-HT2), and others. Upon activation by their ligands these receptors activate second messenger cascades. Some of them, e.g. the EP-receptors are characterized by Gs proteins coupled to the adenylate cyclase–cAMP–protein kinase A (PKA) pathway. Others, e.g. bradykinin receptors, are linked to Gq proteins controlling the pathway phospholipase–IP3–protein kinase C (PKC). In both cases protein kinases, PKA or PKC are at the end of the cascade and phosphorylate membrane channel proteins, e.g. TRPV1 and Nav channels. The resulting sensitization processes are discussed below.

- ◆ **Neurotrophin receptors** are important for the development and maintenance of nociceptor functions. As mentioned earlier, NGF binding to the TrkA-receptor is mandatory for peptidergic nociceptors. A genetic defect of TrkA leads to the long known (rare) *congenital insensitivity to pain with anhidrosis* (CIPA syndrome) (Indo et al. 1996). However, NGF is also known to sensitize nociceptors and to produce hypersensitivity (Lewin et al. 1994).

◆ **Voltage gated sodium channels** are dedicated to the process of transformation, i.e. the generation of action potentials from the generator potential. It has been mentioned that in nociceptors the processes of transduction and transformation take place in parallel in the peripheral axon terminal. Subtypes of voltage dependent $Na^+$ receptors have been described which are specifically expressed in small DRG-neurons of slowly conducting primary afferents: NaV 1.7, NaV 1.8 and NaV 1.9. NaV 1.9 and 1.8 are resistant to the specific antagonist tetrodotoxin, NaV 1.7 is sensitive to this toxin. Under normal conditions NaV 1.8 is responsible for the current generating action potentials. However, NaV 1.7 enhances depolarizing input leading to action potentials. Mutations preventing the expression of NaV 1.7 in man lead to congenital insensitivity to pain (Goldberg et al. 2007). People carrying a mutation leading to a gain of function of NaV 1.7 develop chronic pain diseases, in particular erythromelalgia (Dib-Hajj et al. 2008; Ahn et al. 2010). Polymorphisms of the NaV 1.7 gene may lead to an overexcitability of DRG neurons and hence to altered pain perceptions probably also in muscle pain (Estacion et al. 2009; Reimann et al. 2010). Phosphorylation of NaV 1.8 by protein kinases (PKC or PKA) caused by activation of G-protein coupled receptors of inflammatory mediators, also results in an increase in nociceptor excitability (Amir et al. 2006).

### 4.2.2 Sensitization of nociceptor terminals and the initiation of pathological pain and hyperalgesia

Inflammatory mediators binding to G-protein coupled receptors and initiating second messenger cascades with activation of protein kinases are well known processes of nociceptor sensitization. PKA and PKC phosphorylate transduction channels, e.g. TRPV1, and also spike initiating NaV-channels. In both cases activation thresholds of nociceptors are lowered and suprathreshold stimuli lead to more frequent nerve impulses. In case of acute events, e.g. a short-acting trauma, this process will be reversed after hours or days. Additional mechanisms are required for nociceptor sensitization to become chronic. One such mechanism seems to be the activation of the epsilon isoform of protein kinase C ($PKC_{epsilon}$) by a recently discovered second messenger pathway leading from cAMP through the cAMP-activated guanine exchange factor EPAC to $PKC_{epsilon}$. This pathway is restricted to non-peptidergic (IB4 postitive) nociceptors. In animal experiments sustained mechanical hyperalgesia was induced through this pathway (Hucho et al. 2000).

Agents leading to more chronic changes of nociceptor sensitivity are *neurotrophins*, mentioned above; e.g. NGF is increased in inflamed tissue and has been shown to induce long lasting sensitization of peptidergic nociceptors (Hefti et al. 2006; Rukwied et al. 2010). After binding to the trkA receptor NGF is incorporated by nociceptive nerve endings and transported to the cell bodies where it alters functions of the genome which contribute to long lasting hyperexcitability (Hoheisel et al. 2005; Amir et al. 2006; Murase et al. 2010).

*Cytokines*, which are known to play a major role in the development of arthritis, are also important for chronic inflammatory pain states of ligaments, small joints, muscle, and tendons of the vertebral column. Their role in nociceptive processing has been addressed in a recent review (Schaible et al. 2010). Tumour necrosis factor alpha (TNF-$\alpha$), interleukin 1 and 6 bind to membrane receptors of nociceptors (TNF-R1,2; IL1-R, IL6-R) and mediate long lasting sensitization in the course of inflammation. Their effects include enhancement of prostaglandine effects and upregulation of TRP- and NaV-channels. Increased levels of TNF-$\alpha$ and other cytokines have been detected in herniated disc tissue compared with normal non-degenerated disc tissue (Yamashita et al. 2008; Lee et al. 2009). TNF-α applied to nerve roots produces the pathologic changes observed with nerve root exposure to nucleus pulposus extracts (Igarashi et al. 2000). Furthermore, in an animal model of radiculopathy induced by intervertebral disc material, inhibitors of TNF-α had a moderate effect on the radicular pathology (Norimoto et al. 2008).

There is ample evidence that neurotrophins and cytokines induce not only acute effects, like gating of membrane receptors, but also profound changes in the molecular functions of the nociceptor neurons, such as the expression of membrane receptors. In animal models these effects were particularly prominent in neuropathy models.

## 4.2.3 Neuropathic components of CLBP

CLBP is characterized in many cases by a combination of inflammatory and neuropathic mechanisms (Baron 2009) (see also Chapter 25). This may be a salient reason for the difficulties of finding effective pharmaco-therapies for this kind of chronic pain (see Chapter 25). Neuropathic alterations can be due to mechanical forces, i.e. chronic pressure on nerve roots, but chemical mediators are probably more important, e.g. by the action of the material from disc hernia on the conductile axons. However, also in the absence of a ruptured nucleus pulposus inflammatory cytokines, in particular TNFα released from macrophages, can induce ectopic spike activity from injured and also from uninjured nerve fibres (Sommer 2003; Sorkin et al. 1998). Interestingly, macrophages may accumulate in DRG even when the nerve lesion is located at a distance (Lu et al. 1993).

While chronic inflammatory pain is due to alterations of the transduction and transformation process at the nociceptor terminals, neuropathic changes occur along the conductile membrane of the axons. Several animal models of neuropathic pain have been developed and the results have been described in recent comprehensive reviews (Decosterd and Woolf 2000; Woolf and Salter 2000; Decosterd and Berta 2009; Ossipov and Porreca 2009). In the context of this chapter models of mononeuropathies are most important including loose ligature of a nerve (Bennett and Xie 1988) and partial nerve transection (Decosterd and Woolf 2000).

A large number of cellular changes are the consequence of sustained alterations of the conductile axonal membrane. Partial nerve injury leads to increased levels of messenger RNA for membrane receptors and channels. In particular, sodium channels NaV 1.8 and 1.9 are accumulated at the site of a nerve lesion, and in addition an embryonic channel NaV 1.3 can be expressed (Wood et al. 2004; Omana-Zapata et al. 2005. This can lead to ectopic action potentials. Not only at the lesion site, but also in the cell bodies in the DRG channel expressions are changed. Even more important, altered channel expressions are also found in unaffected neurons. After traumatic nerve injury, redistribution of NaV 1.8 to the axons of uninjured neighbouring nociceptors plays a major role in mechanical hypersensitivity (Amir et al. 2006). The expression of TRPV1 channels at the nerve terminals distal to the lesion site is downregulated after partial nerve lesion but novel expression of TRPV1 in uninjured neighbouring axons has been observed even in myelinated afferents and their ganglion cells (Hudson et al. 2001; Ma et al. 2005). Also receptors which are normally not expressed in primary afferent nociceptive neurons may be produced in spared axons and cell bodies. After a traumatic lesion of a nerve or root, for example, cold sensing TRPM8 (transient receptor potential cation channel, subfamily M, member 8) channels (Obata et al 2005) and alpha adrenoreceptors (Sato and Perl 1991) are expressed in the terminal membrane. There is evidence that the impaired capacity of lesioned axons to take neurotrophins up (e.g. NGF) which are produced in the tissue surrounding the nociceptor terminals leads to 'overfeeding' of spared axons. Since these neurotrophins are taken up by their endings and transported to the cell bodies in the DRG, they can alter the genetic programming in the nucleus leading to the production of increased amounts of mRNA and even altered mRNA fostering the production of signal proteins and their transport to the nerve terminals (Wu et al. 2001).

## 4.3 Altered processing in the central nervous system

### 4.3.1 Synaptic plasticity in the spinal cord dorsal horn

The changes in nociceptor functions following inflammation and axonal damage have profound consequences for pain processing in the central nervous system. Most information is available from animal studies on the changes in the spinal dorsal horn, the first station of central pain processing.

The secondary neurons of the nociceptive pathway are located in the superficial laminae of the dorsal horn. The transmission neurons in lamina I receive more or less specific input from nociceptors (nociception specific neurons), whereas larger multimodal projection neurons are found in lamina V. Both neuronal populations project to higher centres through the classical anterolateral spinothalamic tract and also through multisynaptic projections, relayed through brainstem nuclei.

It has been shown that low-frequency input from muscle nociceptors or even subthreshold synaptic potentials evoked by muscle nociceptors are sufficient to induce a long-lasting hyperexcitability in these neurons (Hoheisel et al. 2007). Important signs of central sensitization are increased neuronal activity to noxious stimuli, expansion of the receptive fields, and spread of excitation to other spinal segments (a phenomenon closely linked with expansion of the peripheral input). If central sensitization is established, innocuous tactile stimuli can become capable of exciting nociceptive projection neurons leading to 'touch-evoked' hyperalgesia (Tal et al. 1994).

Recent reviews provide comprehensive overviews of the plastic changes in nociceptive transmission neurons (Woolf and Salter 2000; Kuner 2010), a short synopsis of the most important mechanisms is given here.

Inflammation or nerve injury causes long-term potentiation in lamina I nociception specific neurons which express the neurokinin 1 receptor for substance P. This synaptic augmentation by a co-transmitter involves activation of T-type voltage gated calcium channels (Ikeda et al. 2003, 2006). Whereas substance P (together with CGRP and neurokinin A) acts as co-transmitter at spinal nociceptive synapses, the main transmitter is glutamate, acting at AMPA, NMDA, and metabotropic receptors. When the postsynaptic neurons are depolarized, a magnesium block of the NMDA-receptors is removed and a more profound depolarization takes place. This leads to short-term enhancement of synaptic transmission which may be the starting point of many longer lasting plastic changes. Whereas NMDA-R always permit $Ca^{++}$ entry upon activation, AMPA-R influence the influx of $Ca^{++}$ in a more subtle way, by expression and inclusion of subunits which cause greater $Ca^{++}$ permeability (Burnashev et al. 1992). It has been shown that this mechanism is crucial for inflammation induced plasticity of spinal transmission (Hartmann et al. 2004; Luo et al. 2008).

A key effect of synaptic plasticity is the increase of intracellular $Ca^{++}$ level which leads to the activation of several calcium-dependent kinases, e.g. CamKII alpha, cyclooxygenase-2 and NO-synthase. Their products, prostaglandin E2 and NO, have been shown to facilitate nociceptive transmission. Another important source of central sensitization is the mitogen-activated protein kinase (MAPK) system, ERK1 and 2 (Ji and Woolf 2001; Kawasaki et al 2004). ERK 1 and 2 can phosphorylate ion channels and thus induce a short term potentiation, but they play also a role in long term sensitization by acting as synapse-to-nucleus communicators changing gene transcription (Garry et al. 2003a, 2003b).

## 4.3.2 **Contribution of glial cells to neuropathic pain**

In recent years increasing evidence has emerged that not only neuronal elements, but also glial cells play an important role in the initiation and maintenance of neuropathic pain. In experimental pain states in animals, astrocytes and microglia are activated by neuronal transmitters including substance P and glutamate (Wieseler-Frank et al. 2005). In turn, glial cells release proinflammatory cytokines and other sensitizing compounds that promote long-lasting spinal hyperexcitability and therefore are key factors for the transition from acute to chronic pain (Chacur et al. 2009). For example, brain-derived neurotrophic factor (BDNF) released from activated glial cells fosters the reduction of the potassium chloride exporter (KCC2) in lamina I neurons. A consequence is an alteration of chloride homeostasis in these cells leading to depolarization. This shift inverts the polarity of currents activated by GABA which become excitatory and thus enhance the sensitization of projecting neurons (Coull et al. 2003, 2005).

## 4.3.3 **Central disinhibition**

The output of the dorsal horn to brain centres depends on a balance of inhibitory and excitatory mechanisms. Hyperalgesia is not only due to hypersensitivity of transmission neurons, but also to a diminished control by inhibitory neurons. Locally, these are mainly GABA-ergic and glycinergic interneurons, apart from the more nociception-specific enkephalinergic and dynorphinergic interneurons of the endogenous opioid system.

It has been proposed that loss of GABAergic interneurons in the spinal dorsal horn after nerve injury causes an imbalance between excitation and inhibition. Peripheral nerve injury may lead to selective apoptosis of GABAergic interneurons in the dorsal horn (Moore et al. 2002; Scholz et al. 2005). For the understanding of the effect of cyclo-oxygenase inhibitors it is important to realise that PGE2 induces protein kinase A-dependent phosphorylation of glycin receptors causing inhibition of these inhibitory interneurons and hence facilitation of nociceptive transmission (Harvey et al. 2004). This important finding has the implication that the effect of COX-inhibiting drugs is not confined to the primary afferents. These drugs have also central actions (see Chapter 25).

Dorsal horn neurons are under a powerful descending control from facilitatory and inhibitory supraspinal brainstem centres. The periaqueductal grey (PAG) and the nucleus raphe magnus and adjacent structures of the rostral ventromedial medulla (RVM) project to the spinal cord dorsal horn. This descending control pathway contains serotonergic neurons and also involves noradrenergic neurons from the locus coeruleus and other noradrenergic brainstem cell groups. Considerable evidence has recently emerged showing modulation of this system in persistent pain conditions due to inflammation or neuropathy. It seems that persistent nociception simultaneously triggers descending facilitation and inhibition from the RVM (Porreca et al. 2002; Heinricher et al. 2009). In models of inflammation, descending inhibition may predominate over facilitation in pain circuits with input from the inflamed tissue, while descending facilitation predominates over inhibition in pain circuits with input from neighbouring tissues, and thus facilitates secondary hyperalgesia (Vanegas and Schaible 2004). Although both descending facilitation and inhibition seem to stem from the RVM, they are probably due to different neuronal pools. According to one hypothesis 'on' and 'off' neurons in this region, i.e. neurons reacting to switching on and off nociceptive input, respectively, are responsible for the balance between facilitation and inhibition. This modulation may be one of the important target mechanisms for the endogenous opioid antinociception (Fields 2000). Because in all models of inflammatory and neuropathic pain descending facilitation and inhibition are triggered simultaneously, it will be important to elucidate why inhibition predominates in some conditions and facilitation in others.

Tipping the balance between descending inhibition and facilitation towards inhibition of chronic pain states is the final goal of centrally-acting pain therapies via serotonin and noradrenaline re-uptake inhibitors, e.g. tricyclic antidepressants (see Chapter 25).

## 4.4 Supraspinal mechanisms of CLBP

### 4.4.1 Functional plasticity

When turning to the supraspinal mechanisms of chronification of LBP, the available evidence on the level of individual neurons and synapses becomes scarce, though some synaptological studies exist, e.g. involving thalamic neurons (Cheong et al. 2008) and neurons in the anterior cingulated gyrus which is regarded as part of the 'medial', affective system (Cao et al. 2009: Jeon et al. 2010).

Most relevant studies are performed in humans suffering from LBP using functional cerebral imaging, mainly functional magnetic resonance imaging (fMRI). These methods have provided an invaluable insight into the cerebral processing of acute and chronic pain. However, one has to keep in mind that they do not allow a direct analysis at the cellular and synaptic level. In the time and in the space domain the resolution is by several orders of magnitude too low for synaptic studies, being typically more than $1mm^3$ and more than 1s in fMRI brain scans. Alternatively, encephalographic (EEG) and magnetoencephalographic (MEG) mappings have been performed which reflect the neuronal mass activity of neuron pools at a high time resolution, but with a limited spatial resolution. These EEG and MEG recordings have also the disadvantage of reflecting only cortical processing.

A thorough discussion of altered cerebral responsiveness in CLBP can be found in this book in Chapter 6. Only a short summary will be given in this chapter for the purpose of discussing pathophysiological implications.

There are numerous studies on pain-related cerebral activation patterns. The majority dealt with the responses of healthy volunteers to experimentally-induced pain. However, some studies tried to compare cerebral processing of CLBP patients and healthy subjects. In an early study, MEG recordings were used (Flor et al. 1997). The experiment employed electrical stimulation of the skin and revealed significant brain activation differences between CLBP patients and healthy controls. Stimulation at the affected back skin lead to a significantly higher potential after about 80ms (N80) in CLBP patients. Since the signal strength and the duration of the chronic pain were positively correlated, the authors reasoned that pain chronification leads to increased and also to more widely spread cortical responses. These results have been confirmed and extended by this group in a newer EEG study employing also intramuscular electrical stimuli (Diers et al. 2007). According to these studies CLBP leads to an expansion of the cortical zone excited by a noxious stimulus in the affected region and to stronger responses, regardless whether the affected tissue or the overlying skin is stimulated.

Later on, fMRI became the predominant tool for those studies. With this method changes in the local blood oxygenation are assessed (BOLD-effect) as an indication of the activation of groups of neurons. The time resolution is 1000-fold lower than in EEG/MEG, but more tonic stimuli can be used and sustained responses can be assessed. Subcortical areas became also accessible with this method. In one such study CLBP patients were compared with controls, and with other painful ailments. Tonic pressure pain was induced in a remote body site (Giesecke et al. 2004), in another study the patients were asked to rate their ongoing back pain in the course of an fMRI session (Baliki et al. 2006). In both studies cortical brain regions were activated which have been often associated with pain perceptions: the somatosensory cortex S1 and S2, the inferior parietal lobe, the insula, and the anterior cingulated gyrus. These regions are often called the 'pain matrix' (Melzack 1999). Prior to the advent of functional brain imaging these cortical regions had been related to pain processing, and in particular to different dimensions of pain perception: a sensory-discriminative dimension which is supposed to be processed by a 'lateral' projection system mainly projecting to the somatosensory projection areas, an affective-emotional dimension which is supposed to be represented in medial and limbic structures, and an evaluative dimension related to frontal cortical fields (Melzack and Casey 1968; Treede et al. 1999). However, more recent fMRI studies raised some doubt, if there is really a 'pain matrix' reflected in the BOLD responses of the above structures. If in normal subjects non-painful tactile stimuli were applied, very similar BOLD activation patterns emerged in the cerebral cortex (Schoedel et al. 2008). In a later study it was shown that the fMRI responses triggered by nociceptive stimuli can be largely explained by a combination of multimodal neural activities (i.e. activities elicited by all stimuli regardless of sensory modality) and somatosensory-specific but not nociceptive-specific neural activities (i.e. activities elicited by both nociceptive and non-nociceptive somatosensory stimuli) (Mouraux et al. 2011). These authors concluded that the BOLD responses in the so-called pain matrix reflect saliency of a stimulus rather than painfulness per se (Legrain et al. 2011). These results do not necessarily imply that the activations in the different elements of the so-called pain matrix have nothing to do with pain processing. Certainly pain, in particular LBP, has a greater saliency for the brain of a chronic pain patient than for a healthy subject, and this greater saliency is part of the pain chronicity. Further, one has to keep in mind that the spatial resolution of present fMRI devices is far too low to allow conclusions about small neuronal circuits in the activated brain regions and their connections.

### 4.4.2 **Structural plasticity**

Two lines of evidence indicate that structural changes also occur in cortical regions as a consequence of CLBP. Flor et al. (Flor et al. 1997; Flor 2002) observed a reorganization of the somatotopy in the primary sensory cortex comparable to that observed in amputees. This cortical re-organization was reversible—at least in part—under successful therapy. Later on, several morphometric MRT studies have been performed which showed consistently that the cortical grey matter was shrinking in the course of the development of chronic pain. This topic is extensively discussed in another chapter of this book (see Chapter 7). It is still unclear which mechanisms are leading to these cortical changes. As far as they are reversible they are possibly not due to the loss of neurons. A loss of dendrites and thus of functional synapses is an intriguing possibility. Future cellular studies will certainly help to fully comprehend this striking phenomenon.

## 4.5 **Conclusions**

CLBP apparently starts with a trauma in the structures in and around the vertebral column. The extension of this trauma is not the salient factor for the development of a chronic pain disease, but a chronification process which is still not fully understood, in spite of the plethora of contributing factors recently discovered which are outlined in this chapter.

Certainly, the special structure of our vertebral column—the continuous stress on it by our upright locomotion combined with a predominantly sedentary way of life in modern times—are disposing factors. However, it is not fully understood why some people get CLBP and others not. Many factors may be genetic and/or psychosocial and will be explained in other chapters of this book.

On a pathophysiological level, the interactions between cerebral cortex, brainstem, spinal cord and the primary afferent system are only incompletely understood. For many questions we have not yet developed a sufficiently powerful scientific repertoire.

# References

**Adriaensen H, Gybels J, Handwerker HO, Van Hees J.** Response properties of thin myelinated (A-delta) fibers in human skin nerves. *J Neurophysiol* 1983; **49**:111–22.

**Ahn HS, Dib-Hajj SD, Cox JJ, et al.** A new Nav1.7 sodium channel mutation I234T in a child with severe pain. *Eur J Pain* 2010; **14**:944–50.

**Amir R, Argoff CE, Bennett GJ, et al.** The role of sodium channels in chronic inflammatory and neuropathic pain. *J Pain* 2006; **7**:S1–29.

**Baliki MN, Chialvo DR, Geha PY, Levy RM, Harden RN, Parrish TB, Apkarian AV.** Chronic pain and the emotional brain: specific brain activity associated with spontaneous fluctuations of intensity of chronic back pain. *J Neurosci* 2006; **26**:12165–73.

**Baron R.** Neuropathic Pain: Clinical. In: Basbaum AI, Bushnell CM (eds) *Science of Pain*. Amsterdam: Elsevier, 2009. pp. 865–900.

**Bennett GJ, Xie YK.** A peripheral mononeuropathy in rat that produces disorders of pain sensation like those seen in man. *Pain* 1988; **33**:87–107.

**Bessou P, Perl ER.** Responses of cutaneous sensory units with unmyelinated fibers to noxious stimuli. *J Neurophysiol* 1969; **32**:1025–43.

**Burnashev N, Monyer H, Seeburg PH, Sakmann B.** Divalent ion permeability of AMPA receptor channels is dominated by the edited form of a single subunit. *Neuron* 1992; **8**:189–98.

**Cao H, Gao YJ, Ren WH, et al.** Activation of extracellular signal-regulated kinase in the anterior cingulate cortex contributes to the induction and expression of affective pain. *J Neurosci* 2009; **29**:3307–21.

**Carr RW, Pianova S, McKemy DD, Brock JA.** Action potential initiation in the peripheral terminals of cold-sensitive neurones innervating the guinea-pig cornea. *J Physiol* 2009; **587**:1249–64.

**Chacur M, Lambertz D, Hoheisel U, Mense S.** Role of spinal microglia in myositis-induced central sensitisation: an immunohistochemical and behavioural study in rats. *Eur J Pain* 2009; **13**:915–23.

**Chemin J, Patel AJ, Duprat F, Sachs F, Lazdunski M, Honore E.** Up- and down-regulation of the mechano-gated K(2P) channel TREK-1 by PIP (2) and other membrane phospholipids. *Pflugers Arch* 2007; **455**:97–103.

**Cheong E, Lee S, Choi BJ, Sun M, Lee CJ, Shin HS.** Tuning thalamic firing modes via simultaneous modulation of T- and L-type Ca2+ channels controls pain sensory gating in the thalamus. *J Neurosci* 2008; **28**:13331–40.

**Coull JA, Beggs S, Boudreau D, et al.** BDNF from microglia causes the shift in neuronal anion gradient underlying neuropathic pain. *Nature* 2005; **438**:1017–21.

**Coull JA, Boudreau D, Bachand K, et al.** Trans-synaptic shift in anion gradient in spinal lamina I neurons as a mechanism of neuropathic pain. *Nature* 2003; **424**:938–42.

**Decosterd I, Berta T.** Animal Models and Neuropathic Pain. In: Basbaum A.I., Bushnell C.M., editors. *Science of Pain*. Amsterdam: Elsevier, 2009. pp. 857–64.

**Decosterd I, Woolf CJ.** Spared nerve injury: an animal model of persistent peripheral neuropathic pain. *Pain* 2000; **87**:149–58.

**Dib-Hajj SD, Yang Y, Waxman SG.** Genetics and molecular pathophysiology of Na(v)1.7-related pain syndromes. *Adv Genet* 2008; **63**:85–110.

**Diers M, Koeppe C, Diesch E, et al.** Central processing of acute muscle pain in chronic low back pain patients: an EEG mapping study. *J Clin Neurophysiol* 2007; **24**:76–83.

**Ellrich J, Makowska A.** Nerve growth factor and ATP excite different neck muscle nociceptors in anaesthetized mice. *Cephalalgia* 2007; **27**:1226–35.

**Estacion M, Harty TP, Choi JS, Tyrrell L, Dib-Hajj SD, Waxman SG.** A sodium channel gene SCN9A polymorphism that increases nociceptor excitability. *Ann Neurol* 2009; **66**:862–6.

**Fields HL.** Pain modulation: expectation, opioid analgesia and virtual pain. *Prog Brain Res* 2000; **122**:245–53

**Flor H.** The modification of cortical reorganization and chronic pain by sensory feedback. *Appl Psychophysiol Biofeedback* 2002; **27**:215–27.

Flor H, Braun C, Elbert T, Birbaumer N. Extensive reorganization of primary somatosensory cortex in chronic back pain patients. *Neurosci Lett* 1997; **224**:5–8.

Garry EM, Moss A, Delaney A, et al. Neuropathic sensitization of behavioral reflexes and spinal NMDA receptor/CaM kinase II interactions are disrupted in PSD-95 mutant mice. *Curr Biol* 2003a; **13**:321–8.

Garry EM, Moss A, Rosie R, Delaney A, Mitchell R, Fleetwood-Walker SM. Specific involvement in neuropathic pain of AMPA receptors and adapter proteins for the GluR2 subunit. *Mol Cell Neurosci* 2003b; **24**:10–22.

Giesecke T, Gracely RH, Grant MA, et al. Evidence of augmented central pain processing in idiopathic chronic low back pain. *Arthritis Rheum* 2004; **50**:613–23.

Gold MS, Gebhart GF. Nociceptor sensitization in pain pathogenesis. *Nat Med* 2010; **16**:1248–57.

Goldberg YP, MacFarlane J, MacDonald ML, et al. Loss-of-function mutations in the Nav1.7 gene underlie congenital indifference to pain in multiple human populations. *Clin Genet* 2007; **71**:311–19.

Handwerker HO. What is a polymodal nociceptor? *J Pain* 2008; **9**:309–10.

Handwerker HO. Primary afferent nociceptors. In: Basbaum Aed (ed) *The Biomedical & Life Sciences Collection*, Henry Stewart Talks Henry Stewart Talks, Ltd, London, 2009.

Handwerker HO. Classification of nociceptors - To what purpose? *Pain* 2010; **148**(3):355–6.

Hartmann B, Ahmadi S, Heppenstall PA, et al. The AMPA receptor subunits GluR-A and GluR-B reciprocally modulate spinal synaptic plasticity and inflammatory pain. *Neuron* 2004; **44**:637–50.

Harvey RJ, Depner UB, Wassle H, et al. GlyR alpha3: an essential target for spinal PGE2-mediated inflammatory pain sensitization. *Science* 2004; **304**:884–7.

Hefti FF, Rosenthal A, Walicke PA, et al. Novel class of pain drugs based on antagonism of NGF. *Trends Pharmacol Sci* 2006; **27**:85–91.

Heinricher MM, Tavares I, Leith JL, Lumb BM. Descending control of nociception: Specificity, recruitment and plasticity. *Brain Res Rev* 2009; **60**:214–25.

Hoheisel U, Reinohl J, Unger T, Mense S. Acidic pH and capsaicin activate mechanosensitive group IV muscle receptors in the rat. *Pain* 2004; **110**:149–57.

Hoheisel U, Unger T, Mense S. Excitatory and modulatory effects of inflammatory cytokines and neurotrophins on mechanosensitive group IV muscle afferents in the rat. *Pain* 2005; **114**:168–76.

Hoheisel U, Unger T, Mense S. Sensitization of rat dorsal horn neurons by NGF-induced subthreshold potentials and low-frequency activation. *A study employing intracellular recordings in vivo. Brain Res* 2007; **1169**:34–43.

Hucho TB, Dina OA, Levine JD. Epac mediates a cAMP-to-PKC signaling in inflammatory pain: an isolectin B4(+) neuron-specific mechanism. *J Neurosci* 2005; **25**:6119–26.

Hudson LJ, Bevan S, Wotherspoon G, Gentry C, Fox A, Winter J. VR1 protein expression increases in undamaged DRG neurons after partial nerve injury. *Eur J Neurosci* 2001; **13**:2105–14.

Igarashi T, Kikuchi S, Shubayev V, Myers RR. (2000). Volvo Award winner in basic science studies: Exogenous tumor necrosis factor-alpha mimics nucleus pulposus-induced neuropathology. Molecular, histologic, and behavioral comparisons in rats. *Spine* **25**:2975–80.

Ikeda H, Heinke B, Ruscheweyh R, Sandkuhler J. Synaptic plasticity in spinal lamina I projection neurons that mediate hyperalgesia. *Science* 2003; **299**:1237–40.

Ikeda H, Stark J, Fischer H, et al. Synaptic amplifier of inflammatory pain in the spinal dorsal horn. *Science* 2006; **312**:1659–62.

Indo Y, Tsuruta M, Hayashida Y, et al. Mutations in the TRKA/NGF receptor gene in patients with congenital insensitivity to pain with anhidrosis. *Nat Genet* 1996; **13**:485–8.

Jeon D, Kim S, Chetana M, et al. Observational fear learning involves affective pain system and Cav1.2 Ca2+ channels in ACC. *Nat Neurosci* 2010; **13**:482–8.

Ji RR, Woolf CJ. Neuronal plasticity and signal transduction in nociceptive neurons: implications for the initiation and maintenance of pathological pain. *Neurobiol Dis* 2001; **8**:1–10.

Kawasaki Y, Kohno T, Zhuang ZY, et al. Ionotropic and metabotropic receptors, protein kinase A, protein kinase C, and Src contribute to C-fiber-induced ERK activation and cAMP response element-binding protein phosphorylation in dorsal horn neurons, leading to central sensitization. *J Neurosci* 2004; **24**:8310–21.

Kruger L. Morphological features of thin sensory afferent fibers: a new interpretation of 'nociceptor' function. *Prog Brain Res* 1988; **74**:253–7.

Kuner R. Central mechanisms of pathological pain. *Nat Med* 2010; **16**:1258–66.

Lee S, Moon CS, Sul D, et al. Comparison of growth factor and cytokine expression in patients with degenerated disc disease and herniated nucleus pulposus. *Clin Biochem* 2009; **42**:1504–11.

Legrain V, Iannetti GD, Plaghki L, Mouraux A. The pain matrix reloaded A salience detection system for the body. *Prog Neurobiol* 2011; **93**(1):111–24.

Lewin GR, Rueff A, Mendell LM. Peripheral and central mechanisms of NGF-induced hyperalgesia. *Eur J Neurosci* 1994; **6**:1903–12.

Lu X, Richardson PM. Responses of macrophages in rat dorsal root ganglia following peripheral nerve injury. *J Neurocytol* 1993; **22**:334–41.

Luo C, Seeburg PH, Sprengel R, Kuner R. Activity-dependent potentiation of calcium signals in spinal sensory networks in inflammatory pain states. *Pain* 2008; **140**:358–67.

Ma W, Zhang Y, Bantel C, Eisenach JC. Medium and large injured dorsal root ganglion cells increase TRPV-1, accompanied by increased alpha2C-adrenoceptor co-expression and functional inhibition by clonidine. *Pain* 2005; **113**:386–94.

Maingret F, Fosset M, Lesage F, Lazdunski M, Honore E. TRAAK is a mammalian neuronal mechano-gated K+ channel. *J Biol Chem* 1999; **274**:1381–7.

Melzack R. From the gate to the neuromatrix. *Pain* 1999; Suppl 6, S121–6.

Melzack R, Casey KL. Sensory, motivational, and central control determinants of pain. In: Kenshalo DR (ed) *The skin senses*. Springfield, IL: Thomas, 1968. pp. 423–43.

Meyer RA, Davis KD, Cohen RH, Treede RD, Campbell JN. Mechanically insensitive afferents (MIAs) in cutaneous nerves of monkey. *Brain Res* 1991; **561**:252–61.

Moore KA, Kohno T, Karchewski LA, Scholz J, Baba H, Woolf CJ. Partial peripheral nerve injury promotes a selective loss of GABAergic inhibition in the superficial dorsal horn of the spinal cord. *J Neurosci* 2002; **22**:6724–31.

Mouraux A, Diukova A, Lee MC, Wise RG, Iannetti GD. A multisensory investigation of the functional significance of the 'pain matrix'. *Neuroimage* 2011; **54**(3):2237–49.

Murase S, Terazawa E, Queme F, et al. Bradykinin and nerve growth factor play pivotal roles in muscular mechanical hyperalgesia after exercise (delayed-onset muscle soreness). *J Neurosci* 2010; **30**:3752–61.

Norimoto M, Ohtori S, Yamashita M, et al. Direct application of the TNF-alpha inhibitor, etanercept, does not affect CGRP expression and phenotypic change of DRG neurons following application of nucleus pulposus onto injured sciatic nerves in rats. *Spine* 2008; **33**:2403–8.

Obata K, Katsura H, Mizushima T, et al. TRPA1 induced in sensory neurons contributes to cold hyperalgesia after inflammation and nerve injury. *J Clin Invest* 2005; **115**:2393–401.

Omana-Zapata I, Khabbaz MA, Hunter JC, Clarke DE, Bley KR. Tetrodotoxin inhibits neuropathic ectopic activity in neuromas, dorsal root ganglia and dorsal horn neurons. *Pain* 1997; **72**:41–9.

Ossipov MH, Porreca F. Neuropathic Pain:Basic Mechanisms (animal). In: Basbaum A.I., Bushnell C.M. (eds) *Science of Pain*. Amsterdam: Elsevier, 2009. pp. 833–55.

Patel AJ, Honore E. Properties and modulation of mammalian 2P domain K+ channels. *Trends Neurosci* 2001; **24**:339–46.

Porreca F, Ossipov MH, Gebhart GF. Chronic pain and medullary descending facilitation. *Trends Neurosci* 2002; **25**:319–25.

Reimann F, Cox JJ, Belfer I, et al. Pain perception is altered by a nucleotide polymorphism in SCN9A. *Proc Natl Acad Sci U S A* 2010; **107**:5148–53.

Richardson JD, Vasko MR. Cellular mechanisms of neurogenic inflammation. *J Pharmacol Exp Ther* 2002; **302**:839–45.

Rukwied R, Mayer A, Kluschina O, Obreja O, Schley M, Schmelz M. NGF induces non-inflammatory localized and lasting mechanical and thermal hypersensitivity in human skin. *Pain* 2010; **148**:407–13.

Sato J, Perl ER. Adrenergic excitation of cutaneous pain receptors induced by peripheral nerve injury. *Science* 1991; **251**:1608–10.

Schaible HG, von Banchet GS, Boettger MK, et al. The role of proinflammatory cytokines in the generation and maintenance of joint pain. *Ann N Y Acad Sci* 2010; **1193**:60–9.

Schaible H-G, Schmidt RF. Responses of fine medial articular nerve afferents to passive movements of knee joints. *J Neurophysiol* 1983; **49**:1118–26.

Schmelz M, Michael K, Weidner C, Schmidt R, Torebjork HE, Handwerker HO. Which nerve fibers mediate the axon reflex flare in human skin? *Neuroreport* 2000; **11**:645–8.

Schmidt R, Schmelz M, Forster C, Ringkamp M, Torebjork E, Handwerker H. Novel classes of responsive and unresponsive C nociceptors in human skin. *J Neurosci* 1995; **15**:333–41.

Schmidt R, Schmelz M, Torebjork HE, Handwerker HO. Mechano-insensitive nociceptors encode pain evoked by tonic pressure to human skin. *Neuroscience* 2000; **98**:793–800.

Schoedel AL, Zimmermann K, Handwerker HO, Forster C. The influence of simultaneous ratings on cortical BOLD effects during painful and non-painful stimulation. *Pain* 2008; **135**:131–41.

Scholz J, Broom DC, Youn DH, et al. Blocking caspase activity prevents transsynaptic neuronal apoptosis and the loss of inhibition in lamina II of the dorsal horn after peripheral nerve injury. *J Neurosci* 2005; **25**:7317–23.

Sluka KA, Kalra A, Moore SA. Unilateral intramuscular injections of acidic saline produce a bilateral, long-lasting hyperalgesia. *Muscle Nerve* 2001; **24**:37–46.

Snider WD, McMahon SB. Tackling pain at the source: new ideas about nociceptors. *Neuron* 1998; **20**:629–32.

Sommer C. Painful neuropathies. *Curr Opin Neurol* 2003; **16**:623–8.

Sorkin LS, Puig S, Jones DL. Spinal bicuculline produces hypersensitivity of dorsal horn neurons: effects of excitatory amino acid antagonists. *Pain* 1998; **77**:181–90.

Taguchi T, Hoheisel U, Mense S. Dorsal horn neurons having input from low back structures in rats. *Pain* 2008; **138**:119–29.

Taguchi T, John V, Hoheisel U, Mense S. Neuroanatomical pathway of nociception originating in a low back muscle (multifidus) in the rat. *Neurosci Lett* 2007; **427**:22–7.

Tal M, Bennett GJ. Extra-territorial pain in rats with a peripheral mononeuropathy: mechano-hyperalgesia and mechano-allodynia in the territory of an uninjured nerve. *Pain* 1994; **57**:375–82.

Torebjörk HE, Schmelz M, Handwerker HO. Functional properties of human cutaneous nociceptors and their role in pain and hyperalgesia. In: Belmonte C, Cervero F (eds) *Neurobiology of Nociceptors*. Oxford: Oxford University Press, 1996. pp. 349–69.

Treede RD, Kenshalo DR, Gracely RH, Jones AK. The cortical representation of pain. *Pain* 1999; **79**:105–11.

Vanegas H, Schaible HG. Descending control of persistent pain: inhibitory or facilitatory? *Brain Res Brain Res Rev* 2004; **46**:295–309.

Walder RY, Rasmussen LA, Rainier JD, Light AR, Wemmie JA, Sluka KA. ASIC1 and ASIC3 play different roles in the development of Hyperalgesia after inflammatory muscle injury. *J Pain* 2010; **11**:210–18.

Wieseler-Frank J, Maier SF, Watkins LR. Immune-to-brain communication dynamically modulates pain: physiological and pathological consequences. *Brain Behav Immun* 2005; **19**:104–11.

Wood JN, Boorman JP, Okuse K, Baker MD. Voltage-gated sodium channels and pain pathways. *J Neurobiol* 2004; **61**:55–71.

Woolf CJ, Ma Q. Nociceptors—noxious stimulus detectors. *Neuron* 2007; **55**:353–64.

Woolf CJ, Salter MW. Neuronal plasticity: increasing the gain in pain. *Science* 2000; **288**:1765–69.

Wu G, Ringkamp M, Hartke TV, et al. Early onset of spontaneous activity in uninjured C-fiber nociceptors after injury to neighboring nerve fibers. *J Neurosci* 2001; **21**:RC140.

Yamashita M, Ohtori S, Koshi T, et al. Tumor necrosis factor-alpha in the nucleus pulposus mediates radicular pain, but not increase of inflammatory peptide, associated with nerve damage in mice. *Spine* 2008; **33**:1836–42.

## Chapter 5

# Dysfunction of the Hypothalamic–Pituitary–Adrenal Axis and Associated Stress Axes in the Development of Chronic Low Back Pain

John McBeth and Andrea Power

## 5.1 Introduction

As discussed in Parts 2 to 4 of this volume, low back pain (LBP) is a complex disorder whose aetiology is associated with a host of factors across multiple domains that include biological, psychological, and individual- and higher-order social factors. By definition *chronic* LBP is LBP that persists beyond the normal healing time required for any insult or injury that may have preceded the onset of symptoms (IASP 2002). That is, for most cases, LBP in the absence of obvious pathology. The challenge then is to identify the factors that are associated with symptom perpetuation, or chronification.

It is clear that to determine the factors that are associated with the transition from acute to chronic LBP, we cannot limit our perspective. Focusing on the role of the biological determinants of chronicity in isolation from psychological and social factors would be meaningless. The interrelationships between risk factors for chronicity can be usefully conceptualized through a traditional biopsychosocial model. However in an excellent theoretical paper (Deary et al. 2007) the biopsychosocial model has been expanded to develop a model of symptom perpetuation that is *autopoietic* (a term borrowed from systems theory and cell biology that literally means 'self-creating') (see Figure 5.1). The core tenet of that model is a multifactorial autopoietic cycle that underlies the perpetuation of symptoms. The strength of this conceptualization is that while across groups of individuals there may be similarities in the factors associated with the chronification of LBP, the model allows for interactions between these factors that may be unique to subgroups or even the individual experience and addresses the important issue of phenotypic heterogeneity. Expanding beyond the original aim of the Deary et al. (2007) paper (to explore the onset and perpetuation of 'medically unexplained' symptoms such as chronic fatigue and irritable bowel syndrome) this model can usefully focus our thoughts on the role of multiple factors in the perpetuation of LBP. The reader is encouraged to place the findings reported below in the context of the model outlined in Figure 5.1.

Stress response systems are notoriously sensitive to multiple factors: prior experience and life stress (Faravelli et al. 2010), psychological distress, cognitive and behavioural factors (Geiss et al. 2005), and body composition (Vicennati et al. 2009) to name a few. In this chapter we will outline the putative role of innate stress response systems in the perpetuation of pain. The main focus will be the primary stress response system in humans the hypothalamic–pituitary–adrenal (HPA) axis. We will also briefly explore the relationship with other related systems; the hypothalamic–pituitary–gonadal (HPG) and hypothalamic–pituitary–growth hormone (HPGH) axes.

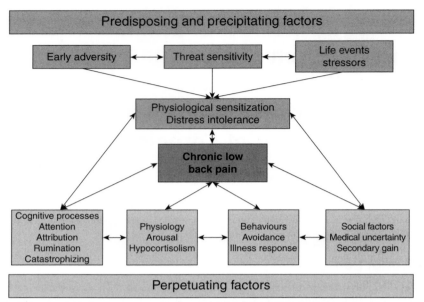

**Fig. 5.1** Autopoietic cycle of low back pain maintenance. This model adapted from Deary et al. (2007) proposes that low back pain is a multifactorial disorder and that pain chronification is associated with a number of predisposing and precipitating factors (early experiences, threat sensitivity, life events) that interact with perpetuating factors (cognitive processes, physiology, behaviours, social) in an autopoietic (self-perpetuating) cycle. This model explains why pain may persist in the absence of physical pathology.

We will argue that these stress response systems may bring about the transition from acute to chronic LBP.

However, while the available data is suggestive, these relationships have not been adequately tested in well-conducted longitudinal epidemiological studies. Data from other disorders that are strongly associated with stress and that have pain as the cardinal symptom will occasionally be included in the discussion where data is not directly available on LBP. We conclude with a research recommendation that outlines a testable hypothesis to establish the true relationship between functioning of stress response systems and the chronification of LBP.

## 5.2 **Allostatic load: the molecular switch from acute to chronic pain?**

*Allostasis* enables the system to maintain stability through adaptation by the activation of different physiological regulatory pathways. These adjustments are homeostatic mechanisms vital for survival; however persistent adaptation of the system to chronic stressors is reported to have a detrimental effect (Chapman et al. 2008). The point at which the system is unable to successfully adapt to this enduring stress is known as the 'allostatic load'. At this point, activity within homeostatic systems appears to be permanently altered, with disruptions to signalling and hence communication between key pathways. Animal models displayed significant alterations within the limbic system following 21 days of stress. Here structural alterations to the hippocampus and amygdale were observed, as well as changes in behaviours such as anxiety and aggression (McEwen 2003; Pham et al. 2003).

In typical situations, activation of the stress pathways discussed below enables physiological adaptation to short term stressors. However, chronic exposure to emotional and physical stress results in the alteration and adaptation of the HPA axis and associated axes to the environment. Although there are sizeable gaps in our knowledge regarding the molecular transition associated with chronic stress states, HPA dysfunctions are usually associated with significant alterations to cortisol regulation. This may eventually manifest as either hypocortisolism or hypercortisolism. For the purpose of this review we will focus on hypocortisolism and examine abnormal communication between the HPA and its surrounding pathways which may influence the transition from acute to chronic pain.

## 5.3 Stress and the HPA axis

### 5.3.1 Normal HPA function

The HPA axis, the central pathway for stress-adaptation, comprises three brain sites: the hypothalamus, the anterior pituitary, and the adrenal cortex (Papadimitriou & Priftis 2009). The upstream component of this pathway, corticotrophin releasing hormone (CRH), is expressed by cells within the paraventricular nucleus (PVN) of the hypothalamus (see Figure 5.2). It is then secreted into the hypophyseal portal system, before being carried to the anterior pituitary, where it stimulates the release of proopiomelanocortin (POMC). POMC is a large molecule which differentially cleaved, produces peptides with a variety of biological functions, such as endogenous opioid, ß-endorphin and ß-melanocyte stimulating hormone (ß-MSH). However, for the purpose of this section, we will concentrate on the cleavage product and stress axis regulator, adrenocorticotropin hormone (ACTH). ACTH subsequently triggers the release of the key stress hormone, cortisol, from the zona reticularis of the adrenal cortex.

On release into the blood system, approximately 90% of cortisol in circulation binds to specialized plasma proteins. The remaining unbound or 'free' cortisol is biologically active. This component, is not only responsible for driving the following stress response, but in sufficient concentrations, suppresses HPA function at both hypothalamic and pituitary levels, and regulates a number of further physiological actions, such as metabolism, immune response and memory consolidation (Harbuz 2002a, 2002b; Henckens et al. 2009; Mussig et al. 2010). Also, by controlling glucose metabolism, cortisol modulates glucose levels within the blood, providing energy substrates for key organs such as the brain and heart. Cortisol is also responsible for the suppression of immune function. It impedes the release of arachidonic acid, a key precursor for numerous inflammatory mediators, preventing the differentiation of mast cells, and the production of nitric oxide, interleukins and gamma interferon (Harbuz 2002b). Furthermore, cortisol exerts its effect on the CNS by directly modulating neuronal electrical activity via type 1 and 2 glucocorticoid receptors, which are widely expressed in the limbic system and hippocampus. Indeed cortisol has demonstrated the ability to reduce hippocampal volume as well as memory (Kumsta et al. 2010; Muller et al. 2002; Patel et al. 2008).

Although CRH, ACTH and cortisol are secreted in small intermittent pulses throughout the day, plasma levels of ACTH and cortisol characteristically peak during early morning, initiated by the release of CRH several hours before waking. Subsequently, plasma ACTH and cortisol levels are at nadir round the time of sleep (Lightman et al. 2000).

### 5.3.2 The impact of acute stress

On receiving stress-associated signals from brain areas, such as the limbic system, cells of the PVN synthesize and release CRH, resulting in cortisol release into the bloodstream (Figure 5.3a).

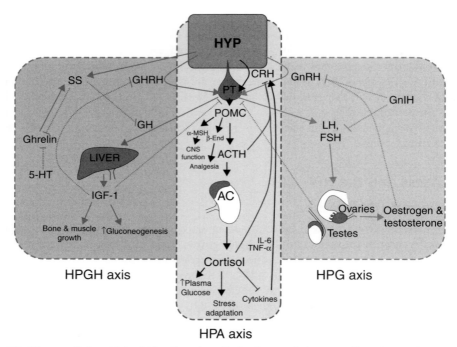

**Fig. 5.2** (Also see Colour Plate 1) The three hypothalamic axes. In humans, the primary stress response system, the hypothalamic pituitary adrenal (HPA) axis (grey), interacts with two other related neuroendocrine pathways, the hypothalamic pituitary growth hormone (HPGH, green) and hypothalamic pituitary gonodal (HPG, blue) axes. Under normal, stress-free conditions, these three hypothalamic pathways function independently and maintain homeostasis through positive (arrows) and negative (bars) regulation. Each axis is driven by hormonal secretion from the pituitary gland (PT). Corticotropin releasing hormone (CRH) released from the hypothalamus (HYP) initiates HPA activity, by stimulating pro-opiomelanocortin (POMC) production from the PT POMC is sequentially cleaved into a number of active components such as adrenocorticotropin hormone (ACTH) β-endorphin (β-E) and α-melanocyte-stimulating hormone (α-MSH). ACTH is responsible for activating the release of downstream element, cortisol, from the adrenal cortex (AC). Cortisol then suppresses HPA function at various levels as well as inhibiting the production of immune system components, such as interleukin-6 (IL-6) and tumour necrosis factor alpha (TNF-α). In comparison, HPGH activity is instigated by the release of gonadotrophin releasing hormone (GnRH) and the subsequent secretion of growth hormone (GH) by the PT Circulating GH then induces the liver to secrete insulin-like growth factor 1 (IGF-1) resulting in bone and muscle growth and gluconeogenesis. HPG activity is prompted by the hypothalamic release of gonadotrophin releasing hormone (GnRH) which stimulates luteinizing hormone (LH) and follicle stimulating hormone (FSH) secretion from the PT This results in the downstream release of oestrogen and testosterone and sequential inhibition of GnRH. Further, control of the HPG pathway is elicited by gonadotrophin inhibitory hormone (GnIH) which inhibits GnRH, LH and FSH secretion.

Under stressful conditions, cortisol re-establishes physiological equilibrium within the organism, by halting the stress response, and consequently initiating the recovery process and coping mechanisms (Olff et al. 1995; Stein-Behrens & Sapolsky 1992; Ursin & Olff 1993). Cortisol impedes further stress response by inhibiting the HPA axis at several levels. Within minutes of cortisol release, CRH and ACTH releasing cells of the PVN and anterior pituitary are suppressed (Steckler et al. 1999). Then, approximately 60–90 minutes later, cortisol inhibits the hippocampal cells responsible for HPA activation (ffrench-Mullen 1995; Young 1995; Young & Vazquez 1996). It therefore makes sense that during acute stress, HPA hyperactivity has been recorded with reported increases in circulating ACTH, urinary cortisol and CSF-CRH (Reul et al. 2000; Steckler et al. 1999; Van Praag 2004).

However slight elevations in basal cortisol levels are sufficient to induce a metabolic response, immunosuppressive effect or alter blood pressure regulation—all of which may be detrimental to the system. In fact, HPA hyperactivity and hypercortisolism has been associated with hypertension, abdominal obesity, diabetes II and osteoporosis (Chiodini et al. 2008; Kudielka et al. 2004; Morelli et al. 2010).

### 5.3.3 The impact of chronic stress

It is difficult to ascertain the juncture at which HPA function is permanently altered by stressors. Persistent exposure to stress down-regulates critical components of the HPA axis, resulting in

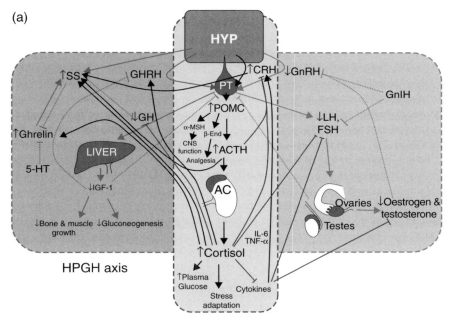

**Fig. 5.3** (Also see Colour Plate 2) The HPA dampens HPGH and HPG activity during acute stress (a), while chronic stress leads to HPA hypoactivity, excessive cytokine production and further down-regulation of the HPGH and HPG axes (b). HYP, hypothalamus; CRH, corticotropin releasing hormone; ACTH, adrenocorticotropin hormone; AC, adrenal cortex; POMC, pro-opiomelanocortin; β-End, β-endorphin; α-MSH, α-melanocyte-stimulating hormones; SS, somatostatin; GnRH, gonadotrophin releasing hormone; LH, luteinizing hormone; FSH, follicle stimulating hormone; GnIH, gonadotrophin inhibitory hormone.

(a) Acute stress up-regulates the production of components within the hypothalamic–pituitary–adrenal (HPA) axis, which then down-regulate both hypothalamic pituitary growth hormone (HPGH) and hypothalamic–pituitary–gonodal (HPG) activity. Cortisol suppresses growth hormone (GH) activity both directly and indirectly (via activation of GH-inhibiting components somatostation (SS) and ghrelin). Cortisol also prevents secretion of gonadotrophin releasing hormone (GnRH), luteinizing hormone (LH) and follicle stimulating hormone (FSH), as well as suppressing the release of immune elements, interleukin-6 (IL-6) and tumour necrosis factor alpha (TNF-α, red bars).

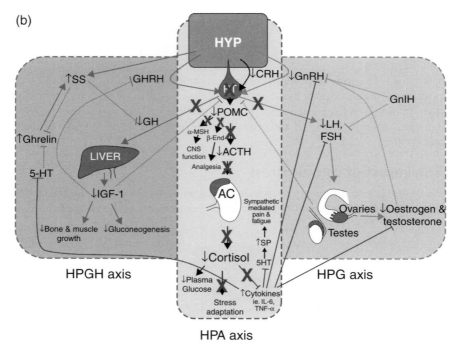

HPA axis

**Fig. 5.3** *(Continued)* (b) HPA activity is severely compromised during chronic stress, resulting in HPA hypoactivity and pituitary gland (PT) desensitization. Reduced cortisol levels fail to regulate cytokine-suppression resulting in the subsequent release of cytokines such as IL-6 and TNF-α. Indeed, these cytokines are responsible for suppressing a variety of components within the HPGH and HPG axes. Cytokines inhibit serotonin (5-HT) production within the HPGH, leading indirectly to reductions in GH, as well as suppression of HPG activity at various levels (red bars). In addition, 5-HT suppression increases CWP-related symptoms, such as sympathetic mediated pain and fatigue, via elevated substance P (SP) levels. Arrows and bars indicate the positive and negative regulation, respectively.

ACTH deficiency and prevents the subsequent secretion of cortisol from the adrenal gland (Figure 5.3b). Hypocortisolism is a deficiency associated with pain disorders, fatigue and enhanced stress sensitivity (Fries et al. 2005; Meeus et al. 2008; Neeck & Crofford 2000). Indeed, patients with fibromyalgia (FM), a disorder characterized by chronic widespread body pain (Wolfe 1990) have reduced levels of urinary and plasma cortisol, cortisol feedback resistance and hypo-responsive pituitary function (Griep et al. 1998b), as well as abnormal immune response. As cortisol is responsible for downstream immune-suppression, hypocortisolism results in atypical elevations in cytokines IL-8, TNF-α, IL-1 and IL-6 (Maier & Watkins 1998). Indeed the excessive levels of cytokines may contribute to pain phenotypes including LBP. Impairments within this axis ultimately impact on communications between the parallel HPG and HPGH pathways.

## 5.4 **Stress and HPG axis function**

### 5.4.1 **Normal function**

Cells containing gonadotropin-releasing hormone (GnRH) project from the olfactory bulb via the hypothalamus and preoptic area to the medial basal hypothalamus (MBH) and median eminence (ME). Ensuing GnRH secretion (Figure 5.2) from the ME stimulates the release of luteinizing hormone (LH) and follicle stimulating hormone (FSH) from gonadotropic cells of the anterior pituitary into the portal system. Circulating LH and FSH bind to receptors of the ovary and testis to up-regulate sex steroid production and gametogenesis. In the testes, LH induces testosterone production from the Leydig cells, FSH induces testicular growth and expression of androgen-binding protein by Sertoli cells, while a combination of these hormones ensures spermatozoa maturation. In the ovaries, LH drives oestrogen and progesterone production and ovulation, FSH regulates the development of the ovarian follicle, and combined LH and FSH control the follicular secretion of oestrogen. LH and FSH then, by directly targeting the pituitary, act as potent negative feedback regulators of the HPG axis exerting homeostatic control (Vadakkadath & Atwood 2005).

### 5.4.2 The impact of acute stress

Gonadotropin inhibitory hormone (GnIH) opposes the action of GnRH, by inhibiting the production of LH and FSH and it has been implicated in stress-mediated reproductive dysfunction (Figure 5.3a). In rodents, GnIH expression occurs within cells of the dorsomedial nucleus of the hypothalamus (DMH). These cells then project to the ME and to the POA, the aforementioned area of GnRH neurons secretion (Kriegsfeld et al. 2006). Receptors homologous to GnIH receptors are expressed in the hypothalamus, pituitary, and testes of other species (Bentley et al. 2008; Yin et al. 2005). In vivo, up-regulation of this receptor or the GnIH ligand, suppress HPG function, LH secretion and sexual activity (Bentley et al. 2006; Calisi et al. 2008; Murakami et al. 2008; Osugi et al. 2004). This perhaps suggests that GnIH acts as a mediator of stressors on mammalian reproduction. Furthermore, GnIH-expressing cells also express stress hormone receptors and as an adrenalectomy prevents increased GnIH expression following stress, it may be that the HPG axis is regulated by stress-induced adrenal hormone release.

The HPA and HPG axes appear to have a bidirectional regulatory relationship. HPG activity is controlled by components of the HPA, and visa-versa. Firstly, both CRH and glucocorticoids are shown to suppress HPG function by altering GnRH production. Whilst CRH inhibits the expression of GnRH from neurons of the arcuate nucleus, glucocorticoids appear to regulate HPG activity on multiple levels. Hence, glucocorticoids not only suppress GnRH production, pituitary secretion of LH and steroidogenesis within the gonads, they also desensitize target tissues to circulating sex-steroids (Rabin et al. 1990; Rivier et al. 1996). In comparison, several components of the HPG axis reportedly activate the HPA. For instance, oestrogen response elements have been identified in the CRH gene promoter region (Vamvakopoulos & Chrousos 1993). Therefore the HPA has an inhibitory effect on the HPG, whist the HPG appears to stimulate HPA activity (Chrousos & Harris 1998; Mastorakos et al. 2006).

### 5.4.3 The impact of chronic stress

The HPG relies on daily signals in CRH and cortisol expression to maintain homeostatic regulation. If, as discussed, chronic stress results in a HPA hypo-function, these daily inhibitory signals fail to adequately control HPG function, the HPG may itself become hypoactive (Figure 5.3b). Availability of sex hormones has been associated with fluctuations in pain. Rheumatoid arthritis tends to improve during pregnancy, during oestrogen replacement therapy and during treatment with oestrogen-containing oral contraceptives (Van Vollenhoven & McGuire 1994), temporomandibular (LeResche et al. 2003) and experimental (Teepker et al. 2010) pain fluctuate over the course of the menstrual cycle, and testosterone has been associated with the amelioration of pain in clinic patients with FM (Dessein et al. 1999). However, the HPG is influenced by a host of factors.

Body weight is an independent regulator of the HPG axis activity. Leptin, an adipose tissue derived hormone (Bray 1997; Mitchell et al. 2005), primarily modulates appetite and energy expenditure within hypothalamic nuclei. It also regulates a variety of functions within the HPG axis, such as the onset of puberty, reproductive capacity and facilitating implantation and pregnancy (Lado-Abeal & Norman 2002; Margetic et al. 2002) This is because adipose tissue metabolizes sex-steroids and therefore significantly alters functionality of the reproductive axis by reducing the levels of circulating sex-steroids (Haffner 2000; Tchernof et al. 2000). Indeed, obesity constitutes as a low-grade inflammatory state (Yudkin 2007) as increased adipose tissue causes enhanced secretion of pro-inflammatory hormones and cytokines, such as TNF-α and IL-6, into the circulation. This imposes systemic chronic inflammatory stress on the body (Tsigos et al. 1999) which is further aggravated by severe reductions in cortisol-mediated and subsequent immune activity.

A further interesting observation is the role of cytokines on HPG function. Pro-inflammatory cytokines, such as TNFα, stimulate HPA axis function via CRH activation, whilst at the same time reducing HPG activity, by preventing GnRH secretion and sex-steroid production (Tsigos et al. 1999). Therefore, prolonged suppression of gonadal function, as a result of abnormal HPA activity, can result in reduced LH and testosterone concentrations in males and menstrual disorders and amenorrhea in females (Meczekalski et al. 2008; Tsutsumi & Webster 2009).

## 5.5 Stress and HPGH axis function

### 5.5.1 Normal function

Growth hormone (GH) is secreted by the anterior pituitary in a pulsatile manner and regulated by the opposing actions of hypothalamic GH releasing hormone (GHRH), and somatostatin (SS)—GHRH stimulates while SS inhibits GH release (Figure 5.2). The secretion of GH into the bloodstream stimulates IGF-I production in many organs, and subsequent elevations in circulating IGF-I. IGF-1 then feeds back to inhibit the axis hence preventing further secretion of GH by the pituitary. Experimentally, administration of exogenous IGF-I lowers GH secretion, and conversely, IGF-I knock-out mice show significant increases in GH secretion (Yakar et al. 2001).

In addition, this pathway is modulated by the regulatory control exerted over SS by key components of this and other pathways. For instance, serotonin (5-HT) diminishes levels of circulating SS while GH, insulin-like growth factor-1 (IGF-1) and CRH individually upregulate SS. Ghrelin, a novel gastric hormone important in appetite regulation has a bi-directional relationship with SS. Whilst ghrelin induces SS expression, SS suppresses ghrelin production, and therefore ghrelin-induced activation of components such as CRH, ACTH, cortisol and vasopressin (Unniappan 2010).

Independently of these control mechanisms, concentrations of circulating GH express diurnal rhythms, peaking during the late night/early morning and at nadir midday (Uchiyama et al. 1998). In bone IGF-I acts on the epiphysial plate, leading to longitudinal bone growth (Kemp 2009; Báez-Saldaña et al. 2009). As illustrated, GH also has direct effects on many organs, including kidney and cartilage, which can be independent of IGF-I action (Gershberg, 1960; Olney, 2009).

### 5.5.2 The impact of acute stress

Interactions between the HPGH and HPA are well documented and occur at both the hypothalamic and pituitary levels (Figure 5.3a). Peaks in CRH or cortisol result in elevation of GHRH, SS and ghrelin and conversely, reduced GH secretion (Maclean & Jackson 1988; Rigamonti et al. 2002).

Additionally, studies have shown that prolonged GH secretion could have a variety of physiological effects such as muscle weakness (Mukherjee et al. 2004).

### 5.5.3 **The impact of chronic stress**

Chronic activation of the HPA axis impedes HPGH activity (Figure 5.3b). In fact, HPA hypofunction due to prolonged stress has been linked to the stress-associated suppression of GH secretion and consequent desensitization of the pituitary gland. In clinical trials fibromyalgia (FM)—a chronic pain disorder characterized by chronic widespread pain that includes axial (often low back) pain (Wolfe et al. 1990)—patients have abnormal HPGH function and basal levels of both GH and IGF-1, while further studies have implicated GH deficiency with depression and other chronic illnesses (Cuatrecasas et al. 2007; Griep et al. 1993).

## 5.6 **Does stress system functioning underpin the transition from acute to chronic LBP?**

While there is robust evidence that links physical, psychological and psychosocial stressors with the chronification of LBP, there is a paucity of data that has examined whether dysfunction of stress response systems underpin these relationships. There are no methodologically robust studies available that have directly tested that hypothesis. The data available and discussed below is 'strongly suggestive', having directly assessed the relationships between markers of stress system functioning and chronic LBP or having assessed the relationship between factors known to be associated with chronicity of acute LBP and stress system functioning.

## 5.7 **Stress system functioning in chronic LBP**

Dysfunction of the HPA axis has been associated with chronic LBP in a number of cross-sectional studies. Compared to healthy pain free individuals those with chronic LBP had lower 24-hour urinary free cortisol (Lentjes et al. 1997), an exaggerated ACTH response to CRH challenge (Griep et al. 1998b) although subsequent cortisol release was identical in those with and without pain (Griep et al. 1998b). While the number of glucocorticoid receptors in circulating mononuclear cells was the same, the binding affinity was lower in those with chronic LBP (Lentjes et al. 1997). These data suggest mild hypocortisolaemia with attenuated feedback resistance similar, although less pronounced, to that observed in patients with FM (Crofford et al. 1994; Griep et al. 1998a), a chronic pain disorder characterized by chronic widespread pain that includes axial (often low back) pain (Wolfe et al. 1990). LBP is associated with the onset of chronic widespread pain and FM (Forseth et al. 1999) and the reported differences in HPA axis functioning may be explained by quantitative differences in pain extent between the two groups. In addition FM is associated with higher rates of psychological distress and other factors (Staud 2009) that could influence HPA function.

Secretion of proinflammatory cytokines including TNF-$\alpha$ (Aoki et al. 2002) and IL-6 (Geiss et al. 2005) have been related to sciatic pain and chronic LBP (Wang et al. 2008), and IL-6 to post-operative pain in patients undergoing surgery for disc herniation (Geiss et al. 2005). Other studies have indirectly suggested an association. Analysis of data from the Third National Health and Nutrition Examination Survey revealed that among 6814 adults aged 20–39 years 1452 (21.3%, weighted for non-response) reported a history of allergic conditions (asthma, hay fever, and allergic reactions) that are associated with increased secretion of pro-inflammatory cytokines including IL-1$\beta$ and altered functioning of the HPA axis (Hurwitz & Morgenstern 1999). Exposure to an allergic reaction was associated with a 53% increase in the odds of reporting LBP (independent of age, sex, race, marital status and employment status) and a three fold increase in the odds of reporting LBP and depression (OR=3.2; 95% CI: 1.4, 7.3).

Women are more likely to report chronic pain when compared to men suggesting a role of female sex hormones in the onset and persistence of symptoms or conversely a protective role of male sex hormones. However the data exploring the role of sex hormones in chronic LBP is unclear. In a prospective survey of women first surveyed when 14 years old 'menstruation' and 'pregnancy' were independent significant predictors of LBP at 38 years old (Harreby et al. 1996). In a population based study of 11,428 women, hormonal and reproductive factors associated with increased oestrogen levels (prolonged menstrual cycle, past—though not current—pregnancy, younger maternal age at first birth, use of oral contraceptives, and use of oestrogens during menopause) were associated with the presence of chronic LBP (Wijnhoven et al. 2006). This is in direct contrast to the hypothesized stress-related reduced availability of oestrogens discussed above. However, in that study hysterectomy was also associated with LBP. Age related declines in oestrogen levels are associated with osteoporosis and osteoporotic fracture which in turn are associated with LBP (Nevitt et al. 1998) with the strength of the association increasing with the number and severity of fractures (O'Neill et al. 2004).

Compared to healthy controls subjects with chronic LBP have poorer overall sleep, increased insomnia symptoms, and less efficient sleep (O'Donoghue et al. 2009) that will impact on production of GH. Serum IGF-I, IGFBP-3, and IGFBP-5 were significantly lower in women with osteoporotic fractures (Yamaguchi et al. 2006). Markers of HPGH axis function have been associated with widespread pain disorders including FM (Bennett 1998; Jones et al. 2007) although the relationship may be explained by higher levels of obesity (McBeth et al. 2009) and the association with LBP remains unclear. Similarly there is a paucity of data examining the relationship with androgen levels although among 119 newspaper employees who were classified according to the presence or absence of neck, shoulder and back pain those with pain had lower levels of serum DHEA-S and testosterone (Schell et al. 2008). After adjustment for age and gender the latter two relationships were no longer significant.

Of course these studies have been conducted on subjects with established LBP and although they suggest a relationship they are unable to establish the temporal relationship between stress mediators and chronic pain.

## 5.8 **The transition from acute to chronic symptoms**

Garofalo and colleagues (Garofalo et al. 2006) recruited 37 patients with acute (<6 months' duration) LBP. Using an algorithm developed by the authors (Gatchel et al. 1995) subjects were classified into 'low' and 'high' risk of developing chronic LBP. All subjects collected two saliva samples (one on wakening and the second 20 minutes later) every day for the first 2 weeks after recruitment. Two measures of cortisol levels were reported: mean cortisol secretions over the first 2 weeks and the difference between wakening and the second sample 20 minutes later. The data suggested that compared to low risk subjects those at high risk had significantly lower mean cortisol concentrations[1] over the first 2 weeks (mean (SD): 0.392 (0.251) and 0.367 (0.131) respectively). These differences were apparent in women but not men. Subjects at high risk also had greater variability in the wakening response when compared to low risk subjects with the former group tending to have a significantly greater secretion 20 minutes after wakening (0.410 (0.209) versus 0.305 (0.214) respectively). The difference in variability in cortisol secretion was

---

[1]  No values for cortisol concentrations are given in the original manuscript

observed in both men and women although the degree of variation was significantly greater in women. The authors concluded that 'patients at high risk for chronic pain were found to exhibit differences in both quantity of cortisol concentrations and variability, relative to low-risk patients' (Garofalo et al. 2006, p. 173).

At this point it would be prudent to further examine the authors' classification system. The classification algorithm was developed on data collected from 324 patients recruited via one occupational health clinic and two orthopaedic clinics (Gatchel et al. 1995). All patients had presented with pain in the lumber spine that had been present for less than 6 weeks (as compared to the six month period in the study described above). At baseline subjects completed a number of assessments: a demographic and medical history form, assessment of psychopathology using the Structured Clinical Interview for DSM-III-R (Spitzer & Williams 1988), and the Million Visual Analog Scale (Million et al. 1982) an occupational based assessment of pain and associated disability that includes 15 items and has a total score of between 0 and 150 with higher scores indicating more pain and associated disability. All subjects were followed up 6 months after initial assessment and classified into one of two groups: not disabled (currently working or vocational training or school/retraining, n=274) and disabled (currently disabled and not working because of the original back injury, n=36). Perhaps unsurprisingly the baseline factors which best discriminated between these two groups were higher levels of baseline pain and disability and the presence of an Axis II personality disorder.

This algorithm identifies subjects with LBP who are distressed and who report considerable pain-related disability. It is perhaps not surprising then that those identified as being at high risk of chronic symptoms were those with derangements of the HPA axis. The study did not follow subjects up. It would have been interesting to know, for example, whether baseline levels of cortisol predicted the chronicity of symptoms, say 6 months later. In a second study from the same group (Garofalo et al. 2007) among subjects with acute (<6 months' duration) LBP, lower cortisol levels were significantly associated with higher reported pain severity. Whether these results simply reflected greater associated distress was unclear.

A more recent pilot study sought to examine the relationship between pain-related coping strategies and functioning of the HPA axis (Sudhaus et al. 2009) and to compare the relationships in subjects with acute to those with chronic LBP. A total of 19 patients with acute and 24 with chronic non-specific LBP with and without distal radiation were recruited. All subjects collected five saliva samples 0, 15, 30, 45, and 60 minutes after waking up in the morning over a 2-day period. The cortisol awakening response was estimated as: (1) the mean value over the 2-day period for each data collection point and (2) the 'area under the curve with respect to ground' ($AUC_G$), an estimation of the total cortisol output which is calculated from repeat measure data with identical time intervals between measurements (Pruessner et al. 2003). Subjects completed the Kiel Pain Inventory (KPI) (Hasenbring et al. 1994) from which three categories of pain-related variables were extracted: 'endurance coping' (EC) comprised measures of behavioural endurance, daily active coping strategies, thought suppression; 'fear avoidance coping' (FAC) included measures of avoidance of social activities, avoidance of physical activities, and helplessness/hopelessness; and 'nonverbal pain behaviour' (NPB). Subjects also completed measures of depression (Beck Depression Inventory (Beck et al. 1961)) and fatigue (General Fatigue Scale of the Multidimensional Fatigue Inventory (Smets et al. 1995)).

For both acute and chronic LBP, mean cortisol levels followed a typical wakening response increasing from wakening through the first 30 minutes and decreasing thereafter (45 and 60 minutes after wakening). However, there were no significant differences between the groups at any time point nor in the total concentration of cortisol over the study period ($AUC_G$ (μg/dl): acute LBP $3.24 \pm 0.85$ and chronic LBP $3.41 \pm 1.55$). Sex, body mass index, smoking or pain intensity did not influence the results. However distinct patterns of association between psychosocial factors and $AUC_G$ cortisol concentrations were observed. Among subjects with acute LBP positive EC strategies (behavioural endurance and daily active coping strategies) were associated with reduced $AUC_G$ cortisol concentrations. Among those with chronic LBP 'maladaptive' FAC strategies (avoidance of social activities, avoidance of physical activity, and helplessness/hopelessness) were associated with reduce $AUC_G$ cortisol concentrations. Importantly, within the chronic LBP group when compared to those subjects with low levels those with high levels of NPB, depression and fatigue had significantly less variation in the wakening cortisol response indicating a blunted or hypofunctioning HPA axis. There were no similar observations among those with acute LBP.

The Swedish Norrtälje Musculoskeletal Intervention Centre study was set up to investigate the role of workplace risk factors in the onset and maintenance of musculoskeletal disorders including LBP (Theorell et al. 2000). A subgroup of subjects who had presented to a 'caregiver' (traditional and alternative) with an episode of acute LBP that had been preceded by 6 months without consultation for LBP were identified (Theorell et al. 2000). 26 women and 19 men (with 85 and 72 respectively gender- and age-matched control subjects identified through a population register) provided two blood samples at 08.00 and 12.00 hours and completed a battery of psychosocial measures: pain and associated disability, decision latitude, job demand, job strain, job satisfaction, and social support. While both male and female cases and controls showed a typical pattern of decreasing cortisol levels from wakening to midday, female cases had a significantly reduced change in cortisol levels when compared to female controls (proportion change in serum cortisol: 7.8% vs. −22.7). Similarly among women, cases had significantly higher midday serum IL-6 levels when compared to controls (pg/ml (95% confidence intervals): 4.4 (3.6–5.4) versus 3.1 (2.6–3.6)). Among men there were no differences between cases and controls on either biomarker although low decision latitude was associated with high IL-6 and higher levels of social support were associated with higher morning cortisol levels. In a follow up study serum IL-6 did not predict persistent pain or subsequent disability at 3 or 6 months post baseline in women. However, among men high IL-6 was associated with persistent pain although this relationship was explained by differences in pain intensity and disability (Hasselhorn et al. 2001)[2]. This is an interesting observation and suggests that the factors driving the transition from acute to chronic LBP are psychosocial independent of the underlying stress axis function.

Together these findings suggest qualitative differences between acute and chronic states in relation to stress axis function. However markers of stress axis dysfunction appear to reflect psychosocial factors and those relationships differ between men and women: lower CSF cortisol levels were associated with more intense or disabling pain in men and with higher levels of anxiety and somatization in men and women (Alaranta et al. 1983), while CSF concentrations of prolactin correlated positively with levels of anxiety and depression (Alaranta et al. 1983) although much of the variation in prolactin levels was explained by sex (Hyyppa et al. 1985). The rate of post-dexamethasone non-suppression in individuals with major depressive disorder was independent of the presence of chronic LBP (France et al. 1987). In a group of 80 patients attending an inpatient pain management programme who had reported daily back pain for 6 months or more 35 (43.8%) satisfied DSM-III criteria for major depression (France & Krishnan 1985). On administration of 1mg dexamethasone 14 (40%) individuals with LBP and major depression failed to suppress (serum cortisol >5μg/dl) while none of the group with LBP in the absence of major

---

[2] No results for the relationship between cortisol levels and subsequent pain and disability were presented although the original paper shows that high IL-6 was associated with low cortisol in this group of subjects.

depression failed to suppress. Among those with LBP and major depression 21 cases were deemed to have an organic cause (physical examination positive for radiculopathy, abnormal radiograph, or positive electromyography) and no organic cause could be found for 11 cases. The rate of post-dexamethasone non-suppression among the latter group was significantly higher (n=7, 63.6%) when compared to those with an organic pathology (n=7, 29.2%). This observation could be explained by higher rates of maladaptive coping strategies in those with non-specific back pain of unknown origin.

Maladaptive coping strategies have been shown to be associated with hypofunctioning of the HPA axis (Abelson et al. 2008, 2010) and potentially with other associated systems such as the HPG axis (Kajantie & Phillips 2006) and proinflammatory cytokines. Patients with lumbar disc herniation and low diurnal cortisol variability had lower levels of physical functioning, lower perceived possibilities of influencing their pain and higher levels of pain related catastrophizing when compared to those with higher diurnal cortisol variability (Johansson et al. 2008). Experimental studies have confirmed the relationship between catastrophizing and stress system functioning. In subjects free of chronic pain the administration of acute painful stimuli (heat, cold and pressure) was associated with post-test IL-6 but not cortisol levels in those with high levels of situation specific catastrophizing (i.e. catastrophic thoughts associated with the administered stimuli) (Edwards et al. 2008). Patients with temporomandibular joint disorder underwent a series of tests to establish response to pressure and thermal stimuli (Quartana et al. 2010). Those with high pain catastrophizing scores had a blunted decline in salivary cortisol levels 20 minutes post-test. Interestingly, a similar relationship was observed in a group of individuals free of pain. These observations in pain free individuals suggest that among those with high levels of catastrophizing exposure to acute painful stimuli may lead to chronic pain via altered functioning of the HPA axis or an increase in pro-inflammatory cytokines. There are a number of putative mechanisms of action including reduced prefrontal cortical modulation of pain signals among those with catastrophic cognitions that may inhibit disengaging and suppressing pain signals (Seminowicz & Davis 2006) or an increased central sensitizaton and sensitivity to stimuli via the action of proinflammatory cytokines in the long-term activation of spinal cord glia and dorsal horn neurons (Diers et al. 2007; Gur & Oktayoglu 2008).

## 5.9 **Causal mechanisms**

There are numerous methodological problems with the studies described above, many of which are acknowledged by the authors, including small sample sizes and the challenge of between and within individual variation in stress biomarkers. But perhaps the most fundamental problem has been the inability of these studies to robustly assess *causality*. The main question remains unanswered: among individuals with acute LBP, does functioning of the HPA and associated axes predict who will go on to develop chronic symptoms? When considering the relationship between a risk factor (stress system function) and outcome (the chronification of acute LBP) we should be mindful that while these factors may be associated with one another an observed association does not necessarily imply causality. In Figure 5.4, a number of possible explanations for the observed associations are outlined: in (a) acute LBP could be associated with chronic LBP directly (dashed line) or via dysfunction of stress response systems (solid lines). Stress system derangement may be pre-existing or may be associated with the high levels of stress and other factors associated with acute LBP that are known to influence chronicity. In (b) both acute LBP and chronic LBP are a consequence of stress system derangement but are independent of each other and not causally related. In (c) acute LBP is causally associated with chronic LBP and stress system derangement is a consequence of chronic LBP. While the true nature of the role of stress system functioning in

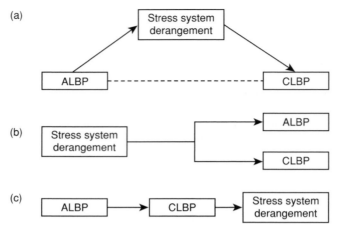

**Fig. 5.4** Pathways of association. In (a) ALBP could be associated with CLBP directly (dashed line) or via dysfunction of stress response systems (solid lines). Stress system derangement may be pre-existing or may be associated with the high levels of stress and other factors associated with ALBP that are known to influence chronicity. In (b) both ALBP and CLBP are a consequence of stress system derangement but are independent of each other and not causally related. In (c) ALBP is causally associated with CLBP and stress system derangement is a consequence of CLBP. ALBP, acute low back pain; CLBP, chronic low back pain.

the transition from acute to chronic LBP awaits rigorous investigation, a small number of prospective studies have investigated the role of altered functioning of the HPA and other axes in the onset and/or perpetuation of more general musculoskeletal pain disorders.

In a two-year prospective study (Wrosch et al. 2008) 184 individuals were asked to report their experience of 12 physical symptoms that included LBP over a 2-day period and to collect five saliva samples (30 minutes after awakening, 14.00 hrs, 16.00 hrs, and before bedtime) on three consecutive days. Baseline cortisol levels predicted an increase in physical symptoms at follow-up but only among those with high levels of negative affect and low sleep efficiency at baseline. Among participants with neck, shoulder or back pain lower levels of serum GH, but not IGF-1, was associated with a worsening of pain 12 months later (Schell et al. 2008). There were no associations with cortisol, DHEA-S, oestradiol, testosterone, or cytokine levels. In individuals free of widespread pain but who were psychologically distressed markers of HPA axis dysfunction predicted the onset of symptoms 12 months later (McBeth et al. 2007). This relationship was not explained by psychological factors although there was no measure of catastrophizing included in the study. Jennifer Glass has elegantly demonstrated the predictive ability of brief exercise cessation in relation to pain onset among healthy people but only among those with a hypofunctioning HPA axis (Glass et al. 2004). Among women who were followed up over a nine year period fluctuations in levels of oestrodial were associated with the development of aches and pains (Freeman et al. 2007).

## 5.10 **Conclusions**

It is unclear whether dysfunction of stress response systems is associated with the transition from acute to chronic LBP. To answer that question a group of individuals with acute LBP need to be identified. Within that group measures of HPA (and other) axis function and other factors known to influence stress system function should be rigorously assessed. All subjects should be followed-up over a reasonable period of time (say, 12 months) to identify those who do and those who do not develop chronic LBP. Only then will the role, if any, of HPA axis function in the chronification of acute LBP become clear. However, the aetiology of LBP is multifactorial. Bringing together multiple levels of causality in a single study is challenging: there is a pay-off between study size and detail in exposure and phenotype measurement. Using novel methodologies (e.g. case-crossover designs, two-stage sampling procedures) and novel statistical methods (e.g. multilevel modelling) will enhance our investigations. We have begun to explain the transition from acute to chronic LBP and although we still need to identify other slices of the 'causal pie' the usefulness of multilevel models in informing interventions across all levels of causality are apparent. In intervention studies of chronic LBP the message is clear; one size does not fit all. The hurdle to developing effective interventions will not be in our conceptualization of the problem to be addressed or how to address it, but in the practicalities of doing so.

## Acknowledgements

John McBeth would like to thank Sarah Parsons for her invaluable help with literature searching, retrieval of manuscripts and, together with Mary Ingram, help with references.

## References

Abelson, J. L., Khan, S., Liberzon, I., Erickson, T. M., & Young, E. A. (2008). Effects of perceived control and cognitive coping on endocrine stress responses to pharmacological activation. *Biol Psychiatry*, **64**(8), 701–7.

Abelson, J. L., Khan, S., Young, E. A., & Liberzon, I. (2010). Cognitive modulation of endocrine responses to CRH stimulation in healthy subjects. *Psychoneuroendocrinology*, **35**(3), 451–9.

Alaranta, H., Hu Báez-Saldaña rme, M., Lahtela, K., & Hyyppa, M. T. (1983). Prolactin and cortisol in cerebrospinal fluid: Sex-related associations with clinical and psychological characteristics of patients with low back pain. *Psychoneuroendocrinology*, **8**(3), 333–41.

Aoki, Y., Rydevik, B., Kikuchi, S., & Olmarker, K. (2002). Local application of disc-related cytokines on spinal nerve roots. *Spin*, **27**(15), 1614–17.

Báez-Saldaña, A., Camacho-Arroyo, I., Espinosa-Aguirre, J.J., et al. (2009). Biotin deficiency and biotin excess: effects on the female reproductive system. *Steroids*, **74**(10–11), 863–9.

Beck, A. T., Ward, C. H., Mendelson, M., Mock, J., & Erbaugh, J. (1961). An inventory for measuring depression. *Arch Gen Psychiatry*, **4**, 561–71.

Bennett, R. M. (1998). Disordered growth hormone secretion in fibromyalgia: a review of recent findings and a hypothesized etiology. *Zeitschrift fur Rheumatologie*, **57**, 72–6.

Bentley, G. E., Kriegsfeld, L. J., Osugi, T., *et al.* (2006). Interactions of gonadotropin-releasing hormone (GnRH) and gonadotropin-inhibitory hormone (GnIH) in birds and mammals. *J Exp Zool A Comp Exp Biol*, **305**(9), 807–14.

Bentley, G. E., Ubuka, T., McGuire, N. L., *et al.* (2008). Gonadotropin-inhibitory hormone and its receptor in the avian reproductive system. *Gen Comp Endocrinol*, **156**(1), 34–43.

Bray, G. A. (1997). Obesity and reproduction. *Hum Reprod*, **12**(Suppl 1), 26–32.

Calisi, R. M., Rizzo, N. O., & Bentley, G. E. (2008). Seasonal differences in hypothalamic EGR-1 and GnIH expression following capture-handling stress in house sparrows (Passer domesticus). *Gen Comp Endocrinol*, **157**(3), 283–7.

Chapman, C. R., Tuckett, R. P., & Song, C. W. (2008). Pain and stress in a systems perspective: reciprocal neural, endocrine, and immune interactions. *J Pain*, **9**(2), 122–45.

Chiodini, I., Francucci, C. M., & Scillitani, A. (2008). Densitometry in glucocorticoid-induced osteoporosis. *J Endocrinol Invest*, **31**(7 Suppl), 33–7.

Chrousos, G. P. & Harris, A. G. (1998). Hypothalamic-pituitary-adrenal axis suppression and inhaled corticosteroid therapy. 1. General principles. *Neuroimmunomodulation*, **5**(6), 277–87.

Crofford, L. J., Pillemer, S. R., & Kalogeras, K. T. (1994). Hypothalamic-pituitary-adrenal axis Pertubations in Patients with Fibromyalgia. *Arthritis Rheum*, **37**, 1583–92.

Cuatrecasas, G., Riudavets, C., Guell, M. A., & Nadal, A. (2007). Growth hormone as concomitant treatment in severe fibromyalgia associated with low IGF-1 serum levels. A pilot study. *BMC Musculoskelet Disord*, **8**, p. 119.

Deary, V., Chalder, T., & Sharpe, M. (2007). The cognitive behavioural model of medically unexplained symptoms: a theoretical and empirical review. *Clin Psychol Rev*, **27**(7), 781–97.

Dessein, P. H., Shipton, E. A., Joffe, B. I., Hadebe, D. P., Stanwix, A. E., & Van der Merwe, B. A. (1999). Hyposecretion of adrenal androgens and the relation of serum adrenal steroids, serotonin and insulin-like growth factor-1 to clinical features in women with fibromyalgia. *Pain*, **83**(2), 313–319.

Diers, M., Koeppe, C., Diesch, E., *et al.* (2007). Central processing of acute muscle pain in chronic low back pain patients: an EEG mapping study. *J Clin Neurophysiol*, **24**(1), 76–83.

Edwards, R. R., Kronfli, T., Haythornthwaite, J. A., Smith, M. T., McGuire, L., & Page, G. G. (2008). Association of catastrophizing with interleukin-6 responses to acute pain. *Pain*, **140**(1), 135–44.

Faravelli, C., Amedei, S. G., Rotella, F., *et al.* (2010). Childhood traumata, Dexamethasone Suppression Test and psychiatric symptoms: a trans-diagnostic approach. *Psychol Med*, **40**, 1–12.

ffrench-Mullen, J. M. (1995). Cortisol inhibition of calcium currents in guinea pig hippocampal CA1 neurons via G-protein-coupled activation of protein kinase C. *J Neurosci*, **15**(1 Pt 2), 903–11.

Forseth, K. O., Husby, G., Gran, J. T., & Forre, O. (1999). Prognostic factors for the development of fibromyalgia in women with self-reported musculoskeletal pain. A prospective study. *Journal of Rheumatology*, **26**(11), 2458–67.

France, R. D. & Krishnan, K. R. (1985). The dexamethasone suppression test as a biologic marker of depression in chronic pain. *Pain*, **21**(1), 49–55.

France, R. D., Krishnan, K. R., Trainor, M., & Pelton, S. (1987). Chronic pain and depression. IV. DST as a discriminator between chronic pain and depression. *Pain*, **28**(1), 39–44.

Freeman, E. W., Sammel, M. D., Lin, H., *et al.* (2007). Symptoms associated with menopausal transition and reproductive hormones in midlife women. *Obstet Gynecol*, **110**(2 Pt 1), 230–40.

Fries, E., Hesse, J., Hellhammer, J., & Hellhammer, D. H. (2005). A new view on hypocortisolism. *Psychoneuroendocrinology*, **30**(10), 1010–16.

Garofalo, J. P., Robinson, R. C., & Gatchel, R. J. (2006). Hypothalamic-pituitary-adrenocortical axis dysregulation in acute temporomandibular disorder and low back pain: A marker for chronicity? *J Applied Biobehav Res*, **11**(3–4), 166–78.

Garofalo, J. P., Robinson, R. C., Gatchel, R. J., & Wang, Z. (2007). A pain severity-hypothalamic-pituitary-adrenocortical axis interaction: The effects on pain pathways. *Applied Biobehav Res,*, **12**(1), 35–42.

Gatchel, R. J., Polatin, P. B., & Kinney, R. K. (1995). Predicting outcome of chronic back pain using clinical predictors of psychopathology: A prospective analysis. *Health Psychol*, **14**, 415–20.

Geiss, A., Rohleder, N., Kirschbaum, C., Steinbach, K., Bauer, H. W., & Anton, F. (2005). Predicting the failure of disc surgery by a hypofunctional HPA axis: evidence from a prospective study on patients undergoing disc surgery. *Pain*, **114**(1–2), 104–17.

Gershberg, H. (1960). Metabolic and renotropic effects of human growth hormone in disease. *J Clin Endocrinol Metab*, **20**, 1107–19.

Glass, J. M., Lyden, A. K., Petzke, F., *et al.* (2004). The effect of brief exercise cessation on pain, fatigue, and mood symptom development in healthy, fit individuals. *Journal of Psychosomatic Research*, **57**(4), 391–8.

Griep, E. N., Boersma, J. W., & de Kloet, E. R. (1993). Altered reactivity of the hypothalamic-pituitary-adrenal axis in the primary fibromyalgia syndrome. *Journal of Rheumatology*, **20**(3), 469–74.

Griep, E. N., Boersma, J. W., Lentjes, E. G., Prins, A. P., Van der Korst, J. K., & de Kloet, E. R. (1998a). Function of the hypothalamic-pituitary-adrenal axis in patients with fibromyalgia and low back pain. *Journal of Rheumatology*, **25**(7), 1374–81.

Griep, E. N., Boersma, J. W., Lentjes, E. G. W. M., Prins, A. P. A., Van der Korst, J. K., & de Kloet, E. R. (1998b). Function of the hypothalamic-pituitary-Adrenal Axis in patients with fibromyalgia and low back pain. *J Rheumatol*, **25**, 1374–81.

Gur, A. & Oktayoglu, P. (2008). Status of immune mediators in fibromyalgia. *Curr Pain Headache Rep*, **12**(3), 175–81.

Haffner, S. M. (2000). Sex hormones, obesity, fat distribution, type 2 diabetes and insulin resistance: epidemiological and clinical correlation. *Int J Obes Relat Metab Disord*, **24**(Suppl 2), S56–58.

Harbuz, M. (2002a). Neuroendocrine function and chronic inflammatory stress. *Exp Physiol*, **87**(5), 519–25.

Harbuz, M. (2002b). Neuroendocrinology of autoimmunity. *Int Rev Neurobiol*, **52**, 133–61.

Harreby, M., Kjer, J., Hesselsoe, G., & Neergaard, K. (1996). Epidemiological aspects and risk factors for low back pain in 38-year- old men and women: a 25-year prospective cohort study of 640 school children. *European Spine Journal*, **5**(5), 312–18.

Hasenbring, M., Marienfeld, G., Kuhlendahl, D., & Soyka, D. (1994). Risk factors of chronicity in lumbar disc patients. A prospective investigation of biologic, psychologic, and social predictors of therapy outcome. *Spine*, **19**(24), 2759–65.

Hasselhorn, H. M., Theorell, T., & Vingard, E. (2001). Endocrine and immunologic parameters indicative of 6-month prognosis after the onset of low back pain or neck/shoulder pain. *Spine*, **26**(3, E24–29.

Henckens, M. J., Hermans, E. J., Pu, Z., Joels, M., & Fernandez, G. (2009). Stressed memories: how acute stress affects memory formation in humans. *J Neurosci*, **29**(32), 10111–19.

Hurwitz, E. L. & Morgenstern, H. (1999). Cross-sectional associations of asthma, hay fever, and other allergies with major depression and low-back pain among adults aged 20–39 years in the United States. *American Journal of Epidemiology*, **150**(10), 1107–16.

Hyyppa, M. T., Alaranta, H., Hurme, M., & Lahtela, K. (1985). Prolactin and cortisol responses to the experience of low back pain. *Pain*, **23**(3), 231–42.

IASP (2002). *Epidemiology of Pain a report of the task force on epidemiology of the International Association of Pain.* Seattle, WA: IASP Press.

Johansson, A. C., Gunnarsson, L. G., Linton, S. J., Bergkvist, L., Stridsbergf, M., Nilsson, O., & Cornefjord, M. (2008). Pain, disability and coping reflected in the diurnal cortisol variability in patients scheduled for lumbar disc surgery. *European Journal of Pain*, **12**(5), 633–40.

Jones, K. D., Deodhar, P., Lorentzen, A., Bennett, R. M., & Deodhar, A. A. (2007). Growth hormone perturbations in fibromyalgia: a review. *Seminars in Arthritis and Rheumatism*, **36**(6), 357–79.

Kajantie, E. & Phillips, D. I. (2006). The effects of sex and hormonal status on the physiological response to acute psychosocial stress. *Psychoneuroendocrinology*, **31**(2), 151–78.

Kemp, S. F. (2009). Insulin-like growth factor-I deficiency in children with growth hormone insensitivity: current and future treatment options. *BioDrugs*, **23**(3), 155–63.

Kriegsfeld, L. J., Mei, D. F., Bentley, G. E., *et al.* (2006). Identification and characterization of a gonadotropin-inhibitory system in the brains of mammals. *Proc Natl Acad Sci U S A*, **103**(7), 2410–15.

Kudielka, B. M., Schommer, N. C., Hellhammer, D. H., & Kirschbaum, C. (2004). Acute HPA axis responses, heart rate, and mood changes to psychosocial stress (TSST) in humans at different times of day. *Psychoneuroendocrinology*, **29**(8), 983–92.

Kumsta, R., Entringer, S., Koper, J. W., van Rossum, E. F., Hellhammer, D. H., & Wust, S. (2010). Working memory performance is associated with common glucocorticoid receptor gene polymorphisms. *Neuropsychobiology*, **61**(1), 49–56.

Lado-Abeal, J. & Norman, R. L. (2002). Leptin and reproductive function in males. *Semin Reprod Med*, **20**(2), 145–51.

Lentjes, E. G. W. M., Griep, E. N., Boersma, J. W., Romijn, F. P. T. H., & de Kloet, E. R. (1997). Glucocorticoid receptors, fibromyalgia and low back pain. *Psychoneuroendocrinology*, **22**(8), 603–14.

LeResche, L., Mancl, L., Sherman, J. J., Gandara, B., & Dworkin, S. F. (2003). Changes in temporomandibular pain and other symptoms across the menstrual cycle. *Pain*, **106**(3), 253–61.

Lightman, S. L., Windle, R. J., Julian, M. D., *et al.* (2000). Significance of pulsatility in the HPA axis. *Novartis Found Symp*, **227**, 244–57.

Maclean, D. B. & Jackson, I. M. (1988). Molecular biology and regulation of the hypothalamic hormones. *Baillieres Clin Endocrinol Metab*, **2**(4), 835–68.

Maier, S. F. & Watkins, L. R. (1998). Cytokines for psychologists: implications of bidirectional immune-to-brain communication for understanding behavior, mood, and cognition. *Psychol Rev*, **105**(1), 83–107.

Margetic, S., Gazzola, C., Pegg, G. G., & Hill, R. A. (2002). Leptin: a review of its peripheral actions and interactions. *Int J Obes Relat Metab Disord*, **26**(11), 1407–33.

Mastorakos, G., Pavlatou, M. G., & Mizamtsidi, M. (2006). The hypothalamic-pituitary-adrenal and the hypothalamic- pituitary-gonadal axes interplay. *Pediatr Endocrinol Rev*, **3**(Suppl 1), 172–81.

McBeth, J., Silman, A. J., Gupta, A., *et al.* (2007). Moderation of psychosocial risk factors through dysfunction of the hypothalamic-pituitary-adrenal stress axis in the onset of chronic widespread musculoskeletal pain - Findings of a population-based prospective cohort study. *Arthritis Rheum*, **56**(1), 360–71.

McBeth, J., Symmons, D. P., Silman, A. J., *et al.* (2009). Musculoskeletal pain is associated with a long-term increased risk of cancer and cardiovascular-related mortality. *Rheumatology*, **48**(1), 74–77.

McEwen, B. S. (2003). Mood disorders and allostatic load. *Biological Psychiatry*, **54**(3), 200–207.

Meczekalski, B., Podfigurna-Stopa, A., Warenik-Szymankiewicz, A., & Genazzani, A. R. (2008). Functional hypothalamic amenorrhea: current view on neuroendocrine aberrations. *Gynecol Endocrinol*, **24**(1), 4–11.

Meeus, M., Nijs, J., Van de, W. N., Toeback, L., & Truijen, S. (2008). Diffuse noxious inhibitory control is delayed in chronic fatigue syndrome: an experimental study. *Pain*, **139**(2), 439–48.

Million, R., Hall, W., Haavik Dilsen, K., Baker, R., & Jayson, M. I. V. (1982). 1981 Volvo Award in Clinical Science - Assessment of the progress of the Back-pain patient. *Spine*, **7**, 204–12.

Mitchell, M., Armstrong, D. T., Robker, R. L., & Norman, R. J. (2005). Adipokines: implications for female fertility and obesity. *Reproduction*, **130**(5), 583–97.

Morelli, V., Masserini, B., Salcuni, A. S., *et al.* (2010). Subclinical hypercortisolism: correlation between biochemical diagnostic criteria and clinical aspects. *Clin Endocrinol (Oxf)*.

Mukherjee, A., Murray, R. D., & Shalet, S. M. (2004). Impact of growth hormone status on body composition and the skeleton. *Horm Res*, **62**(Suppl 3), 35–41.

Muller, M., Holsboer, F., & Keck, M. E. (2002). Genetic modification of corticosteroid receptor signalling: novel insights into pathophysiology and treatment strategies of human affective disorders. *Neuropeptides*, **36**(2–3), 117–31.

Murakami, M., Matsuzaki, T., Iwasa, T., Yasui, T., Irahara, M., Osugi, T., & Tsutsui, K. (2008). Hypophysiotropic role of RFamide-related peptide-3 in the inhibition of LH secretion in female rats. *J Endocrinol*, **199**(1), 105–12.

Mussig, K., Remer, T., & Maser-Gluth, C. (2010). Brief review: Glucocorticoid excretion in obesity. *J Steroid Biochem Mol Biol*, **121**(3–5), 589–93.

Neeck, G. & Crofford, L. J. (2000). Neuroendocrine perturbations in fibromyalgia and chronic fatigue syndrome. *Rheum Dis Clinics North Am*, **26**(4), 989–1002.

Nevitt, M. C., Ettinger, B., Black, D. M., *et al.* (1998). The association of radiographically detected vertebral fractures with back pain and function: A prospective study. *Annals of Internal Medicine*, **128**, 793–800.

O'Donoghue, G. M., Fox, N., Heneghan, C., & Hurley, D. A. (2009). Objective and subjective assessment of sleep in chronic low back pain patients compared with healthy age and gender matched controls: a pilot study. *BMC Musculoskelet Disord*, **10**, 122.

O'Neill, T. W., Cockerill, W., Matthis, C., *et al.* (2004). Back pain, disability, and radiographic vertebral fracture in European women: a prospective study. *Osteoporosis International*, **15**(9), 760–5.

Olff, M., Brosschot, J. F., Godaert, G., *et al.* (1995). Modulatory effects of defense and coping on stress-induced changes in endocrine and immune parameters. *Int J Behav Med*, **2**(2), 85–103.

Olney, R. C. (2009). Mechanisms of impaired growth: effect of steroids on bone and cartilage. *Horm Res*, **72**(S1), 30–5.

Osugi, T., Ukena, K., Bentley, G. E., *et al.* (2004). Gonadotropin-inhibitory hormone in Gambel's white-crowned sparrow (Zonotrichia leucophrys gambelii): cDNA identification, transcript localization and functional effects in laboratory and field experiments. *J Endocrinol*, **182**(1), 33–42.

Papadimitriou, A. & Priftis, K. N. (2009). Regulation of the hypothalamic-pituitary-adrenal axis. *Neuroimmunomodulation*, **16**(5), 265–71.

Patel, P. D., Katz, M., Karssen, A. M., & Lyons, D. M. (2008). Stress-induced changes in corticosteroid receptor expression in primate hippocampus and prefrontal cortex. *Psychoneuroendocrinology*, **33**(3), 360–7.

Pham, K., Nacher, J., Hof, P. R., & McEwen, B. S. (2003). Repeated restraint stress suppresses neurogenesis and induces biphasic PSA-NCAM expression in the adult rat dentate gyrus. *Eur J Neurosci*, **17**(4), 879–86.

Pruessner, J. C., Kirschbaum, C., Meinlschmid, G., & Hellhammer, D. H. (2003). Two formulas for computation of the area under the curve represent measures of total hormone concentration versus time-dependent change. *Psychoneuroendocrinology*, **28**(7), 916–31.

Quartana, P. J., Buenaver, L. F., Edwards, R. R., Klick, B., Haythornthwaite, J. A., & Smith, M. T. (2010). Pain catastrophizing and salivary cortisol responses to laboratory pain testing in temporomandibular disorder and healthy participants. *J Pain*, **11**(2), 186–94.

Rabin, D. S., Johnson, E. O., Brandon, D. D., Liapi, C., & Chrousos, G. P. (1990). Glucocorticoids inhibit estradiol-mediated uterine growth: possible role of the uterine estradiol receptor. *Biol Reprod*, **42**(1), 74–80.

Reul, J. M., Bilang-Bleuel, A., Droste, S., Linthorst, A. C., Holsboer, F., & Gesing, A. (2000). New mode of hypothalamic-pituitary-adrenocortical axis regulation: significance for stress-related disorders. *Zeitschrift fur Rheumatologie*, **59**(Suppl 2), II/22–II/25.

Rigamonti, A. E., Bonomo, S. M., Cella, S. G., & Muller, E. E. (2002). GH and cortisol rebound rise during and following a somatostatin infusion: studies in dogs with the use of a GH-releasing peptide. *J Endocrinol*, **174**(3), 387–94.

Rivier, J., Jiang, G. C., Lahrichi, S. L., *et al.* (1996). Dose relationship between GnRH antagonists and pituitary suppression. *Hum Reprod*, **11**(Suppl 3), 133–47.

Schell, E., Theorell, T., Hasson, D., Arnetz, B., & Saraste, H. (2008). Stress biomarkers' associations to pain in the neck, shoulder and back in healthy media workers: 12-month prospective follow-up. *Eur Spine J*, **17**(3), 393–405.

Seminowicz, D. A. & Davis, K. D. (2006). Cortical responses to pain in healthy individuals depends on pain catastrophizing. *Pain*, **120**(3), 297–306.

Smets, E. M. A., Garssen, B., Bonke, B., & de Haes, J. C. (1995). The Multidimensional Fatigue Inventory (MFI) psychometric qualities of an instrument to assess fatigue. *J Psychosom Res*, **39**(3), 315–25.

Spitzer, R. L. & Williams, J. B. (1988). Revised diagnostic criteria and a new structured interview for diagnosing anxiety disorders. *J Psychiatric Res*, **22**(Suppl 1), 55–85.

Staud, R. (2009). Chronic widespread pain and fibromyalgia: two sides of the same coin?. *Curr Rheumatol Rep*, **11**(6), 433–36.

Steckler, T., Holsboer, F., & Reul, J. M. (1999). Glucocorticoids and depression. *Baillieres Best Pract Res Clin Endocrinol Metab*, **13**(4), 597–614.

Stein-Behrens, B. A. & Sapolsky, R. M. (1992). Stress, glucocorticoids, and aging. *Aging*, **4**(3), 197–210.

Sudhaus, S., Fricke, B., Stachon, A., Schneider, S., Klein, H., von During, M., & Hasenbring, M. (2009). Salivary cortisol and psychological mechanisms in patients with acute versus chronic low back pain. *Psychoneuroendocrinology*, **34**(4), 513–22.

Tchernof, A., Poehlman, E. T., & Despres, J. P. (2000). Body fat distribution, the menopause transition, and hormone replacement therapy. *Diabetes Metab*, **26**(1), 12–20.

Teepker, M., Peters, M., Vedder, H., Schepelmann, K., & Lautenbacher, S. (2010). Menstrual Variation in Experimental Pain: Correlation with Gonadal Hormones. *Neuropsychobiology*, **61**(3), 131–40.

Theorell, T., Hasselhorn, H. M., Vingard, E., Andersson, B., & MUSIC-Norrtalje Study Group (2000). Interleukin 6 and cortisol in acute musculoskeletal disorders: Results from a case-referent study in Sweden. *Stress Medicine*, **16**(1), 27–35.

Tsigos, C., Papanicolaou, D. A., Kyrou, I., Raptis, S. A., & Chrousos, G. P. (1999). Dose-dependent effects of recombinant human interleukin-6 on the pituitary-testicular axis. *J Interferon Cytokine Res*, **19**(11), 1271–76.

Tsutsumi, R. & Webster, N. J. (2009). GnRH pulsatility, the pituitary response and reproductive dysfunction. *Endocr J*, **56**(6), 729–37.

Uchiyama, M., Ishibashi, K., Enomoto, T., *et al.* (1998). Twenty-four hour profiles of four hormones under constant routine. *Psychiatry Clin Neurosci*, **52**(2), 241–43.

Unniappan, S. (2010). Ghrelin: An emerging player in the regulation of reproduction in non-mammalian vertebrates. *Gen Comp Endocrinol*, **167**(3), 340–3.

Ursin, H. & Olff, M. (1993). Psychobiology of coping and defence strategies. *Neuropsychobiology*, **28**(1–2), 66–71.

Vadakkadath, M. S. & Atwood, C. S. (2005). The role of hypothalamic-pituitary-gonadal hormones in the normal structure and functioning of the brain. *Cell Mol Life Sci*, **62**(3), 257–70.

Vamvakopoulos, N. C. & Chrousos, G. P. (1993). Evidence of direct estrogenic regulation of human corticotropin-releasing hormone gene expression. Potential implications for the sexual dimophism of the stress response and immune/inflammatory reaction. *J Clin Invest*, **92**(4), 1896–1902.

Van Praag, H. M. (2004). The cognitive paradox in posttraumatic stress disorder: a hypothesis. *Prog Neuropsychopharmacol Biol Psychiatry*, **28**(6), 923–35.

Van Vollenhoven, R. F. & McGuire, J. L. (1994). Estrogen, progesterone, and testosterone: can they be used to treat autoimmune diseases? *Cleve Clin J Med*, **61**(4), 276–84.

Vicennati, V., Pasqui, F., Cavazza, C., Pagotto, U., & Pasquali, R. (2009). Stress-related development of obesity and cortisol in women. *Obesity*, **17**(9), 1678–83.

Wang, H., Schiltenwolf, M., & Buchner, M. (2008). The role of TNF-alpha in patients with chronic low back pain-a prospective comparative longitudinal study. *Clin J Pain*, **24**(3), 273–8.

Wijnhoven, H. A., de Vet, H. C., Smit, H. A., & Picavet, H. S. (2006). Hormonal and reproductive factors are associated with chronic low back pain and chronic upper extremity pain in women—the MORGEN study. *Spine*, **31**(13), 1496–502.

Wolfe, F. (1990). Fibromyalgia. *Rheum Dis Clinics North Am*, **16**, 681–98.

Wolfe, F., Smythe, H. A., Yunus, M. B., *et al.* (1990). The American College of Rheumatology 1990 Criteria for the Classification of Fibromyalgia. Report of the Multicenter Criteria Committee. *Arthritis and Rheumatism*, **33**(2), 160–72.

Wrosch, C., Miller, G. E., Lupien, S., & Pruessner, J. C. (2008). Diurnal cortisol secretion and 2-year changes in older adults' physical symptoms: the moderating roles of negative affect and sleep. *Health Psychology*, **27**(6), 685–93.

Yakar, S., Liu, J. L., Fernandez, A. M., *et al.* (2001). Liver-specific igf-1 gene deletion leads to muscle insulin insensitivity. *Diabetes*, **50**(5), 1110–18.

Yamaguchi, T., Kanatani, M., Yamauchi, M., *et al.* (2006). Serum levels of insulin-like growth factor (IGF); IGF-binding proteins-3, -4, and -5; and their relationships to bone mineral density and the risk of vertebral fractures in postmenopausal women. *Calcified Tissue International*, **78**(1), 18–24.

Yin, H., Ukena, K., Ubuka, T., & Tsutsui, K. (2005). A novel G protein-coupled receptor for gonadotropin-inhibitory hormone in the Japanese quail (Coturnix japonica): identification, expression and binding activity. *J Endocrinol*, **184**(1), 257–66.

Young, E. A. (1995). Normal glucocorticoid fast feedback following chronic 50% corticosterone pellet treatment. *Psychoneuroendocrinology*, **20**(7), 771–84.

Young, E. A. & Vazquez, D. (1996). Hypercortisolemia, hippocampal glucocorticoid receptors, and fast feedback. *Mol Psychiatry*, **1**(2), 149–59.

Yudkin, J. S. (2007). Inflammation, obesity, and the metabolic syndrome. *Horm Metab Res*, **39**(10), 707–9.

Chapter 6

# Central Imaging of Pain and the Process of Chronicity

Sandra Kamping and Herta Flor

## 6.1 Introduction

Neuroimaging methods were introduced to clinical and experimental pain research only a few decades ago but have had a major impact. In this chapter we will focus on neuroimaging in humans and give a short overview of brain areas involved in the perception and evaluation of pain. We will then discuss functional and structural changes found in patients with chronic back pain (CBP) and will specifically emphasize the role of emotional learning and memory as well as cognitive factors in the chronicity process. This chapter will consider methods ranging from electroencephalography (EEG) and magnetoencephalography (MEG) to functional and structural magnetic resonance imaging (MRI), including magnetic resonance spectroscopy and positron emission tomography (PET). We do not aim to provide an exhaustive review but will highlight key findings and discuss the impact they had on our understanding of CBP and factors that lead to chronicity.

## 6.2 The pain matrix: a short introduction

Brain regions involved in the processing of acute pain have been identified by applying nociceptive stimuli (e.g. heat, electric stimulation, pressure) mostly to the skin of a person. Several key brain regions have been identified, among them the primary (SI) and secondary (SII) somatosensory cortex, the insula, the anterior cingulate cortex (ACC), the prefrontal cortex (PFC), as well as the thalamus (for reviews see Apkarian et al. 2005; Tracey & Mantyh 2007; see also Figure 6.1). Depending on the task of the study or the particular the set of circumstances for the individual, other brain regions such as temporal and parietal areas, the basal ganglia, the cerebellum, the amygdala, and hippocampus are also active.

Traditionally pain has been separated into three components: (1) sensory-discriminative, (2) motivational-affective, and (3) cognitive-evaluative (Melzack & Casey 1968). Activation in SI has been associated with the sensory-discriminative aspect of pain (Bushnell et al. 1999), and most imaging studies showed a robust activation of SI, depending on the type of stimulation and the imaging procedure (e.g. EEG or functional magnetic resonance imaging (fMRI)) that was used. Unfortunately, there are almost as many studies that show activation in SI as there are studies that show no activation (Bingel et al. 2003; Bornhovd et al. 2002; Coghill et al. 1999; Maihofner et al. 2002). It has been suggested that the crucial variable for activation in SI is the amount of spatial and temporal summation (Peyron, Laurent, & Garcia-Larrea 2000).

The secondary somatosensory cortex (SII) plays a role in the sensory analysis of pain, seems to encode the 'painfulness' of the stimulation (e.g. Ringler et al. 2003), is involved in the temporal encoding of the pain experience (Chen et al. 2002) and also contributes to tactile and pain-related

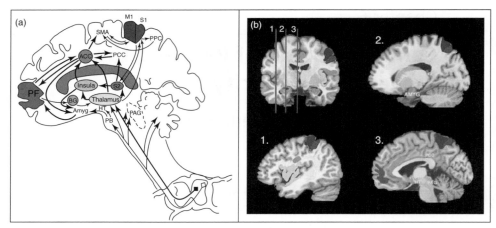

**Fig. 6.1** (Also see Colour Plate 3) Cortical and subcortical regions involved in pain perception. The locations of the regions are superimposed onto an example MRI. The areas primarily involved in pain perception are the primary somatosensory cortex (S1, red), the secondary somatosensory cortex (S2, orange), the anterior cingulate cortex (ACC, green), the insula (light blue), the thalamus (yellow), as well as the basal ganglia (BG, pink), the prefrontal cortex (PF; purple) and the primary motor cortex (M1, blue). Other regions are the supplementary motor area (SMA), the posterior cingulate cortex (PCC), the amygdale (AMYG), the parabrachial nuclei (PB) and the periaqueductal grey (PAG). Reprinted from *Progress in Neurobiology*, **87**(2), A. V. Apkarian, M. N. Baliki, and P. Y. Geha, Towards a theory of chronic pain, pp. 81–97, Copyright (2009), with permission from Elsevier.

memory (Gallace & Spence 2009; Harris, Harris, & Diamond 2001). It seems to be activated via a direct pathway from the thalamus (Ploner, Freund, & Schnitzler 1999) and receives projections via SI. Activation in this region is more frequently and robustly observed than in SI (Ferretti et al. 2003, Peyron, Laurent, & Garcia-Larrea 2000; Treede et al. 2000).

One area that has been consistently activated in imaging studies of pain is the insula. It seems to have an important role in nociceptive processing and can be divided into a posterior and an anterior part. The posterior insula is activated, predominantly contralateral, in response to nociceptive stimuli (Bingel et al. 2003; Brooks et al. 2002) and also encodes temperature (Craig et al. 2000). Activation of the anterior insula is also not specific to pain. It has been described in response to tactile (Baron et al. 1999; Iadarola et al. 1998), vibratory (Coghill et al. 1994), and olfacto-gustatory (Faurion et al. 1999; Small et al. 2004) stimulation. Numerous studies show the involvement of the insula in processes such as memory functions, emotional responses, visceral sensory and motor integration, and self-awareness as well as the processing of painful stimuli. It has also been discussed as the site of the brain that contains the anatomical substrate for self-awareness (Craig 2002, 2009).

The ACC encodes, among others, the affective component of pain (Craig et al. 1996; Rainville et al. 1997). The ACC has been thoroughly investigated and a midcingulate caudal 'cognitive' part and a ventral perigenual cingulate 'emotional' part have been identified. The midcingulate region is activated in all pain studies and most likely related to attentional factors (Davis et al. 1997; Kwan et al. 2000). Activation of the rostral part of the ACC (rACC) seems to be associated with anticipation of pain (Ploghaus et al. 1999). Activations of the perigenual ACC (pACC) and the ventral pACC have been related to pain intensity (Büchel et al. 2002). The rACC seems to play an important role in placebo analgesia. Activity of the rACC during placebo analgesia covaries with subcortical activity in the periaqueductal grey (PAG) and the amygdala and seems to be the cognitive link of the endogenous pain control system (Bingel et al. 2006; Bingel, Schoell, & Buchel 2007). Activations of the anterior ACC are more unspecific and are most likely related to working memory and attentional processes. From the activation of the ACC during various task and stimulations it seems likely that the ACC is a multi-integrative structure: single ACC regions may be involved in several functional networks, and their processing capacities with respect to a given function are probably modulated by other concomitant processes (Apkarian et al. 2005; Lorenz & Casey 2005).

## 6.3 **Brain processes in chronic back pain**

Using painful electric stimulation of the skin at the back or at the finger of CBP patients during a MEG recording, Flor et al. (1997) showed significant brain activation differences between CBP patients and healthy controls. Stimulation at the affected back but not at the finger led to a significantly higher magnetic field in the early time window (<100 ms) for CBP compared to controls. The signal strength in this time window and the duration of pain were positively correlated, suggesting increased cortical responsivity with increasing chronicity. The source of this early activity originated from SI and the localization of the fingers did not differ between patients and controls. However, the localization of the back was more inferior and medial in the patients. This indicates a shift and expansion toward the cortical representation of the leg (see Figure 6.2) suggesting that chronic pain leads to an expansion of the cortical representation zone related to nociceptive input, and that the amount of cortical reorganization increases with pain duration. This is similar to the expansions of cortical representations that have been documented to occur with other types of behaviourally relevant stimulation, but different from the changes that occur with deafferentation where the changes correlate with pain intensity rather than chronicity.

Flor et al (2004) used painful and non-painful electric stimulation to the finger in CBP patients, patients with headache and controls. Only the CBP patients displayed significantly lower pain thresholds and tolerance as well as a reduced habituation, i.e. sensitization. Although the stimulation intensity for the three groups was different (i.e. lower in the CBP group), the CBP patients showed equally high levels of evoked brain responses as assessed by multichannel EEG recordings suggesting also central sensitization. A later study by Diers et al. (2007) expanded these results to intramuscular recordings and observed both higher pain ratings (perceptual sensitization) over the course of the stimulation in the CBP patients and also enhanced central nervous system processing as evidenced by an enhanced N80 component (see Figure 6.3).

Enhanced perceptual sensitization to tonic rather than phasic stimulation was found in CBP patients by Kleinböhl et al. (1999). They used extended heat pain and a behavioral response as indicator of sensitization.

Giesecke et al. (2004) compared chronic low back pain patients, patients with fibromyalgia and healthy controls. During the fMRI measurements they administered two kinds of painful stimulation to the thumbnails of the participants: (1) stimuli of equal pressure and (2) equal subjective pain intensity. The pressure required to produce moderate pain was significantly higher for both patient groups than for the control participants, indicating hyperalgesia. Equal amounts of pressure applied to the thumb revealed activation in five common brain regions for the two patients groups: contralateral SI, bilateral SII, the inferior parietal lobule and the cerebellum. In healthy controls this stimulation resulted only in activation of the contralateral SII. These results can be interpreted as an increased central pain processing in CBP even when the painful stimulus is at a site distant to the region involved in clinical pain. When subjects received a stimulus that resulted

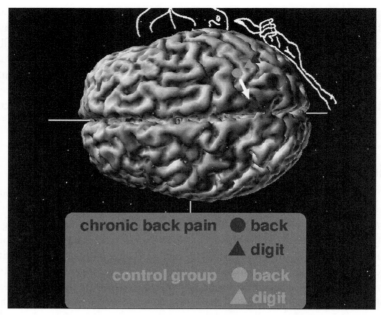

**Fig. 6.2** (Also see Colour Plate 4) Localization of the representation of the digits and the back in primary somatosensory cortex in back pain patients and healthy controls. Stimulation was on the left side of the body, the representations are on the hemisphere contralateral to the stimulation side. Please note the shift of the back representation of the back pain patients into a more medial position (i.e. towards the leg representation). The shift amounted to about 2–3 cm. Reprinted from *Neuroscience Letters*, **224**(1), H. Flor, C. Braun, T. Elbert, and N. Birbaumer, Extensive reorganization of primary somatosensory cortex in chronic back pain patients, pp. 5–8, Copyright (1997), with permission from Elsevier.

in the same amount of pain, all three groups showed activation in the central components of the pain matrix (SI, SII, insula, ACC, inferior parietal lobe), with the magnitude of activation being greater for the two patient groups.

Baliki et al. (2006) examined variations in habitual pain rather than applying acute pain stimuli in patients with CBP. During the fMRI measurements patients were asked to continuously rate their habitual pain level on a scale from 0–10. An increase of spontaneous pain in CBP patients activated regions also seen in acute pain (i.e. the anterior and posterior insula, SII, the mid-cingulate cortex, SI and the cerebellum). However, sustained high pain additionally engaged brain areas involved in emotion, cognition, and motivation such as the medial prefrontal cortex, rostral anterior cingulate cortex, posterior thalami, ventral striatum, and extended amygdala. Insular activity was also present and correlated with pain duration leading the authors to conclude that it may reflect the chronicity of CBP. In contrast, activation of the medial prefrontal cortex correlated with pain intensity ratings.

In a later study Baliki et al. (2008) investigated two groups of chronic pain patients: a group with CBP and a group with osteoarthritis (OA) of the knee. Both groups were placed in the fMRI scanner and rated the intensity of their pain with a finger-span logging device. The CBP patients rated their current pain and its fluctuations and the OA patients rated their pain in response to pressure applied to their knee. During the pain rating task CBP patients reported fluctuations of their spontaneous pain intensity in the absence of any overt experimental stimulus. Activation related

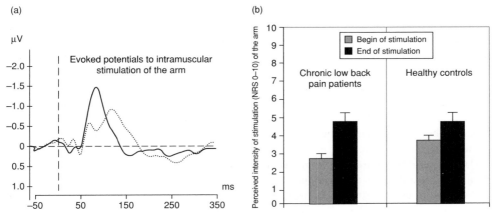

**Fig. 6.3** Central processing and behavioral correlates of acute muscle pain in chronic low back pain patients. Part (a) of the figure shows the pain-related somatosensory evoked potential wave forms for intramuscular stimulation of the left lower arm. The solid line represents the activation in the CBP patients and the dotted line the healthy controls. The analysis revealed significantly higher amplitude of the N80 for the pain patients. Part (b) of the figure displays the differences in perceived intensity of the stimulation of the left lower arm at the beginning and at the end of the stimulation period. Both groups sensitized during the course of the experiment, with the CBP displaying higher sensitization than the healthy controls. Means and standard errors are displayed. Reprinted from *Journal of Clinical Neurophysiology*, **24**(1), M. Diers, C. Koeppe, E. Diesch, *et al*. Central processing of acute muscle pain in chronic low back pain patients: An EEG mapping study. Copyright (2007), with permission from Wolters Kluwer Health.

to these spontaneous fluctuations seemed to be mainly related to emotion/reward mediating areas (i.e. the medial prefrontal cortex and the nucleus accumbens). Activations due to pressure pain in the OA group were found in SII, the insula, the supplementary motor area, the ACC, the medial frontal gyrus, the thalamus, the right putamen and the left amygdala. This activation pattern was similar to that found in healthy participants in response to acute pain (i.e. activation of the pain matrix). In a pre-post design the authors also investigated the activation of brain regions before and after a 2-week treatment with a lidocaine patch applied to the painful body part. On a behavioral level, CBP patients experienced a robust decrease in pain intensity in response to the two week treatment. Before treatment, CBP patients showed increased brain activity mainly in the frontal cortex (including the medial prefrontal cortex, the rostral anterior cingulate cortex, bilateral superior frontal gyrus, and the nucleus accumbens). Increased brain activity was also found in the inferior temporal gyrus, and the left posterior parietal cortex. After treatment the authors reported only one significant cluster of activation that showed increased activity for spontaneous pain, the left motor area (MT). The medial prefrontal cortex was the brain area the correlated best with the treatment effect. The authors conclude that the spontaneous pain occurring in CBP is primarily of an emotional nature and assume that lidocaine treatment decreases mainly emotional pain aspects.

Using PET and noxious heat stimulation Derbyshire et al. (2002) examined 16 CBP patients and 16 matched controls. They were interested in the correlation of pain scores and brain activation patterns. Significant bilateral activation was present in the cerebellum, the midbrain (including the PAG region), the thalamus, the lentiform nucleus, the insula and the midcingulate cortex for both healthy controls and CBP patients. They reported no significant differences between the two groups and concluded that there is no abnormal nociceptive processing in patients with low back pain. Although the authors reported a significant difference in anxiety between the patients and the controls, with the patients being more anxious than the controls, they did not include this difference in their analysis. They also reported a trend towards a difference in depression scores between the two groups, again with the patients being more depressed than the controls and discuss the possible implications of depression on their results.

Thunberg et al. (2005) also used PET in healthy volunteers and injected hypertonic saline into the right m. erector spinae at the level of L3 in an attempt to mimic the pain of low back pain patients. The authors distinguished between two phases: an early acute phase (4min after the start of the infusion), and a late tonic phase (21min after the start of the infusion). They assumed that the latter should be a more realistic model of the chronic muscle pain found in patients. The cerebral response differed in the acute and tonic phase and longer lasting tonic muscle pain resulted in decreases in three clusters (left insula, right insula and right cingulate cortex). Increases in rCBF were only found bilaterally in the occipital cortex. The authors interpret the decrease in subjective levels between the early phase and the late phase as a habituation effect and thus also attribute the changes in brain activity to this habituation. When the late phase was compared with a baseline condition, regions that are implicated in the processing of all three components of pain (sensory-discriminative, motivational-affective, and cognitive-evaluative) were active. These included an increase of activation in the contralateral medial PFC as well as a decrease of activation in the insula, the ACC and the dorsolateral prefrontal cortex of the ipsilateral hemisphere. The authors conclude that this dysfunction of the network may contribute to the development of chronic pain.

Almost all studies on brain imaging revealed that certain brain regions show a deactivation during task performance. This fact has led to the proposal of a 'default mode network' (DMN) of brain function (Raichle et al. 2001). Baliki et al. (2008) suggested that long-term pain alters the functional connectivity of the cortical regions of the DMN, which suggests that chronic pain has a widespread impact on overall brain function and not only on the pain matrix. They studied CBP patients and healthy controls during a simple visual attention task while the blood-oxygen-level-dependent (BOLD) response was measured. Task performance was similar in both groups, but the CBP patients showed a reduced deactivation in the medial prefrontal cortex, amygdalae and PCC. The disruption of the DMN was interpreted as cause of many of the cognitive and behavioral impairments that accompany chronic pain (i.e. depression, anxiety, sleep disturbances, or decision-making abnormalities).

## 6.4 Structural and biochemical changes in the brains of patients with CBP

So far we have only discussed functional changes in patients with CBP. Prolonged and sustained functional changes can, however, also lead to structural changes of the brain (see also Chapter 7). Apkarian et al. (2004) examined the grey matter volume of patients with CBP and healthy using voxel-based morphometry (VBM) as well as alternative methods of structural analyses. With VBM they found a 5.4% decrease in whole-brain neocortical grey matter volume in CBP patients compared to healthy controls. With multiple linear regression they showed that after correcting for age and sex, pain duration was a significant predictor for whole-brain grey matter volume in CBP. A separate analysis of the thalamus showed a significant decrease in grey matter density in the CBP group for the right anterior thalamus. Additionally, the dorsolateral prefrontal cortex was the main region showing local decreases in grey matter density in CBP patients compared to controls. The magnitude of decrease in grey matter volume (between 5–11%) is equivalent to the grey matter volume lost in 10–20 years of normal aging.

Schmidt-Wilcke et al. (2006) also used VBM and demonstrated a reduction of the grey matter of the primary somatosensory cortex and brainstem in individuals with CBP. These decreases were, in contrast, significantly correlated with the unpleasantness and intensity of pain. Increases in grey matter were observed bilaterally in the striatum and the left thalamus. Older adults with CBP showed structural brain changes in the middle corpus callosum, the grey matter of the posterior parietal cortex as well as impaired attention and mental flexibility (Buckalew et al. 2008).

Investigating a slightly different group Valet et al. (2009) studied patients with the DSM-IV diagnosis of pain disorder with VBM. The predominant clinical pain in these patients was either located in the head, neck and shoulder region; the lower back region; the pelvic region; or the lower limbs. Some persons reported more than one predominant pain region. The authors found significant grey matter decreases in structures involved in pain processing (i.e. insula, PPC, OFC, vmPFC), confirming studies of patients with fibromyalgia, chronic tension-type headache and CBP, that also showed these decreases (Schmidt-Wilcke et al. 2005, 2006, 2007).

Magnetic resonance spectroscopy (MRS) monitors biochemical changes in specific regions of the brain. Early studies on patients showed that chronic low back pain is associated with altered brain chemistry (Grachev, Fredrickson, & Apkarian 2000). The authors demonstrated a reduction of two molecules (N-acetyl aspartate (NAA) and glucose) in the dorsolateral prefrontal cortex specifically in CBP patients. A later study by the same authors, however, showed that there was a stronger association of reduced NAA with depression rather than with pain (Grachev et al. 2003). This nicely illustrates that MRS data have to be interpreted carefully since biochemical changes in the brain that may be due to other factors than pain such as depression or medication. Siddall et al. (2006) used a different method of spectral analysis in a study that compared individuals with chronic low back pain and persons without pain. They obtained MR spectra from several brain regions (the ACC, the thalamus and the prefrontal cortex) and analyzed and compared them using a pattern recognition method. With this method they were able to discriminate individuals with low back pain from controls with an accuracy of 97% using the spectrum from the PFC, 99% using the spectrum of the thalamus and 100% using the spectrum of the ACC based only on the regional chemical brain differences. Unfortunately without proper longitudinal studies, the causes and effects for the structural and biochemical changes in the brains of chronic pain patients cannot be untangled. It could be that the structural changes predate the onset of pain and might even be a vulnerability factor (see Chapter 7 for further information).

## 6.5 **The role of learning and memory**

Earlier we have discussed that the brain, and specifically the primary sensory cortex reorganizes in chronic pain (Flor et al. 1997). This reorganization and expansion can be viewed as an implicit learning and memory process where the experience of pain leaves a long-term alteration in the brain, which influences the subsequent processing of painful and non-painful somatosensory stimuli. This non-associative sensitization process may be complemented by operant and respondent conditioning and other associative learning processes and thus a variety of pain associated stimuli and responses may become part of a larger pain-related network that may be maladaptive in the process of chronicity (Apkarian, Baliki, & Geha 2009; Flor 2009; Flor & Diers 2007).

In a series of studies Pincus et al. (1993, 1995, 1996) reported that chronic pain patients not only selectively perceive pain-related words, they also make more pain-related associations to ambiguous words and are more likely to retrieve pain-associated words from memory. In an EEG study, Flor et al. (1997) examined whether CBP patients detect pain- and body-related words earlier, allocate more attention to them, and process them more deeply than neutral words. Additionally they examined peripheral responses (heart rate, muscle tension and skin conductance level). Although the CBP group did not recognize the pain- and body-related words any better or earlier than the healthy controls, they showed selectively enhanced N100 and N200 components in response to pain-related words. This increase in early reactivity was accompanied by enhanced skin conductance levels. Overall, the data confirm the assumption of altered implicit pain memories and selective attention to pain-related materials in chronic pain patients.

Similar results were found for pre-CBP patients by Knost et al. (1997). In contrast to the CBP patients, these individuals reported episodic upper back pain for less than 6 months. Again word recognition performance was not different between the two groups; but a significant enhancement of the N100 component for pain-related words was found in the prechronic pain group. These results suggest that a differential cortical processing of pain-related material may be a vulnerability marker. Montoya et al. (1996) showed that these central differences in word processing may be related to emotional learning. When certain words were associated with painful shock in healthy humans, these subjects showed larger N100 amplitudes and a more negative-going slow wave 400–800 ms after word presentation to shock-related compared to non-shock words. The authors interpreted their results as an activation of cell assemblies representing the memory of the learned word-shock contingency. Furthermore, the increased N100 amplitude can be interpreted as an increased attentive facilitation to aversive pain-related information as a consequence of conditioning.

Another study that examined the role of classical conditioning on muscular responses and EEG measures in chronic pain patients was conducted by Schneider et al. (2004). They used aversive slides as conditioned stimuli, which were followed by intracutaneous electric shocks to the left index finger. The CBP patients already showed an increased muscular response in the preconditioning phase, selective to the area where the shock was later administered. This can be interpreted as an anticipatory muscular response to predicted painful stimuli in CBP patients. In the acquisition phase only the CBP patients showed the expected classical conditioning effect for both the shock site and the right trapezius (i.e. the site of their pain). The results of the extinction phase suggest that the patients generalized the conditioned response (elevated muscular tension) to other stimuli (in this case to the CS). In addition the EEG measures indicated a dysfunctional brain response to the anticipation of the painful stimulus as well as in consequence to it. These results suggest that classical conditioning processes may be important in the development and maintenance of chronic back pain.

Diesch and Flor (2007) examined if non-painful tactile stimuli could serve as conditioned stimuli and could be connected to painful stimuli via classical conditioning in healthy controls. They used innocuous electrical stimuli to one finger as conditioned stimulus and painful electric shock to the lower back as the unconditioned stimulus. They found that muscle tension levels were easily conditioned and that the representation of the finger involved in the conditioning procedure in somatosensory cortex expanded and shifted towards the back representation. These results support the hypothesis that classical conditioning may also be present in the somatosensory system and may evoke pain sensations to normally not painful stimuli. Priming is another form of implicit memory where, for example, repetitions of previously experienced stimuli lead to altered behavior. Dillmann et al. (2000) investigated the effect of different semantic primes on the processing of painful stimuli. Three different categories were used as prime stimuli: somatosensory pain-related words, affective pain-related words and neutral adjectives. While viewing the primes subjects received a painful laser stimulus to their left hand. Painful stimuli applied while the subjects viewed pain-related words (affective and somatosensory words) resulted in larger evoked amplitudes 370ms after stimulus application when compared to neutral words.

The authors interpret this result as a preactivation of pain memory due to the processing of pain-related words.

Whereas respondent conditioning focuses on the development of stimulus associations, operant conditioning deals with the association of responses and reinforcing stimuli. Fordyce (1976) was the first to describe the important role of operant conditioning in chronic pain. He suggested that both positive and negative reinforcement of pain behaviors as well as a lack of reinforcement for well behaviors contribute to chronicity. Although this model had a significant impact on the treatment of chronic pain, there is little experimental evidence on the role of operant factors in chronicity and the underlying brain mechanisms. Flor et al. (2002) examined the role of operant conditioning during acute painful stimulation in CBP patients and healthy controls. EEG, heart rate, skin conductance and muscle tension were concurrently assessed. Half of the chronic pain patients and healthy controls were reinforced for decreased pain reports and the other half were reinforced for increased pain reports. While both groups showed similar learning rates, the CBP group displayed slower extinction of both the verbal and the cortical (N150) pain response. There was no significant correlation between resistance to extinction and pain duration. The authors interpreted this result as evidence that the prolonged operant conditioning effects might precede the onset of chronic pain and might thus be a predisposing factor.

From an operant learning perspective, tensing painful muscles can also be viewed as a learned pain behavior that may be maintained by its consequences (reduced pain impact). Chronic pain patients might have learned to increase their muscle tension in anticipation to painful stimulation, in an attempt to decrease the painfulness of the episode. While this coping behavior might temporarily alleviate pain, it may, however, over time lead to enhanced pain perception as it stimulates and sensitizes nociceptors. Knost et al. (1999) investigated CBP patients, people at high risk for CBP, and healthy controls who received painful electric stimuli to the forearm or lower back, while they had to produce high or low muscle tension levels. The CBP showed significantly elevated and the high risk group a trend to higher N150 and N150/P260 amplitudes when the low muscle tension condition was compared with then high muscle tension condition (see Figure 6.4). These results suggest that operantly conditioned increased muscle tension levels and accompanying cortical network changes contribute to pain chronicity.

Hölzl et al. (2005) devised an operant conditioning design that relies on implicit, non-conscious changes in pain-related reinforcement, which might be very relevant for pain development. They employed a sequence of interconnected trials with tonic heat stimuli applied to the thenar of the dominant hand. Stimulus temperature increased or decreased from trial to trial depending on the participant's adjustment of the heat stimuli in the previous trial and the responses of the subjects were reinforced temperature changes without the subject's knowledge. They showed that increases and decreases in pain sensitivity could be learned implicitly without the participants' awareness.

## 6.6 **The role of cognitive factors**

The role of cognitive factors such as helplessness, lack of coping skills and catastrophizing in the chronicity process has been emphasized for a long time (cf. Turk, Meichenbaum, & Genest 1983). In addition, the fear-avoidance model of chronic back pain by Vlaeyen & Linton (2000) places an emphasis on the mis-interpretation and negative evaluation of acute pain. When pain is (mis-)interpreted and negatively evaluated it can lead to the development of a vicious circle of fear of pain, pain anxiety, avoidance, and depression. Pain catastrophizing has been extensively examined in chronic pain patients and has been consistently associated with disability and enhanced pain behaviours (Peters, Vlaeyen, & Weber 2005; Sullivan, Lynch, & Clark 2005; Turner, Mancl, & Aaron 2004).

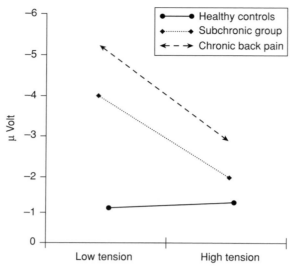

**Fig. 6.4** Mean N150 amplitudes averaged across all electrodes for the painful stimulation (averaged across back and arm stimulation) are displayed. Healthy controls showed no difference in EEG amplitudes between the high and low tension condition, whereas CBP patients displayed a significant difference, with higher amplitudes during the low tension condition. The results of the subchronic group showed a trend towards significance. Reproduced from *Psychophysiology* **36**(6), J. C. Ziegler, A. Benraïss, and M. Besson, From print to meaning: An electrophysiological investigation of the role of phonology in accessing word meaning, pp. 775–85, © 1999 with permission from John Wiley and Sons.

Based on the findings associated with chronicity Lloyd et al. (2008) studied the brain correlates of painful stimulation in patients with high and low levels of clinical indicators of continued chronicity, the so-called non-organic signs and symptoms as first described by Waddell et al. (1980). High scores of Waddell signs (WS) are associated with poor physical performance, increased catastrophizing and poor treatment outcome whereas patients with low scores do not differ from healthy controls. The authors delivered tactile (intense and unpleasant but not painful) stimuli to the back of the participants with high (WS-H) or low Waddell (WS-L) signs. WS-H patients, who have high catastrophizing and disability scores, did not differ in brain activation patters from the healthy controls. In contrast, WS-L patients showed significantly more activation in the left superior parietal lobe and the left extrastriate cortex than the controls. This result is interesting since healthy controls and WS-L patients did not differ in their behavior, but showed differential brain activation in response to pain. When the two patient groups were directly compared, the WS-L patients showed more activation in the posterior cingulate cortex and the extrastriate cortex. The authors note that these regions, which are associated with affective-cognitive processing, might reflect better coping (WS-L group). There were no areas that were more active in the WS-H compared to the WS-L group. A correlation analysis between catastrophizing and the BOLD response was significant in the inferior parietal cortex and the superior parietal lobe.

In accordance with prior findings on chronic back pain patients, Lloyd et al. (2008) found a moderate medial shift of activation (4mm) in primary somatosensory cortex after tactile stimulation of the back for the WS-H compared to the WS-L group. However, patients were allowed to continue their stable medication, including opioids, antiepileptics, and antidepressants. Although medication did not differ between the two patient groups, none of the healthy controls took analgesic medication. Since these drugs directly influence the brain chemistry, some of the differences between the groups examined might be related to this difference. Another variable that needs to be considered is the significant age difference between the healthy controls and the patient groups since age is known to have an influence on brain activation (Abe et al. 2002; Hock et al. 1995; Tumeh et al. 2007).

Gracely et al. (2004) examined the association of catastrophizing independent of depressive symptoms and brain responses to pain in fibromyalgia patients. Activation of the ipsilateral SII was more than twice as large in the persons high on catastrophizing compared to those with a low score. In addition, patients high on catastrophizing scores displayed an additional activation in the contralateral rostral ACC and bilateral lentiform nuclei that was not present in the low catastrophizers. More research is needed to determine the brain mechanisms that underlie catastrophizing in chronic pain.

The effects of attention on pain have been known for a long time and have been investigated in many studies in healthy humans. For example, Miltner et al. (1989) examined effects of attention on pain perception using multichannel EEG. They delivered painful and non-painful stimuli intracutaneously to the tip of the finger while recording somatosensory event-related potentials. In one condition subjects had to attend to the painful stimuli by silently counting them and in the other condition they were told to ignore the stimuli and additionally solve a difficult puzzle. Their results show that the degree of attention a subject pays to a painful stimulus modulates the amplitudes of the later components of the EEG (P200 and P300), which were larger for attended than for unattended stimuli. For example, Bantick et al. (2002) assessed how attention to pain versus distraction from pain (by a cognitively demanding Stroop task) affects central processing of healthy subjects using fMRI. Cognitive distraction reduced activation in a number of areas, e.g. the thalamus, the insula, and the cognitive division of the ACC. Increased activation was found in the affective division of the ACC and orbitofrontal regions related to effects of both pain and distraction. Tracey et al. (2002) showed that in healthy subjects the periaqueductal grey—an area important for opioid analgesia—is also involved in attentional control and thus cognitive functions related to pain. Similar studies in chronic pain patients and those at risk for chronicity are needed.

## 6.7 Imaging and therapeutic interventions

Research about effective treatment strategies for CBP patients has shown that many different behavioural and somatic treatments are effective in interdisciplinary settings (Cherkin et al. 2003; Scascighini et al. 2008). Unfortunately, for CBP patients there are not many studies that investigated the brain changes that occur as an effect of pain reduction. deCharms et al. (2005) used real-time fMRI to teach participants to deliberately control the activation in the rACC, a region involved in pain perception and modulation. During the control condition of the experiment subjects saw a scrolling line chart of the activation of their rACC region next to a visual image of a smaller or larger fire. Participants where then instructed to increase or decrease the activation. After sufficient time for training, subjects received painful heat stimuli to their left palm. During the early trials participants did not rate the pain stimuli any different in the two conditions 'increase' and 'decrease', however at the end of the training stimuli received during the 'increase' condition were rated as significantly more painful than those during the 'decrease' condition.

Using a regression analysis de Charmes et al. (2005) showed that changes in activity in the rACC and changes in pain perception were significantly correlated. Additionally chronic pain patients were examined with the same setup, but without nociceptive stimulation. The authors also reported a significant decrease of the patients' overall pain level after the one day of training. As they pointed out it is necessary for participants to learn control over the activity of a specific brain area, since participants taught to control the activity of the PCC did not show the same decrease in pain perception. Participants presented with a pre-recorded video of the real-time information of an earlier group did also not display any effect. Direct feedback thus seems to be important.

Crawford et al. (1998) used hypnotic instructions during a cold-pressor test training and subsequently examined somatosensory event-related potentials during noxious electrical stimulation. In the first part of the experiment subjects received a hypnotic analgesia instruction (cold pressor pain training) and in the second part they received painful electrical stimuli during two conditions (hypnotic analgesia and attention to the painful stimuli). The participants showed an increased N140 potential in the anterior frontal region during the hypnotic analgesia condition and a pre-stimulus positive-going contingent cortical potential at the same site. A contingent positive variation seems to be a reflection of the participant's effort to inhibit irrelevant movement and is a variation of the contingent negative variation or readiness potential. Additionally, reduced amplitudes of the P200 and P300 components were found and interpreted as a decreased spatiotemporal perception of the painful stimuli. On a behavioural level, the hypnotic analgesia instruction led to a significantly reduced perception of pain and distress. In chronic pain patients a successful transfer of the hypnotic analgesia suggestion into daily life was found. After three experimental sessions the patients reported reduced pain levels, increased well-being and increased quality of sleep. There are no studies available that examined the effects of cognitive-behavioural pain treatment or preventive interventions on brain function in patients with CBP or those at risk.

## 6.8 Conclusions and outlook

We have provided a brief overview over functional and structural changes in the brains of patients with CBP or at high risk for chronicity. We delineated the brain areas involved in the processing of pain and pointed out differences between acute and chronic pain. The examination of the structural and functional neuronal correlates of chronicity is an important task for future research. Longitudinal studies that elucidate the role of emotional learning, and cognitive factors, and their brain correlates could shed light on the causality of the factors involved but are currently lacking.

## Acknowledgements

This work was supported by the Bundesministerium für Bildung und Forschung (grant # 01GW0531) and the Award for Basic Research of the State of Baden-Württemberg to HF.

## References

Abe, O, Aoki, S, Hayashi, N, et al. (2002). Normal aging in the central nervous system: quantitative MR diffusion-tensor analysis. *Neurobiology of Aging*, **23**, 433–41.

Apkarian, AV, Baliki, MN & Geha, PY (2009). Towards a theory of chronic pain. *Progress in Neurobiology*, **87**, 81–97.

Apkarian, AV, Bushnell, MC, Treede, RD & Zubieta, JK (2005). Human brain mechanisms of pain perception and regulation in health and disease. *European Journal of Pain*, **9**, 463–84.

Apkarian, AV, Sosa, Y, Sonty, S, et al. (2004). Chronic back pain is associated with decreased prefrontal and thalamic gray matter density. *Journal of Neuroscience*, **24**, 10410–5.

Baliki, MN, Chialvo, DR, Geha, PY, et al. (2006). Chronic pain and the emotional brain: specific brain activity associated with spontaneous fluctuations of intensity of chronic back pain. *Journal of Neuroscience*, **26**, 12165–73.

Baliki, MN, Geha, PY, Apkarian, AV & Chialvo, DR (2008). Beyond feeling: chronic pain hurts the brain, disrupting the default-mode network dynamics. *Journal of Neuroscience*, **28**, 1398–403.

Baliki, MN, Geha, PY, Jabakhanji, R, Harden, N, Schnitzer, TJ & Apkarian, AV (2008). A preliminary fMRI study of analgesic treatment in chronic back pain and knee osteoarthritis. *Molecular Pain*, **4**, 47.

Bantick, SJ, Wise, RG, Ploghaus, A, Clare, S, Smith, SM & Tracey, I (2002). Imaging how attention modulates pain in humans using functional MRI. *Brain*, **125**, 310–19.

Baron, R, Baron, Y, Disbrow, E & Roberts, TP (1999). Brain processing of capsaicin-induced secondary hyperalgesia: a functional MRI study. *Neurology*, **53**, 548–57.

Bingel, U, Lorenz, J, Schoell, E, Weiller, C & Buchel, C (2006). Mechanisms of placebo analgesia: rACC recruitment of a subcortical antinociceptive network. *Pain*, **120**, 8–15.

Bingel, U, Quante, M, Knab, R, Bromm, B, Weiller, C & Buchel, C (2003). Single trial fMRI reveals significant contralateral bias in responses to laser pain within thalamus and somatosensory cortices. *Neuroimage*, **18**, 740–8.

Bingel, U, Schoell, E & Buchel, C (2007). Imaging pain modulation in health and disease. *Current Opinions in Neurology*, **20**, 424–31.

Bornhovd, K, Quante, M, Glauche, V, Bromm, B, Weiller, C & Buchel, C (2002). Painful stimuli evoke different stimulus-response functions in the amygdala, prefrontal, insula and somatosensory cortex: a single-trial fMRI study. *Brain*, **125**, 1326–36.

Brooks, JC, Nurmikko, TJ, Bimson, WE, Singh, KD & Roberts, N (2002). fMRI of thermal pain: effects of stimulus laterality and attention. *Neuroimage*, **15**, 293–301.

Buchel, C, Bornhovd, K, Quante, M, Glauche, V, Bromm, B & Weiller, C (2002). Dissociable neural responses related to pain intensity, stimulus intensity, and stimulus awareness within the anterior cingulate cortex: a parametric single-trial laser functional magnetic resonance imaging study. *Journal of Neuroscience*, **22**, 970–6.

Buckalew, N, Haut, MW, Morrow, L & Weiner, D (2008). Chronic pain is associated with brain volume loss in older adults: preliminary evidence. *Pain Medicine*, **9**, 240–8.

Bushnell, MC, Duncan, GH, Hofbauer, RK, Ha, B, Chen, JI & Carrier, B (1999). Pain perception: is there a role for primary somatosensory cortex? *Proceedings of the National Academy of Sciences*, **96**, 7705–9.

Chen, JI, Ha, B, Bushnell, MC, Pike, B & Duncan, GH (2002). Differentiating noxious- and innocuous-related activation of human somatosensory cortices using temporal analysis of fMRI. *Journal of Neurophysiology*, **88**, 464–74.

Cherkin, DC, Sherman, KJ, Deyo, RA & Shekelle, PG (2003). A review of the evidence for the effectiveness, safety, and cost of acupuncture, massage therapy, and spinal manipulation for back pain. *Annals of Internal Medicine*, **138**, 898–906.

Coghill, RC, Sang, CN, Maisog, JM & Iadarola, MJ (1999). Pain intensity processing within the human brain: a bilateral, distributed mechanism. *Journal of Neurophysiology*, **82**, 1934–43.

Coghill, RC, Talbot, JD, Evans, AC, et al. (1994). Distributed processing of pain and vibration by the human brain. *Journal of Neuroscience*, **14**, 4095–108.

Craig, AD (2002). How do you feel? Interoception: the sense of the physiological condition of the body. *Nature Reviews Neuroscience*, **3**, 655–66.

Craig, AD (2009). How do you feel—now? The anterior insula and human awareness. *Nature Reviews Neuroscience*, **10**, 59–70.

Craig, AD, Chen, K, Bandy, D & Reiman, EM (2000). Thermosensory activation of insular cortex. *Nature Neuroscience*, **3**, 184–90.

Craig, AD, Reiman, EM, Evans, A & Bushnell, MC (1996). Functional imaging of an illusion of pain. *Nature*, **384**, 258–60.

Crawford, HJ, Knebel, T, Kaplan, L, et al. (1998). Hypnotic analgesia: 1. Somatosensory event-related potential changes to noxious stimuli and 2. Transfer learning to reduce chronic low back pain. *International Journal of Clinical and Experimental Hypnosis*, **46**, 92–132.

Davis, KD, Taylor, SJ, Crawley, AP, Wood, ML & Mikulis, DJ (1997). Functional MRI of pain- and attention-related activations in the human cingulate cortex. *Journal of Neurophysiology*, **77**, 3370–80.

deCharms, RC, Maeda, F, Glover, GH, et al. (2005). Control over brain activation and pain learned by using real-time functional MRI. *Proceedings of the National Academy of Sciences*, **102**, 18626–31.

Derbyshire, SW, Jones, AK, Creed, F, et al. (2002). Cerebral responses to noxious thermal stimulation in chronic low back pain patients and normal controls. *Neuroimage*, **16**, 158–68.

Diers, M, Koeppe, C, Diesch, E, et al. (2007). Central processing of acute muscle pain in chronic low back pain patients: an EEG mapping study. *Journal of Clinical Neurophysiology*, **24**, 76–83.

Diesch, E & Flor, H (2007). Alteration in the response properties of primary somatosensory cortex related to differential aversive Pavlovian conditioning. *Pain*, **131**, 171–80.

Dillmann, J, Miltner, WH & Weiss, T (2000). The influence of semantic priming on event-related potentials to painful laser-heat stimuli in humans. *Neuroscience Letters*, **284**, 53–6.

Faurion, A, Cerf, B, Van De Moortele, PF, Lobel, E, Mac Leod, P & Le Bihan, D (1999). Human taste cortical areas studied with functional magnetic resonance imaging: evidence of functional lateralization related to handedness. *Neuroscience Letters*, **277**, 189–92.

Ferretti, A, Babiloni, C, Gratta, CD, et al. (2003). Functional topography of the secondary somatosensory cortex for nonpainful and painful stimuli: an fMRI study. *Neuroimage*, **20**, 1625–38.

Flor, H (2009). Extinction of Pain Memories: Importance for the Treatment of Chronic Pain. in J Castro-Lopes (ed.), *Current Topics in Pain: 12th World Congress on Pain*, IASP Press, Seattle, 221–44.

Flor, H, Braun, C, Elbert, T & Birbaumer, N (1997). Extensive reorganization of primary somatosensory cortex in chronic back pain patients. *Neuroscience Letters*, **224**, 5–8.

Flor, H & Diers, M (2007). Limitations of pharmacotherapy: behavioral approaches to chronic pain. *Handbook of Experimental Pharmacology*, **177**, 415–27.

Flor, H, Diers, M & Birbaumer, N (2004). Peripheral and electrocortical responses to painful and non-painful stimulation in chronic pain patients, tension headache patients and healthy controls. *Neuroscience Letters*, **361**, 147–50.

Flor, H, Knost, B & Birbaumer, N (1997). Processing of pain- and body-related verbal material in chronic pain patients: central and peripheral correlates. *Pain*, **73**, 413–21.

Flor, H, Knost, B & Birbaumer, N (2002). The role of operant conditioning in chronic pain: an experimental investigation. *Pain*, **95**, 111–8.

Fordyce, WE (1976) Behavioral concepts in chronic pain and illness. in PO Davidson (ed.), *The behavioral treatment of anxiety, depression and pain*, Bruner & Mazel, New York, 147–88.

Gallace, A & Spence, C (2009). The cognitive and neural correlates of tactile memory. *Psychological Bulletin*, **135**, 380–406.

Giesecke, T, Gracely, RH, Grant, MA, et al. (2004). Evidence of augmented central pain processing in idiopathic chronic low back pain. *Arthritis and Rheumatism*, **50**, 613–23.

Gracely, RH, Geisser, ME, Giesecke, T, et al. (2004). Pain catastrophizing and neural responses to pain among persons with fibromyalgia. *Brain*, **127**, 835–43.

Grachev, ID, Fredrickson, BE & Apkarian, AV (2000). Abnormal brain chemistry in chronic back pain: an in vivo proton magnetic resonance spectroscopy study. *Pain*, **89**, 7–18.

Grachev, ID, Ramachandran, TS, Thomas, PS, Szeverenyi, NM & Fredrickson, BE (2003). Association between dorsolateral prefrontal N-acetyl aspartate and depression in chronic back pain: an in vivo proton magnetic resonance spectroscopy study. *Journal of Neural Transmission*, **110**, 287–312.

Harris, JA, Harris, IM & Diamond, ME (2001). The topography of tactile working memory. *Journal of Neuroscience*, **21**, 8262–9.

Hock, C, Muller-Spahn, F, Schuh-Hofer, S, Hofmann, M, Dirnagl, U & Villringer, A (1995). Age dependency of changes in cerebral hemoglobin oxygenation during brain activation: a near-infrared spectroscopy study. *Journal of Cerebral Blood Flow and Metabolism*, **15**, 1103–8.

Iadarola, MJ, Berman, KF, Zeffiro, TA, et al. (1998). Neural activation during acute capsaicin-evoked pain and allodynia assessed with PET. *Brain*, **121**, 931–47.

Kleinbohl, D, Holzl, R, Moltner, A, Rommel, C, Weber, C & Osswald, PM (1999). Psychophysical measures of sensitization to tonic heat discriminate chronic pain patients. *Pain*, **81**, 35–43.

Knost, B, Flor, H, Birbaumer, N & Schugens, MM (1999). Learned maintenance of pain: muscle tension reduces central nervous system processing of painful stimulation in chronic and subchronic pain patients. *Psychophysiology*, **36**, 755–64.

Knost, B, Flor, H, Braun, C & Birbaumer, N (1997). Cerebral processing of words and the development of chronic pain. *Psychophysiology*, **34**, 474–81.

Kwan, CL, Crawley, AP, Mikulis, DJ & Davis, KD (2000). An fMRI study of the anterior cingulate cortex and surrounding medial wall activations evoked by noxious cutaneous heat and cold stimuli. *Pain*, **85**, 359–74.

Lloyd, D, Findlay, G, Roberts, N & Nurmikko, T (2008). Differences in low back pain behavior are reflected in the cerebral response to tactile stimulation of the lower back. *Spine*, **33**, 1372–7.

Lorenz, J & Casey, KL (2005). Imaging of acute versus pathological pain in humans. *European Journal of Pain*, **9**, 163–5.

Maihofner, C, Kaltenhauser, M, Neundorfer, B & Lang, E (2002). Temporo-spatial analysis of cortical activation by phasic innocuous and noxious cold stimuli—a magnetoencephalographic study. *Pain*, **100**, 281–90.

Melzack, R & Casey, KL (1968). Sensory, motivational, and central control determinants of pain. in DR Kenshalo (ed.), *The skin senses*, Charles C. Thomas, Springfield (IL), 423–39.

Miltner, W, Johnson, R, Jr., Braun, C & Larbig, W (1989). Somatosensory event-related potentials to painful and non-painful stimuli: effects of attention. *Pain*, **38**, 303–12.

Montoya, P, Larbig, W, Pulvermuller, F, Flor, H & Birbaumer, N (1996). Cortical correlates of semantic classical conditioning. *Psychophysiology*, **33**, 644–9.

Peters, ML, Vlaeyen, JW & Weber, WE (2005). The joint contribution of physical pathology, pain-related fear and catastrophizing to chronic back pain disability. *Pain*, **113**, 45–50.

Peyron, R, Laurent, B & Garcia-Larrea, L (2000). Functional imaging of brain responses to pain. A review and meta-analysis (2000). *Clinical Neurophysiology*, **30**, 263–88.

Pincus, T, Pearce, S, McClelland, A & Isenberg, D (1995). Endorsement and memory bias of self-referential pain stimuli in depressed pain patients. *British Journal of Clinical Psychology*, **34** (Pt 2), 267–77.

Pincus, T, Pearce, S, McClelland, A & Turner-Stokes, L (1993). Self-referential selective memory in pain patients. *British Journal of Clinical Psychology*, **32** (Pt 3), 365–74.

Pincus, T, Pearce, S & Perrott, A (1996). Pain patients' bias in the interpretation of ambiguous homophones. *British Journal of Medical Psychology*, **69** (Pt 3), 259–66.

Ploghaus, A, Tracey, I, Gati, JS, et al. (1999). Dissociating pain from its anticipation in the human brain. *Science*, **284**, 1979–81.

Ploner, M, Freund, HJ & Schnitzler, A (1999). Pain affect without pain sensation in a patient with a postcentral lesion. *Pain*, **81**, 211–4.

Raichle, ME, MacLeod, AM, Snyder, AZ, Powers, WJ, Gusnard, DA & Shulman, GL (2001). A default mode of brain function. *Proceedings of the National Academy of Sciences*, **98**, 676–82.

Rainville, P, Duncan, GH, Price, DD, Carrier, B & Bushnell, MC (1997). Pain affect encoded in human anterior cingulate but not somatosensory cortex. *Science*, **277**, 968–71.

Ringler, R, Greiner, M, Kohlloeffel, L, Handwerker, HO & Forster, C (2003). BOLD effects in different areas of the cerebral cortex during painful mechanical stimulation. *Pain*, **105**, 445–53.

Scascighini, L, Toma, V, Dober-Spielmann, S & Sprott, H (2008). Multidisciplinary treatment for chronic pain: a systematic review of interventions and outcomes. *Rheumatology (Oxford)*, **47**, 670–8.

Schmidt-Wilcke, T, Leinisch, E, Ganssbauer, S, et al. (2006). Affective components and intensity of pain correlate with structural differences in gray matter in chronic back pain patients. *Pain*, **125**, 89–97.

Schmidt-Wilcke, T, Leinisch, E, Straube, A, et al. (2005). Gray matter decrease in patients with chronic tension type headache. *Neurology*, **65**, 1483–6.

Schmidt-Wilcke, T, Luerding, R, Weigand, T, et al. (2007). Striatal grey matter increase in patients suffering from fibromyalgia—a voxel-based morphometry study. *Pain*, **132** (Suppl 1), S109–16.

Schneider, C, Palomba, D & Flor, H (2004). Pavlovian conditioning of muscular responses in chronic pain patients: central and peripheral correlates. *Pain*, 112, 239–47.

Siddall, PJ, Stanwell, P, Woodhouse, A, et al. (2006). Magnetic resonance spectroscopy detects biochemical changes in the brain associated with chronic low back pain: a preliminary report. *Anesthesia & Analgesia*, 102, 1164–8.

Small, DM, Voss, J, Mak, YE, Simmons, KB, Parrish, T & Gitelman, D (2004). Experience-dependent neural integration of taste and smell in the human brain. *Journal of Neurophysiology*, 92, 1892–903.

Sullivan, MJ, Lynch, ME & Clark, AJ (2005). Dimensions of catastrophic thinking associated with pain experience and disability in patients with neuropathic pain conditions. *Pain*, 113, 310–5.

Thunberg, J, Lyskov, E, Korotkov, A, et al. (2005). Brain processing of tonic muscle pain induced by infusion of hypertonic saline. *European Journal of Pain*, 9, 185–94.

Tracey, I & Mantyh, PW (2007). The cerebral signature for pain perception and its modulation. *Neuron*, 55, 377–91.

Tracey, I, Ploghaus, A, Gati, JS, et al. (2002). Imaging attentional modulation of pain in the periaqueductal gray in humans. *Journal of Neuroscience*, 22, 2748–52.

Treede, RD, Apkarian, AV, Bromm, B, Greenspan, JD & Lenz, FA (2000). Cortical representation of pain: functional characterization of nociceptive areas near the lateral sulcus. *Pain*, 87, 113–9.

Tumeh, PC, Alavi, A, Houseni, M, et al. (2007). Structural and functional imaging correlates for age-related changes in the brain. *Seminars in Nuclear Medicine*, 37, 69–87.

Turk, DC, Meichenbaum, D & Genest, M (1983). *Pain and behavioral medicine: A cognitive-behavioral perspective*, Guilford Press, New York.

Turner, JA, Mancl, L & Aaron, LA (2004). Pain-related catastrophizing: a daily process study. *Pain*, 110, 103–11.

Valet, M, Gundel, H, Sprenger, T, et al. (2009). Patients with pain disorder show gray-matter loss in pain-processing structures: a voxel-based morphometric study. *Psychosomatic Medicine*, 71, 49–56.

Vlaeyen, JW & Linton, SJ (2000). Fear-avoidance and its consequences in chronic musculoskeletal pain: a state of the art. *Pain*, 85, 317–32.

Waddell, G, McCulloch, JA, Kummel, E & Venner, RM (1980). Nonorganic physical signs in low-back pain. *Spine*, 5, 117–25.

Chapter 7

# Structural Brain Changes in Patients with Chronic Back Pain

Arne May and A. Vania Apkarian

## 7.1 Introduction

In the past decade of pain research, a network of pain transmitting areas within the CNS has been established, based on both animal studies (Wall and Melzack 2006) and findings from functional imaging studies in humans (Peyron et al. 2000). Consequently, the neurobiology of pain is increasingly understood as an integration of activity in distinct neuronal structures. Evidence of altered local brain chemistry (Grachev et al. 2000) and functional reorganization in chronic back pain (CBP) patients (Flor et al. 1997) supports the idea that chronic pain could be understood not only as an altered functional state, but also as a consequence of central plasticity (Flor 2003).

Recent neurobiological findings suggest cortical reorganization on a functional level (Grusser et al. 2004). For example, amputation of a limb is very often accompanied by phantom pain. In these patients, the deafferentation leads to cortical reorganization where the representational fields of adjacent areas move into the into the representation zone of the deafferented limb (Pons et al. 1991; Flor et al 2006). This 'functional reorganization' was not only detected in patients suffering from phantom limb pain (Flor et al. 1995), but also in CBP patients (Flor et al. 1997). Regarding CBP, increased cortical activity and a shift of the cortical representation of the back, which was interpreted as an expansion of the back's representation into the neighbouring foot and leg area (Flor et al. 1997), was found. In patients with chronic regional pain syndrome (CRPS Type I), a shrinkage of the representational field of the affected arm was found and the extent of shrinkage correlated highly with the intensity of pain and the magnitude of mechanical hyperalgesia (Maihofner et al. 2003; Pleger et al. 2004). It is noteworthy, that the functional changes in CRPS (Maihofnere et al. 2004) and in phantom pain (Flor et al. 2001) were dynamic, (i.e. cortical reorganization reversed coincident with clinical improvement).

Currently, chronic pain states are attributed to abnormal nociceptive/antinociceptive function on different levels of the neuroaxis (Wall and Melzack 2006) with a normal brain structure. However, any significant challenge that requires a specific function, including learning a specific task, has the potential to alter brain structure (May et al. 2007). Given that the initiation of chronification of pain involves nociceptive input, one would expect that neuroplasticity would probably occur in modulatory areas of nociception—namely, the antinociceptive system.

An alternative view of the cumulative human brain imaging studies regarding pain is that we have firmly established that various brain regions are activated in a reproducible pattern for acute and experimental pain conditions. Yet, brain activity for chronic pain is distinct from acute pain (Apkarian et al. 2005). Moreover, the 'pain matrix' assumed to underlie pain in general in fact corresponds to spinothalamic inputs to the cortex and as such identifies brain areas involved in acute nociception. Even for acute pain, the involvement of primary somatosensory cortex (S1) remains unresolved. Multiple evoked potential studies assert its role while functional brain imaging, primarily functional magnetic resonance imaging (fMRI), studies often fail to find activity in appropriate parts of S1, however, with some exception (Bingel 2004). Animal studies have shown that the S1 body map is dynamic and reorganizes with body part use or neglect, as well as with peripheral nerve injuries. Recently, this was also shown for humans (Flor et al. 1995, 1997, 2002). Thus, changes in somatotopy in S1, which have been described in various chronic pain conditions and which were determined mainly for non-painful tactile stimuli, may be a consequence of behavioural modifications of body use due to coping strategies necessary for living with chronic pain.

There is now accumulating evidence that brain activity for acute and chronic pain (especially for fluctuations of spontaneous pain) are distinct from each other, and that brain activity for various clinical chronic pain conditions are also distinct from each other (Apkarian et al. 2009). For example, in CBP patients, activity in the medial prefrontal cortex (mPFC) identifies the intensity of patients' pain with a predictive power larger than 80% (Baliki et al. 2006). When in the same patients brain activity for acute thermal pain is examined, applied on the back at a location closest to the back pain, the mPFC activity show no related activity, and instead parts of the insula code the perceived intensity at a comparable predictive level as the mPFC for spontaneous pain. Moreover, the brain activations for acute thermal pain in CBP engages the same brain regions as seen in healthy subjects, and contrasting these activations between the two groups shows no brain region to be more active or less active in either group, thus demonstrating that acute thermal pain brain activity does not differ between CBP and normals, and spontaneous pain of CBP activates distinct pattern.

Brain activity for spontaneous pain was also reported for patients with chronic postherpetic neuralgia (PHN) (Geha et al. 2007), a prototypical neuropathic chronic pain condition. The PHN patients were studied in the same lab as CBP patients, using the same methods and similar analyses, thus the result can be directly compared. In PHN spontaneous pain activated a more elaborate set of brain regions, but most importantly parts of the basal ganglia and amygdala, and these regions best reflected the intensity as well as multiple questionnaire based properties of PHN pain. It therefore seems that brain activity for spontaneous pain engages distinct brain regions in different chronic pain conditions. We should add, however, that the mPFC is a brain region tightly connected to basal ganglia and amygdala, and in the CBP patients' study these structures were also activated but at a lower statistical level.

The PHN patients' study also examined the effects of a therapy on brain activity, and the same therapy effects were also recently reported in CBP patients for their spontaneous pain (Baliki et al. 2008). Both studies examined the effects of 5% lidocaine patch application on the painful body part (a sodium channel blocker that should only be effecting neural transmission for the tissue just underneath the patch), and correlated the change in pain perception with that of brain activity determined for spontaneous pain. In both studies decreased pain perception was accompanied with decreased brain activity, and in each group the brain regions involved were distinct and corresponded to those best reflecting spontaneous pain, that is, lidocaine therapy decreased activity in mPFC in CBP patients while in PHN patients it decreased activity in basal ganglia and amygdala. These results and similar accumulating evidence (Apkarian et al. 2009) question the utility of the notion of the 'pain matrix' and imply that chronic pain conditions need to be investigated as distinct entities with unique brain properties.

## 7.2 **Structural brain imaging**

In the past, studies of brain morphology completely depended on autopsy material. Fortunately, chronic pain is not a life limiting factor, and given that the common assumption of chronic pain has been that it is simply pain sustained over a long time, there was no urge to examine the anatomy of autopsies of patients suffering from chronic pain. This situation changed with the advent of modern *in vivo* imaging methods, in particular magnetic resonance (MR) imaging. All quantitative MR-based methods are subsumed under the heading of MR morphometry of the brain and are based on the idea of using a common coordinate system or atlas. Normally, three-dimensional, high-resolution, T1-weighted MR images acquired with conventional 1.5 T MR scanners and 1 mm$^3$ voxels provide sufficient detail and contrast (Ashburner et al. 2003) whereas scanners with higher field strength (3 Tesla, 7 Tesla) allow for higher spatial resolution. Images from several subjects can be grouped together and analysed by mapping them onto a standardized coordinate space. Voxel-based morphometry (VBM) is the most commonly applied technique. It is relatively simple to use, has moderate demands on computational resources and is available in common software packages like FSL (FSL;, Smith et al. 2004) or SPM (Friston et al. 1999).

As a non-invasive procedure, MR morphometry is the ideal tool for finding the morphological substrates of diseases, deepening our understanding of the relationship between brain structure and function, and even to monitor therapeutic interventions. It has to be said that most studies focus on cohort or cross-sectional studies, leading to the question of cause and consequence. Important contributions to the exact causes of structural changes will come from studies that look at the time parameters of these changes and include independent factors (i.e. electrophysiology or genetics). Moreover, the exact cause of lesion- and training-related morphological changes in the adult brain is still not known. A decrease in the brain grey matter, such as has been described in chronic pain patients, does not necessarily mean neuronal destruction. Potential correlates of the observed morphometric changes include a simple change in cell size, shrinkage or atrophy of neurons or glia, as well as changes in the intra-cortical axonal architecture (synaptic loss) (May and Glaser 2006).

The analysis of the cortical surface complements voxel-based methods. For these approaches, the cortical surface is extracted from brain scans and further computations are applied to then calculate parameters such as cortical thickness (Fjell et al. 2006) or complexity (Thompson et al. 2005). More recently, this has also allowed the local three-dimensional computation of the gyrification index as a measure of the degree of folding of a given cortical area (Luders et al. 2006). An advantage over VBM and DBM is the improved reduction of intersubject variability in cortical folding patterns (Argall et al. 2006). However, the extraction of the cortical surface imposes high demands on computational resources and crucially depends on the quality of surface extraction, which sometimes requires additional manual correction or interaction.

A disadvantage of all of the methods described is that they are insensitive to changes in white matter, where diffusion tensor imaging (DTI) is the method of choice. DTI takes advantage of water diffusion along axons and allow the study of the integrity and structural connectivity of the white matter (Beaulieu 2002). By fitting a diffusion tensor model to DTI measurements at each voxel, one can measure fractional anisotropy (FA) and its three principle diffusivities (eigenvalues l1, l2, and l3), all of which characterize the microenvironment of the white matter tissue (Beaulieu 2002; Buchel et al. 2004). With the development of novel computational techniques during the last few years and increasing image resolution, the era of MRI-based morphometry has begun to expand. Recent findings and further methodological developments should lead to scientific breakthroughs that will change how we think of the brain (May 2011).

## 7.3 **Structural imaging in chronic back pain**

The mechanisms of chronification are the subject of intense research and debate and several studies have investigated the possible functional changes in back pain (Grachev et al. 2000;

Apkarian et al. 2001, 2004a). As sophisticated structural brain imaging methods became available, the question emerged whether the brain of patients experiencing chronic back pain (CBP) may be different from healthy controls. The pioneering work by Apkarian et al. used VBM methods in 17 patients with CBP and demonstrated a significant but spatially restricted brain atrophy in these patients. The authors were again able to show that these morphological changes are correlated with the clinical parameters of the condition (duration of pain) and suggested that the patho-physiology of chronic pain includes thalamo-cortical processes (Apkarian et al. 2004b). Specifically, this study found a decrease in grey matter in the dorsolateral prefrontal cortices (DLPFC) (a region outside of the spinothalamic projections to the cortex) bilaterally and a decrease in grey matter in the right thalamus (implicating involvement of spinothalamic projections). The authors suggested that neurodegeneration—rather than tissue shrinkage—without a substantial impact on neuronal properties may be the cause of this finding, based on an earlier observation that N-acetyl-aspartate concentrations are decreased in DLPFC in back pain (Grachev et al. 2000).

The Apkarian et al. study was in part replicated by Schmidt-Wilcke et al. (Schmidt-Wilcke et al. 2006), who investigated 18 patients with matched healthy controls and also found a decrease in grey matter in the DLPFC. However, this study also found an increase in thalamic grey matter and an additional decrease in the dorsolateral pons and the somatosensory cortex. Interestingly, the correlation analyses suggested that the grey matter decrease in the brainstem does not correlate with pain duration, but rather with pain intensity and pain unpleasantness experienced at the time of scanning, thus possibly accounting for the degree of impaired antinociception at that time. The differences between the studies by Apkarian et al. and Schmidt-Wilcke et al. are not easy to interpret. One explanation is the relatively small sample sizes used in these studies, so that negative findings have little meaning. However, Schmidt-Wilcke et al. only included patients without radiating pain, including radiculopathy, whereas Apkarian studied a mixture of patients with and without neurological manifestations as well as patients with pain outside of his region (for example, in the upper back). Moreover, in the Apkarian study the clinical properties of back pain could be related to the extent of grey matter decrease in DLPFC: the amount of this regional decrease was significantly larger for back pain with radiculopathy in contrast to back pain without radiculopathy. In a subsequent study where brain activity for spontaneous pain was studied in back pain patients and mPFC activity identified, the authors demonstrated that activity in DLPFC was negatively correlated with that of mPFC (Baliki et al. 2006), leading to the suggestion that the anatomical changes in DLPFC may underlie the increased activity in mPFC and thus lead to a more emotional perception of the pain of back pain. In summary, chronic back pain is accompanied by specific morphological alterations in structures known to play a crucial role in either antinociception or in the control of complex responses to the pain specifically in emotional control for back pain, which may correlate to the intensity and unpleasantness of pain (May 2011).

## 7.4 Are the brain changes in chronic back pain specific?

The morphometric data in CBP patients have to be seen in relation to nearly a dozen morpho-metric studies done in different chronic pain diseases (May 2008). All studies showed local morphologic alterations of the brain in areas ascribable to the transmission of pain in patients with phantom pain (Draganski et al. 2006), irritable bowl syndrome (Davis 2000), fibromyalgia (Kuchinad et al. 2007; Schmidt-Wilcke et al. 2007), tension type headache (Schmidt-Wilcke et al. 2005), migraine (Granziera et al. 2006; Rocca et al. 2006; Kin et al. 2008; Schmidt-Wilcke et al. 2008; Valfre et al. 2008), chronic vulvar pain (Schweinhardt et al. 2008), chronic complex regional pain syndrome (CRPS) (Geha et al. 2008), and chronic pain following thoracic spinal damage

(Wrigley et al 2008). These alterations were different for each pain syndrome, but most studies showed a decrease in grey matter in the cingulate cortex, the parts of the prefrontal cortex and the anterior insula (May 2008). These regions are suggested to function as multi-integrative structures during the experience and the anticipation of pain.

As neither pain related inactivity (Draganski et al. 2006), nor pain medication (Apkarian et al. 2004b; Schmidt-Wilcke et al. 2005; Kuchinad et al. 2007) explain these findings, the *in vivo* demonstration of a loss of brain grey matter in patients experiencing chronic pain compared to age- and sex-matched healthy controls could represent the heavily discussed neuroanatomical substrate for pain memory. These alterations were different for the different pain syndromes, but, in terms of functional systems, overlapped to an astounding extent. It is, however, crucial to stress that this phenomenon, which coincides with the chronicity of pain does not act in isolation. It influences and is influenced by nociceptive and spinal events. The plasticity and dynamic inter-action among nociceptors (Woolf and Salter 2000), neurotransmitters (Koltzenburg 1999), glial, neuronal and endothelial cells (Gordh et al. 2006), receptive fields (Suzuki et al. 2000) and the immune system (Marchand et al. 2005) as well as higher cognitive functions (Flor et al. 2002; Gureje 2007) needs to be considered. They comprise a complex collection of many discrete, but interacting, systems (Melzack et al. 2001). However, although the complexity of pain percep-tion involves many levels of the neuraxis, cortical plasticity is certainly not restricted to functional changes.

The data indicating that the cingulate cortex is affected in chronic pain raises some speculation on the neuronal pathways of chronic pain. The anterior cingulate cortex and the anterior insulae function as multi-integrative structures during the experience and the anticipation of pain (Peyron et al. 2000; Porro et al. 2002). The anterior cingulate cortex, including the perigenual part, is of particular interest, since it plays a deterministic role in pain modulation and analgesia. The analgesic/modulating effect is mediated through the interaction with other structures, such as the orbitofrontal cortex, the amygdala and the PAG (Zhang et al. 1997). All of these structures also showed alteration in some of the studies mentioned here. The collective evidence for the rACC as a crucial site for endogenous pain control has been observed in the context of pain modulation by attention, anticipation of pain and placebo analgesia (for a review see (Kupers et al. 2005) and also studies of neurostimulation for pain relief (Davis 2006)). A recent study by Apkarian and colleagues raise novel questions as to the role of ACC and of insulae in acute nociception (Baliki et al 2009). The temporal properties of ACC activity for acute thermal pain seem to closely correspond to that for the amygdalae, with both activations preceding the peak thermal stimulus, which is consistent with their role in pain anticipation rather than encoding its properties.

The insular activity, on the other hand, was segregated into two functionally distinct portions one activated early and closely related to the stimulus properties (encoding nociceptive input) while the other was activated later, encoded perceived subjective pain, and was an area that equally well encoded the size of bars presented visually (representing magnitude estimation). Thus, depending on the specific part of the insula showing decreased grey matter one would reach very different underlying reasons and implications regarding processing pain and other sensory or cognitive events. Moreover, given the distinct brain activity patterns associated with various clinical pain conditions, the interaction between brain morphology, morphological reorganiza-tion and brain activity needs to be studied far more intensively.

The decrease of grey matter in brain regions which are highly associated with pain suppression could certainly lead to dysfunction in effective antinociception. Abnormal modulation of brain nociceptive systems, at first transient, but becoming permanent with continuing illness, could in part explain the shift from acute to chronic pain. Very recently, and using a different methodological approach, Davis et al. were able to show that patients suffering from irritable bowel syndrome (IBS) show a significant cortical thinning of the ACC, a finding which has striking similarity to the findings discussed above (Davis et al. 2008).

## 7.5 Relating brain grey matter changes to white matter connectivity

Grey matter morphological changes in back pain (Apkarian et al. 2004) and in CRPS (Geha et al. 2008) were studied in the same lab using similar imaging and data analysis techniques. The results indicate that the two clinical conditions affect non-overlapping brain regions, and yet in both the changes are correlated with duration and/or intensity of the pain. In the CRPS patients, DTI analyses were used to examine relationship between grey matter decreased density and white matter connectivity. The study generally indicates that brain regions where grey matter is reduced is also accompanied with a general decrease in white matter connectivity, although in some cases this was also accompanied with target specific increased connectivity as well. This is the first study linking grey matter changes to white matter properties and the results are consistent with the general idea of loss of neurons, but also suggest that it is a result of competitive reorganization of connectivity across brain regions. More importantly this study demonstrates the power of combining various brain anatomical imaging techniques to begin to unravel the processes underlying brain reorganization with chronic pain.

## 7.6 Brain changes in chronic pain: cause or consequence?

As chronic pain patients may have a common 'brain signature' in areas known to be involved in pain control, the question arises whether the central reorganization processes in chronic pain syndromes could involve a 'degeneration' of specific brain areas. This question is not redundant, as a degenerative process is irreversible. Although many VBM studies demonstrate changes in grey matter, the neurobiological basis of these structural alterations on a microscopic level are not well defined (May and Gaser 2006). VBM detects changes in grey matter concentration per voxel as well as changes in the classification of individual voxels (e.g. from white to grey matter (Good et al. 2001) and probably a combination of both). In general, a decrease in grey matter could be due to a simple decrease in cell size, neural or glial cell apoptosis, a decrease in spine density or even changes in blood flow or interstitial fluid. Unfortunately, all available studies compared cohorts of patients and therefore no statement regarding dynamic changes can be made.

It is not understood why only a relatively small proportion of humans develop a chronic pain syndrome, considering that pain is a universal experience. As the adult human brain may change its structure in response to environmental demands (Flor et al. 2001; Draganski et al. 2004), the question arises whether in some humans a (possibly genetically) structural difference in central pain transmitting systems may act as a diathesis for chronic pain. What argues against the assumption that the people with chronic pain have a priori a different brain structure and thus are susceptible to chronicity is the fact, that people experiencing phantom pain and chronic pain following spinal cord damage show some similar brain changes as, for example, people with CBP. Moreover, a recent study showed in patients with chronic hip pain that these changes are in part reversible (Rodriguez-Raecke et al. 2009). On the other hand the opposite argument has just as convincing data, namely, brain activity for spontaneous pain seems distinct for diverse clinical chronic pain conditions and brain morphometric changes, especially between CRPS and back pain.

A recent study aimed to investigate how repeated painful stimulation over several days is proc-essed, perceived and modulated in the healthy human brain and whether repeated painful stimu-lation may lead to structural changes of the brain. A standardized nociceptive heat paradigm for 8 consecutive days is reflected in increased grey matter in brain areas ascribable to the transmis-sion of sensory input and pain perception (Teutsch et al. 2008). This data is in line with most morphometric studies investigating structural brain plasticity as a result of exercise and learning (Flor et al. 2001; Gaser et al. 2003; Draganski et al. 2004; Boyke et al. 2008). Moreover, these find-ings of structural changes follow the previously described functional pattern (Bingel et al. 2007) precisely (i.e. a significant change during the protocol that reverses to pre-stimulation levels at the fourth time-point, namely, after 1 year (Bingel et al. 2008).

However, it is an intriguing fact that chronic pain patients have constant pain, but seem not to develop an increase in grey matter in somatosensory areas (in fact the bulk of the data points to decreased grey matter in areas outside of the somatosensory regions), although several studies showed that exercise is accompanied by an increase of grey matter in the regions which are specific for the respective task (for review see (Friston et al. 1996)).

One explanation for this lack of grey matter increase in chronic pain patients is that they do not have a significant noxious input to explain the pain experience (any more, although there is no real convincing data for this notion; for spontaneous pain of back pain a transient afferent nociceptive input has been described (Baliki et al. 2006)). In that case the experience of constant pain would be mostly driven by the brain itself and the afferent (peripheral noxious) input is no longer needed for this experience. Another possibility is, that a given task-specific exercise will only increase grey matter in corresponding brain areas until the task is learned and that this change recedes once the task is learned sufficiently.

There is no conclusive data regarding the cause or the consequence of the different cortical and subcortical morphological changes, although the correlation of pain duration and degree of grey matter decrease in most studies suggests that the morphological changes are at least in part secondary to constant pain. This notion is also consistent with the evidence of the same brain region showing decreased metabolite concentration as well as decreased white matter connectiv-ity for the same regions that also show decreased grey matter density. Still, thorough longitudinal studies need to address whether the morphological changes reverse when the disproportionate amount of nociceptive stimulation (i.e. following sufficient pain treatment) stops. The idea of structural maladaptive plasticity however, serves certainly well as a good model for structural cortical/subcortical reorganization following chronic input of nociceptive information.

# References

Apkarian AV, Krauss BR, Fredrickson BE, Szeverenyi NM. Imaging the pain of low back pain: functional magnetic resonance imaging in combination with monitoring subjective pain perception allows the study of clinical pain states. *Neurosci Lett* 2001; **299**(1–2):57–60.

Apkarian AV, Sosa Y, Krauss BR, *et al.* Chronic pain patients are impaired on an emotional decision-making task. *Pain* 2004; **108**(1–2):129–36.

Apkarian AV, Sosa Y, Sonty S, *et al.* Chronic back pain is associated with decreased prefrontal and thalamic gray matter density. *J Neurosci* 2004; **24**(46):10410–5.

Apkarian AV, Bushnell MC, Treede RD, Zubieta JK. Human brain mechanisms of pain perception and regulation in health and disease. *Eur J Pain* 2005; **9**(4):463–84.

Argall BD, Saad ZS, Beauchamp MS. Simplified intersubject averaging on the cortical surface using SUMA. *Hum Brain Mapp* 2006; **27**(1):14–27.

Apkarian AV, Baliki MN, Geha PY. Towards a theory of chronic pain. *Prog Neurobiol* 2009; **87**(2):81–97.

Ashburner J, Csernansky JG, Davatzikos C, Fox NC, Frisoni GB, Thompson PM. Computer-assisted imaging to assess brain structure in healthy and diseased brains. *Lancet Neurol* 2003; **2**(2):79–88.

Baliki MN, Chialvo DR, Geha PY, *et al.* Chronic pain and the emotional brain: specific brain activity associated with spontaneous fluctuations of intensity of chronic back pain. *J Neurosci* 2006; **26**(47): 12165–73.

Baliki MN, Geha PY, Jabakhanji R, Harden N, Schnitzer TJ, Apkarian AV. A preliminary fMRI study of analgesic treatment in chronic back pain and knee osteoarthritis. *Mol Pain* 2008; **4**:47.

Baliki MN, Geha PY, Apkarian AV. Parsing pain perception between nociceptive representation and magnitude estimation. *J Neurophysiol* 2009; **101**(2):875–87.

Beaulieu C. The basis of anisotropic water diffusion in the nervous system - a technical review. *NMR Biomed* 2002; **15**:435–55.

Bingel U, Lorenz J, Glauche V, *et al.* Somatotopic organization of human somatosensory cortices for pain: a single trial fMRI study. *Neuroimage* 2004; **23**(1):224–32.

Bingel U, Herken W, Teutsch S, May A. Habituation to painful stimulation involves the antinociceptive system—a 1-year follow-up of 10 participants. *Pain* 2008; **140**(2):393–4.

Bingel U, Schoell E, Herken W, Buchel C, May A. Habituation to painful stimulation involves the antinociceptive system. *Pain* 2007; **131**(1–2):21–30.

Boyke J, Driemeyer J, Gaser C, Büchel C, May A. Training induced brain structure changes in the Elderly. *J Neuroscience* 2008; **28**:7031–35.

Buchel C, Raedler T, Sommer M, Sach M, Weiller C, Koch MA. White matter asymmetry in the human brain: a diffusion tensor MRI study. *Cereb Cortex* 2004; **14**(9):945–51.

Davis KD. The neural circuitry of pain as explored with functional MRI. *Neurol Res* 2000; **22**(3):313–7.

Davis KD, Pope G, Chen J, Kwan CL, Crawley AP, Diamant NE. Cortical thinning in IBS: implications for homeostatic, attention, and pain processing. *Neurology* 2008; **70**(2):153–4.

Draganski B, Gaser C, Busch V, Schuierer G, Bogdahn U, May A. Neuroplasticity: Changes in grey matter induced by training. *Nature* 2004; **427**(6972):311–12.

Draganski B, Moser T, Lummel N, *et al.* Decrease of thalamic gray matter following limb amputation. *Neuroimage* 2006; **31**(3):951–7.

Fjell AM, Walhovd KB, Reinvang I, *et al.* Selective increase of cortical thickness in high-performing elderly—structural indices of optimal cognitive aging. *Neuroimage* 2006; **29**(3):984–94.

Flor H. The modification of cortical reorganization and chronic pain by sensory feedback. *Appl Psychophysiol Biofeedback* 2002; **27**(3):215–27.

Flor H. Cortical reorganisation and chronic pain: implications for rehabilitation. *J Rehabil Med* 2003(41 Suppl):66–72.

Flor H, Elbert T, Knecht S, *et al.* Phantom-limb pain as a perceptual correlate of cortical reorganization following arm amputation. *Nature* 1995; **375**(6531):482–4.

Flor H, Braun C, Elbert T, Birbaumer N. Extensive reorganization of primary somatosensory cortex in chronic back pain patients. *Neurosci Lett* 1997; **224**(1):5–8.

Flor H, Denke C, Schaefer M, Grusser S. Effect of sensory discrimination training on cortical reorganisation and phantom limb pain. *Lancet* 2001; **357**(9270):1763–4.

Flor H, Knost B, Birbaumer N. The role of operant conditioning in chronic pain: an experimental investigation. *Pain* 2002; **95**(1–2):111–18.

Flor H, Nikolajsen L, Staehelin Jensen T. Phantom limb pain: a case of maladaptive CNS plasticity? *Nat Rev Neurosci* 2006; **7**(11):873–81.

Friston KJ, Holmes AP, Ashburner J, Poline J-B. SPM99. World Wide Web 1999; http://www.fil.ion.ucl. ac.uk/spm

FSL: http://www.fmrib.ox.ac.uk/fsl/

Gaser C, Schlaug G. Brain structures differ between musicians and non-musicians. *J Neurosci* 2003; **23**(27):9240–5.

**Geha PY, Baliki MN, Chialvo DR, Harden RN, Paice JA, Apkarian AV.** Brain activity for spontaneous pain of postherpetic neuralgia and its modulation by lidocaine patch therapy. *Pain* 2007; **128**(1–2):88–100.

**Geha PY, Baliki MN, Harden RN, Bauer WR, Parrish TB, Apkarian AV.** The brain in chronic CRPS pain: abnormal gray-white matter interactions in emotional and autonomic regions. *Neuron* 2008; **60**(4):570–81.

**Good CD, Johnsrude IS, Ashburner J, Henson RN, Friston KJ, Frackowiak RS.** A voxel-based morphometric study of ageing in 465 normal adult human brains. *Neuroimage* 2001; **14**(1 Pt 1):21–36.

**Gordh T, Chu H, Sharma HS.** Spinal nerve lesion alters blood-spinal cord barrier function and activates astrocytes in the rat. *Pain* 2006; **124**(1–2):211–21.

**Grachev ID, Frederickson BE, Apkarian AV.** Abnormal brain chemistry in chronic back pain; an in vivi proton magnetic resonance spectroscopy study. *Pain* 2000; **89**:7–18.

**Granziera C, Dasilva AF, Snyder J, Tuch DS, Hadjikhani N.** Anatomical alterations of the visual motion processing network in migraine with and without aura. *PLoS Med* 2006; **3**(10):e402.

**Grusser SM, Muhlnickel W, Schaefer M, Villringer K, Christmann C, Koeppe C, Flor H.** Remote activation of referred phantom sensation and cortical reorganization in human upper extremity amputees. *Exp Brain Res* 2004; **154**(1):97–102.

**Gureje O.** Psychiatric aspects of pain. *Curr Opin Psychiatry* 2007; **20**(1):42–6.

**Kim JH, Suh SI, Seol HY, et al.** Regional grey matter changes in patients with migraine: a voxel-based morphometry study. *Cephalalgia* 2008; **28**(6):598–604.

**Koltzenburg M.** The changing sensitivity in the life of the nociceptor. *Pain* 1999; Suppl **6**:S93–102.

**Kuchinad A, Schweinhardt P, Seminowicz DA, Wood PB, Chizh BA, Bushnell MC.** Accelerated brain gray matter loss in fibromyalgia patients: premature aging of the brain? *J Neurosci* 2007; **27**(15):4004–7.

**Kupers R, Faymonville ME, Laureys S.** The cognitive modulation of pain: hypnosis- and placebo-induced analgesia. *Prog Brain Res* 2005; **150**:251–69.

**Luders E, Thompson PM, Narr KL, Toga AW, Jancke L, Gaser C.** A curvature-based approach to estimate local gyrification on the cortical surface. *Neuroimage* 2006; **29**(4):1224–30.

**Maihofner C, Handwerker HO, Neundorfer B, Birklein F.** Patterns of cortical reorganization in complex regional pain syndrome. *Neurology* 2003; **61**(12):1707–15.

**Maihofner C, Handwerker HO, Neundorfer B, Birklein F.** Cortical reorganization during recovery from complex regional pain syndrome. *Neurology* 2004; **63**(4):693–701.

**Marchand F, Perretti M, McMahon SB.** Role of the immune system in chronic pain. *Nat Rev Neurosci* 2005; **6**(7):521–32.

**May A.** Chronic pain may change the structure of the brain. *Pain* 2008; **137**(1):7–15.

**May A.** Structural Brain imaging: A window into chronic pain. *The Neuroscientist* 2011; **17**:209–20.

**May A, Gaser C.** Magnetic resonance-based morphometry: a window into structural plasticity of the brain. *Curr Opin Neurol* 2006; **19**(4):407–11.

**May A, Hajak G, Ganssbauer S, et al.** Structural brain alterations following 5 days of intervention: dynamic aspects of neuroplasticity. *Cereb Cortex* 2007; **17**(1):205–10.

**Melzack R, Coderre TJ, Katz J, Vaccarino AL.** Central neuroplasticity and pathological pain. *Ann N Y Acad Sci* 2001; **933**:157–74.

**Peyron R, Laurent B, Garcia-Larrea L.** Functional imaging of brain responses to pain. A review and meta-analysis (2000). *Neurophysiol Clin* 2000; **30**(5):263–88.

**Pleger B, Tegenthoff M, Schwenkreis P, et al.** Mean sustained pain levels are linked to hemispherical side-to-side differences of primary somatosensory cortex in the complex regional pain syndrome I. *Exp Brain Res* 2004; **155**:115–19.

**Pons TP, Garraghty PE, Ommaya AK, Kaas JH, Taub E, Mishkin M.** Massive cortical reorganization after sensory deafferentation in adult macaques. *Science* 1991; **252**(5014):1857–60.

**Porro CA, Baraldi P, Pagnoni G, et al.** Does anticipation of pain affect cortical nociceptive systems? *J Neurosci* 2002; **22**(8):3206–14.

Rocca MA, Ceccarelli A, Falini A, *et al.* Brain gray matter changes in migraine patients with T2-visible lesions: a 3-T MRI study. *Stroke* 2006; **37**(7):1765–70.

Rodriguez-Raecke R, Niemeier A, Ihle K, Ruether W, May A. Brain gray matter decrease in chronic pain is the consequence and not the cause of pain. *J Neurosci* 2009; **29**(44):13746–50.

Schmidt-Wilcke T, Leinisch E, Straube A, *et al.* Gray matter decrease in patients with chronic tension type headache. *Neurology* 2005; **65**(9):1483–6.

Schmidt-Wilcke T, Leinisch E, Ganssbauer S, *et al.* Affective components and intensity of pain correlate with structural differences in gray matter in chronic back pain patients. *Pain* 2006; **125**(1–2):89–97.

Schmidt-Wilcke T, Luerding R, Weigand T, *et al.* Striatal grey matter increase in patients suffering from fibromyalgia - A voxel-based morphometry study. *Pain* 2007; **132**(Suppl 1):S109–16.

Schmidt-Wilcke T, Ganssbauer S, Neuner T, Bogdahn U, May A. Subtle grey matter changes between migraine patients and healthy controls. *Cephalalgia* 2008; **28**(1):1–4.

Schweinhardt P, Kuchinad A, Pukall CF, Bushnell MC. Increased gray matter density in young women with chronic vulvar pain. *Pain* 2008; **140**(3):411–19.

Smith SM, Jenkinson M, Woolrich MW, *et al.* Advances in functional and structural MR image analysis and implementation as FSL. *Neuroimage* 2004; **23** Suppl 1:S208–19.

Suzuki R, Kontinen VK, Matthews E, Williams E, Dickenson AH. Enlargement of the receptive field size to low intensity mechanical stimulation in the rat spinal nerve ligation model of neuropathy. *Exp Neurol* 2000; **163**(2):408–13.

Teutsch S, Herken W, Bingel U, Schoell E, May A. Changes in brain gray matter due to repetitive painful stimulation. *Neuroimage* 2008; **42**(2):845–9.

Thompson PM, Lee AD, Dutton RA, *et al.* Abnormal cortical complexity and thickness profiles mapped in Williams syndrome. *J Neurosci* 2005; **25**(16):4146–58.

Valfre W, Rainero I, Bergui M, Pinessi L. Voxel-based morphometry reveals gray matter abnormalities in migraine. *Headache* 2008; **48**(1):109–17.

Wall P, Melzack R. *Textbook of pain.* Edinburgh, Churchill Livingstone, 2006.

Woolf CJ, Salter MW. Neuronal plasticity: increasing the gain in pain. *Science* 2000; **288**(5472):1765–9.

Wrigley PJ, Gustin SM, Macey PM, *et al.* Anatomical changes in human motor cortex and motor pathways following complete thoracic spinal cord injury. *Cereb Cortex* 2008; **19**(1):224–32.

Zhang YQ, Tang JS, Yuan B, Jia H. Inhibitory effects of electrically evoked activation of ventrolateral orbital cortex on the tail-flick reflex are mediated by periaqueductal gray in rats. *Pain* 1997; **72**(1–2):127–35.

# Chapter 8

# The Psychophysiology of Chronic Back Pain Patients

Kati Thieme and Richard H. Gracely

## 8.1 Introduction

Psychophysiological methods investigate peripheral and central physiological responses provoked by stressors, cognitions, emotions, and behaviours. These methods involve physiology, functional anatomy, and neuroscience as well as general and physiological psychology. Studies of medical conditions, including cardiology, psychiatry, sleep, and chronic pain, use psychophysiological methods to determine mechanisms mediating diseases and treatments. In contrast to simple physiological theories, pain can be considered to be a modulated complex of physiological and psychological processes (Birbaumer and Schmidt 1996). These processes are modulated by factors such as sensitization and both classical and operant conditioning. While the psychophysiological experiments of the past focused on one selected physiological system such as muscle tension, present studies record a complex of interrelated physiological systems. The goal of the multimethod assessment approach is to determine individual-specific stress reactivity and symptom-specific stress responses that may initiate and maintain pathological processes.

Psychophysiological pain treatment includes biofeedback (e.g. Guzman et al. 2007 ; Ostelo et al. 2005), deep brain stimulation (IBS; Coffey et al. 2001), and brain–computer interface (BCI; Birbaumer and Flor 1999; Birbaumer et al. 1999a; DeCharms et al. 2005). These are usually combined with behavioural-oriented psychological treatments such as operant and cognitive-behavioural therapies (e.g. Glombiewski et al. 2010; Newton-Jon 1995). Common modalities for biofeedback include surface electromyography, respiration rate and depth, skin surface temperature, cardiovascular reactivity, and electrodermal response. Clinical biofeedback therapy broadly involves the direct feedback learning model as a therapeutic stress-management biofeedback model, which emphasizes the need to understand each patient as an individual. EMG-biofeedback has been used for the treatment of low back pain, tension headache, temporomandibular joint disorders, migraine, brain blood flow, temperature-biofeedback for migraine, and Raynaud syndrome.

Electric neurostimulation includes approved and investigational therapies directed at the spinal cord, thalamus, periaqueductal, or periventricular grey (PAG or PVG) matter, motor cortex, and peripheral nerves and has provided short-term relief for untreatable deafferentation and cancer pain (Coffey et al. 2001). Although preliminary studies support the utility of neurostimulation methods, randomized control trials with extended follow-up periods are needed. The interactive method of BCI enables individuals to gain voluntary control over activation in a specific brain region such as anterior cingulate cortex. These effects can be powerful, providing relief for severe, chronic clinical pain (DeCharms et al. 2005), possible because the effects of psychophysiological methods extend beyond palliative coping to the actual amelioration of the pathological mechanisms mediating pain disease (Birbaumer and Schmidt 1996).

## 8.1.1 **Biomechanical models**

Back pain may result from physically demonstrable chronic back pain (CBP) disease such as: (1) *degenerative disorders* with degeneration of the intervertebral disc(s), spondylolisthesis and osteoarthritis (Hirsch 1966); (2) *structural abnormalities* with spina bifida occulta, hyperlordosis, kyphosis, scoliosis (Cailliet 1981); and (3) *muscular and ligamentous dysfunctions* with fibrositis or ligamentous ruptures associated with muscle spasm and muscle degeneration (Jinkins 2003). These degenerative processes, structural abnormalities and ligamentous ruptures have often been considered to be pathological entities and possible causal factors for back pain (e.g. Cailliet 1981; Chataigner et al. 1998, Toyone et al. 1994). However, these physical findings can be found also in individuals who do not report back pain and accumulating evidence does not support the role of biomechanical factors as the sole relevant cause of pain (e.g. Beattie and Meyers 1998; Hult 1954; Jinkins 2004,). For example, the physical findings of muscle spasm and atrophy following ligamentous ruptures are usually viewed as a consequence, not a cause of the pain, spinal derangements, or postural faults (e.g. Jinkins 2003).

The *biomechanical model* proposes that CBP may be a result of abnormally low levels of muscle activity during movement or right-left movement asymmetries revealed by electromyographic (EMG) recording. In this model, abnormal EMG activity patterns result from poor posture and guarding that develops in response to the original insult (Cram and Steger 1983). Proponents of this model believe that irregular muscle activity provides abnormal support for the spine, which in turn becomes unstable and this instability facilitates infringement upon nerve endings and resultant pain (Ahern et al. 1988; Dolce and Raczynski 1985; Wolf et al. 1982). There is some experimental support for the biomechanical model. For example, patients with CBP have been found to display lower EMG levels compared to controls during movement (Ahern et al. 1988; Collins et al. 1982, Wolf et al. 1982). In addition, greater EMG asymmetries for CBP patients have been found compared to controls reported by Cram and Steger (1983). Greater asymmetries have been observed while sitting, but not while standing (Hoyt et al. 1981) or during dynamic movements (Ahern et al. 1988). Other studies contradict the predictions of the biomechanical model and provide evidence that supports the reflex-spasm model.

The link between pain and muscle activity is the basis of a *reflex-spasm model* of pain. This model describes a cycle that typically begins with an injury that produces reflex-muscle activity. If sustained, this activity produces more pain and more muscle spasms in a self-perpetuating cycle (Cobb et al. 1975; Collins et al. 1982). Many of the treatments for CBP, such as heat, cold, transcutaneous electrical nerve stimulation, and relaxation training, are thought to provide relief by interrupting the cycle, reducing both muscle activity and pain.

Two competing reflex-spasm hypotheses of CBP define different aetiological factors. One emphasizes the importance of physical stressors, while the other focuses on psychophysiological factors that underlie the development of CBP. Regardless of whether the initial damage is caused by physical or psychophysiological factors, both hypotheses agree that eventually a reflex spasm determines pain (Cobb et al. 1975; deVries 1966; Dolce and Raczynski 1985; Miller 1985; Nouwen and Bush 1984).

Those traditional medical approaches to chronic pain are characterized by a somatosensory model that focuses on mechanical factors. These perspectives effectively ignore the physical heterogeneity of CBP, the presence or non-presence of physical injuries, the association and non-association between physical changes and pain, and varying levels of muscle activity. These models narrowly consider pain to be a purely sensory event that is assumed to be directly proportional to peripheral damage. Several factors support the inadequacy of these reflex-spasm models, in particular the many instances of pain without discernible peripheral damage (e.g. McCabe et al. 2005; van Dieën et al. 2003) and the clinical reports of the absence of pain expression despite severe injury (e.g. Beattie and Meyers 1998; Harris 1999; Jensen et al. 1994; Jinkins 2004).

Medical research tends to disregard the psychosocial antecedents and consequences of CBP (Flor and Turk 1984). Linton (2000) and Pincus and colleagues (2002), have emphasized in their reviews the considerable evidence that psychological factors influence CBP. Stress, affective distress, anxiety, cognitive functioning and pain behaviour significantly impact the magnitude of CBP (Linton 2000). CBP is also modulated by learning and conditioning. A number of psychobiological process-sensitization, cognitive-affective factors (catastrophizing, depression), classical conditioning, (Gentry and Bernal 1977) and operant conditioning (Flor et al. 2002; Fordyce 1976) influence the interaction among physiological and psychological factors in persistent pain (Flor et al. 1990).

## 8.1.2 Psychological models of chronic pain

Psychological factors are implicated when there is no empirical evidence to support an isomorphic relationship between the physiological factors such as inflammatory processes, degenerative changes, structural deformities, traumatic incidents, and muscular or ligamentous strain (Loeser 1980), and CBP (e.g. Harris et al. 1999; Jinkins et al. 2004; McCabe et al. 2005). More recently, the lack of association between CBP and physical factors has focused attention on the interaction between physiological and psychological factors, including subconscious learning and cognitive-affective variables. Flor et al. (1990) proposed that the development and maintenance of chronic pain is a function of several interacting components: (1) a predisposition to respond with a specific bodily system; (2) external or internal aversive stimulation; (3) maladaptive information processing of and coping with pain-related social and/or physiological stimuli, and (4) operant, respondent, and observational learning processes. These authors defined *psychobiological mechanisms* that impact the development and maintenance of somatosensory and affective pain memory in chronic pain patients (see also, Gracely et al. 2002, 2004). The various models of learning and their relationship to CBP are presented below.

### Sensitization

The term 'sensitization' has specific meanings in pain physiology and psychology. It is used by physiologists to describe an increased peripheral and/or central response to a pain stimulus. Birbaumer and Schmidt (1996), and Flor et al. (1990), have used the term to describe augmented pain reports and behaviour caused by a range of factors that include operant and classical conditioning, as well as maladaptive pain cognitions such as catastrophizing and helplessness. We use this latter meaning in this section.

### Classical conditioning

Gentry and Bernal (1977) have proposed a respondent model of CBP in which classical conditioning of pain and muscle tension may occur in acute pain states, leading to a pain-tension cycle and subsequent chronic back pain. The pain may be exacerbated by conditioned fear of movement, leading to avoidance of activity and immobilization, (e.g. Lethem et al. 1983). Some preliminary tests of the assumptions of the respondent model have been conducted with mixed results. For example, several investigators have reported that in comparison to pain-free participants, CBP patients demonstrated higher EMG levels in various body positions, or even during relaxation (e.g. Hoyt et al. 1981; Kravitz et al. 1981) suggesting a diminished recovery of muscle tension, although decreased lower back EMG levels have been reported in certain body positions (Collins et al. 1982).

## Operant conditioning

The general assumptions of the operant pain model posit that pain, even though originally a reflex, is modulated through reinforcement controlled by operant conditioning (Fordyce 1976; 1988). The negative consequences of operant learning are 'pain behaviours' that become automatic and subconscious through positive (e.g. excessive solicitous spouse response to pain) and negative (e.g. avoidance of unpleasant activities) reinforcement. Pain behaviours that coincide with the perception of increased pain intensity provoke the development of pain memory (Flor et al. 2002). Operant learning increases avoidance behaviour, such as reducing activities in multiple life areas that leads in turn to physical problems such as muscular deconditioning (Smeets et al. 2006), medication misuse (Turk et al. 1997), muscle tension and immobility (Flor and Birbaumer 1994), and finally to mental problems such as anxiety and mood disorders (e.g. Atkinson et al. 1991; Waxman et al. 2008).

## Cognitive-behavioural approach

Cognitive-behavioural approaches to chronic pain emphasize the important role of patients' cognitions (e.g. appraisals, beliefs, expectancies) as mediators between situational stimuli and emotional and behavioural responses (Turner and Chapman 1982). Among the cognitive variables related to individual self-statements, *catastrophizing, psychosocial distress, anger,* and *fear* have received considerable attention in the last decade of CBP research (Flor et al. 1997; Gracely et al. 2004; Sullivan et al. 2001; Vlaeyen et al. 1995). Maladaptive self-appraisals are associated with pain expectation (e.g. Gracely et al. 2004; Sullivan et al. 2001). Patients with chronic pain are viewed as having negative *expectations* about their own ability to control certain motor skills such as performing specific physical activities (e.g. climbing stairs, lifting objects, bending over). They tend to attribute their disabilities to a reality characterized by *loss of control*. The pain expectations are strongly associated with situation-specific self-statements about the inability to exert control over aversive sensations (Turk et al. 1983) and may reinforce the experience of demoralization, inactivity, and overreaction to nociceptive stimulation (Flor and Turk 1988). The expectations have been associated with lower pain tolerance and higher ratings of pain intensity (Gracely et al. 2002, 2004). Cognitions can also reduce pain. From the psychophysiological view, the conviction of personal *control over pain* can ameliorate the experience of experimentally induced nociception by learning to exert deliberate, voluntary control over the activation in the rostral anterior cingulate cortex (rACC; deCharms et al. 2005; LaChapelle et al. 2001). Both self-statements like catastrophizing vs. coping and situation-specific self-statements like loss of control over pain are associated with anger, fear, and psychosocial distress and can contribute to significant changes in perceived pain.

## Diathesis–stress model

Flor and Turk (1984) proposed a diathesis–stress model of CBP that integrates many of the disparate findings noted above. The model postulates that CBP may result from the interaction of personally relevant stressful events with a predisposing organic or psychological condition. Intense or recurrent potentially aversive stimulation in a predisposed individual with maladaptive or inadequate coping abilities is hypothesized to lead to extensive and sustained reactions of the back muscles. The diathesis–stress model suggests that this increased muscle tension might lead to ischemia, reflex muscle spasms, oxygen depletion, and the release of pain-eliciting substances (e.g. histamine, substance P). The augmented pain may act as a new stressor provoking a vicious circle. The development of movement-related anticipatory anxiety and subsequent immobility and the reinforcement of pain behaviours may exacerbate the pain problem. Moreover, the anticipatory anxiety may produce hyperactivity (muscle tension) and may further exacerbate nociception and, subsequently, pain.

The diathesis–stress model (Turk and Flor 1984) predicts that CBP patients will exhibit elevated and prolonged reactions of the back musculature to stress in comparison to healthy controls or other pain patients. It predicts that muscular reactions to stress will *only* occur in response to personally relevant stressors. Additionally, the model hypothesizes that these muscular hyper-reactions will be predicted best by psychological variables (e.g. anxiety, helplessness) rather than by organic variables (e.g. amount of degenerative damage, number of surgeries, duration of the pain problem) and that anxiety levels and immobility are related in CBP patients.

### 8.1.3 Psychophysiological models

Physiological responses to stress may be partially responsible for the development and mainte-nance of chronic pain disorders. Traditional models of the impact of stress on physiological func-tions assumed the principle of a universal stress response, *'concept of general activation'* (e.g. Selye, 1956). Alternative models present a more specific view. The *'concept of response specificity'* (Lacey and Lacey 1958) describes psychophysiological response patterns characterized by a series of multiple autonomic functions with varied levels of involvement. The autonomic function with the greatest involvement defines a stress-reactivity that may be important for the aetiopathogen-esis of the disease.

The 'concept of response specificity' (Lacey and Lacey 1958) describes three different psycho-physiological response patterns. In the first *stimulus-specific response* pattern, a defined stimulus provokes a similar response in different individuals. In the second, *individual-specific response pattern*, identical psychophysiological response patterns are provoked by different stress stimuli, for example mental (mental arithmetic), social (exam), physical (heat or cold), or pain stimuli (electrical, pressure, thermal). In the third *'motivation-specific response pattern'*, different indi-viduals produce different patterns independent of the type of stimulus. These patterns are consid-ered to be reproducible if found in a comparable state that uses the same external experimental setting and provokes comparable internal variables such as motivation and evaluation of the situ-ation (Ax 1964; Fahrenberg 1986; Lacey et al. 1953).

Perhaps the earliest description of a *stimulus-specific response* was outlined by James (1884) in the 'theory of emotion'. In this theory, special emotions are provoked by specific physiological response patterns. This theory was supported by Ax (1953) who investigated the emotions anger and anxiety—highly relevant for CBP patients—as well as their physiological responses. Anger was associated with a cardiovascular response pattern of increased diastolic blood pressure (BP) due to a hypothesized higher norepinephrine production. Anxiety was associated with an increase in heart rate (HR) and systolic BP attributed to higher epinephrine production. This seminal study was partially replicated by Berntson and co-workers (1998, 2003) who confirmed the car-diovascular response pattern for anxiety but not the mediating epinephrine hypothesis (Berntson et al. 1998). This group also provided mechanistic evidence for the role of norepinephrine, anxi-ety and pharmacological management. They proposed mediating mechanisms that include noradrenergic projections from the nucleus of the tractus solitarius and the locus coeruleus both to the amygdala in memory processes, and the basal forebrain in the processing of anxiety-related information (Berntson et al. 2003). These studies used only cardiovascular variables to define anxiety or anger response patterns. Other important parameters (i.e. muscle tension, breathing, or skin conductance level) were not examined. The concept of a stimulus-specific response pat-tern offers a new approach that describes the interaction between emotion, cardiovascular system and pain perception. The empirical results supporting the stimulus-specific response pattern suggest that psychophysiological response patterns are determined mainly by phylogenetically significant conditions such as fright, sexual arousal, or pain.

The *individual-specific response* pattern may reflect increased or decreased response systems. Lacey and colleagues (1953) defined the increased response system in stress situation as '*response stereotypy*', proposing a connection to causes of the disease. The individual-specific response indicates that an individual shows the same stereotypical physiological response pattern (e.g. sympathetic or parasympathetic) to varied stressors such as cold pressure, mental arithmetic, hyperventilation, word-association (Lacey et al 1953). The organ with the most frequent responses in these different stress situations has the highest risk for development of a disease (Lacey et al. 1953).

An important study reported by Malmo and Shagass (1949) showed that painful stimulation activated the same functional systems that mediate clinical symptoms in psychophysiological disorders, for example cardiovascular disorders or tension headache. The authors termed this specific response as a '*symptom specificity*' that describes the *reactivity* of one functional system. Hodapp et al. (1975) and Johannes et al. (2003) demonstrated that patients with hypertension respond with higher BP increases in stress situations compared to normotensive individuals. This symptom specificity is not limited to psychophysiological disorders. Patients with non-psychophysiological diseases, such as the inflammatory rheumatic diseases of rheumatoid arthritis and systemic lupus erythematosus, also respond with BP reactivity and showed a highly significant correlation with pain sensitivity. Johannes and colleagues (2003), who examined BP and additionally HR, skin conductance level (SCL), electromyogram (EMG) and voice pitch found four psychophysiological response patterns.

Thieme and Turk (2006) used a similar design as Johannes et al. (2003) to investigate the stress reactivity of fibromyalgia (FM) patients and healthy controls. They replicated the same four response patterns with high BP, low BP, high SCL, and high EMG-reactivity identified by Johannes et al. Further, this psychophysiological study found that only BP reactivity in patients with chronic musculoskeletal pain appears to be positively related to pain intensity (Thieme et al. submitted). These results were confirmed by Bragdon et al. (2002) and Bruehl et al. (2002, 2005) who found chronic pain-related alterations in the BP–pain sensitivity relationship in patients with chronic pain. Several studies of patients suffering from CBP and temporomandibular joint disorders (TMJD) show an EMG-reactivity at the site of pain but not at distal sites (e.g. Burns 1997; Flor et al. 1992; Peters and Schmidt 1991). This EMG-reactivity is highly associated with pain sensitivity. Similar to the psychophysiological results in FM, Flor and Turk (1995) found that baseline levels are not generally elevated in chronic pain patients. They concluded that the presence of symptom-specific psychophysiological responses is more commonly observed. The intriguing results on psychophysiological reactivity patterns (e.g. Flor et al. 1992; Johannes et al. 2003; Thieme and Turk 2006) suggest that stress-related symptom specificity associated with the main symptom may indicate the aetiology of the painful condition, for example, EMG-reactivity with pain in CBP or BP-reactivity with pain in FM.

## 8.2 Assessment of stress-related psychophysiological reactions

### 8.2.1 Psychological factors in chronification of pain

As noted, stress may facilitate the development of chronic pain states, irrespective of aetiology (Jensen et al. 1991; Passatore and Roatta 2006). This 'chronification' of pain is influenced by psychological factors such as expectations, cognitive self-statements, learning and by comorbidity associated with stressful situations reviewed above. Based on the assumptions above, stress is the interaction between the person's psychological and physiological response to a stressor.

The following considers the stressors of patients suffering from CBP such as psychosocial risk factors at work, pain behaviours, cognitions, and comorbidity.

## Psychosocial stressors in CBP

CBP stressors include work disability due to physical impairment, reduced free-time, and pain-related interference in family and social relationships. A growing body of evidence for *psychosocial risk factors at work* highlights high task demands, lack of support from colleagues, low job control, and low influence. The evidence for high job strain, low supervisor support, conflicts at work, low job security, and limited rest periods is inconclusive (Ariëns et al. 2001). There is interesting evidence for a relation between mental stress at work and upper extremity complaints (Malchaire et al. 2001; Bongers et al. 2002). An important mental stressor is related to 'mobbing/bullying' that is defined as psychological terror that involves hostile and unethical communication, social exclusion, active and passive obstruction in demanding working tasks. Bullying/mobbing can initiate and maintain a helpless and defenceless position, usually over a long period of time (statistical definition: at least 6 months of duration) (Lehmann 1996).

Bullying/mobbing and a loss of social support are thought to increase the risk of developing a CBP and other musculoskeletal disorders frequently in the neck/shoulder region, particularly in occupations of low physical demand (Wærsted 2000).

The primary consequences of psychosocial stressors are reduced activity and absence from work, interpreted as pain-avoidance behaviours mediated by fear and anger (Anderson 1999) associated with an increased cardiovascular stress response (Berntson et al. 2003). The 1988 National Health Interview Survey (1985–88) indicated that women with CBP experienced 56% days of restricted activity (Praemer et al 1992). Patients returning to work after 6 months absence had 68% lost work days (Rossignol et al. 1988). Interestingly, the precipitating event, diagnosis, and prescribed treatment do not influence treatment outcome, while a specific aetiological diagnosis, older age, previous back pain, and psychosocial distress and psychological disturbance and disorder are negatively associated with recovery (Van Doorn 1995; Greenough, 1993). Compensation that is only loosely linked to the presence of physical pathology has been show to prolong disability in numerous studies. For example, in a retrospective cohort study of 300 patients in Adelaide, Australia, the average time off work for men with compensation was a year versus a week for men with no compensation, despite comparable levels of objective pathology. For women with comparable injuries, the corresponding off-work periods were 15 months versus 2 weeks (Greenough et al. 1993). The location of symptom onset is also influential, work-related back symptoms result in longer absence from work than non-work-related symptoms, even after controlling for the influence of the physical work environment (Leavitt 1992).

It is not surprising that social problems at the workplace and the associated financial problems, anger, fear and maladaptive pain cognitions provoke distress in the family (Pienimäki et al. 2002; Schneider et al. 2005). Chronic pain has a negative impact on relationship satisfaction (Cano 2000, 2004; Flor et al. 1987, 1992; Kerns 1990). This association is bidirectional; the quality of relationships may affect pain experience associated with psychophysiological responses (Cano 2004a, Flor et al. 1987, Kerns and Turk 1987) such as increased cortisol and blood pressure response (Carels et al. 1998; Heffner et al. 2004). Psychological distress impairs activities of daily life (Ryan et al. 2010) and decreases amount of free-time, affecting individual-specific stress reactivity.

## Personality

A pain- or CBP-personality has not been identified. A specific complex of behaviours seems to be reflective rather of a general chronification syndrome (Hildebrandt and Franz 1988).

Interestingly, many of these behaviours would be described by patients as 'good' behaviours. Using a qualitative analyses of both anamnestic and standardized questionnaires data in 104 CBP patients, Hildebrandt and Franz (1988) identified three behavioural patterns that appear as if they would characterize healthy behaviours yet actually maintain chronic pain: (1) consistent performance; (2) readiness to help others; and (3) avoidance of conflicts. Performance pressure and suppressing of emotions to avoid conflicts are strongly associated with psychophysiological stress responses such as increased skin conductance level (SCL), heart rate (HR) and BP (see also, Johannes et al. 2003; Thieme et al. 2006).

These patients described themselves as 'always busy', hard-working employees with high performance expectations and their identity is related strongly to their work. They characterized their lives by early acceptance of responsibility, destitution, and fighting to survive. The fixation on work as the centre of their life reduced their enjoyment of success and relaxation. Eighty per cent of the CBP patients ranked 'ready to help others' as a primary goal. The prevalent 'helper role' was associated with needs that are ignored and not perceived, and rejecting help from others. These patients failed to present an adequate, self-protective and assertive approach to environmental demands. Yet, the patients view themselves in a positive way, as they avoid conflicts by excessive adaptation or by adapting a helper-role. The tendency to avoid conflicts suggests inhibition and deficits in social competence that has been confirmed by standardized test inventories (e.g. Asmundson et al. 1995; Hildebrandt et al. 1997). Psychophysiological experiments using social conflicts to provoke a temporary emotional deprivation showed an increase of EMG, BP, and HR in those participants who avoided the expression of emotions. In contrast, participants with lower psychophysiological responses were able to perceive and express anger and fear necessary to solve social conflicts (Flor et al. 1995; Shapiro et al. 1996). The connection of pain and the cardiovascular system is described below.

## Cognitions

Cognitions powerfully influence pain perception. Prominent cognitions in CBP include pain-related fear (Leeuw et al. 2007; Woby et al. 2007), catastrophizing (Cano 2004; Vowles et al. 2007) and control over pain (Haythornthwaite et al. 1998; LaChapelle et al. 2001). In comparison to a number of biomedical indices, Waddell et al. (1993) reported that *fear-avoidance beliefs* about work comprised the most specific and powerful factor accounting for disability and work loss. These pain related avoidance beliefs are related to fear of movements, fear of pain, and fear of work-related activities. CBP patients may have high or minimal levels of kinesiophobia. Fear of movement is strongly connected with the presence of pain behaviours as an expression of operant conditioning. The different level of subconscious learning in patients with chronic pain suggests the heterogeneity of chronic pain that may be manifest not only in physical but also in pain-specific fear-avoidance beliefs.

Catastrophizing describes a cognitive style that attributes the most negative interpretation among a range of possible interpretations of an event. Flor and Turk (1988) found that the combination of situation-specific variables such as *catastrophizing* and general cognitive variables explained between 32–60% of the variance in pain and disability, respectively. Turner et al (2002) replicated these results and reported that pain coping and catastrophizing explain an additional 29% of the variance in pain intensity and 30% of the variance in psychological distress. Hanley et al. (2008) found that increases in catastrophizing and lack of belief in one's ability to control pain were each significantly associated with greater pain interference and poorer psychological functioning. In contrast, changes in specific coping strategies and social support were not predictors of changes in pain, interference, or psychological functioning (Hanley et al. 2008), particularly social support provided by someone who is involved in a patient's daily life. Of course, not all styles of partner support are adaptive!

Perceived control, independent of other variables, is associated with greater use of cognitive and social coping strategies (i.e. asking for assistance, seeking social support and coping self-statements) (LaChapelle et al. 2001). Coping self-statements and reinterpreting pain sensations predicted greater perceptions of control over pain, whereas ignoring pain sensations predicted lower perceptions of control over pain (Haythornthwaite et al. 1998).

## Psychosocial adaptation

Several studies have generally replicated the psychosocial subgroups determined originally by Turk's (1996) cluster analysis of responses to the Multidimensional Pain Inventory (MPI). Asmundson et al. (1997) found three groups: One group, labelled *dysfunctional* (34.9%), experienced higher than average pain severity, pain interference, affective distress, higher solicitous response from their spouses, and lower levels of self-efficacy and general activity. A second subgroup comprised 24.3% of the CBP patients. This *interpersonally distressed* group reported moderate pain severity and lower perceived social support by significant others who instead responded with more punishing responses. This group had fewer solicitous or distracting responses from their spouses and highest levels of activity and affective distress. The third group, *adaptive copers* (40.8%), was characterized by lower pain severity, pain interference and affective distress, and higher levels of self-efficacy and general activity. Spousal behaviour was characterized as distracting more than solicitous.

An analysis of patients with spinal cord injuries (SCI) also found 3 subgroups (Widerström-Noga et al. 2007). In addition to the dysfunctional and an adaptive patterns found by Turk et al (1996), this analysis found an *interpersonally supported* (33%), instead of an interpersonally distressed, subgroup characterized by moderately high pain severity, higher life control, support from significant others with more distracting and solicitous responses, and higher activities scores. In that injury condition, negative or punishing spouse responses were not observed.

Carels et al. (1998) reported significant increases in BP after stress associated with recalling a marital conflict. Heffner et al. (2004) who also investigated sympathetic responses in 'healthy' couples identified a relationship between lower spousal support satisfaction and higher affective distress as well as higher cortisol production associated with BP reactivity.

Asmundson et al. (1997) showed that psychosocial adaptation is associated with different dimensions of pain-specific cognitions regarding fear and avoidance. In contrast to interpersonally-distressed and adaptive copers, patients with dysfunctional strategies reported greater *pain-specific cognitive fear*, e.g. 'I can't think straight when in pain', and cognitions regarding *physiological anxiety*, e.g. 'I begin trembling when engaged in an activity which increases pain', more cognitions of *escape/avoidance behaviour*, e.g. 'When I feel pain I try to stay as still as possible', and elevated *fearful appraisals of pain*, e.g. 'When I feel pain, I am afraid something terrible will happen'. In contrast, negative responses by a partner that provoke less active coping (Thieme et al. 2004) are frequently associated with depression and both were found to mediate the association between pain and relationship satisfaction, with negative responses emerging as the most important mediator (Waxman et al. 2008). Considering that cognitions influence pain behaviours, the heterogeneity of cognitions in CBP patients suggests heterogeneous pain perception and avoidance behaviour that determines different subgroups based on those cognitions and behaviours.

## Pain behaviour

Pain behaviours are influenced by significant others and by dysfunctional strategies. Solicitous responses by significant others have been found to be positively associated with higher ratings of pain severity, greater disability, decreased activity levels, and more pain and avoidance behaviours (Flor et al. 1995; Lousberg et al. 1992). Vlaeyen et al. (1995) proposed that avoidance, arising from beliefs that activity will produce pain and suffering, leads to a vicious cycle characterized by decreased self-efficacy, fear, and further avoidance as well as disability. This cycle is maintained by the momentary reduction of anxiety attained through avoidance of feared and/or undesirable activities. Flor and colleagues (1987) have shown that CBP patients with a solicitous partner show higher pain behaviour than patients with a distracting or punishing spouse.

CBP patients with dysfunctional strategies reported more pain-specific fear and avoidance as well as catastrophizing than did those classified as interpersonally distressed or as adaptive copers (Asmundson et al. 1997). The lower activity in the dysfunctional subgroup is associated with disuse and deconditioning. The presence of persistent low back pain leads to avoidance of daily activities, which may lead to physical deconditioning, both generally such as loss of cardiovascular capacity and as specifically such as loss of strength and endurance of paraspinal muscles (Smeets et al. 2006, Verbunt et al. 2003), linked with increased muscular and cardiovascular responses in physical stress situations. Pain catastrophizing and fear of physical activity exacerbate pain, promoting a self-perpetuating cycle of avoidance, hypervigilance, depression, disuse, and pain (Vlaeyen et al. 1995). Catastrophizing is related to higher SCL and HR response (Bartley and Rhudy 2008). These deconditioning models are based on classical and operant conditioning, and the influence of cognitive, affective, and physical variables (Thieme et al. 2004; Turk and Okifuji 1997).

In conclusion, similar to cognitions and psychosocial adaptation, heterogeneous pain behaviours result from different psychobiological mechanisms. These differences likely provide a rational basis for classification of subgroups in CBP.

## Comorbidity

CBP is associated with comorbid anxiety (30.9–95%), depression (32–54%) and addictive behaviour (64–95%). The first episode of major depression follows pain onset in 58.1% of patients (Atkinson et al. 1991; Polatin et al. 1993), commencing within the first 2 years of established pain. Anxiety disorders followed a similar pattern in terms of rates of onset before or after pain, and of increased risk of 'new' cases during the 2 years immediately following back injury. Alcohol use disorder usually precedes pain onset considerably. However, the pooled life time prevalence of psychiatric illnesses in chronic pain patients is not significantly different than that of non-pain subjects. There is little evidence for factors that differentiate depressed from non-depressed chronic pain patients (Haley et al. 1985; Sullivan et al. 2000). Further studies are needed to examine the relationship between comorbidity and pain. The data suggest that substance abuse and anxiety disorders precede chronic low-back pain, whereas depression may develop before or after onset (Andersson 2000).

Since patients with physical comorbidities appear to adapt to CBP, the presence of psychiatric disorders likely interferes with this adaptation. Increasing evidence suggests that the tendency to fear pain and to avoid pain and pain-related situations is mediated in part by anxiety sensitivity (Asmundson and Norton 1995; Asmundson and Taylor 1996), a dispositional trait-like tendency to respond fearfully to anxiety-related symptoms, and also to social situations (Asmundson et al. 1996; Vlaeyen 1999).

## Summary

Stress variables influencing CBP are *psychosocial risk factors at work* such as high quantitative demands, lack of support from colleagues, low job control and low influence, *cognitions* such as fear-avoidance beliefs, catastrophizing vs. active coping, and *pain and avoidance behaviours* reinforced by spousal responses at home and causing disuse and deconditioning. These pain-related variables can be exacerbated by psychiatric disorders such as depression, anxiety, and substance dependence. The next section presents their relationship to physiological responses.

## 8.2.2 **Psychophysiological variables**

### Static and dynamic postures

Presently, the high incidence of muscular (myalgia-type) disorders in individuals employed in light industrial work has no satisfactory explanation. The biomechanical model assumes that static and dynamic posture influence muscle tension and pain perception, and predicts an increased EMG associated with the experience of pain after physical activity.

Of 38 studies reviewed, only 17 evaluated both static and dynamic postures (Table 8.1). A concordance between surface electromyographic (sEMG) responses of both conditions was reported in 52.9% of the studies. Forty-seven per cent reported that sEMG of CBP and pain-free control participants were similar during static postures such as standing but different during dynamic postures such as flexion and extension. These results suggest that subgroups based on movement sEMG may be relevant for diagnosis and treatment. Thirty-five studies reported sEMG responses during static and dynamic postures. Surprisingly, only 29% of these reported significantly higher sEMG-responses in CBP patients during dynamic postures (highlighted in grey in Table 8.1), however 43% showed less erector spinae activity in CBP patients than in pain-free controls, and 29% could not find any differences in muscle tension between CBP patients and pain-free controls during both static and dynamic postures. Arena et al. (1989) divided the CBP sample into spondylarthritis, intervertebral disc disorder, and unspecified musculoskeletal backache, and found that spondylarthritis patients and PFCs had lower muscle tension during dynamic postures in comparison to intervertebral disc disorder and unspecified musculoskeletal backache patients. The presence of diagnostic subgroups in CBP may explain these varied EMG responses.

The findings of sEMG-reactivity after dynamic postures in 30% of the studies in Table 8.1 suggest that the reflex-spasm-approach may be relevant for one subgroup of CBP patients. Unfortunately, sEMG and pain intensity were associated in only one study (Ahern et al. 1988) that observed a positive correlation between sEMG and pain (Table 8.1). Physiological maladaptations may be the reason: the agonist muscle contractions were still maintained while antagonist muscles were already activated (Radebold et al 2000, 2001). The agonist muscles did not show the expected pattern of sEMG responses during trunk rotation, most likely because of restricted range of motion and/or compensatory posturing as pain-maintaining sEMG-pattern (Ahern et al. 1988). Patients with higher sEMG maintained an increased level of muscle activity after lifting objects (Soderberg et al. 1983). In addition, most patients were not capable to show different EMG-responses in flexion or relaxation conditions.

Moseley et al. (2004) proposed an altered postural mechanism as a further explanation for the transition from acute to chronic pain. They suggest that these alterations serve to protect the spine in the short-term, but increased vulnerability to injury in the long-term. They showed an increased activity of superficial trunk muscles during anticipation of experimental back pain in healthy subjects. Moseley et al. (2004) concluded that the anticipation of back pain could evoke a protective posture that stiffens the spine.

The postural changes are associated with expectations. Anticipatory postural adjustments (APAs) of trunk-stabilizing muscles result in a feed-forward function in lateral abdominal muscles during rapid arm movements. (Hodges et al. 2001). Sprott and colleagues used a new method for the non-invasive determination of abdominal muscle feed-forward activity based on tissue Doppler imaging (TDI, Mannion et al. 2008) as shown in Figure 8.1. The patients with CBP did not have a delayed-onset of feed-forward activation but rather an earlier activation of abdominal muscle activity. Further, the onset of muscle activity was not associated with clinical variables (pain, disability, etc.). The authors proposed that APAs depend on the postural set, therefore the individual's perception of their steady-state postural equilibrium and quality of external support

**Table 8.1** EMG measured during static (SP) and dynamic postures (DP)

| Study | Sample size | Stressor | Baseline CBP vs HC | EMG-reactivity CBP vs HC | Relationship between pain and baseline | Relationship between Pain and EMG- reactivity | Comorbidity |
|---|---|---|---|---|---|---|---|
| Ahern et al. 1988 | CBP=40 HC=40 | Standing, flexion/ extension, rotation | ns | SP: CBP<HC DP: CBP>HC | na | yes | Pain behaviour |
| Alexiev, 1994 | CBP=40 (acute) HC=40 | Standing, isometric muscle activity | na | SP: ns DP: ns higher EMG on painful site | na | na | na |
| Ambroz et al. 2000 | CBP=30 HC=30 | Standing, flexion/ extension | na | SP: CBP > HC DP: CBP > HC | na | na | na |
| Arena et al. 1989 | CBP=178 (3 groups: SA, IDD, UMB) HC=29 | Standing, bending, rising, unsupported sitting, supported sitting, and prone | EMG HC< IDD, UMB | SP: CBP > HC DP: IDD, UMB > HC, SA | na | na | na |
| Arena et al. 1990 | CBP=29 HC=20 | Standing, bending, rising, unsupported sitting, supported sitting, and prone during two testing sessions | na | SP: ns DP: ns | na | na | na |
| Arena et al. 1991 | CBP=46 (2 groups : IDD, UMB) HC=20 | Standing, bending, rising, unsupported sitting, supported sitting, and prone. CBP were tested while having high and low pain | na | SP: CBP > HC DP: IDD > HC UMB ns HC CBP with low compared to high pain: ns | na | na | na |
| Capodaglio and Nilsson, 1996 | CBP=4 HC=4 | Isometric contraction | na | SP: na DP: ns | na | na | na |

| Study | Sample | Task | | Results | | | |
|---|---|---|---|---|---|---|---|
| Cassisi et al. 1993 | CBP=21 HC=12 | Sitting, maximal isometric exertion | na | SP: CBP < HC / DP: CBP < HC | na | na | na |
| Cram and Steger 1983 | CBP=33 (3 groups: UBP, LBP, MBP) HA=12 | flexion/extension, rotation | ns | SP: ns / DP: CBP > HA / For bilateral levels in lumbar and cervical paraspinal muscle groups / DP: CBP < HA / For bilateral levels in frontalis and masseter groups | na | na | na |
| Elfing et al 2003 | CBP=57 HC=55 | Seated isometric trunk extension | na | SP: na / DP: ns | na | na | na |
| Hoyt et al. 1981 | CBP= HC= | flexion/extension, rotation | EMG ns | SP: na / DP: CBP > HC | na | na | na |
| Jalovaara et al. 1995 | CBP=18 HC=11 | Standing | na | SP: CBP > HC DP: na | na | na | na |
| Kankaanpää et al. 1998 | CBP=20 HC=15 | Isometric contraction | na | SP: na / DP: ns | na | na | na |
| Klein et al. 1991 | CBP=8 HC=17 | Isometric contraction | na | SP: na / DP: ns | na | na | na |
| Kravitz et al. 1981 | CBP= HC= | flexion/extension, rotation | EMG ns | SP: na / DP: CBP > HC | na | na | na |
| Lee et al. 1992 | CBP=8 HC=10 | Prone, isometric holds with torso unsupported | na | SP: na / DP: ns | na | na | na |
| Leinonen et al. 2001 | CBP=20 HC=15 | Expected and unexpected loading of the upper extremities while sitting and standing | na | SP: ns / DP: ns / ns between expected and nonexpected loading in CBP | na | na | na |

*(Continued)*

**Table 8.1** (continued) EMG measured during static (SP) and dynamic postures (DP)

| Study | Sample size | Stressor | Baseline CBP vs HC | EMG-reactivity CBP vs HC | Relationship between pain and baseline | Relationship between Pain and EMG- reactivity | Comorbidity |
|---|---|---|---|---|---|---|---|
| Lisiński, 2000 | CBP=62 HC=31 | Prone, isometric hold for 2 seconds with torso unsupported | | SP: na DP: CBP < HC | na | na | na |
| Lofland et al, 2000 | CBP (high)=18 CBP (low)=33 HC=30 | Standing | na | SP: CBP (high) > CBP (low) and CBP (high) > HC DP: na | na | na | na |
| Lu et al. 2001 | CBP=20 HC=20 | Standing in postural restraint device, performing lifts with and without trunk rotation | na | SP: ns DP: CBP > HC | na | na | na |
| Mayer et al. 1989 | CBP=10 HC=11 | Prone, isometric hold for 15 seconds with torso unsupported. Two 10-consecutive-trial sessions | na | SP: ns DP: CBP < HC | na | na | na |
| Miller, 1985 | CBP=11 HC=11 | Sitting, standing, active sitting | na | SP: ns DP: ns | na | na | na |
| Ng et al. 2002 | CBP=12 HC=12 | Axial rotation while standing at different levels of effort | na | SP: na DP: CBP < HC | na | na | na |
| Pääsuke et al. 2002 | CBP=12 HC=12 | Prone, isometric hold with torso unsupported | na | SP: na DP: CBP < HC Lower time endurance in CBP | na | na | Fatigue |
| Peach and McGill, 1998 | CBP=21 HC=18 | Semistanding | na | SP: na DP: ns | na | na | na |

| Study | Sample | Task | | SP/DP | | | |
|---|---|---|---|---|---|---|---|
| Robinson et al. 1992 | CBP=16 HC=12 | Sitting, repetitive concentric and eccentric contractions with light and heavy resistance | na | SP: ns<br>DP: CBP < HC | na | na | na |
| Roy et al. 1989 | CBP=12 HC=12 | Standing, isometric muscle activity | na | SP: ns<br>DP: CBP < HC | na | na | na |
| Roy et al. 1990 | CBP=6 HC=17 | Standing, isometric muscle activity | na | SP: ns<br>DP: CBP < HC<br>CBP had higher recovery time | na | na | na |
| Roy et al. 1995 | A : CBP=28 HC=42<br>B : CBP=57 HC=6 | Standing, isometric muscle activity | na | SP: ns<br>DP: CBP < HC | na | na | na |
| Shirado et al. 1995 | CBP=20 HC=25 | Flexion and extension | na | SP: na<br>DP: CBP < HC | na | na | na |
| Silvonen et al. 1991 | CBP=87 HC=25 | Flexion and extension | na | SP: na<br>DP: CBP > HC | na | na | na |
| Silvonen et al. 1998 | Pregnant CBP=21 Pregnant HC=32 | Flexion and extension | na | SP: CBP > HC<br>DP: CBP > HC | na | na | na |
| Soderberg and Barr 1983 | CBP=25 HC=20 | Flexion and extension | CBP>HC | SP: na<br>DP: CBP < HC | na | na | na |
| Suter and Lindsay, 2001 | CBP=25 HC=16 | Prone, isometric hold with torso unsupported | na | SP: na<br>DP: CBP < HC | na | na | na |
| Watson et al. 1997 | CBP=70 HC=20 | Flexion and extension | ns | SP: na<br>DP: CBP < HC | na | na | na |

(Continued)

**Table 8.1** (continued) EMG measured during static (SP) and dynamic postures (DP)

| Study | Sample size | | Stressor | Baseline CBP vs HC | EMG-reactivity CBP vs HC | Relationship between pain and baseline | Relationship between Pain and EMG- reactivity | Comorbidity |
|---|---|---|---|---|---|---|---|---|
| Collins et al. 1982 | CBP=11 | HC=11 | flexion/extension, rotation | ns | SCL DP: CBP > HC | na | na | na |
| Radebold et al. 2000 | CBP=17 | HC=17 | Standing, supported with feet off the ground | na | Slower muscle recovery time in CBP in agonist and antagonist muscles | na | na | na |
| Radebold et al. 2001 | CBP=16 | HC=14 | Standing, supported with feet off the ground | na | | na | na | na |

na: no assessed, ns: non-significant, SA: spondyloarthritis, IDD: intervertebral disc disorder, UMB: unspecified musculoskeletal backache, UBP : upper back pain, LBP : low back pain, MBP : mixed back pain, HA : headache

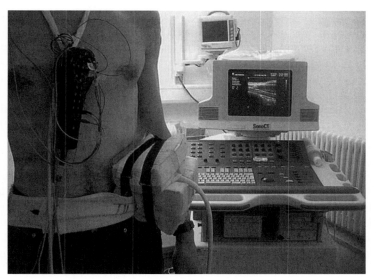

**Fig. 8.1** (Also see Colour Plate 5) Tissue Doppler imaging (TDI).

(Cordo et al. 1982), and that modifications to APAs are centrally mediated (Morris et al. 2006). Hence, it is conceivable that factors such as fear of pain, fear of movement, weakness, etc.— factors that might lead patients with CBP to expect that they will be less able to withstand challenges to postural stability—could precipitate the earlier APAs (Gubler et al. 2010).

The neurophysiological consequence of posture appears to be influenced by both neuropsychological and endocrine variables. Kravitz et al. (1980) showed that a flexed posture is associated with serotonin production and an extended posture is associated with octopamine production. An increased serotonin production is connected with emotional factors such as affective distress and anxiety that can influence the posture. A consequence of postural changes is muscle fatigue that is associated with significantly shorter endurance time and declining of sEMG spectral mean power frequency during performance of isometric contractions (Pääsuke et al. 2002). Two further studies of recovery time in agonist and antagonist muscles found that CBP need 30% more time than HC for recovery (Radebold et al. 2000, 2001).

These findings of enhanced sEMG activity during postural changes and an extended time for recovery provide support for the biomechanical model of chronic pain in only one subgroup of CBPs. The heterogeneous sEMG activity and earlier APAs indicate the need for further research pertaining to movement-related lumbar muscle activity and implicate the influence of cognitions and pain behaviour associated with pain-maintaining central changes (Aherns et al. 1988; Flor et al. 2002).

An extension to the myogenic model considered variables of HR and SCL as well as frontalis sEMG in addition to paraspinal sEMG. Those measures were recorded while CBP patients and pain-free controls were tested by three conditions of different postures, physiological and mental stress. Though differences were found between different postural categories, the CBP group exhibited similar or significantly less paraspinal muscle activity than the pain-free control group. In contrast, frontalis sEMG and skin conductance were significantly higher in the CBP group. SCL in CBP patients was enhanced by mental arithmetic and cold pressor stimulation. This study provides no support for the biomechanical reflex spasm theory of CBP suggesting an alternative explanation of an increased arousal response and altered ability to respond to demanding tasks, leading to pain and eventually to decreased paraspinal muscle activity (Collins et al. 1982).

In summary, there is a considerable incidence of myalgia-type disorders in light industrial work. In 38 studies of static and dynamic postures, less than 30% confirmed the assumption of increased muscle tension and pain as a reflex-spasm. Differences in sEMG activity in static and dynamic postures, in diagnoses of CBP, and the heterogeneity of stress-reactivity in sEMG and in other variables such as SCL challenge the assumption of a homogenous group of CBP. These differences and the further findings of altered APAs, the influence of attention and subconscious operant and classical conditioning, and the association of muscle tension and pain intensity strongly suggest that the population of CBP patients can be divided into several distinct subgroups.

## Symptom-specific psychophysiological response

Heterogeneous sEMG-responses in response to postural change suggest that the determining variables extend beyond physical workload to include psychological distress related to time pressure, low job satisfaction and lack of control of muscular tension (Waersted et al. 1991). To fully understand the high prevalence of musculoskeletal disorders associated with stressful work, it is important to explore the relationship between muscle activity and psychophysiological stress responses.

**Field studies** Rissén et al. (2000) evaluated trapezius sEMG activity, HR, BP, and levels of urinary catecholamines and salivary cortisol among 31 female supermarket employees suffering from neck and shoulder disorders. The participants had increased endocrine responses with elevated epinephrine, norepinephrine, and cortisol values. They also showed higher BP and HR and slightly enhanced sEMG and self-reported variables during a 2-hour work period in comparison to 1-hour defined rest period. The sEMG activity during work was significantly associated with self-reported negative stress (r=0.38–0.43) and with systolic BP (r=0.38). Associations were found also between BP and workload (r=0.43–0.57) as well as BP and urinary epinephrine (r=0.40) and norepinephrine (r=0.46) during work. No associations were found between sEMG activity and pain or workload defined as the numbers of customers and as the number and weight of the items that the participant lifted. Thus, perceived negative stress, but not workload, may have a specific influence on muscle activity. Further, the data showed a lack of association between clinical pain before work and higher sEMG activity during work. The association between workload and stress-induced sEMG may be mediated by a noradrenergic mechanism that impacts the BP response (e.g. Johannes et al 2003). Future studies may clarify the association between BP and pain in CBP.

The association between sEMG and negative stress is supported by other field studies. A 2-year prospective study (Heydari et al. 2010) investigated the association of CBP with sEMG variables over time in 120 healthcare workers. After 2 years, 17.2% of the group with no history of CBP deteriorated as measured by time off work, disability, reported pain and self-assessment rating. Several EMG variables were significantly associated with the outcome measures. The value of the EMG variable half-width (HW, measured as the width of the spectrum at half the maximum power) at inception demonstrated significant association with changes in outcome measures and self-assessments of CBP at follow up. CBP patients with a HW of greater than 56Hz were at threefold greater risk, and those with an initial median frequency greater than 49Hz were at a 5.8-fold greater risk of developing back pain.

The finding of increased low-level and long-lasting work-related muscle activity is often interpreted as representing solely biomechanical muscle load, ignoring the possibility of extra muscle activation due to nonbiomechanical factors (Waersted 2000). Several studies tend to support this assumption but the experimental data remain inconclusive (Waersted et al. 1991; Westgaárd and Bjøklund 1987).

**Experimental studies** Flor and Turk (1989) reviewed 59 studies published during 1975–1989 that evaluated psychophysiological responses of patients with chronic pain. This review included 8 studies with CBP patients that evaluated physical variables such as posture and psychological variables such as maladaptive cognitions. Only 30% of the studies reported an EMG-reactivity in CBP (Table 8.2). In one study (Flor et al. 1985), pain-free patients and patients with CBP or other pain disorders were asked to recall a very painful episode and a stressful event. Responses during this recall were compared to two other conditions: reciting the alphabet backwards and performing mental arithmetic. In comparison to controls, only the condition of recalling a pain episode and a stressful event was sufficient to increase the muscle tension of the erector spinae muscle in CBP patients. Frontalis-sEMG, HR and SCL were not significantly different among the three groups. In addition, tasks with high personal relevance, but not low personal relevance, provoked a muscular stress response, a finding described as 'muscular response stereotypy' (Flor et al. 1985).

In contrast to this important result of a symptom-specific stress response related to an emotional highly relevant individual state, two studies (Cohen et al. 1986; Collins et al. 1982) found similar or less paraspinal muscle activity in CBP and pain-free controls. Both studies used mental arithmetic as the psychological stressor. The participants did not receive any positive or negative responses that minimized the personal relevance of this task. This result supports previous data (Flor et al. 1985) that only personally important states provoke a symptom-specific psychophysiological response. The results suggest that social and emotional factors at work exert a much greater influence on maintenance of CBP symptoms than the level of work intensity. Collin's results (1982) also support the heterogeneity of CBP. Increased SCL, not sEMG, was associated with pain, suggesting that increased arousal response and altered ability to respond to demanding tasks leads to pain and to decreased paraspinal muscle activity.

The different sEMG and SCL responses, both at baseline and evoked by physical and psychological stressors, further suggest heterogeneity in CBP. There was little evidence for the hypothesis that varied CBP subgroups can be differentiated by levels of muscular activity. Baseline levels of activity, regardless of type of physiological measure, are not generally elevated in chronic pain patients, while symptom-specific stress-related psychophysiological responses are commonly observed. Future studies should examine if the baseline level is increased in the subgroup with muscular symptom-specific stress response in comparison to the subgroup with sudomotor stress response.

## Individual-specific psychophysiological response

What mediates individual psychophysiological responses to emotionally relevant stressors? Candidate mediators include anger, fear, and pain behaviour.

*Anger* appears to be an important consideration in the understanding of chronic pain. Over 70% of CBP patients report angry feelings (Okifuji et al. 1999). Most commonly, patients report that they are angry with themselves (74%) and with healthcare professionals (62%). The relevance of anger to chronic pain experience seems to vary across targets. Anger toward oneself is significantly associated with pain and depression, whereas overall anger is significantly related to perceived disability (Okifuji et al. 1999).

It is not just the experience of anger that is important for pain perception, but also the manner in which anger is typically managed (Burns et al. 1998; Kerns et al. 1994). Two styles of anger management have received particular attention: anger-in, the tendency to suppress anger when it is experienced, and anger-out, the tendency to express anger through verbal or physical means (Spielberger et al. 1985). In comparisons with non-pain participants, CBP patients have elevated levels of anger (Burns 1997; Fernandez and Turk 1995). Kerns et al. (1994) found that both

**Table 8.2** EMG measured during mental, physical and physiological stressors as well as pain induction and during sleep

| Study | Sample size | Stressor | Baseline CBP vs HC | Stress-reactivity CBP vs HC | Relationship between pain and baseline | Relationship between Pain and Stress reactivity | Comorbidity |
|---|---|---|---|---|---|---|---|
| **Controlled studies** | | | | | | | |
| Bonnet et al. 2004 | D-CBP=9 ND-CBP=9 D-HC=9 ND-HC=9 | Acoustic stimulation | SCL ND-CBP>rest | SCL ND-CBP>rest HC> D-CBP | Yes in D-CBP | Yes in D-CBP | Depression |
| Bruehl et al. 2006 | CBP=43 HC=45 | Pressure pain Ischemic pain Opioid blockade (8mg Naloxon) Placebo blockade | na | Absence of Opioid-Analgesia in CBP | na | yes | Anger-Out |
| Cohen et al. 1986 | CBP=13 HC=13 | Dynamic postures Mental arithmetic Cold pressure | ns | EMG ns | na | no | no psychiatric comorbidity |
| Collins et al. 1982 | CBP=11 HC=11 | Dynamic postures Mental arithmetic | ns | SCL CBP > HC | na | na | no psychiatric comorbidity |
| DeGood et al. 1994 | CBP=20 (disabling, non-disabling) HC=12 | Mental stress | ns | EMG CBP > HC (disabling) | na | na | na |
| Fischer and Chang 1985 | CBP=9 HC=12 | Sleep | na | EMG CBP > HC | na | na | na |
| Flor et al. 1985 | CBP=17 HC=17 | Talk about stress Talk about pain Mental arithmetic Reciting an alphabet | EMG CBP > HC | EMG CBP > HC | no | yes | Depression |
| Lundberg et al. 1999 | CBP=50 HC=22 | Mental Arithmetic STROOP Cold Pressure Test Test contractions | na | EMG | na | na | Stress |

| Study | Sample | Task / Stimulus | | | | | |
|---|---|---|---|---|---|---|---|
| Peters and Schmidt 1991 | CBP=20 HC=20 | Pressure pain stimuli | SCL CBP > HC | SCL CBP > HC | no | Yes for HC | na |
| Peters and Schmidt 1999 | CBP=20 HC=20 | Pressure pain | EMG ns. | EMG CBP < HC | no | no | Anxiety Depression |
| Sjörs et al. 2009 | CBP=18 HC=30 | Baseline rest Repetitive low-force work Trierer Stress–Test Recovery | EMG CBP > HC | EMG CBP > HC | no | yes | Anxiety |
| Tousignant-Laflamme and Marchand, 2006 | f-CBP=14 m-CBP=16 | Pressure pain as clinical pain Thermal pain as experimental pain | HR ns SCL ns | HR f < m SCL f > m | na | yes (HR) no (SCL) | na |
| Vlaeyen et al. 1999 | HF-CBP=16 LF-CBT=15 | Fear-eliciting video presentation vs. neutral nature documentary | EMG ns | EMG ns | na | yes | Fear Negative Affectivity |
| **Uncontrolled studies** | | | | | | | |
| Burns et al. 1997 | CBP=107 | Mental Arithmetic Anger recall interview | EMG | EMG Stress > Baseline | no | yes | Depression |
| Burns 1997 | CBP=102 | Mental Arithmetic Anger recall interview | EMG | EMG Stress > Baseline | no | yes | Anger Hostility |
| Geisser at al. 1995 | CBP=21 | Field study (8.1 h) Physical activity Psychosocial Stress | na | EMG | na | no | na |
| Rissen et al 2000 | CBP=31 | Field study: Repetitive physical work | EMG | EMG Stress > Baseline | na | no | Negative Stress at work |

na: not assessed, ns: non-significant, D-CBP: depressed CBP, ND-CBP: non-depressed CBP, D-HC: depressed HC, ND-HC: non-depressed HC, f-CBP: female CBP, m-CBP: male CBP, HF-CBP: high-fear CBP, LF-CBP: low-fear CBP 'anger-in' (toward self) and 'anger-out' (toward external agents or events) showed significant positive associations with ratings of pain intensity in a sample of CBP patients. High levels of anger-out have been shown to be associated with low levels of improvement in lifting capacity, and high levels of anger-in with low levels of improvement in activity levels among chronic pain patients undergoing multidisciplinary pain treatment (Burns et al. 1998). Psychophysiological studies with pain-free controls showed that experimental induced anger was associated with increased pain sensitivity to ischemic pain induction, and less control of anger has associated with lower pain and tolerance thresholds (Gehlkopf et al. 1997; Janssen et al. 2001). Overall, the available data strongly suggest that anger and anger management style may affect pain and functioning in chronic pain sufferers.

Anger style influences muscle reactivity. Higher levels of anger-out were associated with greater increases in lower paraspinal muscle activity, but not trapezius muscle activity, during an anger recall interview among men with chronic LBP (Burns 1997). Thus, anger-out could influence the development or maintenance of chronic pain through selective effects of increased muscle tension at the site of injury or disorder. In contrast, Janssen et al. (2001) found another type of symptom-specific stress reactivity to anger. They observed increased cardiovascular reactivity in pain-free subjects after anger induction by harassing comments presented in computer tasks. The cardiovascular measures and pain sensitivity were higher during harassment than during the neutral situation. Harassment appears to inhibit pain through physiological mechanisms. This effect is consistent with evidence that high BP reactivity is associated with lower sensitivity to pain, possibly resulting from baroreceptor stimulation. According to the results of studies that show diminished baroreceptor sensitivity in chronic pain patients, CBP patients with cardiovascular stress reactivity in anger situations should experience increased pain related to anger.

The relationship between anger and both acute and chronic pain sensitivity may be related to endogenous opioid dysfunction. Subjects with higher anger exhibit impaired endogenous opioid inhibition of cardiovascular responses to a painful stressor (Bruehl et al. 1996). The high anger-out scores were associated with an absence of opioid analgesia during acute pain tasks; low anger-out scores were associated with effective opioid analgesia–similar to that of pain-free controls. These findings suggest that anger-in and anger-out affect pain sensitivity through different mechanisms. Anger-out may be mediated by endogenous opioid dysfunction (Bruehl et al. 2002a). Anger-in may result from depressed affect (Tschannen et al. 1992) and its biochemical sequelae. These results are consistent with the hypothesis that anger-related variables may affect pain through an association with endogenous opioid dysfunction and impair the psychological adaptation to chronic pain.

**Fear and pain avoidance behaviour** The 'fear-avoidance model of exaggerated pain perception' (Lethem et al. 1983), and the more recent 'cognitive model of fear of movement/(re)injury' address the important topic of pain-related fear and avoidance behaviour (Vlaeyen et al. 1995). The central concept of these models is fear of pain, or the more specific fear that physical activity will cause (re)injury. Two opposing behavioural responses to these fears are confrontation and avoidance (Crombez et al. 1999). 'Confrontation' may lead to adaptive responses which may lead to the reduction of fear and the promotion of recovery. In contrast, 'avoidance' leads to the maintenance or exacerbation of fear, possibly resulting in a phobic state. Avoidance behaviour is strongly connected with fear-avoidance beliefs associated with higher pain perception and less range of motion seen during a procedure involving a passive but painful straight leg raising test (McCracken et al. 1992). Fear-avoidance beliefs about work are strongly related to disability in daily living and lost work days in the past year, and less related to pain variables such as anatomical pattern of pain, time pattern, and pain severity (Waddell et al. 1993). Using the Tampa-Scale for Kinesiophobia (TSK), Vlaeyen et al. (1995) found that fear of movement/(re)injury was the most powerful predictor of the performance in a simple weight lifting task. Patients were asked to stand and lift a 5.5-kg bag with the dominant arm and hold it until pain or physical discomfort made it impossible for the patient to continue. This performance test showed differences in behavioural performance between patients with lower and higher fear of movement, with lower behavioural performance related to higher fear of movement/(re)injury. Interestingly, fear was higher after the performance test than before the test. Consistent with the delayed perception of fear, no significant correlations were found between changes in the psychophysiological variables of heart rate and skin conductance and fear beliefs. A systematic increase in heart rate and skin conductance was not observed. Similarly, no significant differences in heart rate and skin conductance were found between patients with low and high levels of fear beliefs. One possible explanation is that behavioural avoidance occurred before psychophysiological arousal levels increased, i.e. patients may think that short-term avoidance of movement prevents injury or an increase in pain, a process of 'cognitive avoidance'. Patients showed avoidance behaviour before they noticed their anxious feelings. In addition, higher avoidance behaviour was associated with prolonged pain complaints, possibly because delayed perception of fear permits a subconscious avoidance behaviour associated with increased pain. Both feelings of fear and psychophysiological stress responses may be delayed, explaining why pain is perceived only after physical activities. These results are consistent with classical conditioning models in which pain is associated with a fear response and an urge to avoid the pain. Avoidance and pain behaviour may also be explained by operant conditioning. An experiment with 30 CBP patients and 30 matched healthy controls investigated learning rates and extinction of verbal and cortical pain responses after operant conditioning. Half of each group was reinforced for increased, and half for decreased, pain reports during recording of EEG and muscle tension. Both groups showed similar learning rates, however, the CBP patients displayed slower extinction of both the verbal and the cortical (N150) pain response. In addition, the CBP group displayed prolonged elevated EMG levels to the task. These data suggest that CBP patients are more easily influenced by operant conditioning factors than healthy controls and this susceptibility may add to the maintenance of the chronic pain problem (Flor et al. 2002).

In summary, musculoskeletal pain is often exacerbated by mental and social stress and psychophysiological mechanisms may play an important role in the development and maintenance of chronic pain states. The heterogeneity of pain behaviours, anger expression, and fear beliefs in CBP patients likely leads to different levels of classical and operant conditioning.

## 8.3 Interaction between pain regulatory and cardiovascular systems: a new approach

Several studies indicate that resting BP levels may be elevated in patients with CBP (Brody et al. 1997, Lundberg et al. 1999, Nilsson et al. 1997) including pharmacological studies with the exclusion criteria of 'hypertension' in CBP patients (Ongley et al. 1987). In a study of 300 patients with chronic pain and 300 patients in a non-pain group, 39% of the pain patients were diagnosed with clinical hypertension, compared with 21% in the non-pain group (Bruehl et al. 2005). Within chronic pain patients, higher systolic blood pressure, along with higher BMI and more pronounced metabolic disturbances have been observed with more intense pain (Nilsson et al. 1997). BP is associated with muscle tension in patients suffering from neck and shoulder pain, and with levels of norepinephrine which plays an important role in BP homeostasis (Lundberg et al. 1999). These studies support the role of BP in pain chronification.

An important component of the pain regulatory system is the interaction of pain sensitivity and cardiovascular response. This interaction is influenced by baroreceptor activity, which inhibits activity in the ascending reticular activating system. The net result is modulation of pain inhibition by multiple factors (Angrilli et al. 1997 ; Bruehl et al. 2004 ; Droste et al. 1994; Dworkin et al. 1994 ; Maixner 1991; Mini et al. 1995; Rau and Elbert 2001).

In healthy individuals, there is a *functional* interaction between the cardiovascular and pain regulatory systems that results in an inverse relationship between resting blood pressure levels and acute pain sensitivity (Dworkin et al. 1994; Myers et al. 2001; Zamir and Schuber 1980). Baroreceptor activation leads to the activation of descending pain inhibitory systems that decreases acute pain sensitivity and result in progressive adaptation to repeated pain stimuli (Villanueva and Bars 1995; Kleinboehl et al. 1999; Peters et al. 1989; Millan 2002). This *baroreflex mechanism* may explain hypertensive hypoalgesia in normotensive individuals (e.g. Bruehl et al. 1992; Ghione et al. 1996).

In contrast, patients with CBP display a lack of the inverse relationship between BP and pain intensity (Bragdon et al. 2002; Bruehl et al. 2002; Maixner et al. 1997). This lack of inverse relationship may be related to: (1) impairments in the descending pain inhibitory pathways normally activated by increased baroreceptor stimulation (Maixner et al. 1995; Millan 2002); (2) increased activity in descending facilatory mechanisms; or (3) diminished baroreceptor sensitivity (Bruehl and Chung 2004).

While coordinated cardiovascular-pain regulatory responses may be part of an adaptive mechanism that helps the body to face stressful events in pain-free individuals, the *dysfunctional* inverse relationship of BP and pain has been found to be maladaptive with central sensitization and increased wind-up (Eide 2000; Kleinboehl et al. 1999; Li et al. 1999; Peters et al. 1989), consistent with *diminished descending pain inhibition* (Kosek and Orderberg 2000). Brain regions involved in descending pain facilitation appear to include the periaqueductal grey (PAG; Berrino 2001), the nucleus raphne magnus (NRM, Wiertelak 1997), the nucleus tractus solitarius (NTS, Wiertelak 1997), and the rostroventromedial medulla (RVM, Pertovaara 1998). Descending pain inhibition is likely mediated by both endogenous opioids (Bruehl et al. 2004a) and by nonopioid mechanisms such as central noradrenergic mechanisms. The alterations of the BP—pain sensitivity relationship are not related to a dysfunction in opioid analgesic systems (Bruehl et al. 2002). However, in more disabled CBP patients with higher level of expressed anger (Bruehl et al. 2003), an endogenous opioid antinociceptive impairment may elevate acute and chronic pain sensitivity (Bruehl et al. 2004a). Impairments in alpha-2 noradrenergic inhibitory pathways evoked by stress and anxiety may be of particular relevance for understanding chronic pain-related alterations in the BP/pain sensitivity relationship (Bruehl et al. 2004).

The net effect of descending modulation reflects the combined effects of descending inhibition and facilitation. *Increased descending facilatory activity* may be triggered by baroreceptor activation via mechanisms involving substance P (Millan 2002; Randich and Gebhardt 1992). This increased facilitatory activity results in central sensitization and increased temporal summation (Watkins and Mayer 1999, 1999a) and is also involved in cardiovascular regulation (Ku et al. 1998; Seagard et al. 2000). Substance P pathways and brainstem regions such as NTS and NRM that are involved in the BP—pain sensitivity modulation appear to overlap, and substance P has effects on both pain regulation and baroreflex control of cardiovascular function (Gamboa-Esteves 2001; Wiertelak et al. 1997).

A third contributor of the BP/pain sensitivity relationship is related to alterations of baroreceptor sensitivity (BRS). Changes in BRS sensitivity may alter pain regulatory processes (Maixner et al. 1995). This effect could be due to an altered threshold for baroreceptor firing or altered CNS gain associated with this firing. The functional consequences of diminished BRS include impaired inhibition of sympathetic nervous system arousal and impaired activation of parasympathetic nervous system inhibitory responses evoked by stressful stimuli (Randich and Maixner, 1984). Only one study activated baroreceptors (by external carotid suction) in CBP patients, showing an increased sensitivity to electrical pain stimuli (Brody et al. 1997). In contrast, pain-free normo-tensives respond with analgesia to the same manipulation of baroreceptors (Rau and Elbert 2001). Altered BRS function may have both psychological and physiological consequences. Decreased BRS is associated with increased anxiety levels (Watkins et al 2002) and increased acute (Dito et al 1990; Steptoe et al. 1993) and chronic stress (Lawler et al. 1991; Qian et al. 1997). The decrease in BRS in chronic pain may be due to altered central noradrenergic activity (Lawler et al. 1991; Mitchell and Lawler 1989). Possible interactive effects of substance P and alpha-2 adrenergic activity in baroreceptor-mediated cardiovascular regulation are combined with chronic pain-related changes in pathways mediated by these neurochemicals. That might also suggest a role for baroreceptor changes in the altered BP/pain sensitivity relationship in chronic pain. Baroreceptor sensitivity can be diminished by acute and chronic stress, and therefore, pain-related stress might be expected to lead to similar diminished BRS. The resulting non-inverse BP–pain sensitivity relationship in chronic pain may reflect multiple potential pathways such as baroreceptor, opioid, norepinephrine, and dopamine pathways, and others located at the brain stem level (Bruehl and Chung 2004).

## 8.3.1 CNS and baroreceptor sensitivity

Maixner and co-workers (1995a) suggested that impairments in baroreceptor mediated regula-tion of nociception may contribute to the development of chronic musculoskeletal pain disorder by disinhibition of the ascending reticular activating system. This system is a non-specific, cortical projecting system (Randich and Maixner 1984; Dworkin et al. 1994) that originates from a diverse number of nuclear groups in the brain stem and basal forebrain (e.g. parabrachial nucleus, locus coeruleus, raphe system, nucleus basalis) and plays an important role in sculpting sensory, motor, and autonomic responses to somatosensory input (Rau et al. 1993, Steriade 1988; Steriade and Llinas 1988). The rostral part of the reticular formation has been described as the head of the autonomic nervous system (Rohen 1978) from which ascending input is transmitted to the lateral prefrontal and insular cortices (Bornhovd et al. 2002). The hypothalamus receives direct input from the nucleus tractus solitarius, but also visceral information via the thalamus. The thalamus receives baroreceptor input via the reticular formation. Rutecki (1990) suggests that the connec-tion between the thalamus and the insular cortex mediates important visceral reflexes and this connection has been mentioned as the possible link to conscious perception of visceral sensations (Elbert and Schandry 1998).

Specific cardiovascular information reaches cortical areas mainly via the thalamus, the hypoth-alamus and the tegmentum. In addition to widespread innervation through the reticular forma-tion, additional regions such as the prefrontal cortex, the insula, and multiple somatosensory areas process specific cardiovascular input. Of particular interest is the experimental demonstra-tion that the activity of the ascending reticular formation is regulated, at least in part, by baro-receptor input: The ascending reticular activating system is normally inhibited by baroreceptor stimulation and can be disinhibited by deafferentation of baroreceptor pathways (Randich and Maixner 1984). Disinhibition of this system, by diminishing the efficacy of baroreceptor afferent input, may contribute to the mosaic of chronic, maladaptive psychological, sensory, motor, auto-nomic, and neuroendocrine changes associated with CBP. In addition to altering the ascending reticular activating system, impairments in baroreceptor mediated regulation of nociception may result in a suppression of descending inhibitory pathways that tonically inhibit trigeminal and dorsal horn neurons that respond to muscle and cutaneous nociceptive inputs (Mense 1993; Yu and Mense 1990).

Taken together, these data indicate that stress may activate noradrenergic, serotonergic, and dopaminergic pathways that diminish baroreceptor sensitivity and thus disinhibit the ascending reticular activating system that: (1) activates prefrontal cortex, the insula, and somatosensory via thalamic areas resulting in higher blood pressure and pain perception, and (2) inhibits trigeminal and dorsal horn neurons resulting in increased EMG response. Thus the heterogenous EMG-response and the heterogeneous relationship between muscle tension and pain sensitivity may be mediated by stress-related diminished BRS and enhanced blood pressure. The different patterns of pain processing in hypotensive persons compared with normotensive (Angrili et al. 1997) suggest that CBP patients with a decreased cardiovascular response will have a lower pain perception than CBP patients with higher BP response. The hypotensive stress pattern may be associated with increased baroreceptor sensitivity, decreased muscular response and decreased pain inhibition.

### 8.3.2 Learning

In addition to these direct physiological effects, psychobiological mechanisms such as operant and classical conditioning may influence baroreceptor activation. For example, the *operant conditioning* of chronic pain articulated by Fordyce (1976) emphasized the influence of social context on pain perception. This type of operant learning may mediate decreased pain perception in hypertensive men with parental history of hypertension (Al'Absi 2005; Sandkuehler 2000; Thieme 2005). There is some evidence that the BP is operantly conditionable, in particular in patients with a predisposition for essential hypertension (Elbert et al. 1988; Goldstein et al. 1977; Rau and Elbert 2001). A negative reinforcement of pain behaviour by hypertensive parents may provoke an operant conditioned increase of baroreceptor sensitivity (Rau and Elbert 2001).

Elbert and co-workers (1994a) investigated the influence of daily life stress on baroreceptor sensitivity and suggested a *classical conditioning* mechanism. They found that the increase of BP was proportional to self-assessed daily life stress. Among the participants reporting the greatest amount of stress, the pain inhibition effect accounted for more than 80% of the BP variance. These results support the hypothesis that the reduction in perceived stress produced by baroreceptor stimulation reinforces increased BP.

Multiple types of learning likely activate multiple pathways of chronic pain. Perceived pain after operant conditioning is associated with increased activation of the anterior insula, medial frontal cortex and cerebellum (Ploghaus et al. 1999). In contrast, classical conditioning activates a different network involving entorhinal cortex of hippocampus, perigenual cingulum and medial insula (Ploghaus et al. 2001). Classical conditioning is also related to alterations in the primary somatosensory cortex (SI) that contributes to memory process in associative learning (Diesch and Flor 2007).

## 8.4 Conclusion

Psychophysiological studies have disproved the biomechanical model of CBP that proposed that pain may result from physically demonstrable CBP disease and from poor posture caused by reflex spasm connected with high muscle tension. Studies that tested static and dynamic postures found only 29% of the CBP patients with significantly higher sEMG-responses during dynamic postures in comparison with pain-free controls. Only one study could report a connection between higher sEMG responses and pain perception.

Studies of anticipatory postural adjustments of trunk-stabilizing muscles showed that postural changes are connected with expectations that lead to an earlier centrally mediated activation of abdominal muscle activity caused by fear of pain and movement.

In contrast to the myogenic model, psychophysiological studies showed an important influence of stress on the aetiopathogenesis of CBP. Classical and operant conditioning as well as cognitions are relevant factors that play an important role in stress at work and in the partnership.

According to the symptom-specific response pattern, increased muscle tension has also been proposed to be responsible for maintenance of CBP. However, only 30% of psychophysiological studies could confirm the assumption of higher muscle tension in CBP. Personally important situations provoke a symptom-specific psychophysiological response. The results suggest that social and emotional factors at work exert a much greater influence on maintenance of CBP symptoms than the level of work intensity.

Studies that reported higher SCL, HR or BP instead of higher EMG suggest psychophysiological heterogeneity. Higher SCL suggests an increased arousal response influenced by anger, fear, and comorbidity. A further individual-specific stress responses can be related to higher BP responses that propose an interaction between cardiovascular and pain system. An inverse relationship between BP and pain based on diminished baroreceptor sensitivity in CBP patients is assumed as a further psychophysiological response pattern besides sudomotor (SCL) and muscular response pattern.

The heterogeneity of the psychophysiological studies with CBP patients is determined by different groups of characteristics. Physical characteristics such as diagnosis, association, and non-association between physical changes and pain allow the definition of physical subgroups. Varying levels of muscle activity and psychophysiological response pattern may similarly contribute to the determination of psychophysiological subgroups. The role of personal relevant stressors, comorbidity, and close relationships in learned pain behaviour are consistent with previously described psychosocial subgroups (Turk et al. 1996).

### 8.4.1 Future implications

Recent results suggest that future studies may investigate different psychophysiological subgroups with assumed EMG, SCL and BP reactivity as well as their connection to psychosocial subgroups characterized by pain, cognitions, emotions and behaviour to define different pathways of CBP.

## References

Ahern, D. K., Follick, M.J., Council, J.R., Laser-Wolston, N., Litchman, H. (1988). Comparison of lumbar paravertebral EMG patterns in chronic low back pain patients and non-patient controls. *Pain* **34**(2): 153–60.

Al' Absi, M., France, C.R., Ring, C., et al. (2005). Nociception and baroreceptor stimulation in hypertension-prone men and women. *Psychophysiology* **42**: 83–91.

Alexiev, A.R. (1994). Some differences of the electromyographic erector spinae activity between normal subjects and low back pain patients during the generation of isometric trunk torque. *Electromyography and Clinical Neurophysiology* **34**: 495–99.

Ambroz, C., Scott, A., Ambroz, A., Talbott, E.O. (2000). Chronic low back pain assessment using surface electromyography. *Journal of Occupational Environmental Medicine* **42**:660–9.

Anderson, G. B. J. (1999). Epidemiological features of chronic low-back pain. *Lancet* **354**: 581–5.

Angrilli, A., Mini, A., Mucha, R.F., Rau, H. (1997). The influence of low blood pressure and baroreceptor activity on pain responses. *Physiological Behavior* **62**: 391–97.

Arena, J. G., Sherman, R.A., Bruno, G.M., Young, T.R. (1989). Electromyographic recordings of 5 types of low back pain subjects and non-pain controls in different positions. *Pain* **37**(1): 57–65.

Arena, J. G., Sherman, R.A., Bruno, G.M., Young, T.R. (1990). Temporal stability of paraspinal electromyographic recordings in low back pain and non-pain subjects. *International Journal of Psychophysiology* **9**(1): 31–7.

Arena, J. G., Sherman, R.A., Bruno, G.M., Young, T.R. (1991). Electromyographic recordings of low back pain subjects and non-pain controls in six different positions: effect of pain levels. *Pain* **45**: 23–8.

Ariëns, G. A., van Mechelen, W., Bongers, P.M., Bouter, L.M., van der Wal, G. (2001). Psychosocial risk factors for neck pain: a systematic review. *American Journal of industrial medicine* **39**(2): 180–93.

Asmundson, G. J. G., Norton, G.R. (1995). Anxiety sensitivity in patients with physically unexplained chronic back pain: a preliminary report. *Behaviour Research and Therapy* **33**(7): 771–7

Asmundson, G. J. G., Norton, G.R., Allerdings, M.D. (1997). Fear and avoidance in dysfunctional chronic back pain patients. *Pain* **69**: 231–6.

Asmundson, G. J. G., Norton, G.R. and Jacobson, S.J. (1996). Social, blood/injury, agoraphobic fears in patients with physically unexplained chronic pain: are they clinically significant? *Anxiety* **2**: 28–33.

Asmundson, G. J. G., Taylor, S. (1996). Role of anxiety sensitivity in pain related fear and avoidance. *Journal of Behavioral Medicine* **19**: 573–82.

Atkinson, J. H., Slater, M.A., Patterson, T.L., Grant, I., Garfin, S.R. (1991). Prevalence, onset, and risk of psychiatric disorders in men with chronic low back pain: a controlled study. *Pain* **45**(2): 111–21.

Ax, A. F. (1953). The physiological differentiation between fear and anger in humans. *Psychosomatic Medicine* **75**: 433–42.

Ax, A. F. (1964). Goal and methods of psychophysiology. *Psychophysiology* **1**: 8–25.

Bartley, E.J., Rhudy, J.L. (2008). The influence of pain catastrophizing on experimentally induced emotion and emotional modulation of nociception. *Journal of Pain*. **9**(5): 388–96.

Beattie, P. F., Meyers, S.P. (1998). Magnetic resonance imaging in low back pain: general principles and clinical issues. *Physical Therapy* **78**(7): 738–53.

Berntson, G. G., Sarter, M., Cacioppo, J.T. (1998). Anxiety and cardiovascular reactivity: the basal forebrain cholinergic link. *Behavioral Brain Research* **94**(2): 225–48.

Berntson, G. G., Sarter, M., Cacioppo, J.T. (2003). Ascending visceral regulation of cortical affective information processing. *The European Journal of Neuroscience* **18**(8): 2103–9.

Berrino, L., Oliva, P., Rossi, F., Palazzo, E., Nobili, B., Maione, S. (2001). Interaction between metabotropic and NMDA glutamate receptors in the periaqueductal grey pain modulation system. *Naunyn Schmiedebergs Archive of Pharmacology* **364**: 437–43.

Birbaumer, N., Flor, H. (1999). Applied psychophysiology and learned physiological regulation. *Applied psychophysiology and biofeedback* **24**(1): 35–7.

Birbaumer, N., Ghanayim, N., Hinterberger, T., et al. (1999a). A spelling device for the paralyzed. *Nature* **25**(398(6725)): 297–8.

Birbaumer, N., Murguialday, A.R., Cohen, L. (2008). Brain-computer interface in paralysis. *Current Opinion in Neurology* **21**(6): 634–8.

Birbaumer, N., Schmidt, R.F. (1996). *Biological Psychology [Biologische Psychology]*. Berlin, Heidelberg, New York, Springer.

Bongers, PM, Kremer, A.M., ter Laak J. (2002). Are psychosocial factors, risk factors for symptoms and signs of the shoulder, elbow, or hand/wrist? : A review of the epidemiological literature. *American Journal of Industrial Medicine* **41**: 315–42.

Bonnet, A., Naveteur, J. (2004). Electrodermal activity in low back pain patients with and without co-morbid depression. *International Journal of Psychophysiology* **53**(1): 37–44.

Bornhovd, K., Quante, M., Glauche, V., Bromm, B., Weiller, C., Buchel, C. (2002). Painful stimuli evoke different stimulus-response functions in the amygdala, prefrontal, insula and somatosensory cortex: a single-trial fMRI study. *Brain* **125**: 1326–36.

Bragdon, E. E., Light, K.C., Costello, N.L., et al. (2002). Group differences in pain modulation: pain-free women compared to pain-free men and to women with TMD. *Pain* **96**: 227–37.

Brody, S., Angrilli, A., Weiss, U., Birbaumer, N., Mini, A., Veit, R., Rau, H. (1997). Somatosensory evoked potentials during baroreceptor stimulation in chronic low back pain patients and normal controls. *International Journal of Psychophysiology* **25**: 201–10.

Bruehl, S., Burns, J.W., Chung, O.Y., Ward, P., Johnson, B. (2002a). Anger and pain sensitivity in chronic low back pain patients and pain-free controls: the role of endogenous opioids. *Pain* **99**(1–2): 223–33.

Bruehl, S., Carlson, C.R., McCubbin, J.A. (1992). The relationship between pain sensitivity and blood pressure in normotensives. *Pain* **48**: 463–7.

Bruehl, S., Chung, O. Y., Ward, P., Johnson, B., McCubbin, J. A. (2002). The relationship between resting blood pressure and acute pain sensitivity in healthy normotensives and chronic back pain sufferers: the effects of opioid blockade. *Pain* **100**: 191–201.

Bruehl, S., Chung, O.Y. (2004). Interactions between the cardiovascular and pain regulatory systems: an updated review of mechanisms and possible alterations in chronic pain. *Neuroscience and Biobehavioral Reviews* **28**(4): 395–414.

Bruehl, S., Chung, O.Y., Burns, J.W. (2006). Anger expression and pain: an overview of findings and possible mechanisms. *Journal of behavioral medicine* **29**(6): 593–606.

Bruehl, S., Chung, O.Y., Burns, J.W. (2006). Trait anger and blood pressure recovery following acute pain: evidence for opioid-mediated effects. *International journal of behavioral medicine* **13**(2): 138–46.

Bruehl, S., Chung, O.Y., Burns, J.W., Biridepalli, S. (2003). The association between anger expression and chronic pain intensity: evidence for partial mediation by endogenous opioid dysfunction. *Pain* **106**(3): 317–24.

Bruehl, S., Chung, O.Y., Jirjis, J.N., Biridepalli, S. (2005). Prevalence of clinical hypertension in patients with chronic pain compared to nonpain general medical patients. *Clinical Journal of Pain* **21**(2): 147–53.

Bruehl, S., Chung, O.Y., Ward, P., Johnson, B. (2004a). Endogenous opioids and chronic pain intensity: Interactions with level of disability. *Clinical Journal of Pain* **20**(5): 283–92.

Bruehl, S., McCubbin, J.A., Carlson, C.R., et al. (1996). The psychobiology of hostility: possible endogenous opioid mechanisms. *International Journal of Behavioral Medicine* **3**:163–76.

Burns, J.W., Johnson, B.J., Devinem J, Mahoney, N., Pawl, R. (1998). Anger manger management style and prediction of treatment outcome among male and female chronic pain patients. *Behavior and Research Therapy* **36**:1051–62.

Burns, J. W., Wiegner, S., Derleth, M., Kiselica, K., Pawl, R. (1997). Linking symptom-specific physiological reactivity to pain severity in chronic low back pain patients: a test of mediation and moderation models. *Health Psychology* **16**(4): 319–26.

Cailliet, R. (1981). *Low Back Syndrome*. Philadelphia, PA, Davis.

Cano, A. (2004a). Pain catastrophizing and social support in married individuals with chronic pain: The mediating role of pain duration. *Pain* **110**: 656–64.

Cano, A., Gillis, M., Heinz, W., Geisser, M., Foran, H. (2004). Marital functioning, chronic pain, and psychological distress. *Pain* **107**:99–106.

Cano, A., Weisberg, J., Gallagher, M. (2000). Marital satisfaction and pain severity mediate the association between negative spouse responses to pain and depressive symptoms in a chronic pain patient sample. *Pain Med* **1**:35–43.

Capodaglio, P., Nilsson, J. (1996). Functional correlates in the rehabilitation of occupational low back pain. *Gioliane Italiano di Medicina del Lavoro* **18**:35–9.

Carels, R.A., Szczepanski, R., Blumenthal, J.A., Sherwood, A. (1998). Blood pressure reactivity and marital distress in employed women. *Psychosomatic Medicine* **60**:639–43.

Cassisi, J.E., Robinson, M.E., O'Connor, P., MacMillian, M. (1993). Trunk strength and lumbar paraspinal muscle activity during isometric exercise in chronic low-back pain patients and controls, *Spine* **18**: 245–51.

Chataigner, H., Onimus, M., Polette, A. (1998). Surgery for degenerative lumbar disc disease. Should the black disc be grafted? *Revue de chirurgie orthopedique et reparatrice de'l appareil moteur* **84**(7): 583–9.

Cobb, C. R., DeVries, H.A., Urban, R.T., Luekens, C.A., Bagg, R.J. (1975). Electrical activity in muscle pain. *American Journal of Physical Medicine* **54**: 80–7.

Coffey, P. J., Girman, S., Wang, S.M., et al. (2001). Long-term preservation of cortically dependent visual function in RCS rats by transplantation. *Nature Neuroscience* **5**(1): 53–6.

Cohen, M. J., Swanson, G.A., Naliboff, B.D., Schandler, S.L., McArthur, D.L. (1986). Comparison of electromyographic response patterns during posture and stress tasks in chronic low back pain patterns and control. *Journal of Psychosomatic Research* **30**(2): 135–41.

Collins, G., Cohen, M., Naliboff, B.D., Schandler, S.L. (1982). Comparative analysis of paraspinal and frontalis EMG, heart rate and skin conductance in chronic low back pain patient and normals to various postures and stress. *Scandinavian Journal of Rehabilitative Medicine* **14**(1): 39–46.

Cordo, P.J., Nashner, L.M. (1982). Properties of postural adjustments associated with rapid arm movements. *Journal of Neurophysiology* **47**:287–302.

Cram, J. R., Steger, J.C. (1983). EMG scanning in the diagnosis of chronic pain. *Applied Psychophysiology and Biofeedback* **8**(2): 229–41.

Crombez, G., Vlaeyen, J.W.S., Heuts, P.H.T.G., Lysens, R. (1999). Pain-related fear is more disabling than pain itself: evidence on the role of pain-related fear in chronic back pain disability, *Pain* **80**: 329–39.

DeCharms, R. C., Maeda, F., Glover, G.H., et al. (2005). Control over brain activation and pain learned by using real-time functional MRI. *Proceedings of the National Academy of Sciences of the United States of America* **102**(51): 18626–31.

DeCharms, R. C., Maeda, F., Glover, G.H., Ludlow, D., Pauly, J.M., Soneji, D., Gabrieli, J.D., Mackey, S.C. (2005). Control over brain activation and pain learned by using real-time functional MRI. *Proceedings of the National Academic of Science of the United States of America* **102**: 18626–31.

DeGood, D.E., Stewart, W.R., Adams, L.E., Dale, J.A. (1994). Paraspinal EMG and autonomic reactivity of patients with back pain and controls to personally relevant stress, *Percept Mot Skills* **79**:1399–409.

DeVries, H. A. (1966). Quantitative electromyographic investigation of the spasm theory of muscle pain. *Journal of physical medicine* **45**: 119–34.

Diesch, E., Flor, H. (2007). Central processing of acute muscle pain in chronic low back pain patients: an EEG mapping study. *Journal of clinical neurophysiology* **24**(1): 76–83.

Ditto, B., France, C. (1990). Carotid baroreflex sensitivity at rest and during psychological stress in offspring of hypertensives and non-twin sibling pairs. *Psychosomatic Medicine* **52**: 610–20.

Dolce, J. J., Raczynski, J. M. (1985). Neuromuscular activity and electromyography in painful backs: Psychological and biomechanical models in assessment and treatment. *Psychological Bulletin* **97**: 502–20.

Droste, C., Kardos, A., Brody, S., Greenlee, M.W., Roskamm, H., Rau, H. (1994). Baroreceptor stimulation: pain perception and sensory thresholds. *Biological Psychology* **37**: 101–13.

Dworkin, B. R., Elbert, T., Rau, H., et al. (1994). Central effects of baroreceptor activation in humans: Attenuation of skeletal reflexes and pain perception. *Proceedings of the National Academy of Sciences of the United States of America* **91**(14): 6329–33.

Eide, P. K. (2000). Wind-up and the NMDA receptor complex from a clinical perspective. *European Journal of Pain.* **4**: 5–17.

Elbert, T., Dworkin, B.R., Rau, H., Pauli, P., Birbaumer, N., Droste, C., Brunia, C.H. (1994). Sensory effects of baroreceptor activation and perceived stress together predict long-term blood pressure elevations. *International Journal of Behavioral Medicine* **1**: 215–28.

Elbert, T., Ray, W.J., Kowalik, Z.J., Skinner, J.E., Graf, K.E., Birbaumer, N. (1994a). Chaos and physiology: deterministic chaos in excitable cell assemblies. *Physiological Review* **74**: 1–47.

Elbert, T., Rockstroh, B., Lutzenberger, W., Kessler, M., Pietrowsky, R. (1988). Baroreceptor stimulation alters pain sensation depending on tonic blood pressure. *Psychophysiology* **25**(1): 25–9.

Elbert T, Schandry, R.I.E. (1998). Wechselwirkungen zwischen kardiovaskulärem und zentralnervösem System [Interactions between cardiovascular and central nervous system]. *Enzyklopädie der Psychologie, Serie Biologische Psychologie [Encyclopedia of Psychology, Biological Psychology]*. F. Roesler. Göttingen, Hogrefe: 427–77.

Elfving, B., Dedering, A., Németh, G. (2003). Lumber muscle fatigue and recovery in patients with long-term back trouble–electromyography and health-related factors, *Clin Biomech* **18**:619–30.

Fahrenberg, J. (1986). Psychophysiological individuality. A pattern analytic approach to personality research and psychosomatic medicine. *Advances in behavioral research and therapy* **8**: 43–100.

Fernandez, E., Turk, D.C. (1995). The scope and significance of anger in the experience of chronic pain. *Pain* **61**:165–75.

Fisher, A. A., Chang, C.H. (1985). Electromyographic evidence of muscle spasm during sleep in patients with low back pain. *Clinical Journal of Pain* **1**: 147–54.

Flor, H., Birbaumer, N. (1994). Acquisition of chronic pain: Psychophysiological mechanisms. *American Pain Society Journal* **3**: 119–27.

Flor, H., Birbaumer, N., Schugens, M.M., Lutzenberger, W. (1992). Symptom-specific psychophysiological responses in chronic pain patients. *Psychophysiology* **29**(4): 452–60.

Flor, H., Birbaumer, N., Turk, D. (1990). The psychobiology of chronic pain. *Advances in Behaviour Research and Therapy* **12**(2): 47–84

Flor, H., Braun, C., Elbert, T., Birbaumer, N. (1997). Extensive reorganization of primary somatosensory cortex in chronic back pain patients. *Neuroscience Letters* **224**(1): 5–8.

Flor, H., Breitenstein, C., Birbaumer, N., Fürst, M.A. (1995). A psychophysiological analysis of spouse solitousness towards pain behaviors, spouse interaction and pain perception. *Behavioral Therapy* **26**: 255–72.

Flor, H., Haag, G., Turk, D.C. and Koehler, H. (1983). Efficacy of EMG biofeedback, pseudotherapy and medical treatment for chronic rheumatic back pain. *Pain* **17**: 21–31.

Flor, H., Kerns, R.D., Turk, D.C. (1987). The role of spouse reinforcement, perceived pain, and activity levels of chronic pain patients. *Journal of Psychosomatic Research* **31**: 251–9.

Flor, H., Knost, B., Birbaumer, N. (2002). The role of operant conditioning in chronic pain: an experimental investigation. *Pain* **95**(1–2): 111–18.

Flor, H., Turk, D., Birbaumer, N. (1985). Assessment of stress-related psychophysiological reactions in chronic back pain patients. *Journal of Consulting and Clinical Psychology* **53**(3): 354–64.

Flor, H., Turk, D.C. (1984). Etiological Theories and Treatments for Chronic Back Pain. I. Somatic Models and Interventions. *Pain* **19**: 105–21.

Flor, H., Turk, D.C. (1988). Chronic Back Pain and Rheumatoid Arthritis: Predicting Pain and Disability from Cognitive Variables. *Journal of Behavioral Medicine* **11**(3): 251–65.

Flor, H., Turk, D.C. (1989). Psychophysiology of chronic pain: do chronic pain patients exhibit symptom-specific psychophysiological responses? *Psychological Bulletin* **105**: 215–9.

Fordyce, W. E. (1976). *Behavioral Methods for Chronic Pain and Illness.* St. Louis, MO, C V Mosby Co.

Gamboa-Esteves, F.O., Kaye, J.C., McWilliam, P.N., Lima, D., Batten, T.F.C. (2001). Immunohistochemical profiles of spinal lamina I neurons retrogradely labeled from the nucleus tractus solitarii in rat suggest excitatory projections. *Neuroscience* **104**: 523–38.

Gelkopf, M. (1997). Laboratory pain and styles of coping with anger. *Journal of Psychology* **131**:121–3.

Geisser, M.E., Robinson, M.E., Richardson, C. (1995). A time series analysis of the relationship between ambulatory EMG, pain, and stress in chronic low back pain. *Biofeedback Self Regul.* **20**(4): 339–55.

Gentry, W.D., Bernal, A. (1977). Chronic pain. *Behavioral approaches to medical treatment* . In W. D. Genty and R.B. Williams (eds). New York, Ballinger: 173–91.

Ghione, S. (1996). Hypertension-associated hypalgesia. Evidence in experimental animals and humans, pathophysiological mechanisms, and potential clinical consequences. *Hypertension* **28**: 494–504.

Glombiewski, J.A., Hartwich-Tersek, J., Rief, W. (2010). Two psychological interventions are effective in severely disabled, chronic back pain patients: a randomised controlled trial. *International Journal of Behavioral Medicine* **17**(2): 97–107.

Goldstein, D.S., Harris, A.H., Brady, J.V. (1977). Baroreflex sensitivity during operant blood pressure conditioning. *Biofeedback Self Regulation* **2**(2): 127–38.

Gracely, R.H., Geisser, M.E., Giesecke, T., et al. (2004). Pain catastrophizing and neural responses to pain among persons with fibromyalgia. *Brain* **127**: 835–43.

Gracely, R.H., Petzke, F., Wolf, J.M., Clauw, D.J. (2002). Functional magnetic resonance imaging evidence of augmented pain processing in fibromyalgia. *Arthritis & Rheumatism* **46**: 1333–43.

Greenough, C.G. (1993). Recovery from low back pain. 1–5 year follow-up of 287 injury-related cases. *Acta Orthopedica Scandinavia* **64:** (suppl 254): 1–64.

Gubler, D., Mannion, A.F., Schenk, P., et al. (2010). Ultrasound tissue Doppler imaging reveals no delay in abdominal muscle feed-forward activity during rapid arm movements in patients with chronic low back pain. *Spine* (Phila Pa 1976). **35**(16): 1506–13.

Guzman, J., Esmail, R., Karjalainen, K.A., Malmivaara, A., Irvin, E., Bombardier, C. (2007). Withdrawn: Multidisciplinary bio-psycho-social rehabilitation for chronic low-back pain (Review). *Cochrane Database of Systematic Reviews (Online)* **18**(2): CD000963.

Haley, W. E., Turner, J.A., Romano, J.M. (1985). Depression in chronic pain patients: relation to pain, activity, and sex differences. *Pain* **23**(4): 337–43.

Hanley, M. A., Raichle, K., Jensen, M., Cardenas, D.D. (2008). Pain catastrophizing and beliefs predict changes in pain interference and psychological functioning in persons with spinal cord injury. *Journal of Pain* **9**(9): 863–71.

Harris, A. J. (1999). Cortical origins of pathological pain. *Lancet* **354**: 1464–66

Haythornthwaite, J. A., Menefee, L.A., Heinberg, L.J., Clark, M.R. (1998). Pain coping strategies predict perceived control over pain. *Pain* **77**(1): 33–39.

Heffner, K.L., Kiecolt-Glaser, J.K., Loving, T.J., Glaser, R., Malarkey, W.B. (2004). Spousal support satisfaction as a modifier of physiological responses to marital conflict in younger and older couples. *Journal of Behavioral Medicine* **27**(3): 233–54.

Heydari, A., Nargol, A.V., Jones, A.P., Humphrey, A.R., Greenough, C.G. (2010). EMG analysis of lumbar paraspinal muscles as a predictor of the risk of low-back pain. *European Spine Journal* **19**:1145–52.

Hildebrandt, J., Franz, C. (1988). Low back pain - pathophysiology of so called 'idiopathic' low back pain. [Kreuzschmerz - Zur Pathophysiologie des sogenannten 'idiopathischen' Rueckenschmerzes]. In: Sehathi-Chafai, G.H. (Editor) *Pathophysiology, diagnostic and therapy of low back pain* [Pathophysiologie, Diagnostik und Therapie des Kreuzschmerzes. Winkler, Bochum, 11.

Hildebrandt, J., Pfingsten, M., Saur, P., Jansen, J. (1997). Prediction of success from a multidisciplinary treatment program for chronic low back pain. *Spine* **22**(9): 990–1001.

Hirsch, C. (1966). Low back pain etiology and pathogenesis. *Applied Therapy* **8**: 857–62.

Hodapp, V., Weyer, G., Becker, J. (1975). Situational stereotypy in essential hypertension patients. *Journal of psychosomatic research* **19**(2): 113–21.

Hodges, P.W. (2001). Changes in motor planning of feedforward postural responses of the trunk muscles in low back pain. *Experimental Brain Research* **141**: 261–6.

Hoyt, W. H., Hunt, H.H., Depauw, M.A., et al. (1981). Electromyographic assessment of chronic low-back pain syndrome. *Journal of the American Osteopathic Association* **80**: 728–30.

Hult, L. (1954). Cervical, dorsal, and lumbar spinal syndromes. A field investigation of a non-selected material of 1200 workers in different occupations with special reference to disc degeneration and so-called muscular rheumatism. *Acta orthopedica stand* **17** (Suppl): 1–102.

Jalovaara, P., Niinimäki, T., Vanharanta, H. (1995). Pocket-size, portable surface EMG device in the differentiation of low back pain patients. *European Spine J* **4**:210–12.

James, W. (1984). What is an emotion? *Mind* **9**: 188–205.

Janssen, S.J., Spinhoven, P., Brosschot, J.F. (2001). Experimentally induced anger, cardiovascular reactivity, and pain sensitivity. *Journal of Psychosomatic Research* **51**:479–85.

Jensen, M. C., Brant-Zawadzki, M.N., Obuchowski, N., et al (1994). Magnetic resonance imaging of the lumbar spine in people without back pain. *New England Journal of Medicine* **14**(331(2)): 69–73.

Jensen, M.P., Turner, J.A., Romano, J.M., Karoly, P. (1991). Coping with chronic pain: a critical review of the literature. *Pain* , **47**:249–83.

Jinkins, J. R. (2003). Lumbosacral interspinous ligament rupture associated with acute intrinsic spinal muscle degeneration. *JBR-BTR: Organe de la societe royal belge de radiologie (SRBR)* **86**(4): 226–30.

Jinkins, J. R. (2004). Acquired degenerative changes of the intervertebral segments at and suprajacent to the lumbosacral junction. A radioanatomic analysis of the nondiscal structures of the spinal column and perispinal soft tissues. *European Journal of Radiology* **50**(2): 134–58.

Johannes, B., Salnitski, V.P., Thieme, K., Kirsch, K.A. (2003). Differences in the autonomic reactivity pattern to psychological load in patients with hypertension and rheumatic diseases. *Aerospace and environmental Medicine* **37**(1): 28–42.

Kankaanpää, M., Taimela, S., Laaksonen, D., Hannien, O., Airksinen, O. (1998). Back and hip extensor fatigability in chronic low back pain patients and controls. *Arch Phys Med Rehabil* **79**:412–17.

Kerns, R.D., Haythornthwaite, J., Southwick S., Giller, E. L. (1990). The role of marital interaction in chronic pain and depressive symptom severity. *Journal of Psychosomatic Research* **34**(4): 401–8.

Kerns, R.D. Rosenberg R, Jacob MC. (1994). Anger expression and chronic pain. *Journal of Behavioral Medicine* **17**:57–67.

Kerns, R.D., Turk, D.C. (1984). Depression and chronic pain: The mediating role of the spouse. *Journal of Marriage and Family* **46**: 845–52.

Klein, A.B., Snyder-Mackler, L., Roy, S.H., DeLuca, C.J. (1991). Comparison of spinal mobility and isometric trunk extensor forces with electromyographic spectral analysis in identifying low back pain, *Phys Ther* **71**:445–54.

Kleinbohl, D., Holzl, R., Moltner, A., Rommel, C., Weber, C., Osswald, P.M. (1999). Psychophysical measures of sensitization to tonic heat discriminate chronic pain patients. *Pain* **81**(1–2): 35–43.

Kosek, E., Orderberg, G. (2000). Lack of pressure pain modulation by heterotopic noxious conditioning stimulation in patients with painful osteoarthritis before, but not following, surgical pain relief. *Pain* **88**: 69–78.

Kravitz, E. A., Moore, M.E., Glaros, A. (1981). Paralumbar muscle activity in chronic low back pain. *Archives of Physical Medicine and Rehabilitation* **62**: 172–6.

Kravitz, E. A. Glusman, S., Harris-Warrick, R.M., Livingstone, M.S., Schwarz, T., Goy, M.F. (1980). Amines and a peptide as neurohormones in lobsters: actions on neuromuscular preparations and preliminary behavioural studies. *The Journal of experimental biology* **98**:159–75.

Ku, Y. H., Tan, L., Li, L.S., Ding, X. (1998). Role of corticotropin-releasing factor and substance P in pressor responses of nuclei controlling emotion and stress. *Peptides* **19**: 677–82.

Lacey, J., Lacey, B. (1958). Verification and extension of the principle of autonomic response-sterotype. *American Journal of Psychology* **71**: 50–73.

Lacey, J. I., Bateman, D.E., Van Lehn, R. (1953). Autonomic response specificity: An experimental study. *Psychosomatic medicine* **15**: 8–21.

LaChapelle, D. L., Hadjistavropoulos, H.D., McCreary, D.R., Asmundson, G.J. (2001). Contributions of pain-related adjustment and perceptions of control to coping strategy use among cervical sprain patients. *European Journal of Pain* **5**(4): 405–13.

Lawler, J. E., Sanders, B.J., Cox, R.H., O'Connor, E.F. (1991). Baroreflex function in chronically stressed borderline hypertensive rats. *Physiological Behavior* **49**: 539–42.

Leavitt, F. (1992). The physical exertion factor in compensable work injuries: a hidden flaw in previous research. *Spine* **17**: 307–10.

Lee, D.J., Stokes, M.J., Taylor, R.J., Cooper, R.G. (1992). Electro and acoustic myography for noninvasive assessment of lumbar paraspinal muscle function, *Eur J Appl Physiol Occup Physiol* **64**:199–203.

Leeuw, M., Houben, R.M.A., Severeijns, R., et al. (2007). Pain-related fear in low back pain: A prospective study in the general population. *European Journal of Pain* **11**: 256–66.

Lehmann, H. (1996). The content and development of mobbing at work. *European Journal of Work and Organizational Psychology* **5**(2): 165–84.

Leinonen, V., Kankaanpää, M., Luukkonen, M., Hänninen, O., Airaksinen, O., Taimela, S. (2001). Disc herniation-related back pain impairs feed-forward control of paraspinal muscles. *Spine* **26**: E367–72.

Lethem, J., Slade, P.D., Troup, J.D., Bentley, G. (1983). Outline of a Fear-Avoidance Model of exaggerated pain perception—I. *Behaviour Research and Therapy* **21**(4): 401–8.

Li, J., Simone, D.A., Larson, A.A. (1999). Windup leads to characteristics of central sensitization. *Pain* **79**: 75–82.

Linton, S. J. (2000). A review of psychological risk factors in back and neck pain. *Spine* 25: 1148–56.

Lisiński, P. (2000). Surface EMG in chronic low back pain. *Eur Spine J* **9**:559–62.

Loeser, J. D. (1980). *Low back pain*. New York, Raven Press.

Lofland, K.R., Cassisi, J.E., Levin, J.B., Palumbo, N.L., Blonsky, E.R. (2000). The incremental validity of lumbar surface EMG, behavioral observation, and a symptom checklist in the assessment of patients with chronic low-back pain. *Appl Psychophysiol Biofeedback* **25**:67–78.

Lousberg, R., Schmidt, A.J., Groenman, N.H. (1992). The relationship between spouse solicitousness and pain behavior: searching for more experimental evidence. *Pain* **51**: 75–9.

Lu, W.W., Luk, K.D., Cheung, K.M., Wong, Y.W., Leong, J.C. (2001). Back muscle contraction patterns of patients with low back pain before and after rehabilitation treatment: an electromyographic evaluation. *J Spinal Disord* **14**:277–82.

Lundberg, U., Dohns, I.E., Melin, B., et al. (1999). Psychophysiological stress responses, muscle tension, and neck and shoulder pain among supermarket cashiers. *Journal of Occupational Health Psychology* **4**(3): 245–55.

Maixner, W. (1991). Interactions between cardiovascular and pain modulatory systems: physiological and pathophysiological implications. *Journal of Cardiovascular Electrophysiology* **2**: S3–S12.

Maixner, W., Fillingim, R., Booker, D., Sigurdsson, A. (1995). Sensitivity of patients with painful temporomandibular disorders to experimentally evoked pain. *Pain* **63**: 341–51.

Maixner, W., Fillingim, R.B., Kincaid, S., Sigurdsson, A. Harris, M.B. (1997). Relationship between pain sensitivity and resting arterial blood pressure in patients with painful temporomandibular disorders. *Psychosomatic Medicine* **59**: 503–11.

Maixner, W., Sigurdsson, A., Fillingim, R.B., Lundeen, T., Booker, D.K. (1995a). Regulation of acute and chronic orofacial pain. *Orofacial pain and temporomandibular disorders*. D. R. Fricton JR. New York, Raven Press.

Malchaire, J., Cock, N., Vergracht, S. (2001). Review of the factors associated with musculoskeletal problems in epidemiological studies. *International Archives of Occupational Environmental Health* **74**: 79–90.

Malmo, R. B., Shagass, C. (1949). Physiologic studies of reaction to stress in anxiety and early schizophrenia. *Psychosomatic Medicine* **11**: 9–24.

Mannion, A. F., Pulkovski, N., Schenk, P., et al. (2008). A new method for the noninvasive determination of abdominal muscle feedforward activity based on tissue velocity information from tissue Doppler imaging. *Journal of Applied Physiology* **104**(4): 1192–201.

Mayer, T.G., Kondraske, G., Mooney, V., Carmichael, T.W., Butsch, R. (1989). Lumbar myoelectric spectral analysis for endurance assessment. A comparison of normals with deconditioned patients. *Spine* **14**: 986–91.

McCabe, C. S., Haigh, R.C., Halligan, P.W. Blake, D.R. (2005). Simulating sensory–motor incongruence in healthy volunteers: implications for a cortical model of pain. *Rheumatology (Oxford)* **44**: 509–16.

McCracken, L.M., Zayfert, C., Gross, R.T. (1992). The Pain Anxiety Symptoms Scale: development and validation of a scale to measure fear of pain. *Pain* **50**: 63–7.

Mense, S. (1993). Nociception from skeletal muscle in relation to clinical muscle pain. *Pain* **54**: 241–89.

Millan, M. J. (2002). Descending control of pain. *Progressive Neurobiology* **66**: 355–474.

Miller, D. J. (1985). Comparison of electromyographic activity in the lumbar paraspinal muscles of subjects with and without chronic low back pain. *Physical Therapy* **65**(9): 1347–54.

Mini, A., Rau, H., Montoya, P., Palomba, D., Birbaumer, N. (1995). Baroreceptor cortical effects, emotions, and pain. *International Journal of Psychophysiology* **19**(1): 67–77.

Mitchell, V. P., Lawler, J.E. (1989). Norepinephrine content of discrete brain nuclei in acutely and chronically stressed borderline hypertensive rats. *Brain Research Bulletin* **22**: 545–47.

Morris, S.L., Allison, G.T. (2006). Effects of abdominal muscle fatigue on anticipatory postural adjustments associated with arm raising. *Gait Posture* **24**:342–8.

Myers, C. D., Robinson, M. E., Riley, J.L. 3rd, Sheffield, D. (2001). Sex, gender, and blood pressure: contributions to experimental pain report. *Psychosomatic Medicine* **63**: 545–50.

Newton-John, T. R., Spence, S.H., Schotte, D. (1995). Cognitive-behavioural therapy versus EMG biofeedback in the treatment of chronic low back pain. *Behavior Research and Therapy* **33**(6): 691–7.

Ng, J.K. -F., Richardson, C.A., Parnianpour, M., Kippers, V. (2002). EMG activity of trunk muscles and torque output during isometric axial rotation exertion: a comparison between back pain patients and matched controls. *Journal of Orthopedic Research* **20**:112–21.

Nilsson, P. M., Kandell-Collen, A., Andersson, H.I. (1997). Blood pressure and metabolic factors in relation to chronic pain. *Blood Pressure* **6**: 294–8.

Nouwen, A., Bush, C. (1984). The relationship between paraspinal EMG and chronic low back pain. *Pain* **20**: 109–23.

Okifuji, A., Turk, D.C., Curran, S.L. (1999). Anger in chronic pain: investigations of anger targets and intensity. *Journal of Psychosomatic Research* **47**:1–12.

Ongley, M. J., Klein, R.G., Dorman, T.A., Eek, B.C., Hubert, L.J. (1987). A new approach to the treatment of chronic low back pain. *Lancet* **18**(2(8551)): 143–6.

Ostelo, R. W., van Tulder, M.W., Vlaeyen, J.W., Linton, S.J., Morley, S.J., Assendelft, W.J. (2005). Behavioural treatment for chronic low-back pain. *Cochrane Database of Systematic Reviews* **25**(1): CD002014.

Passatore, M., Roatta, S. (2006). Influence of sympathetic nervous system on sensorimotor function: whiplash associated disorders (WAD) as a model. *European Journal of Applied Physiology* **98**: 423–49.

Pääsuke, M., Johanson, E., Proosa, M., Ereline, J., Gapeyeva, H. (2002). Back extensor muscle fatigability in chronic low back pain patients and controls: Relationship between electromyogram power spectrum changes and body mass index. *Journal of Back Musculoskeletal Rehabilitation* **16**:17–24.

Peach, J.P., McGill, S.M. (1998). Classification of low back pain with the use of spectral electromyogram parameters. *Spine* **23**:1117–23.

Pertovaara, A. (1998). A neuronal correlate of secondary hyperalgesia in the rat spinal dorsal horn is submodality selective and facilitated by supraspinal influence. *Experimental Neurology* **149**: 193–202.

Peters, M. L., Schmidt, A.J.M. (1991). Psychophysiological responses to repeated acute pain stimulation in chronic low back pain patients. *Journal of Psychosomatic Research* **35**(1): 59–74.

Peters, M. L., Schmidt, A.J.M., Van den Hout, M.A. (1989). Chronic low back pain and the reaction to repeated pain stimulation. *Pain* **39**: 69–76.

Pienimäki, T., Tarvainen, T., Siira, P., Malmivaara, A., Vanharanta, H. (2002). Associations between pain, grip strength, and manual tests in the treatment evaluation of chronic tennis elbow. *Clinical Journal of Pain* **18**(3): 164–70.

Pincus, T., Burton, A.K., Vogel, S., Field, A.P. (2002). A systematic review of psychological factors as predictors of chronicity/disability in prospective cohorts of low back pain. Review. *Spine* **27**(5): E109–20.

Ploghaus, A., Narain, C., Beckmann, C.F., et al. (2001). Exacerbation of pain by anxiety is associated with activity in a hippocampal network. *Journal of Neuroscience* **21**(24): 9896–903.

Ploghaus, A., Tracey, I., Gati, J.S., et al. (1999). Dissociating pain from its anticipation in the human brain. *Science* **284**(5422): 1979–81.

Polatin, P. B., Kinney, R.K., Gatchel, R.J., Lillo, E., Mayer, T.G. (1993). Psychiatric illness and chronic back pain. *The mind and the spine—which goes first? Spine* **18**: 66–71.

Praemer, A., Furnes, S., Rice, D.P. (1992). *Musculoskeletal conditions in the United States.* Rosemont, AAUS.

Qian, Z.M., X. D., Huang, W.Q., Tang, P.L., Xu, B. (1997). Central ANG II receptor involved in carotid sinus reflex resetting in chronically stressed rats. *Physiological Behavior* **62**: 241–7.

Radebold, A., Cholewicki, J., Panjabi, M., Patel, T. (2000). Muscle response pattern to sudden trunk loading in healthy individuals and in patients with chronic low back pain. *Spine* **25**: 947–54.

Radebold, A., Cholewicki, J., Polzhofer, G.K., Greene, H.S. (2001). Impaired postural control of the lumbar spine is associated with delayed muscle response times in patients with chronic idiopathic low back pain. *Spine* **26**: 724–30.

Randich, A., Gebhart, G.F. (1992). Vagal afferent modulation of nociception. *Brain Research Brain Research Reviews* **17**(2): 77–99.

Randich, A., Maixner, W. (1984). Interactions between cardiovascular and pain regulatory systems. *Neuroscience & Biobehavioral Review* **8**: 343–67.

Rau, H., Elbert, T. (2001). Psychophysiology of arterial baroreceptors and the etiology of hypertension. *Biological Psychiatry* **57**: 179–201.

Rau, H., Pauli, P., Brody, S., Elbert, T., Birbaumer, N. (1993). Baroreceptor stimulation alters cortical activity. *Psychophysiology* **30**: 322–5.

Rissén, D., Melin, B., Sandsjö, L., Dohns, I., Lundberg, U. (2000). Surface EMG and psychophysiological stress reactions in women during repetitive work. *European Journal of Applied Psychology* **83**(2–3): 215–22.

Robinson, M.E., Cassisi, J.E., O'Connor, P.D., MacMillian, M. (1992). Lumbar iEMG during isotonic exercise: chronic low back pain patients versus controls. *Journal of Spinal Disorder* **5**: 8–15.

Rohen, J. W. (1978). *Functional anatomy of nervous system.* Stuttgart, Schattauer.

Rossignol, M., Suissa, S., Abenhaim, L. (1988). Working disability due to occupational back pain: three-year follow-up of 2300 compensated workers in Quebec. *Journal of Occupational Medicine* **30**: 502–5.

Roy, S.H., De Luca, C.J., Casavant, D.A. (1989). Lumbar muscle fatigue and chronic lower back pain. *Spine* **14**:992–1001.

Roy, S.H., De Luca, C.J., Emley, M., Buijs, R.J. (1995). Spectral electromyographic assessment of back muscles in patients with low back pain undergoing rehabilitation, *Spine* **20**:38–48.

Roy, S.H., De Luca, C.J., Snyder-Mackler, L., Emley, M.S., Crenshaw, R.L., Lyons, J.P. (1990). Fatigue, recovery, and low back pain in varsity rowers. *Medical Science of Sports Exercises* **22**: 463–69.

Rutecki, P. (1990). Anatomical, physiological, and theoretical basis for the antiepileptic effect of vagus nerve stimulation. *Epilepsia* **31**: S1–S6.

Ryan, C. G., Gray, H.G., Newton, M., Granat, M.H. (2010). The relationship between psychological distress and free-living physical activity in individuals with chronic low back pain. *Manual therapy* **15**(2): 185–9.

Sandkuehler, J. (2000). Learning and memory in pain pathways. *Pain* **88**: 113–18.

Shirado, O., Ito, T., Kaneda, K., Strax, T. (1995). Flexion-relaxation phenomenon in the back muscles: a comparative study between healthy subjects and patients with chronic low back pain. *American Journal of Physical and Medical Rehabilitation* **74**:139–44.

Schneider, S., Schmitt, H., Zoller, S., Schiltenwolf, M. (2005). Workplace stress, lifestyle and social factors as correlates of back pain: a representative study of the German working population. *International Archives of Occupational and Environmental Health* **78**(4): 253–69.

Seagard, J.L., Dean, C., Hopp, F.A. (2000). Modulation of the carotid baroreceptor reflex by substance P in the nucleus tractus solitarius. *Journal of Autonomic Nervous System* **78**: 77–85.

Selye, H. (1956). *Stress and disease.* New York, McGraw-Hill.

Shapiro, D., Goldstein, I.B., Jamner, L.B. (1996). Effects of cynical hostility, anger out, anxiety, and defensiveness on ambulatory blood pressure in black and white college students. *Psychosomatic Medicine,* **58**: 354–64.

Sihvonen, T., Huttunen, M., Makkonen, M., Airaksinen, O. (1998). Functional changes in back muscle activity correlate with pain intensity and prediction of low back pain during pregnancy. *Archive of Physical and Medical Rehabilitation* **79**:1210–12.

Sihvonen, T., Partanen, J., Hänninen, O., Soimakallio, S. (1991). Electric behavior of low back muscles during lumbar pelvic rhythm in low back pain patients and healthy controls, *Archive of Physical and Medical Rehabilitation* **72**:1080–7.

Sjörs, A., Larsson, B., Dahlman, J., Falkmer, T., Gerdle, B. (2009). Physiological responses to low-force work and psychosocial stress in women with chronic trapezius myalgia. *BMC_Musculoskeletal disorders* **7**(10): 63.

Smeets, R. J., Wade, D., Hidding, A., Van Leeuwen, P.J., Vlaeyen, J.W., Knottnerus, J.A. (2006). The association of physical deconditioning and chronic low back pain: a hypothesis-oriented systematic review. *Disability and Rehabilitation* **28**(11): 673–93.

Soderberg, G.L., Cook, T.M. (1983). An electromyographic analysis of quadriceps femoris muscle setting and straight leg raising. *Physical Therapy* **63**(9): 1434–8.

Spielberger, C.D., Johnson, E.H., Russell, S.F., Crane, R.J., Jacobs, G.A., Worden, T.J. (1985). The experience and expression of anger: construction and validation of an anger expression scale. In: Chesney MA, Rosenman RH, editors. Anger and hostility in cardiovascular and behavioral disorders, Washington, DC: Hemisphere Publishing, 1985. pp. 5–30.

Steriade, M. (1988). New vistas on the morphology, chemical transmitters and physiological actions of the ascending brainstem reticular system. *Archives Italiennes de Biologie* **126**(4s): 225–38.

Steriade, M., Llinas, R.R. (1988). The functional states of the thalamus and the associated neuronal interplay. *Physiology Review* **68**: 649–742.

Sullivan, M. J. L., Rodgers, W.M., Kirsch, I. (2001). Catastrophizing, depression and expectancies for pain and emotional distress. *Pain* **91**(1–2): 147–54.

Suter, E., Lindsay, D. (2001). Back muscle fatigability is associated with knee extensor inhibition in subjects with low back pain. *Spine* **26**: E361–66.

Thieme, K., Rose, U., Pinkpank, T., Spies, C., Turk, D.C., Flor, H. (2006). Psychophysiological responses in patients with fibromyalgia syndrome. *Journal of Psychosomatic Research* **61**(5): 671–79.

Thieme, K., Spies, C., Sinha, P., Turk, D.C., Flor, H. (2005). Predictors of pain behaviors in fibromyalgia syndrome. *Arthritis & Rheumatism* **53**(3): 343–50.

Thieme, K., Turk, D.C. (2006). Heterogeneity of psychophysiological stress responses in fibromyalgia syndrome patients. *Arthritis Research & Therapy* **8**(1): R9.

Thieme, K., Turk, D.C., Gracely, R.H., Maixner, W., Flor, H. Interaction of psychological and psychophysiological characteristics in fibromyalgia patients. Submitted.

Thieme, K., Turk, D.C., Flor, H. (2004). Comorbid depression and anxiety in fibromyalgia syndrome: relationship to somatic and psychosocial variables. *Psychosomatic Medicine* **66**(6): 837–44.

Tousignant-Laflamme, Y., Marchand, S. (2006). Sex differences in cardiac and autonomic response to clinical and experimental pain in LBP patients. *European Journal of Pain* **10**:603–14.

Toyone T, T. K., Kitahara H, Yamagata M, Murakami M, Moriya H. (1994). Vertebral bone-marrow changes in degenerative lumbar disc disease. An MRI study of 74 patients with low back pain. *Journal of Bone and Joint Surgery* **46**(5): 757–64.

Tschannen, T.A., Duckro, P.N., Margolis, R.B., Tomazic, T.J. (1992). The relationship of anger, depression, and perceived disability among headache patients. *Headache* **32**:501–3.

Turk, D. C., Flor, H. (1984). Etiological theories and treatments for chronic back pain. II. Psychological models and interventions. *Pain* **19**(3): 209–33.

Turk, D. C., Meichenbaum, D., Oenest, M. (1983). *Pain and Behavioral Medicine. A Cognitive-Behavioral Perspective.* New York, Guilford Press.

Turk, D. C., Okifuji, A. (1997). What factors affect physicians' decisions to prescribe opioids for chronic noncancer pain patients? *Clinical Journal of Pain* **13**(4): 330–6.

Turk, D. C., Okifuji, A. (1997a). Evaluating the role of physical, operant, cognitive, and affective factors in the pain behaviors of chronic pain patients. *Behavioral Modification* **21**: 259–80.

Turk, D. C., Okifuji, A., Starz, T.W., Sinclair, J.D. (1996). Effects of type of symptom onset on psychological distress and disability in fibromyalgia syndrome patients. *Pain* **68**(2–3): 423–30.

Turner, J. A., Chapman, C. R. (1982). Psychological interventions for chronic pain: A critical appraisal. II. Operant conditioning, hypnosis, and cognitive-behavior therapy. *Pain* **12**: 23–46.

Turner, J. A., Jensen, M.P., Warms, C.A., Cardenas, D.D. (2002). Catastrophizing is associated with pain intensity, psychological distress, and pain-related disability among individuals with chronic pain after spinal cord injury. *Pain* **98**(1–2): 127–34.

van Dieën, J. H., Selen, L.P.J., Choloewicki, J. (2003). Trunk muscle activation in low-back pain patients, an analysis of the literature. *Journal of Electromyography and Kinesiology* **13**(4): 333–51.

van Doorn, T. W. C. (1995). Low back disability among self-employed dentists, veterinarians, physicians and physical therapists in the Netherlands. *Acta Orthopedica Scandinavia* **66** (suppl 263): 1–64.

Verbunt, J. A., Seelen, H.A., Vlaeyen, J.W., et al. (2003). Disuse and deconditioning in chronic low back pain: concepts and hypotheses on contributing mechanisms. Review. *European Journal of Pain* 7(1): 9–21.

Villanueva, L., Le Bars, D. (1995). The activation of bulbo-spinal controls by peripheral nociceptive inputs: diffuse noxious inhibitory controls. *Biological Research* 28: 113–25.

Vlaeyen J.W.S., Crombez G. (1999). Fear of movement/(re)injury, avoidance and pain disability in chronic low back pain patients. *Manual Therapy* 4(4): 187–95.

Vlaeyen, J. W. S., Kole-Snijders, A.M.J., Boeren, R.G.B., van Eek H. (1995). Fear of movement/(re)injury in chronic low back pain and its relation to behavioral performance. *Pain* 62(3): 363–72.

Vowles, K. E., McCracken, L.M., Eccleston, C. (2007). Processes of change in treatment for chronic pain: The contributions of pain, acceptance, and catastrophizing. *European Journal of Pain* 11: 779–87.

Waddell, G., Newton, M., Henderson, I., Somerville, D., Main, C.J. (1993). A fear-avoidance beliefs questionnaire (FABQ) and the role of fear avoidance beliefs in chronic low back pain and disability. *Pain* 52: 157–68.

Waersted, M. (2000). Human muscle activity related to non-biomechanical factors in the workplace. *European Journal of applied physiology* 83(2–3): 151–8.

Waersted, M., Bjøklund, R., Westgaard, R.H. (1991). Shoulder muscle tension induced by two VDT-based tasks of different complexity. *Ergonomics* 34: 137–50.

Watkins, L. R., Maier, S.F. (1999). *Cytokines and pain: progress in inflammation research.* Boston, Birkhauser.

Watkins, L. R., Maier, S.F. (1999a). Implications of immune-to-brain communication for sickness and pain. *Proceedings of the National Academy of Sciences of the United States of America* 96: 7710–13.

Watkins, L.L., Blumethal, J.A., Carney, R.M. (2002). Association of anxiety with reduced baroreflex cardiac control in patients after acute myocardial infarction. *American Heart Journal* 143:460–6.

Watson, P. J., Booker, C.K., Main, C.J., Chen, A.C. (1997). Surface electromyography in the identification of chronic low back pain patients: the development of the flexion relaxation ratio. *Clinical Biomechanics* 12(3): 165–71.

Waxman, S. E., Tripp, D.A., Flamenbaum, R. (2008). The mediating role of depression and negative partner responses in chronic low back pain and relationship satisfaction. *Journal of Pain* 9(5): 434–42.

Westgaard, R. H., Bjørklund, R. (1987). Generation of muscle tension additional to postural muscle load. *Ergonomics* 30(6): 911–23.

Widerström-Noga, E.G., Felix, E.R., Cruz-Almeida, Y., Turk, D.C. (2007). Psychosocial subgroups in persons with spinal cord injuries and chronic pain. *Archives of Physical Medicine and Rehabilitation* 88(12): 1628–35.

Wirtelak, E.P., Roemer, B., Maier, S.F., Watkins, L.R. (1997). Comparison of the effects of nucleus tractus solitarius and ventral medial medulla lesions on illness-induced and subcutaneous formalin-induced hyperalgesia. *Brain Research* 748:143–50.

Woby, S., Urmston, M., Watson, P. (2007). Self-efficacy mediates the relation between pain-related fear and outcome in chronic low back pain patients. *European Journal of Pain* 11(7): 711–18.

Wolf, S.L., Nacht, M., Kelly, J.R. (1982). EMG feedback training during dynamic movement for low back pain patients. *Behavioral Therapy* 13: 395–406.

Yu, X.M., Mense, S. (1990). Response properties and descending control of rat dorsal horn neurons with deep receptive fields. *Neuroscience* 39(3): 823–31.

# Part 3

# Risk Factors of Chronic Back Pain and Disability: Biomechanical Mechanisms

# Chapter 9

# Electromyographically-Determined Muscular Fatigue in Low Back Pain

Anne F. Mannion and David O'Riordan

## 9.1 The theoretical basis for a link between back muscle function and back pain

The back muscles initiate and control all movements of the vertebral column: they are involved in minor active movements of the spine, such as the initiation of manoeuvres that are later assisted by gravity; they contribute to the maintenance of posture when, for example, the movement of other body segments acts to displace the centre of gravity; and they contribute to major movements during forward bending and lifting (Bogduk and Twomey 1991). By controlling these movements, the back muscles also act to stabilize and protect the underlying osteoligamentous spinal structures from potentially harmful stresses that might otherwise be experienced by movements made beyond their optimal functional range and/or for protracted periods of time (Adams and Hutton, 1986). It is not difficult, therefore, to imagine the potential consequences associated with malfunctioning of this muscle group.

Over the last two decades many studies have documented an association between suboptimal back muscle function and the presence of low back pain (LBP). Deficits in the cross-sectional area (Hultman et al. 1993), muscle density (Hultman et al. 1993), maximal force production (Klein et al. 1991; Mooney et al. 1997; Elfving et al. 2003; Lariviere et al. 2003a; Crossman et al. 2004) and local muscular endurance (or fatigue-resistance) (Nicolaisen and Jorgensen 1985; Jorgensen and Nicolaisen 1987; Roy et al. 1989; Mayer et al. 1989; Biedermann et al. 1991; Klein et al. 1991; Cooper et al. 1993; Tsuboi et al. 1994; Roy et al. 1995; Candotti et al. 2008) of the muscles have all been observed, particularly in association with chronic pain. However, despite intensive investigation, a definitive answer to the age-old question of cause and effect—'what comes first, the back pain or the muscle dysfunction?'—remains elusive. From a theoretical point of view, it certainly seems conceivable that inadequate muscular *strength* could predispose to the development of LBP.

The application of a load to the hands requires that the back extensors generate an appropriate antiflexion moment to balance or raise the load against the force of gravity. If sufficient force cannot be generated by active muscle contraction, then the loading may be inadvertently displaced to the passive tissues integrated within and surrounding the osteoligamentous spine. The reduced joint protection, stability, and support may be even more pronounced under conditions of uncontrolled or sudden loading (Wilder et al. 1996), which can be a prominent feature of many manual handling environments. The back extensors are primarily 'slow' postural muscles (Mannion et al. 1997c), with a well-developed capacity to *sustain* static forces, but at the expense of reaction time and speed of contraction (see later). Particularly when loading is applied unexpectedly, these muscles may be unable to generate the required force rapidly enough to prevent excessive bending or twisting of the spine. Rapid trunk flexion movements will generate particularly high bending moments on the spine, because spinal tissues are viscoelastic and resist rapid deformations more vigorously than slow ones (Adams and Dolan 2005).

Despite the plausible hypothesis implicating inadequate back muscle strength in the development of first-time back pain, there is little evidence to support it (Biering-Sorenson 1984; Mostardi et al. 1992; Kujala et al. 1996; Adams et al. 2005). This may be because inappropriate tests of maximal strength have been used, or it might simply suggest that strength requirements are highly job-specific and that the situations in which the back muscles fail to adequately perform their supporting role are mostly random and unpredictable, occurring in connection with accidental events.

The mechanism by which back muscle *fatigability* could be causally associated with the development of LBP is essentially analogous to that discussed above for insufficient strength, in so far as fatigued muscles are actually temporarily weakened (Mannion and Dolan 1996b) and slower (Duchateau and Hainaut 1984) muscles. Thus, during repetitive lifting, the fatigued back muscles may be less effective in generating the required extensor moment, forcing the intervertebral discs and ligaments to withstand a relatively greater bending stress and thereby rendering them more susceptible to injury. Three studies have shown that there is a progressive increase in the degree to which the lumbar spine is flexed during repetitive lifting (Van Doorn 1995; Sparto et al. 1997b; Dolan and Adams 1998), sometimes to an extent that affords only a narrow margin of safety with regards to potential mechanical injury to the intervertebral discs (Dolan and Adams 1998). Further, with back muscle fatigue significant changes have been reported in the angular displacements at the knee, hip, trunk, and elbow during lifting, and these biomechanical changes were associated with increased peak torque and forces at the L4–L5 vertebral segment (Bonato et al. 2003).

Other reports have demonstrated that back muscle fatigue is accompanied by an alteration in anticipatory postural adjustments (Allison and Henry 2002), a reduction in accuracy when trying to generate a given force (Sparto et al. 1997a), impaired sensory (positional) acuity (Taimela et al. 1999), delayed responses to sudden loading (Magnusson et al. 1996), reduced active muscle stiffness necessitating increased antagonist co-contraction (and hence greater spinal compression) to maintain spinal stability (Granata et al. 2004), and an altered coordination of trunk muscle activities, with reduced precise motor control, such that the spine is loaded in a more injury prone pattern (Parnianpour et al. 1988). Each of these could render the lumbar spine more vulnerable to injury during repetitive lifting. Whilst people are often aware of their absolute strength limitations, and can make a considered judgement as to whether they should attempt a given manoeuvre or not, the same is probably not true in the case of muscle fatigue, the onset and consequences of which can be considerably more difficult to predict. This is nicely demonstrated by the familiar scenario in which we judge the weight of a load and deem it manageable to carry, only to realize a short time later—whilst struggling to sustain the effort—that we have failed to account for the continuously declining capacity of the fatiguing muscles. The inability to accurately anticipate fatigue may thus result in individuals being 'caught off guard' at a time when they can least afford to be.

All these findings supported the hypothesis that readily fatigable back muscles might predispose to LBP or be part of a vicious circle in which LBP leads to suboptimal muscle function (consequent to inactivity, disuse or continuous overactivity/overload) which in turn leads to inadequate protection of the osteoligamentous spine, rendering the individual more liable to subsequent episodes of pain or the development of chronic symptoms (Figure 9.1). The evidence supporting this role for back muscle fatigability in LBP will be considered later, once the methods used for its assessment have been discussed.

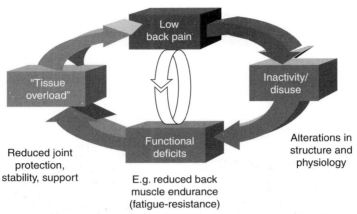

**Fig. 9.1** The vicious circle of the 'deconditioning syndrome', originally described by Mayer et al. (1985). For more information see Mayer et al. (1985).

## 9.2 **Measurement of back muscle fatigue**

Some of the earliest studies examining the predictive role of back muscle endurance and fatigability in LBP involved the use of the now well-known Biering-Sorensen test (Biering-Sorenson 1984). The test is shown in Figure 9.2. Basically, it involves placing the individual in a prone position on an examination couch with the lower body (i.e. from the anterior superior iliac spine distally) strapped firmly to the couch. Individuals attempt to maintain the unsupported upper body in a horizontal position until they are no longer able to overcome the force of gravity. As soon as the upper body ceases to be horizontal, and the person is unable to rectify the situation when urged to do so, the test is terminated. Verbal encouragement is typically given throughout, and the endurance time for the test is recorded to the nearest whole second. Variations on the method (Demoulin et al. 2006) concern the positioning of the arms and hands, the equipment used for the test, and the extent to which correct positioning is assessed.

Other methods for assessing the endurance capacity involve the initial determination of the maximum voluntary contraction (MVC) of the back extensors, using either commercial devices or custom-built equipment (e.g. Figure 9.2), and the subsequent maintenance of a proportion of this maximum for as long as the individual can endure. However, when applied to the clinical population, the need for a maximum contraction in order to set the submaximal load can be problematic, since issues such as fear of (re)injury, pain, etc., can lead to suboptimal performance and hence inaccurate load-setting for the submaximal test. Since the endurance time during a fatiguing task is dependent on the relative force output (Hagberg 1981; Mannion and Dolan 1996b), this has important implications when comparing individuals: if they have not been set the same test to start with, then the comparison of their endurance capacity is futile. Moreover, since measurement of MVC may pose a real risk of injury (Hansson et al. 1984), the use of such tests is necessarily accompanied by various ethical considerations.

Since its introduction, the definition of fatigue as 'the inability to maintain a predetermined exercise intensity' (Ciba Foundation 1981) has been widely accepted—particularly in the study of metabolic mechanisms responsible for human skeletal muscle fatigue. However, it is not entirely satisfactory, especially in relation to the conditions typically encountered in the clinical situation. The definition implies that fatigue is an event that occurs at a specific point in time and it therefore fails to consider the changing conditions within the muscle that ultimately precipitate that failure point. It also necessitates that one be able to drive oneself to this failure point in order to

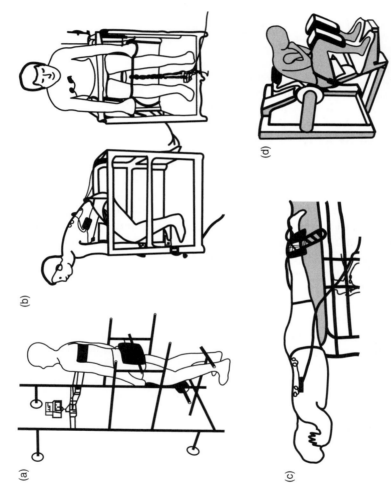

**Fig. 9.2** The four test positions most commonly used for performing back muscle fatigue tests: a) upright standing, pushing backwards; b) standing with flexed trunk pulling up on a bar attached to a load cell between the feet; c) prone, Biering-Sorensen test; d) seated, hips and knees flexed, using back extension machine.

make the assessment. In practice, when measuring an individual's ability to sustain a given force or power output, the endurance time is influenced not only by the intrinsic physiological qualities of the muscle but also by factors such as motivation, boredom, tolerance of the discomfort of fatiguing muscles, and in the clinical situation perhaps also by actual pain or fear of pain. It therefore adopts a psychological dimension.

Although it may be of importance to know the maximum length of time that an individual can sustain a contraction, it is also useful to assess the changes in the muscle that lead up to the eventual failure point, not least in order to predict when it might occur. In some studies, this has been done by monitoring the changing metabolic status of the muscle during contraction (e.g. the increasing lactate concentration, or declining pH and intracellular potassium ion concentrations). However, such measures require invasive techniques or the use of sophisticated equipment such as 31P-NMR, and are hence not suitable for clinical studies. For these reasons, the use of surface electromyography became an increasingly popular tool for monitoring the progressively declining capacity of the muscles during fatiguing contractions (De Luca 1997; Jurell 1998). The technique typically involves examination of the change in the frequency distribution of the power density spectrum of the electromyographic (EMG) signal, obtained by fast Fourier transform of the EMG signal.

During sustained isometric contraction, a compression of the spectrum to lower frequencies is observed (Figure 9.3), and this is tracked using a characteristic component of the spectrum, such as its median frequency (MF) or mean power frequency (MPF), plotting this against time using linear regression techniques. The slope of the decline in MF (in either Hz/s or %/s, normalized to the initial MF, i.e. the intercept of the regression curve) is then taken to indicate the fatigability of the muscle. Previous work has shown that the rate of decline in MF is highly correlated with endurance time (Hagberg 1981; Mannion and Dolan 1994) and also with the accumulation of certain muscle metabolites that have been implicated in the development of muscle fatigue (Bouissou et al. 1989; Brody et al. 1991; Vestergaard-Poulsen et al. 1992). The EMG power spectral

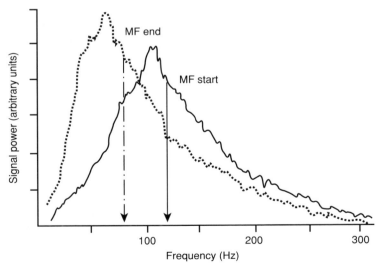

**Fig. 9.3** EMG power spectrum at the start and end of a fatiguing contraction, showing the reduction in median frequency (i.e. the frequency that splits the power spectrum in two parts containing equal power).

statistics can hence be used to indirectly monitor the development of these underlying metabolic changes in the muscle, even in the absence of any decline in its given mechanical output.

It has been shown that the decline in EMG MF reflects the muscle's inability to generate its *maximal* force (Mannion and Dolan 1996b) (Figure 9.4). Therefore, it can be stated that the decline in EMG MF can be used to monitor fatigue, where fatigue is defined as the inability to generate the maximum force that can be produced by the muscle in its fresh state. The definition is similar to that originally proposed by Bigland-Ritchie and Woods (1984).

EMG indices other than the MF or MPF are sometimes used in attempts to monitor the development of back muscle fatigue. The rise in the average or integrated EMG signal has been measured (Cooper et al. 1993), as has the power in the low frequency bands (Dolan et al. 1995;

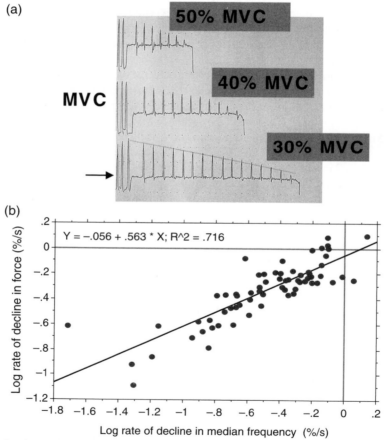

**Fig. 9.4** Decline in maximum force-generating capacity of the knee extensors at different force levels (a) and relationship between rate of decline in median frequency of the rectus femoris and rate of decline in quadriceps isometric maximal force output during sustained contraction (b) (for further details see Mannion and Dolan 1996b). With kind permission from Springer Science+Business Media: *European Journal of Applied Physiology and Occupational Physiology*, Relationship between myoelectric and mechanical manifestations of fatigue in the quadriceps femoris muscle group, 74(5), 1996, Anne F. Mannion.

Kramer et al. 2005), the spectral power 'high to low ratio' (Bradl et al. 2005) and the 'half-width' of the EMG power spectrum signal (Oliver et al. 1996; Nargol et al. 1999; Humphrey et al. 2005). Further, some studies have used nonlinear time series analysis (Sung et al. 2005), wavelet analyses (Sparto et al. 1999), short-time Fourier transforms, or non-linear recurrence quantification analysis (Liu et al. 2004) of the EMG signal in order to obviate the difficulties caused by non-stationary signals, especially when analysing dynamic movements. However, it is not always clear how such measures (or their changes with fatigue) are to be interpreted on a physiological or anatomical basis; as such, they are less helpful in establishing the nature of the deficit and the type of intervention required to remedy it (see later). Of all the EMG parameters, only the slope of the reduction in MF or MPF of the EMG power spectrum has been linked to known metabolic indices of fatigue (Bouissou et al. 1989; Brody et al. 1991) and/or the muscle fibre type composition (Kupa et al. 1995; Mannion et al. 1998).

The establishment of EMG-based indices of back muscle fatigue initially generated great optimism that a measure had been found that was free of the subjectivity of voluntary effort and would represent an ideal test to assess LBP-related deficiencies in clinical practice. However, initial enthusiasm was dampened somewhat by later reports that challenged the true objectivity of these measures. First, it became apparent that the power spectral changes were not entirely independent of test contraction time, because the decline in MF was not always linear (Mayer et al. 1989; Mannion and Dolan 1994; Dedering et al. 2000); hence, during an exercise bout of submaximal duration, the choice of test-length became an issue. The initial hope had been that, with a linear rate of decline in the spectral indices, the test duration would be immaterial, as long as sufficient data points could be collected to allow accurate enough determination of the slope of the regression. Ultimately, it was recommended that, in order to circumvent this problem, the endurance test should be carried out as far as possible to the individual's endurance limit (Mayer et al. 1989; Mannion and Dolan 1994; Dedering et al. 2000). In practice, a shortfall of perhaps up to 20–30 seconds on a 2–3-minute test would, however, be unlikely to lead to grossly inaccurate values.

Another issue concerned the relative loading chosen for the test, for which still no optimal solution exists: if the load is set as a percentage maximum voluntary contraction (Lariviere et al. 2003a; Crossman et al. 2004), then it becomes dependent on the generation of a true maximum in the first place, which can be a challenge in the clinical population (see earlier); if it is expressed as an absolute force (i.e. the same load for all alike) (Biedermann et al. 1991), then this is disadvantageous for the smaller or weaker individuals in the group. If it is set using one's own body-weight supported against gravity (e.g. as in the Biering-Sorensen (Biering-Sorenson 1984), Roman chair test (Mayer et al. 1989)), then it is dependent on the individual's anthropometric characteristics and their upper body load (Suuden et al. 2008) as a proportion of their maximum back strength. There is no satisfactory answer to this problem, although the Biering-Sorensen test might arguably be considered the 'best of a bad lot', since it has the greatest potential for providing a load-challenge in proportion to the individual's own body dimensions. Further, even if it *does* place some 'atypically proportioned' individuals at a disadvantage, those same unfavourable biomechanics that prevail during performance of the test prevail also during everyday activities involving repeated or prolonged bending and lifting activities; in this sense, performance in the Biering-Sorensen test may be considered to better reflect the response of the muscles to the demands placed upon them in daily life and hence represent a measure of 'functional fatigability' (Mannion et al. 1997a).

The aforementioned methodological shortcomings should be considered carefully when seeking to interpret the results of the various clinical studies on back muscle fatigue. This will be discussed in more detail later in this chapter.

## 9.3 **Reliability of EMG measurements of back muscle fatigue**

If EMG-fatigue indices are to be used to monitor individual performance and its change over time (e.g. to examine deterioration accompanying the development of a 'chronic' back problem, or improvement following rehabilitation) then it is extremely important that the methods demonstrate adequate test-retest reliability (i.e. low measurement error). A search in PubMed of studies concerned with EMG measures of back muscle fatigue (search terms 'EMG and low back and fatigue' or 'EMG and lumbar and muscle fatigue'; search date, 13 August 2008) revealed many studies on the reliability of the established EMG indices of muscle fatigue (rate of decline in MF/MPF), in both control and LBP patients. Their main findings are summarized in Table 9.1. The studies report differing degrees of reliability, which is likely influenced by the test type, duration of contraction, test equipment, muscles monitored, number of subjects, time between repeated test sessions, etc. Notably, the data of patients with LBP were just as reliable as those of controls.

Reliability will always be compromised if good technique following established guidelines (e.g. Hermens et al. 2000; and www.seniam.org) is not adhered to and if attention is not paid to factors such as maintaining consistent and accurate electrode alignment between sessions. It is not easy to condense the findings of the various reliability studies into overarching practical recommendations; however, in general, it would appear that measures are most reliable when using tests that demand moderately high force outputs (50–60% MVC), performed for at least 60–90 seconds, with electrodes positioned more medially (i.e. overlying the multifidi muscles) at lower lumbar levels (between L3 and L5), using the average of multiple recording sites on both sides of the body. Whether the MF or MPF data are normalized to the initial value of the MF or MPF (intercept of the regression of MF/MPF against time) does not appear to make a large difference (Table 9.1). Following the above recommendations, intraclass correlation coefficients (ICCs) of over 0.8 appear to be achievable, with smallest detectable differences of approx 30% of the absolute mean value for the given index. The latter figure is particularly important since it influences the sensitivity of the measure to differences between individuals and individual change over time. If the error of measurement is large, then only interventions with extremely large effect sizes will be able to be evaluated by the method (i.e. the signal would need to be very large in comparison to the noise).

As can be seen from Table 9.1, many studies report that the initial median frequency (IMF) is highly reliable. However, the relevance of this measure per se within the context of muscle fatigue is uncertain. Certainly it would appear to have more to do with the size, length, relative force output, and (possibly) relative fibre type sizes of the muscle (Mannion and Dolan 1996a; Mannion et al. 1998), as well as the degree of subcutaneous fat interposed between the electrodes and the muscle (Mannion and Dolan 1996a), than with muscle fatigue.

## 9.4 **Physiological/anatomical factors governing fatigability/ muscle endurance**

Compared with the number of studies that have examined either the reliability of EMG measures of back muscle fatigue (see above) or their ability to distinguish between individuals with LBP and 'normal' healthy controls (see later), relatively few studies have been carried out to better understand the cause of the changes in the power spectrum and hence the mechanisms that might underlie any observed differences between groups, following disuse, or upon training/rehabilitation. If preventive strategies are to be developed in relation to first-time LBP or its deterioration from the acute to the chronic condition, then such information must be considered indispensable.

**Table 9.1** Summary of results of studies examining the test-retest reliability of EMG-measures of back muscle fatigue using the rate of decline of median or mean power frequency

| Author year | No. subjects | LBP (Y/N) | Test condition | Measures (muscle and EMG index) | Retest interval | MF or MPF slope (Hz/s or %/s) | IMF or IMPF (Hz) | Other measures | Authors' comments |
|---|---|---|---|---|---|---|---|---|---|
| Roy et al. (1989) | 4 (4M) | N | Upright standing extension. 80% MVC for 30s | Longiss L1, iliocost L2 and multif L5<br><br>IMF, MFslope (Hz/s) | 15 min | ICC 0.94 | ICC 0.98 | | Technique highly reliable |
| Biedermann et al. (1990) | 31 | N | Upright standing, weight of 11.6 lbs in outstretched arms 45s | Multif, iliocost<br><br>IMF, IRMS | 5 days | | **Test/retest correl** Multifidus 0.90 (L), 0.95 (R) Iliocostalis 0.79 (L), 0.76(R) | **IRMS (retest correl)** Multifidus 0.92 (L), 0.86 (R) Iliocostalis 0.93 (L), 0.86 (R) | Test/retest reliability is better for the multifidus than the iliocostalis. |
| Mannion and Dolan (1994) | 5 (2F, 3M) | N | Biering Sorensen test to exhaustion | Erector spinae, unilateral T10 and L3<br><br>MF init, MF slope (%/s) | 1–2 wks | ICC 0.82–0.98 CV 14.0–23.3% | ICC 0.70–0.77 CV 7.0–9.1% | Greatest MF slope %/s, either region ICC 0.97, CV 9.7% | MF slope is a suitable technique for monitoring back muscle fatigue. |
| Ng and Richardson (1996) | 12 (M) | N | Biering-Sorensen test 60s | Iliocost, L2; multif, L5<br><br>IMF, MFslope (Hz/s) | 3 days | **Iliocost** ICC 0.56, CV 33.0% **Multif** ICC 0.78, CV 27.5% | **Iliocost** ICC 0.86, CV 8.5% **Multif** ICC 0.79, CV 7.0% | | Reliable method if use adequate measures to minimize cross-talk. Better reliability for the multifidus |

*(continued)*

**Table 9.1** (continued) Summary of results of studies examining the test–retest reliability of EMG-measures of back muscle fatigue using the rate of decline of median or mean power frequenc

| Author year | No. subjects | LBP (Y/N) | Test condition | Measures (muscle and EMG index) | Retest interval | MF or MPF slope (Hz/s or %/s) | IMF or IMPF (Hz) | Other measures | Authors' comments |
|---|---|---|---|---|---|---|---|---|---|
| van Dieen and Heijblom (1996) | 9 (M) | N | Sitting lumbar extension (Biodex); 80%MVC to exhaustion | Multif, iliocost and longiss. <br><br> RAEMG (rectified & ave EMG, µV/s) <br> MPF slope (%/s) | ≥2 days | ICC 0.84–0.91 <br> SDD (%) 25–71 | | RAEMG slope <br> ICC 0.31–0.91 <br> SDD (%) 61–188 | Reproducibility of MPF superior to RAEMG. ICCs tended to be high, but smallest detectable difference large, limiting clinical applicability. |
| Oliver et al. (1996) | 10 (M) | N | Standing pulling up with trunk flexed 30°. 33% and 66% MVC for 30s | Erector spinae, bilat L4–5 (NB electrodes widely spaced) <br><br> IMF <br> MF slope (Hz/s) <br> Spectral half-width <br> Total power slope | 1 day–4 wks | **33% MVC test** <br> ICC 0.44 <br> **66% MVC test** <br> ICC 0.72 | **33% MVC test** <br> ICC 0.92 <br> SDD (Hz) 8.5 <br> **66% MVC test** <br> ICC 0.96 <br> SDD (Hz) 6.3 | **Half-width** <br> **33%, 66% MVC** <br> ICC 0.92, 0.94 <br> **Power slope** <br> **33%, 66% MVC** <br> ICC 0.18, 0.43 | At 33% and 66% of MVC, MF init and half-width were reproducible; slopes of the increase in power and decrease in median frequency were not reproducible |
| Mannion et al. (1997a) | 10 (4M, 6F) | N | 1) Standing pulling up at 60%MVC isom trunk extension, lumbar spine 60–70% of max ROF 2) Biering-Sorensen test. | Erector spine, bilateral T10 L3 MF init MF slope (%/s) | ≥1 day | **60% MVC** <br> Indiv muscles ICC 0.73–0.96 <br> mean ICC T10, 0.72 <br> mean ICC L3, 0.95 <br> **BS test** <br> Indiv muscles ICC 0.97–0.99 | **60% MVC** <br> Indiv muscles ICC 0.80–0.98 <br> **BS test** <br> Indiv muscles ICC 0.59–0.94 | Greatest MF slope %/s <br> **60% MVC test** <br> ICC 0.94 <br> **BS test** <br> ICC 0.97 | Recommend recording from more than one site. MF slope, excellent technique for objectively monitoring fatigability of the erector spinae muscles during sustained isometric contractions |

| Study | n (sex) | | Task | Muscles / Measures | Interval | Results | Results | Results | Comments |
|---|---|---|---|---|---|---|---|---|---|
| | | | Each to exhaustion. | | | | mean ICC T10, 0.99 mean ICC L3, 0.98 | | Good reproducibility of the spectral indices |
| Kankaanpaa et al. (1997) | 10 (8M, 2F) | N | Sitting, submax 30 reps/min isoinertial trunk flex/ext on a David Back Clinic 110 machine | Paraspinal muscles, L3–4 and L5/S1 — MF slope (%/min) MPF slope (%/min) Recorded over: 60s, 90s, 120s | 1 day | Both sides, all levels: **Over 60s (MF)** ICC 0.36–0.77 **Over 90s (MF)** ICC 0.58–0.89 **Over 120s (MF)** ICC 0.70–0.94 (MPF similar) | | | |
| Peach et al. (1998) | 16 (2 grps × 8 (3M, 5F in each)) | N | Semi-standing 30s isometric contraction at 60% MVC | Erector spinae T9 and L3 levels, multifidus L5 level — IMF MF slope (Hz/s) REC | (1) every day for 1wk; (2) 1 day/ wk for 4 wks | ICC over all sites, both groups, R & L −0.138–0.656 | ICC over all sites, both groups, R & L 0.380–0.975 ICC L3, L5 sites, day group L & R 0.889–0.975 | REC ICC over all sites R & L L −.045–0.377 | Apart from IMF, spectral parameters not very reliable within a subject. Experimental condition must have sufficiently large changes in MF to constitute a valid measure (signal>noise). |
| Elfving et al. (1999) | 11 (3M, 8F) | N | Sitting, knee and hips flexed, 80% MVC isometric trunk extension, David Back 110, 45s | Erector spinae L1 and L5 levels — IMF MF slope, %/s | Ave 5 (range 2–13) days | **80% MVC test** ICC 0.04–0.45 SEM all sites R & L 0.20–0.27%/s (CV 35–75%) | **80% MVC test** ICC 0.41–0.70 SEM all sites R & L 4.4–5.5 Hz (CV approx 10%) | **Borg scale** ICC 0.84 SEM 0.8 CV 17% | The 95% CIs for the variables were: IMF ± 10 Hz, slope ± 0.4–0.5%/s. Slope may be of limited value because of its large variability |

*(continued)*

**Table 9.1** (continued) Summary of results of studies examining the test–retest reliability of EMG-measures of back muscle fatigue using the rate of decline of median or mean power frequenc

| Author year | No. subjects | LBP (Y/N) | Test condition | Measures (muscle and EMG index) | Retest interval | MF or MPF slope (Hz/s or %/s) | IMF or IMPF (Hz) | Other measures | Authors' comments |
|---|---|---|---|---|---|---|---|---|---|
| Dedering et al. (2000) | 10 (2M,8F) | N | Biering-Sorensen test to exhaustion. | Erector spinae L1 and L5 levels<br><br>IMF<br>MF slope, Hz/s, %/s | ≥ 1 day | **Raw, Hz/s** ICC 0.70–0.87 SEM 0.014–0.022 CV%, 14.4–26.2% **Normalized, %/s** ICC 0.65–0.90 SEM 0.015–0.025 CV%, 12.0–23.9% | ICC 0.73–0.84 SEM 4.6–7.8 Hz CV%, 7.2–8.9% | Endurance time ICC 0.89 | Protocol proved to be reliable and is recommended for further use |
| Koumantakis et al. (2001) | 16 (7M, 9F) | N | 1) Standing pulling up isometric trunk extension at 60% MVC 2) Biering-Sorensen test each for 60s | Erector spinae L2/3, multifidi L4/5<br><br>IMF<br>MF slope Hz/min<br>MF slope %/min<br>RMS | 3 wks | **60% MVC all sites** **MF Hz/min** ICC 0.62–0.91 SDD 36–69% **MF %/min** ICC 0.73–0.92 SDD 33–53% **BS test all sites** **MF Hz/min** ICC 0.53–0.87 SDD 46–82% **MF %/min** ICC 0.52–0.84 SDD 49–71% | **60% MVC test** all sites, R & L ICC 0.89–0.96 SDD 12–25% **BS test** all sites, R & L ICC 0.79–0.97 SDD 10–27% | 60% MVC, all sites RMS (%/min) ICC 0.38–0.89 SDD 86–170% BS test, all sites RMS (%/min) ICC 0.51–0.74 SDD 350–467% | Reproducibility of IMF excellent for both tests. Normalized MF slope (%/min) more reliable with 60% MVC than BS test. Both MFinit and MFslope can have clinical applicability. RMS amplitude had a very large between-day error for both tests |

| Study | N | LBP | Protocol | Muscles / Indices | Interval | Results | Conclusions |
|---|---|---|---|---|---|---|---|
| Ebenbichler et al. (2002) | 14 (all M) | N | Standing, knees flexed: static lifting at 80% MVC for 30s; 12 dynamic box-lifts (13kg)/min for 4.5 min | Paravertebral back muscles L5, L2, T10 / Instantaneous median frequency (IMDF) dynamic. MF time trends | 2 hrs and 2 wks | **MF time trends** all data sampled ICC 0.73–0.95; **IMDF (dynamic)** all data sampled ICC 0.62–0.90 | Static and dynamic lifting MDF time dependent changes, good to excellent reliability |
| Lariviere et al. (2002) | 40 (M) | Y (20cLBP) | Standing 75% MVC fatigue test for 30s | Bilateral longiss L1 and T10, iliocost L3, multif L5 — IMF Hz, MFslope Hz/s, %/s, RMSslope  µV/s, REC (recovery of MF) | ≥ 2 days | **MF slope** **Control** Indiv muscles ICC 0.26–0.77; mean (SD) of all 0.64 (0.14) Indiv muscles **SEM** 22–71%; mean (SD) of all, 35 (18)% **CLBP** Indiv muscles **ICC** 0.43–0.76; mean (SD) of all 0.64 (0.10) Indiv muscles **SEM** 34–87%; mean (SD) of all, 47(16)% (values for MF %/s; MF Hz/s similar) / **IMF** **Control** Indiv muscles, **ICC** 0.47–0.85; mean (SD) all muscles 0.76 (0.13) Indiv muscles **SEM** 6–12%; mean (SD) all muscles, 7 (2)% **CLBP** Indiv muscles, ICC 0.52–0.89; mean (SD) all muscles 0.82 (0.12) Indiv muscles SEM 6–16%; mean (SD) all muscles 8 (3)% / **Power in 20–60 Hz band (µV².Hz)/s)** **Control** Indiv muscles, ICC 0.54–0.90; mean (SD) of all 0.78 (0.13) Indiv muscles, SEM 49–89% Mean (SD) of all, 59 (12)% **CLBP** Indiv muscles, ICC 0.40–0.68; mean (SD) of all 0.52 (0.10) Indiv muscles, SEM 6–16%; mean (%) 74–159; mean (SD) of all, 114 (26) | Reliable EMG indices obtainable for both controls and cLBP patients. Better reliability with the medial muscles of the back. The reliability of EMG indices might be increased by averaging across recording sites and over repeated measurements. |

*(continued)*

**Table 9.1** (continued) Summary of results of studies examining the test–retest reliability of EMG-measures of back muscle fatigue using the rate of decline of median or mean power frequenc

| Author year | No. subjects | LBP (Y/N) | Test condition | Measures (muscle and EMG index) | Retest interval | MF or MPF slope (Hz/s or %/s) | IMF or IMPF (Hz) | Other measures | Authors' comments |
|---|---|---|---|---|---|---|---|---|---|
| Arnall et al. (2002) | 10 (6M, 4F) | N | Standing pulling up at 40, 50 & 60% MVC isom trunk extension, trunk flexed 30° to vertical, 60s | Paraspinal muscles L2/3 and L4/5 bilaterally. <br><br> IMF (Hz) <br> MFslope (Hz/s and %/s) <br> RMSincline (μV/s and %/min) | 3 days | **50%MVC test** ICC 0.26–0.77 SEM 4. 2–8.3%/min <br> **60%MVC test** ICC 0.24–0.53 SEM 3.8–9.1%/min (values for MF %/s; MF Hz/s similar) No measurable EMG-fatigue at 40%MVC | **50%MVC test** ICC 0.74–0.86 SEM 4.2–12.0 Hz **60%MVC test** ICC 0.70–0.89 SEM 4.1–11.2 Hz | **RMS./min** **50%MVC test** ICC 0.70–0.83 SEM 11.3–25.5%/min **60%MVC test** ICC s 0.30–0.87 SEM 6.3–15.7%/min (values for RMS %/s; μV/s similar) | Measures at 50% MVC most reliable. IMF and RMS values more reliable than MFslope. **Overall, reliability better at L4/5 than L2/3.** At L4/5 level all parameters acceptably reliable at 50% MVC |
| Lariviere et al. (2003a) | 40 (M) | Y(20M), N (20 M) | Standing isometric trunk extension fatigue test 75% MVC for 30s | Longiss T10, L1, Illiocost L3, Multif L5. <br><br> IMF <br> MFslope, Hz/s | ≥2 days | **Bilateral average, medial muscles** ICC 0.68–0.91 SEM 5–35% **Average of all** ICC 0.77–0.91 SEM 5–30% | ICC 0.68–0.91 SEM (%) ≤10 | Greatest MF slope, any muscle ICC 0.74–0.79 SEM (%) 21–26 | Similar reliability, controls and patients. RMS slope not eliable. Averaging MF slope over all sites increased reliability. Bilateral medial recording sites most reliable. |

| Elfving et al. (2003) | 20 | Y (20) | Sitting, knee and hips flexed, 80% MVC isometric trunk extension, David Back 110, 45s | Erector spinae L1, L5 ――― IMF, MF slope %/s, REC | 1–6 days | ICC 0.45–0.71 (L1 mean 0.49, L5 mean 0.63) SEM 0.16–0.23%/s (L1 mean 0.17, L5 mean 0.21) | ICC 0.78–0.89 SEM 3.9–6.0 Hz | REC **ICC 0–0.36** | Reliability of IMF good; MF slope less so. ICC's higher for patients than (in previous study) controls; SEM similar for both. REC not reliable enough for individual assessment. |

ICC, intraclass correlation coefficient; IMF, initial MF at the beginning of the fatigue test; MF, median frequency; MPF, mean power frequency; REC, recovery of median frequency after fatigue test; RMS, root mean squared amplitude; IRMS, RMS amplitude at the beginning of the fatigue test; SDD, smallest detectable difference; SEM, standard error of measurement. Longiss, longissimus; iliocost, iliocostalis; multif, multifidus.

The fatigue-resistance of skeletal muscles is typically governed by their fibre type area distribution, capillary density, and enzyme activities and associated metabolism (Saltin and Gollnick 1983). All adult mammalian skeletal muscles contain at least three distinct fibre types, classified on the basis of their functional and metabolic properties as type I (or 'slow twitch'), type IIA ('fast twitch oxidative'), or type IIX ('fast twitch glycolytic') (in previous nomenclature, referred to as the type IIB fibre; Sant'Ana Pereira et al. 1997). The type I fibre possesses low ATPase activity, a prolonged twitch duration (hence, 'slow twitch') and a low maximal velocity. In addition, it contains a higher mitochondrial content and a greater oxidative enzyme complement than the type II fibre. Type II fibres are characterized by higher ATPase activities and correspondingly shorter isometric twitch durations and are better endowed with enzymes that support the regeneration of ATP through anaerobic mechanisms. The type IIX fibre is generally more 'extreme' in each of these respects than the type IIA. During sustained isometric contraction, muscles that possess a predominance of slow twitch type I fibres contract more 'economically' (i.e. they utilize less energy to maintain the same relative force for the same time, compared with muscles in which the fast twitch fibre predominates). This reduces the rate of development of inhibitory metabolic end-products, which have often been implicated in the fatigue process (Bouissou et al. 1989; Laurent et al. 1993). As such, a greater fatigue-resistance is bestowed upon the 'slow twitch' muscle, which allows for a protracted contraction time (whilst maintaining the same relative force output) in comparison with 'faster' muscle. By virtue of variations in their fibre-type proportions and relative fibre-type sizes, skeletal muscles have the potential to be specialized for specific types of movement or function. The back extensors have evolved as primarily postural muscles, with a predominance of large slow twitch fibres and a superior endurance capacity compared with other skeletal muscles.

As mentioned previously, the rate of decline in the EMG power spectrum MF shows a high correlation with the force being sustained (Figure 9.5), the task endurance time, and the rate of reduction of the muscle's maximum force-generating capacity (Figure 9.4) (Mannion and Dolan 1996b). This indicates that—even if the common denominator remains elusive—there

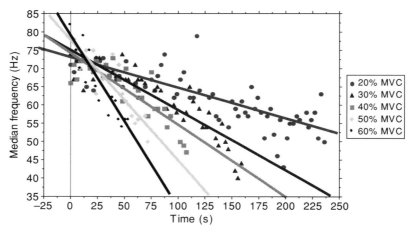

**Fig. 9.5** (See also Colour Plate 6) Rate of decline in median frequency at differing submaximal contraction force outputs (% MVC) for the quadriceps femoris muscle. See Mannion and Dolan (1996b) for details. With kind permission from Springer Science+Business Media: *European Journal of Applied Physiology and Occupational Physiology*, Relationship between myoelectric and mechanical manifestations of fatigue in the quadriceps femoris muscle group, **74**(5), 1996, A. F. Mannion.

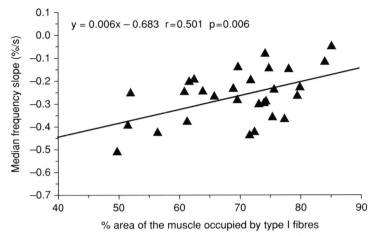

**Fig. 9.6** Relationship between proportional area of the muscle occupied by type I fibres and the slope of the decline in EMG median frequency (for details see Mannion et al. 1998). Reproduced from Mannion, A.F., Dumas, G.A., Stevenson, J.M. and Cooper, R.G. The influence of muscle fiber size and type distribution on electromyographic measures of back muscle fatigability. *Spine*, **23**, pp. 576–84. © 1998, Lippincott, Williams, and Wilkins.

exists a close association between myoelectric and mechanical indices of fatigue for specific tasks. As the muscle's fibre type composition influences the rate of build-up of inhibitory metabolites and these, in turn, seem to be responsible for changes in the muscle's mechanical function (twitch tension, rate of rise of twitch tension, twitch relaxation time, etc.) (Sahlin 1992), it is to be expected that there would also be some relationship between the muscle's fibre type composition and its myoelectric manifestations of fatigue. Our own studies conducted on healthy controls in the late 1990s showed that the greater the relative area of the muscle occupied by type I (slow twitch) fibres, the less rapid was the decline in MF and (generally) the longer was the contraction sustained (Mannion et al. 1998) (Figure 9.6). In two recent studies (Kaser et al. 2001; Crossman et al. 2004) this relationship was confirmed also in LBP patients. If, as suggested, changing metabolic conditions within the muscle are responsible for eliciting the EMG power spectral shift, then this would explain the observed association between the decline in MF and the muscle fibre type area distribution. The correlation appears to be crucially dependent on the relative *size* of the muscle fibre types, in addition to their distribution by number.

   In one of the above studies, the relationship between the percentage type I area and the EMG fatigability of the muscle was shown to remain relatively constant before and after 3 months of exercise therapy (Kaser et al. 2001). The findings of a relatively consistent fatigue level associated with a given proportional area of the muscle occupied by type I fibres were also supported by the study of Crossman et al. (2004), in which the values observed for percentage type I fibre area and the MF decline during fatigue were almost identical in a group of patients with chronic LBP and in controls.

## 9.5 **The evidence for back muscular fatigue as a predictor of back pain**

At this stage in our examination of the role of EMG-fatigue in LBP, we can conclude that: (1) there are good theoretical arguments as to why fatigable back muscles might be associated with LBP;

(2) EMG-fatigue can be measured sufficiently reliably; (3) any differences in EMG-determined back muscle fatigability are likely related to differences in the underlying muscle fibre type size and composition. The next two sections will examine the evidence for a role of back muscular fatigability in LBP.

Using the Biering-Sorensen test, three prospective studies have shown that poor back muscle endurance is associated with an increased risk of developing first-time low back pain (Biering-Sorenson 1984; Luoto et al. 1995; Adams et al. 1999). However, as mentioned earlier, the 'time to fatigue' during isometric endurance tests is influenced by certain psychological factors, and since some of these may themselves be independent determinants of the risk of developing LBP (Bigos et al. 1992; Mannion et al. 1996), this rather complicates things. In one study of risk factors for first-time LBP, 'psychological disturbance' was assessed by questionnaire (a combined score from the Zung depression questionnaire and the Modified Somatic Perception Questionnaire (Greenough and Fraser 1991) and the scores were examined in relation to performance on the Biering-Sorensen test (Mannion et al. 1996). For each individual, the time completed on the endurance test was deducted from the time that would have been predicted on the basis of the corresponding EMG changes in the back muscles, using the relationship between the greatest decline in MF at any recording site versus endurance time for the group (Figure 9.7).

The extent to which the endurance time either exceeded or fell short of the predicted time showed a significant correlation with psychological 'disturbance' (Mannion et al. 1996), which itself was one of the most significant predictors of first time significant LBP (Adams et al. 1999). Thus, in risk factor studies in which muscle endurance has been examined in isolation, its importance may have been overestimated and it may have earned its role in predictive models by virtue of its relationship with some of the important psychological factors. Using a similar 'performance

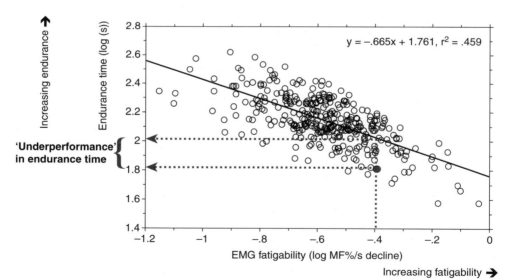

**Fig. 9.7** (See also Colour Plate 7) Plot of the endurance time versus EMG-MF slope for individuals participating in a study of risk factors for LBP (for details, see Mannion et al. 1996). Using the slope of the relationship between these two measures, it was possible to predict the endurance time associated with a given EMG fatigability. The subject's actual performance (e.g. filled circle at approx. −0.4%/s below) could then be calculated in relation to his predicted endurance time (using the regression equation) and expressed as the number of seconds of either 'under-performance' or 'over-performance' compared with his/her peers.

discrepancy score' for the Biering-Sorensen test, a group of 148 patients with chronic LBP were categorized as either underperformers (or 'discomfort-intolerant') or over-performers ('discomfort-tolerant') compared with their contemporaries (Mannion et al. submitted). In bivariate analyses, underperformers had significantly higher scores for Roland–Morris disability (Roland and Morris 1983), Back Beliefs (Symonds et al. 1996), psychological disturbance (Zung and MSPQ) (Greenough and Fraser 1991), catastrophizing (Rosenstiel and Keefe,1983), and exercise self-efficacy (Schwarzer 1993); their scores for Fear Avoidance Beliefs were of borderline significance (p=0.055) Underperformers were also older, and more likely to be female. Interestingly, body mass index (BMI), maximum rate of decline in MF per second ('intrinsic' fatigability), average and worst back pain intensity, duration of LBP and frequency of back pain did not differ significantly between the groups. In multiple stepwise linear regression analysis to predict the 'expected minus actual endurance time', female gender, psychological disturbance and 'negative' back beliefs were significant predictors of 'underperformance' in the model (adj R-squared, 22.3%; p <0.001). Once again, this highlights the fact that performance in the Biering-Sorensen, as measured by endurance time alone, reflects much more than just the intrinsic physiological fatigability of the trunk musculature and this must be borne in mind when interpreting the results of studies based on this measure. A similar conclusion was reached in a recent review of the test for spinal muscle evaluation (Demoulin et al. 2006).

No studies to date have shown that the 'intrinsic' physiological fatigability of the back musculature (measured using EMG-techniques) influences the likelihood of developing LBP. In the aforementioned study of predictors of first-time LBP (Adams et al. 1999), endurance time was significantly (though weakly) associated with the development of LBP in bivariate analyses (albeit failing to make a significant contribution in a multivariate model including the psychological variables), but the objective EMG-indices of fatigability failed to reach significance at any of the many follow-ups, in either bivariate or multivariate analyses. Thus, despite the convincing theoretical arguments, there is actually little evidence to support the notion that back muscle fatigability (as distinct from endurance capacity) is a significant risk factor for the development of low back pain.

## 9.6 **The evidence for changes in back muscular fatigue as a consequence of back pain**

From the foregoing discussion, it would appear that any associations between muscle fatigability and LBP are likely the consequence rather than the cause of the development of first-time LBP. Conceivably, they might be 'causal' in relation to the recurrence of LBP, via the vicious circle of pain, inactivity and altered muscular function described in Figure 9.1, but this has not been well investigated. In examining any such relationships, the use of objective EMG measures is absolutely essential. As discussed earlier, if only the endurance time for the contraction is measured, then poor achievers may be demonstrating nothing more than an unwillingness to perform, or a particularly low pain/discomfort tolerance.

In the PubMed search of the literature referred to earlier (see earlier section 'Reliability of EMG measurements of back muscle fatigue'), more than 20 studies were identified in which the rate of decline in MF (or MPF) was compared in groups of patients with LBP and healthy controls. Brief methodological details and the main findings of these studies are shown in Table 9.2, ordered by the date of publication. Interestingly, the first seven studies, carried out between 1989 and 1994 (many of them small studies, on males only, and from the same research group), all showed that groups of individuals with LBP were significantly more fatigable than controls, and that individuals could be classified accurately into their groups based on their EMG-spectral characteristics

**Table 9.2** Summary of results of studies examining the difference between groups of controls and groups of patients with LBP using the rate of decline of the EMG median (or mean) power frequency.

| Author (year) | Groups | Test procedure | Findings for differences in MF slope (EMG fatigability) |
|---|---|---|---|
| Roy et al. (1989) | 12 LBP, 12 control (all male) | Back Analysis System (standing isometric extension, 40%, 60%, 80% MVC for max 60s; 15min between efforts); bilateral EMG at L1 longiss, L2 iliocost, L5 multifid | LBP > control (at L2, L5 80% MVC only) |
| Mayer et al. (1989) | 10 LBP (8M, 2F) 11 control (8M, 3F) | Upper torso unsupported (Roman Chair) for successive fixed-time trials; EMG, erector spinae L3 | LBP > control |
| Roy et al. (1990) | 6 LBP, 17 control (all male) | Back Analysis System (standing isometric extension, 80% MVC for max 30s); bilateral EMG at L1 longiss, L2 iliocost, L5 multifid | LBP > control |
| Klein et al. (1991) | 8 LBP, 17 control (all male) | Back Analysis System (standing isometric extension, 80% MVC for max 30s); bilateral EMG at L1 longiss, L2 iliocost, L5 multifid | LBP > control |
| Biedermann et al. (1991) | 25 LBP (13M, 11F) 22 cont (10M, 12F) | Standing, in reference frame. Arms outstretched, holding a free weight (2×5lb). EMG MF, L2–3, L4–5. Patients classified as 'avoiders' or 'confronters' using Pain Behaviour Checklist | LBP > control avoiders > confronters |
| Cooper et al. (1993) | 11 LBP (4M, 7F) 28 cont (15M,13F) | Biering-Sorensen test; unilat erector spinae at L4; iEMG rate of change | LBP > control |
| Tsuboi et al. (1994) | 9 LBP, 10 cont (all male) | Biering-Sorensen test, trunk with lifted further 5 degrees, 120s; same but with loading of 30% MVC; EMG L1, L2, L4, L5 | LBP > control (but no stat analyses for the difference) |
| Kankaanpaa et al. (1998) | 20 LBP (F), 15 cont (F) | Seated, trunk flexed 30 deg, 50% MVC isometric back extension (David Back 100) to fatigue; EMG erector spinae (L3/4 and L5/S1) | LBP = control |
| Peach and McGill (1998) | LBP 21 (13M, 8F) Cont 18 (3M, 10F). NB age 48 (14) and 22 (2) respectively | Isometric trunk extension with harness around the torso. 30 second fatigue test at 60% MVC; EMG T9, L3 (erector spinae), L5 (multifidus) | LBP < control |
| Suter and Lindsay (2001) | 25Y, 16N (all male) | BS test; EMG bilat erector spinae at T12 and L4–L5. | LBP = control |
| Ng et al. (2002) | LBP 12, Cont 12 (all male) | Fatigue test in standing, 80% MVC, right and left axial rotation. EMG bilat, illiocostalis lumborum L2, multifidus L5 (plus rectus abdominus, ext & int oblique, latissimus dorsi) | LBP = control |
| Elfving et al. (2003) | 57 LBP (27M, 30F) 55 controls (28M, 27F) | EMG bilat erector spinae, L1 and L5 Seated 80% max isometric extension torque for 45s | LBP < control (in females only; in males no difference) |

*(continued)*

**Table 9.2** (continued) Summary of results of studies examining the difference between groups of controls and groups of patients with LBP using the rate of decline of the EMG median (or mean) power frequency.

| Author (year) | Groups | Test procedure | Findings for differences in MF slope (EMG fatigability) |
|---|---|---|---|
| Lariviere et al. (2003a) | LBP 20 controls 20 (all male) | Standing, static trunk extension 75% MVC for 30s; EMG bilaterally longissimus T10 and L1, illiocostalis L3, and multifidus L5; (also rectus abdominus, external oblique, internal oblique) | LBP < control (for all sites) |
| Crossman et al. (2004) | LBP 35, controls 32 (all male) | Biering-Sorensen and standing pulling up 60% MVC fatigue tests; EMG bilat erector spinae, L4/5 | LBP=control (both tests) |
| Kankaanpaa et al. (2005) | LBP 17, controls 12 (all male) | Seated, trunk flexed 30°, submax (wt & ht-based) dynamic back extension (David Back 100); 30 reps/min for max 90s; EMG bilat erector spinae (L4/5) | LBP=control |
| da Silva et al. (2005) | LBP 13, controls 15 (all male) | Standing upright, standing trunk flexed (each 50% MVC), Biering-Sorensen test; EMG bilat longiss (T10 and L1), iliocostalis (L3), multifidus (L5) | LBP=control (all tests) |
| Kramer et al. (2005) | LBP 31, control 31 | Seated, trunk flexed 30°, 60% MVC isometric back extension (David Back 100) for 60s; EMG bilateral multifidus (L4/5 and T11/12) and erector spinae (L4/5/&T11/12) | LBP < control (signif. for multifidus, L4/5 and T11/12) |
| Humphre y et al. (2005) | LBP 145 (chronic), 30 history, control 175 | Standing, trunk flexed, pulling up at 66% MVC for 30; EMG bilat paraspinal muscles L4/5 | LBP=control |
| Candotti et al. (2008) | LBP 30, control 30 (gender not given) | Lying prone, 80% max extensor force for 35s; EMG bilateral longiss (L1) iliocostalis (L2) | LBP > controls (for left side muscles only) |
| Suuden et al. (2008) | LBP 20 (10M, 10F) control 20 (10M, 10F) | Biering-Sorensen test to fatigue; EMG bilat erector spinae, L3 | LBP=controls |
| Sung et al. (2009) | LBP 40 control 40 (gender distrib not given) | Biering-Sorensen test for max 60s; EMG bilat erector spinae (approx T12, L5) | Methods and results not clear |

during a fatiguing task. These findings in relation to fatigability were compatible with altered muscle fibre type characteristics in LBP patients, in the direction of an increase in the proportional area of the muscle occupied by fast twitch type II fibres. Such an increase could occur due to either reflex inhibition of the musculature or pain-induced inactivity and disuse following the initial acute episode of LBP. In other musculoskeletal systems, it is known that injury to a joint is associated with a reduction in alpha-motoneuron activity to the muscles surrounding that joint

(Morrissey 1989). It has also been shown that cessation of normal repetitive low-level activity patterns and stretch, which otherwise serve to maintain the slow twitch fibre population, results in a transformation of the muscle towards a faster, more fatigable type (Goldspink et al. 1994). It was hence quite feasible that the observed fatigability of the back muscles of patients reflected muscular adaptations, consequent to the onset of back pain.

These findings, in turn, stimulated various interventional studies attempting to 're-condition' the deconditioned muscles (see later). However, in the years that followed the initial cross-sectional studies, few research groups were able to reproduce the findings. A series of studies carried out throughout the late 1990s up to the present day—using varying types of test position, test contractions, and electrode recording sites, and some with very large group sizes (making type II errors unlikely)—reported either no difference between LBP patients and controls, or even the reverse of the earlier findings, namely LBP patients being less fatigable than controls (Table 9.2). In all studies reporting the latter, the submaximal load had been set as a %MVC, and it was questioned whether a true MVC had been obtained in the first place; if not, then the load-challenge would have been less in the patients, and the fatigue rate naturally lower for these reasons alone. It is not easy to verify the maximality of voluntary efforts in back strength tests in patients: twitch interpolation techniques (Mannion et al. 1997b) are not entirely practical and predictive models based on anthropometric dimensions are not accurate enough, generally explaining only 30–40% variance in strength (Mannion et al. 1999; Lariviere et al. 2003b; Wang et al. 2005). Thus, the uncertainties surrounding an individual's true maximum strength continue to represent a confounder in any assessments of muscle fatigue that use submaximal contractions set as a %MVC.

As can be seen in Table 9.2, in all the studies in which the Biering-Sorensen test was used to assess fatigability, there was no statistically significant difference between the EMG-MF slopes of patients and controls. Although this test is not without its own limitations, it probably represents the best available option for making non-MVC-dependent measures of fatigability (see earlier). Further, one might expect that the 'trunk fat-mass to lean-mass ratio' of the theoretically 'inactive, overweight, and weaker' patient might, if anything, put them at a disadvantage during performance of this test. The finding that their back muscles do not fatigue more rapidly than controls hence indicates that they are definitely not more fatigable, and may even be less fatigable, than controls.

Possible explanations for the discrepancies of these findings with those of the earlier studies include the fact that the latter used generally quite athletic LBP-sufferers (that may have been atypical compared with clinical populations); that generally only men were included; that too many EMG-variables were used for the classification procedure, such that the model was over-fitted statistically; and the fact that many of the variables included in the classification models were actually not related to fatigue per se (e.g. the initial MF; see earlier). Either way, it seems that the only clear conclusion emerging from the last 20 years' research on the association between LBP and EMG-fatigability is that the relationship is highly inconsistent.

## 9.7 Changes in fatigability through exercise training and their clinical relevance

In acknowledgement of the early findings on back muscle fatigability in LBP patients, some studies sought to examine the response of the muscles to various types of training or rehabilitation (Thompson et al. 1992; Moffroid et al. 1993; Roy et al. 1995; Wood et al. 1997; Kankaanpaa et al. 1999; Mannion et al. 2001b; Sung 2003). In some studies a post-training improvement in endurance time was recorded without any corresponding change in the EMG-determined muscle fatigability (Moffroid et al. 1993; Wood et al. 1997; Mannion et al. 2001b) or muscle fibre type distributional area (Mannion et al. 2001b). This perhaps indicates a determination on the behalf of the patient to do better after therapy, despite the lack of any real accompanying physiological change in their muscles enabling them to do so. Some of the research groups that had originally reported overly-fatigable muscles in LBP patients also reported improvements following exercise training (Mayer et al. 1989; Thompson et al. 1992; Roy et al. 1995,). Decreases in the steepness of the MF-slope lasting up to 6 months after therapy, were similarly reported by Kankaanpaa et al. (1999), although their cross-sectional studies had not shown excessive fatigability in connection with LBP at baseline, and values for the MF-slope were unrelated to patients' self-ratings of pain or disability (Kankaanpaa et al. 1998).

As pointed out by Elfving et al. (2003), in all these studies the submaximal load for the fatigue test remained the same pre- and post-therapy; any improvements in strength would therefore have rendered the given force less demanding post-therapy, perhaps explaining the reduced fatigability. Later studies failed to reproduce the findings of these earlier studies, sometimes even finding a post-therapy *increase* in EMG-determined fatigability in some test situations, commensurate with an increased ability to activate the muscles and drive them to fatigue (Mannion et al. 2001b; Sung 2003,). The finding that an increased MF-slope might indicate a 'back-healthier' condition was also suggested by the study of Elfving et al. (2003) in which the ability to achieve a decline in the MF during a sustained contraction was significantly associated with lower scores for disability in everyday activities.

Few intervention studies have addressed the ultimate question, critical in relation to the clinical relevance of back muscle fatigability, as to whether improvements observed after therapy are actually associated with a corresponding reduction in the patient's self-rated pain and disability. Ultimately, it is these factors, which influence the quality of life, that drive the patient back into the clinic and give rise to the enormous societal costs associated with the management of LBP. There is good reason to suppose that *disability* might be decreased following active rehabilitation, but the question of whether an improved muscular capacity should translate to a reduction in *pain* is perhaps more complicated. If the muscular deficits are intricately linked with the source of pain—for example, by their failure to stabilize an injured or unstable joint—then an improvement in muscular support accompanied by a gradual relief from the pain may indeed be anticipated. If, however, the decline in muscle function is simply the result of general disuse, then improvements would not necessarily be expected to relieve the existing pain—although they may certainly offer a protective effect against the chances of 'reinjury' and repeated episodes of low back pain in the future.

One of the biggest difficulties in interpreting the results of rehabilitation studies concerns identification of the 'active element' of the programme. Typical active therapy programmes include various elements that aim to 'recondition' the patient, some of which are carefully introduced into the programme and others of which inadvertently accompany it. Specially designed exercises may aim to restore a particular aspect of physical function, and these may indeed be effective; however, regular attendance at therapy may coincidentally elicit feelings of well-being and accomplishment in achieving an improved physical fitness (Nutter, 1988) as well as antidepressive effects in connection with the release of natural endorphins (Ransford 1982; Dey 1994). Each of these elements could independently modify the perception and reporting of pain, and possibly even the degree of disability that patients allow it to create. In this sense, the recording of group changes in both function and clinical status does not necessarily confirm that the clinical changes followed the functional changes; instead, it is necessary to examine comparison groups in which clinical but no functional changes occurred or to examine the concordance of findings on an individual basis (i.e. whether improvements in fatigability and clinical status occur in the same subjects, and whether the magnitude of change in each is related). Even if a correlation between the changes in two variables can be established, this still doesn't necessarily prove the existence of a causal relationship; the converse, however—a reduction in symptoms or disability in the *absence* of any significant change in muscle function, or vice versa—would certainly imply that the two were unrelated. Though difficult, identifying the active ingredient in muscle reconditioning programmes is of paramount importance in concluding the case for the clinical significance of back muscle fatigability in LBP.

Only one study has directly addressed this issue, by examining changes in back muscle EMG-fatigability after different active therapies for chronic LBP in relation to corresponding changes in pain and disability (Mannion et al. 2001a). The findings were not supportive of any clinical relevance for back muscle fatigability. Firstly, there was no relationship between individual measures of EMG-fatigability (isometric or dynamic) and self-rated disability at baseline, and no relationship between the changes in back muscle fatigability and changes in self-rated disability after therapy (Mannion et al. 2001a). Pain and disability were reduced to a similar extent in each of the three active therapy groups, despite their differing nature (mainly strengthening/reconditioning vs. aerobic vs. physiotherapeutic). There were no significant changes in the MF slope during the BS test, and though the MF slope during a dynamic fatigue test changed after therapy (*increased*), it did so in a manner unrelated to the changes in pain or disability. No significant changes in the size or structure of the paraspinal muscles were observed (Kaser et al. 2001). Overall, the results indicated that neither the intrinsic fatigability of the back muscles, nor the structural characteristics that determined it, bore any meaningful relationship to measures of LBP disability. The clinical significance of these measures hence remains obscure. Future studies should investigate whether these aspects of muscle function (and their changes with training) are associated with future episodes of LBP, either in their frequency, duration or intensity.

In summary, there are many convincing hypotheses linking fatigable back muscles with LBP. Fatigability of the back muscles, as measured by the rate of decline in the mean or median frequency of the EMG power spectrum, can be measured with acceptable reliability if the basic principles of EMG are adhered to, and optimized sampling methods are used. The rate of decline in MF is correlated with the rate of decline in maximum force-generating capacity and is (at least in part) dependent on the underlying muscle fibre characteristics. The findings on differences in EMG-determined fatigability in patients with LBP and healthy controls are conflicting, as are those concerned with changes in EMG-fatigability after rehabilitation or exercise therapy. Back muscle fatigability does not relate to subjective ratings of pain or disability in LBP patients, and does not change in parallel to changes in these clinical variables after therapy. Hence, the clinical significance of EMG-determined back muscle fatigability remains obscure. Future studies should focus on its potential role in relation to predicting LBP recurrence/chronification.

## References

Adams, M.A. and Dolan, P. (2005). Spine biomechanics. *J Biomechanics,* **38**, 1972–83.

Adams, M.A. and Hutton, W.C. (1986). Has the lumbar spine a margin of safety in forward bending? *Clinical Biomechanics,* **1**, 3–6.

Adams, M.A., Mannion, A.F. and Dolan, P. (1999). Personal risk factors for first-time low back pain. *Spine,* **24**, 2497–505.

Adams, S.A., Matthews, C.E., Ebbeling, C.B., Moore, C.G., Cunningham, J.E., Fulton, J. and Hebert, J.R. (2005). The effect of social desirability and social approval on self-reports of physical activity. *American Journal of Epidemiology,* **161**, 389–98.

Allison, G.T. and Henry, S.M. (2002). The influence of fatigue on trunk muscle responses to sudden arm movements, a pilot study. *Clinical Biomechanics,* **17**, 414–17.

Arnall, F.A., Koumantakis, G.A., Oldham, J.A. and Cooper, R.G. (2002). Between-days reliability of electromyographic measures of paraspinal muscle fatigue at 40, 50 and 60% levels of maximal voluntary contractile force. *Clinical Rehabilitation, 16*, 761–71.

Biedermann, H.J., Shanks, G.L. and Inglis, J. (1990). Median frequency estimates of paraspinal muscles: reliability analysis. *Electromyography Clinical Neurophysiology, 30*, 83–8.

Biedermann, H.J., Shanks, G. L., Forrest, W.J. and Inglis, J. (1991). Power spectrum analyses of electromyographic activity discriminators in the differential assessment of patients with chronic low back pain. *Spine, 16*, 1179–84.

Biering-Sorenson, F. (1984). Physical measurements as risk indicators for low-back trouble over a one-year period. *Spine, 9*, 106–19.

Bigland-Ritchie, B. and Woods, J.J. (1984). Changes in muscle contractile properties and neural control during human muscular fatigue. *Muscle Nerve, 7*, 691–9.

Bigos, S.J., Battie, M.C., Spengler, D.M., *et al.* (1992). A longitudinal, prospective study of industrial back injury reporting. *Clinical Orthopaedics and Related Research, 279*, 21–33.

Bogduk, N. and Twomey, L.T. (1991). *Clinical anatomy of the lumbar spine and sacrum* (2nd edn.). London: Churchill Livingstone.

Bonato, P., Ebenbichler, G.R., Roy, S.H., et al. (2003). Muscle fatigue and fatigue-related biomechanical changes during a cyclic lifting task. *Spine, 28*, 1810–20.

Bouissou, P., Estrade, P.V., Goubel, F., Guezennec, C.Y. and Serrurier, B. (1989). Surface EMG power spectrum and intramuscular pH in human vastus lateralis muscle during dynamic exercise. *Journal of Applied Physiology, 67*, 1245–9.

Bradl, I., Morl, F., Scholle, H.C., Grassme, R., Muller, R. and Grieshaber, R. (2005). Back muscle activation pattern and spectrum in defined load situations. *Pathophysiology, 12*, 275–80.

Brody, L.R., Pollock, M.T., Roy, S.H., DeLuca, C.J. and Celli, B. (1991). pH induced effects on median frequency and conduction velocity of the myoelectric signal. *Journal of Applied Physiology, 71*, 1878–85.

Candotti, C.T., Loss, J.F., Pressi, A.M., *et al.* (2008). Electromyography for assessment of pain in low back muscles. *Physical Therapy, 88*, 1061–7.

Ciba Foundation (1981). *Human muscle fatigue: physiological mechanisms*. London: Pitman Medical.

Cooper, R.G., Stokes, M.J., Sweet, C., Taylor, R.J. and Jayson, M.I.V. (1993). Increased central drive during fatiguing contractions of the paraspinal muscles in patients with chronic low back pain. *Spine, 18*, 610–16.

Crossman, K., Mahon, M., Watson, P.J., Oldham, J.A. and Cooper, R.G. (2004). Chronic low back pain-associated paraspinal muscle dysfunction is not the result of a constitutionally determined 'adverse' fiber-type composition. *Spine, 29*, 628–34.

da Silva, R.A., Jr., Arsenault, A.B., Gravel, D., Lariviere, C. and de Oliveira, E., Jr. (2005). Back muscle strength and fatigue in healthy and chronic low back pain subjects: a comparative study of 3 assessment protocols. *Archives of Physical Medicine Rehabilitation, 86*, 722–9.

De Luca, C. (1997). The use of surface electromyography in biomechanics. *Journal of Applied Biomechanics, 13*, 135–63.

Dedering, A., Roos af Hjelmsater, M., Elfving, B., Harms-Ringdahl, K. and Nemeth, G. (2000). Between-days reliability of subjective and objective assessments of back extensor muscle fatigue in subjects without lower-back pain. *Journal of Electromyography and Kinesiology 10*, 151–8.

Demoulin, C., Vanderthommen, M., Duysens, C. and Crielaard, J.M. (2006). Spinal muscle evaluation using the Sorensen test: a critical appraisal of the literature. *Joint Bone Spine, 73*, 43–50.

Dey, S. (1994). Physical exercise as a novel antidepressant agent: possible role of serotonin receptor subtypes. *Physiology and Behaviour, 55*, 323–29.

Dolan, P. and Adams, M.A. (1998). Repetitive lifting tasks fatigue the back muscles and increase the bending moment acting on the lumbar spine. *Journal of Biomechanics, 31*, 713–21.

Dolan, P., Mannion, A.F. and Adams, M. (1995). Fatigue of the erector spinae muscles: A quantitative assessment using 'frequency banding' of the surface electromyography signal. *Spine, 20*, 149–59.

Duchateau, J. and Hainaut, K. (1984). Training effects on muscle fatigue in man. *European Journal of Applied Physiology and Occupational Physiology*, **53**, 248–52.

Ebenbichler, G.R., Bonato, P., Roy, S.H., *et al*. (2002). Reliability of EMG time-frequency measures of fatigue during repetitive lifting. *Medicine and Science in Sports and Exercise*, **34**, 1316–23.

Elfving, B., Nemeth, G., Arvidsson, I. and Lamontagne, M. (1999). Reliability of EMG spectral parameters in repeated measurements of back muscle fatigue. *Journal of Electromyography and Kinesiology*, **9**, 235–43.

Elfving, B., Dedering, A. and Nemeth, G. (2003). Lumbar muscle fatigue and recovery in patients with long-term low-back trouble—electromyography and health-related factors. *Clinical Biomechanics*, **18**, 619–30.

Goldspink, G., Gerlach, G. F., Jaenicke, T. and Butterworth, P. (1994). In Lyall, F., El Haj, A.J. (Eds.) *Biomechanics and cells*, pp. 81–95. Cambridge: Cambridge University Press.

Granata, K. P., Slota, G. P. and Wilson, S. E. (2004). Influence of fatigue in neuromuscular control of spinal stability. *Human Factors*, **46**, 81–91.

Greenough, C.G. and Fraser, R.D. (1991). Comparison of eight psychometric instruments in unselected patients with back pain. *Spine*, **16**, 1068–74.

Hagberg, M. (1981). Muscular endurance and surface electromyogram in isometric and dynamic exercise. *Journal of Applied Physiology*, **51**, 1–7.

Hansson, T.H., Bigos, S.J., Wortley, M.K. and Spengler, D.M. (1984). The load on the lumbar spine during isometric strength testing. *Spine*, **9**, 720–4.

Hermens, H.J., Freriks, B., Disselhorst-Klug, C. and Rau, G. (2000). Development of recommendations for SEMG sensors and sensor placement procedures. *Journal of Electromyography and Kinesiology* **10**, 361–74.

Hultman, G., Nordin, M., Saraste, H. and Ohlsen, H. (1993). Body composition, endurance, strength, cross-sectional area, and density of MM erector spinae in men with and without low back pain. *Journal of Spinal Disorders*, **6**, 114–23.

Humphrey, A., Nargol, A.V., Jones, A.P., Ratcliffe, A.A. and Greenough, C. (2005). The value of electromyography of the lumbar paraspinal muscles in discriminating between chronic-low-back-pain sufferers and normal subjects. *European Spine Journal*, **24**, 175–84.

Jorgensen, K. and Nicolaisen, T. (1987). Trunk extensor endurance: determination and relation to low back trouble. *Ergonomics*, **30**, 259–67.

Jurell, K.C. (1998). Surface EMG and fatigue. *Physical Medicine and Rehabilitation Clinics of North America*, **9**, 933–46.

Kankaanpaa, M., Taimela, S., Webber, C.L., Airaksinen, O. and Hanninen, O. (1997). Lumbar paraspinal muscle fatigability in repetitive isoinertial loading: EMG spectral indices, Borg scale and endurance time. *European Journal of Applied Physiology*. 76, 236–42.

Kankaanpaa, M., Taimela, S., Laaksonen, D., Hanninen, O. and Airaksinen, O. (1998). Back and hip extensor fatigability in chronic low back pain patients and controls. *Archives of Physical Medicine and Rehabilitation* **79**, 412–17.

Kankaanpaa, M., Taimela, S., Airaksinen, O. and Hanninen, O. (1999). The efficacy of active rehabilitation in chronic low back pain. Effect on pain intensity, self-experienced disability, and lumbar fatigability. *Spine*, **24**, 1034–42.

Kaser, L., Mannion, A.F., Rhyner, A., Weber, E., Dvorak, J. and Muntener, M. (2001). Active therapy for chronic low back pain: part 2. Effects on paraspinal muscle cross-sectional area, fiber type size, and distribution. *Spine*, **26**, 909–19.

Kankaanpaa, M., Colier, W.N., Taimela, S., *et al*. (2005). Back extensor muscle oxygenation and fatigability in healthy subjects and low back pain patients during dynamic back extension exertion. *Pathophysiology* **12**, 267–73

Klein, A. B., Snyder Mackler, L., Roy, S.H. and DeLuca, C.J. (1991). Comparison of spinal mobility and isometric trunk extensor forces with electromyographic spectral analysis in identifying low back pain. *Physical Therapy*, **71**, 445–54.

Koumantakis, G.A., Arnall, F., Cooper, R.G. and Oldham, J.A. (2001). Paraspinal muscle EMG fatigue testing with two methods in healthy volunteers. Reliability in the context of clinical applications. *Clinical Biomechanics* **16**, 263–6.

Kramer, M., Ebert, V., Kinzl, L., Dehner, C., Elbel, M. and Hartwig, E. (2005). Surface electromyography of the paravertebral muscles in patients with chronic low back pain. *Archives Physical Medicine Rehabilitation*, **86**, 31–6.

Kujala, U.M., Taimela, S., Viljanen, T., *et al.* (1996). Physical loading and performance as predictors of back pain in healthy adults. A 5-year prospective study. *European Journal Applied Physiology Occupational Physiology*, **73**, 452–8.

Kupa, E.J., Roy, S.H., Kandarian, S.C. and De Luca, C.J. (1995). Effects of muscle fiber morphology on the EMG signal. *Annals of Biomedical Engineering*, **23**, S112.

Lariviere, C., Arsenault, A.B., Gravel, D., Gagnon, D. and Loisel, P. (2002). Evaluation of measurement strategies to increase the reliability of EMG indices to assess back muscle fatigue and recovery. *Journal of Electromyography and Kinesiology* **12**, 91–102.

Lariviere, C., Arsenault, A.B., Gravel, D., Gagnon, D. and Loisel, P. (2003a). Surface electromyography assessment of back muscle intrinsic properties. *Journal of Electromyography and Kinesiology* **13**, 305–18.

Lariviere, C., Gravel, D., Gagnon, D., Arsenault, A.B., Loisel, P. and Lepage, Y. (2003b). Back strength cannot be predicted accurately from anthropometric measures in subjects with and without chronic low back pain. *Clinical Biomechanics*, **18**, 473–9.

Laurent, D., Portero, P., Goubel, F. and Rossi, A. (1993). Electromyogram spectrum changes during sustained contraction related to proton and diprotonated inorganic phosphate accumulation: A 31P nuclear magnetic resonance study on human calf muscles. *European Journal Applied Physiology Occupational Physiology*, **66**, 263–68.

Liu, Y., Kankaanpaa, M., Zbilut, J.P. and Webber, C.L., Jr. (2004). EMG recurrence quantifications in dynamic exercise. *Biological Cybernetics*, **90**, 337–48.

Luoto, S., Heliovaara, M., Hurri, H. and Alaranta, H. (1995). Static back endurance and the risk of low-back pain. *Clinical Biomechanics*, **10**, 323–24.

Magnusson, M.L., Aleksiev, A., Wilder, D.G., *et al.* (1996). Unexpected load and asymmetric posture as etiologic factors in low back pain. *European Spine Journal*, **5**, 23–35.

Mannion, A.F. and Dolan, P. (1994). Electromyographic median frequency changes during isometric contraction of the back extensors to fatigue. *Spine*, **19**, 1223–9.

Mannion, A.F. and Dolan, P. (1996a). The effects of muscle length and force output on the EMG power spectrum of the erector spinae. *Journal of Electromyography and Kinesiology* **6**, 159–68.

Mannion, A.F. and Dolan, P. (1996b). Relationship between myoelectric and mechanical manifestations of fatigue in the quadriceps femoris muscle group. *European Journal Applied Physiology Occupational Physiology*, **74**, 411–19.

Mannion, A.F., Dolan, P. and Adams, M.A. (1996). Psychological questionnaires: do 'abnormal' scores precede or follow first-time low back pain? *Spine*, **21**, 2603–11.

Mannion, A.F., Connolly, B., Wood, K. and Dolan, P. (1997a). The use of surface EMG power spectral analysis in the evaluation of back muscle function. *Journal of Rehabilitation Research and Development* **34**, 427–39.

Mannion, A.F., Dolan, P., Adam, G.G., Adams, M.A. and Cooper, R.G. (1997b). Can maximal back muscle strength be predicted from submaximal efforts? *Journal of Back and Musculoskeletal Medicine*, **9**, 49–51.

Mannion, A.F., Weber, B. R., Dvorak, J., Grob, D. and Muntener, M. (1997c). Fibre type characteristics of the lumbar paraspinal muscles in normal healthy subjects and in patients with low back pain. *Journal of Orthopaedic Research*, **15**, 881–7.

Mannion, A.F., Dolan, P. and Adams, M.A. (1996). Psychological questionnaires: do 'abnormal' scores precede or follow first time low back pain? *Spine*, **21**, 2603–2611.

Mannion, A.F., Dumas, G.A., Stevenson, J.M. and Cooper, R.G. (1998). The influence of muscle fiber size and type distribution on electromyographic measures of back muscle fatigability. *Spine*, **23**, 576–84.

Mannion, A.F., Adams, M.A., Cooper, R.G. and Dolan, P. (1999). Prediction of maximal back muscle strength from indices of body mass and fat-free body mass. *Rheumatology, 38*, 652–5.

Mannion, A.F., Junge, A., Taimela, S., Muntener, M., Lorenzo, K. and Dvorak, J. (2001a). Active therapy for chronic low back pain: part 3. Factors influencing self-rated disability and its change following therapy. *Spine, 26*, 920–9.

Mannion, A.F., Taimela, S., Muntener, M. and Dvorak, J. (2001b). Active therapy for chronic low back pain: part 1. Effects on back muscle activation, fatigability, and strength. *Spine, 26*, 897–908.

Mannion, A.F., O'Riordan, D., Dvorak, J., Masharawi, Y. The dependence of back muscle endurance time on psychological factors. (Submitted)

Mayer, T.G., Gatchel, R. J., Kishino, N., *et al.* (1985). Lumbar myoelectric spectral analysis for endurance assessment. A comparison of normals with deconditioned patients. *Spine, 10*, 482–93.

Mayer, T.G., Kondraske, G., Mooney, V., Carmichael, T.W. and Butsch, R. (1989). Lumbar myoelectric spectral analysis for endurance assessment. A comparison of normals with deconditioned patients. *Spine, 14*, 986–91.

Moffroid, M.T., Haugh, L.D., Haig, A.J., Henry, S.M. and Pope, M.H. (1993). Endurance training of trunk extensor muscles. *Physical Therapy, 73*, 3–10.

Mooney, V., Gulick, J., Perlman, M., *et al.* (1997). Relationships between myoelectric activity, strength, and MRI of lumbar extensor muscles in back pain patients and normal subjects. *Journal of Spinal Disorders, 10*, 348–56.

Morrissey, M.C. (1989). Reflex inhibition of thigh muscles in knee injury. Causes and treatment. *Sports Medicine, 7*, 263–76.

Mostardi, R.A., Noe, D.A., Kovacik, M.W. and Porterfield, J.A. (1992). Isokinetic lifting strength and occupational injury. A prospective study. *Spine, 17*, 189–93.

Nargol, A.V.F., Jones, A.P.C., Kelly, P.J. and Greenough, C.G. (1999). Factors in the reproducibility of electromyographic power spectrum analysis of lumbar paraspinal muscle fatigue. *Spine, 24*, 883–8.

Ng, J.K.F. and Richardson, C.A. (1996). Reliability of electromyographic power spectral analysis of back muscle endurance in healthy subjects. *Archives of Physical Medicine and Rehabilitation, 77*, 259–64.

Ng, J.K., Richardson, C.A., Parnianpour, M. and Kippers, V. (2002). Fatigue-related changes in torque output and electromyographic parameters of trunk muscles during isometric axial rotation exertion: an investigation in patients with back pain and in healthy subjects. *Spine, 27*, 637–46.

Nicolaisen, T. and Jorgensen, K. (1985). Trunk strength, back muscle endurance and low-back trouble. *Scandinavian Journal of Rehabiltation Medicine, 17*, 121–27.

Nutter, P. (1988). Aerobic exercise in the treatment and prevention of low back pain. *Occupational Medicine, 3*, 137–45.

Oliver, C.W., Tillotson, K.M., Jones, A.P.C., Royal, R.A. and Greenough, C.G. (1996). Reproducibility of lumbar paraspinal surface electromyogram power spectra. *Clinical Biomechanics, 11*, 317–21.

Parnianpour, M., Nordin, M., Kahanovitz, N. and Frankel, V. (1988). The triaxial coupling of torque generation of trunk muscles during isometric exertions and the effect of fatiguing isoinertial movements on the motor output and movement patterns. *Spine, 13*, 982–92.

Peach, J.P. and McGill, S.M. (1998). Classification of low back pain with the use of spectral electromyogram parameters. *Spine, 23*, 1117–23.

Peach, J.P., Gunning, J. and McGill, S.M. (1998). Reliability of spectral EMG parameters of healthy back extensors during submaximum isometric fatiguing contractions and recovery. *Journal of Electromyography and Kinesiology 8*, 403–10.

Ransford, C.P. (1982). A role for amines in the antidepressant effect of exercise:a review. *Medicine & Science in Sports & Exercise 14*, 1–10.

Roland, M. and Morris, R. (1983). A study of the natural history of back pain. Part 1: Development of a reliable and sensitive measure of disability in low-back pain. *Spine, 8*, 141–4.

Rosenstiel, A.K. and Keefe, F.J. (1983). The use of coping strategies in chronic low back pain patients: relationship to patient characteristics and current adjustments. *Pain, 17*, 33–44.

Roy, S.H., De Luca, C.J. and Casavant, D.A. (1989). Lumbar muscle fatigue and chronic lower back pain. *Spine,* **14**, 992–1001.

Roy, S.H., De Luca, C.J., Snyder-Mackler, L., Emley, M.S., Crenshan, R.L. and Lyons, J.P. (1990). Fatigue, recovery and low back pain in varsity rowers. *Medicine & Science in Sports & Exercise,* **22**, 463–9.

Roy, S.H., De Luca, C.J., Emley, M. and Buijs, R.J.C. (1995). Spectral electromyographic assessment of back muscles in patients with low back pain undergoing rehabilitation. *Spine,* **20**, 38–48.

Sahlin, K. (1992). Metabolic factors in fatigue. *Sports Medicine,* **13**, 99–107.

Saltin, B. and Gollnick, P. (1983). *Skeletal muscle adaptability: significance for metabolism and performance.* Washington, DC: American Physiological Society.

Sant'Ana Pereira, J.A.A., Ennion, S., Sargeant, A.J., Moorman, A.F.M. and Goldspink, G. (1997). Comparison of the molecular, antigenic and ATPase determinants of fast myosin heavy chains in rat and human: a single-fibre study. *Pfluegers Archives - European Journal Physiology,* **435**, 151–63

Schwarzer, K.A. (1993). *Measurement of perceived self-efficacy.* Berlin: Forschung an der Freien Universitaet.

Sparto, P.J., Parnianpour, M., Marras, W.S., Granata, K.P., Reinsel, T.E. and Simon, S. (1997a). Neuromuscular trunk performance and spinal loading during a fatiguing isometric trunk extension with varying torque requirements. *Journal of Spinal Disorders,* **10**, 145–56.

Sparto, P.J., Parnianpour, M., Reinsel, T.E. and Simon, S. (1997b). The effect of fatigue on multijoint kinematics and load sharing during a repetitive lifting test. *Spine,* **22**, 2647–54.

Sparto, P.J., Parnianpour, M., Barria, E.A. and Jagadeesh, J.M. (1999). Wavelet analysis of electromyography for back muscle fatigue detection during isokinetic constant-torque exertions. *Spine,* 24, 1791–8.

Sung, P.S. (2003). Multifidi muscles median frequency before and after spinal stabilization exercises. *Archives of Physical Medicine and Rehabilitation,* **84**, 1313–8.

Sung, P.S., Zurcher, U. and Kaufman, M. (2005). Nonlinear analysis of electromyography time series as a diagnostic tool for low back pain. *Medical Science Monitor,* **11**, CS1–5.

Sung, P.S., Lammers, A.R. and Danial, P. (2009). Different parts of erector spinae muscle fatigability in subjects with and without low back pain. *Spine Journal,* **9,** 115–20.

Suter, E. and Lindsay, D. (2001). Back muscle fatigability is associated with knee extensor inhibition in subjects with low back pain. *Spine,* **26**, E361–6.

Suuden, E., Ereline, J., Gapeyeva, H. and Paasuke, M. (2008). Low back muscle fatigue during Sorensen endurance test in patients with chronic low back pain: relationship between electromyographic spectral compression and anthropometric characteristics. *Electromyography and Clinical Neurophysiology* **48**, 185–92.

Symonds, T.L., Burton, A.K., Tillotson, K.M. and Main, C.J. (1996). Do attitudes and beliefs influence work loss due to low back trouble? *Occupational Medicine,* **46**, 25–32.

Taimela, S., Kankaanpaa, M. and Luoto, S. (1999). The effect of lumbar fatigue on the ability to sense a change in lumbar position. *Spine,* **24**, 1322–27.

Thompson, D.A., Biedermann, H.J., Stevenson, J.M. and MacLean, A.W. (1992). Changes in paraspinal electromyographic spectral analysis with exercise: two studies. *Journal of Electromyography and Kinesiology,* **2**, 179–86.

Tsuboi, T., Satou, T., Egawa, K., Izumi, Y. and Miyazaki, M. (1994). Spectral analysis of electromyogram in lumbar muscles: fatigue induced endurance contraction. *European Journal of Applied Physiology* **69**, 361–6.

van Dieen, J.H. and Heijblom, P. (1996). Reproducibility of isometric trunk extension torque, trunk extensor endurance, and related electromyographic parameters in the context of their clinical applicability. *Journal of Orthopaedic Research,* **14**, 139–43.

Van Doorn, J.W.C. (1995). Low back disability among self-employed dentists, veterinarians, physicians and physical therapists in the Netherlands. A retrospective study over a 13-year period (N = 1,119) and an early intervention program with 1-year follow-up (N = 134). *Acta Orthopaedica Scandinavica, Supplement,* **263**, 1–64.

Vestergaard-Poulsen, P., Thomsen, C., Sinkjaer, T., Stubgaard, M., Rosenfalck, A. and Henriksen, O. (1992). Simultaneous electromyography and 31P nuclear magnetic resonance spectroscopy – with application to muscle fatigue. *Electroencephalography and Clinical Neurophysiology,* **85**, 402–11.

Waddell, G., Newton, M., Henderson, I., Somerville, D. and Main, C.J. (1993). Fear-Avoidance Beliefs Questionnaire (FABQ) and the role of fear-avoidance beliefs in chronic low back pain and disability. *Pain,* **52**, 157–68.

Wang, M., Leger, A.B. and Dumas, G.A. (2005). Prediction of back strength using anthropometric and strength measurements in healthy females. *Clinical Biomechanics* **20**, 685–92.

Wilder, D., Aleksiev, A.R., Magnusson, M.L., Pope, M.H., Spratt, K.F. and Goel, V.K. (1996). Muscular response to sudden load. A tool to evaluate fatigue and rehabilitation. *Spine,* **21**, 2628–39.

Wood, K.A., Standell, C.J., Adams, M.A., Dolan, P. and Mannion, A.F. (1997). Exercise training to improve spinal mobility and back muscle fatigability: a possible prophylaxis for low back pain? Physical Medicine Research Foundation Symposium: 'Clinical Approaches to Spinal Disorders' Prague, Czech Republic.

Chapter 10

# Unmasking the Deconditioning Paradigm for Chronic Low Back Pain Patients

Jeanine Verbunt, Rob J.E.M. Smeets, and Harriet Wittink

## 10.1 Introduction

Physical activity is behaviour. Like all behaviours it varies widely between (healthy) people and tends to decrease as people age or develop health impairments. Physical activity and physical fitness are interrelated; physical activity influences fitness, which in turn may modify the level of physical activity. Health-related fitness consists of those components of physical fitness that are affected by habitual physical activity and that are related to health status. An adequate level of health-related fitness has been defined as a state of being able to perform daily activities with vigour, and traits and capacities that are associated with a low risk of premature development of hypokinetic diseases and conditions (Bouchard and Shephard 1994).

The components of health-related fitness are defined as morphological (body composition and bone strength), muscular (muscular strength, muscular endurance, and flexibility), motor (postural control), cardiorespiratory and metabolic fitness (carbohydrate and lipid metabolism) (Bouchard and Shephard 1994; Skinner and Oja 1994). A decrease in the volume and intensity of physical activities may therefore reduce physical fitness and the capacity for physical activity, thus creating a downward spiral resulting in physical deconditioning. Physical deconditioning is defined as an integrated physiological response of the body to a reduction in metabolic rate; that is, to a reduction in energy use or exercise level (Greenleaf 2004) and affects all aspects of health related fitness.

Physical inactivity and the resultant physical deconditioning have been hypothesized to be associated with both the aetiology and consequence of chronic pain (Verbunt et al. 2003). Physical inactivity, however, has not only become a topic in chronic pain management, but also in public health. In developed countries, physical inactivity is associated with considerable economic burden, accounting for 1.5–3.0% of the total direct healthcare costs (Oldridge 2008). This may give rise to the question whether patients with chronic low back pain (CLBP) exceed the general population concerning their level of physical inactivity. The extent of the problem of deconditioning in CLBP and its specific perpetuating role in chronicity still seems unclear. Despite this, the restoration of function (i.e. health related fitness) through intensive physical rehabilitation intervention continues to form the basis of many physiotherapy-guided training programmes as well as comprehensive pain management programs. This approach is in part based on the hypothesis of the 'deconditioning syndrome' in which deconditioning itself is seen as a factor contributing to the intolerance to physical activities and subsequent loss of function and disability in patients with chronic pain (Mayer et al. 1985, 1986; Vlaeyen and Linton 2000).

A second theoretical model, in which the role of disuse is included as one of the perpetuating factors of pain is the fear-avoidance model (Vlaeyen and Linton 2000). According to the fear-avoidance model, patients may interpret their pain as threatening (catastrophizing about their pain) and this can result in pain-related fear, of which fear of movement/(re)injury is the most salient. Both this fear and expectation of adverse consequences from keep on performing or increasing activities may cause avoidance of these physical activities. In the long run, avoidance behaviour might result in disability, depression and the loss of physical activities in daily life of which loss of aerobic fitness is a consequence.

Although the influence of pain-related fear on the perceived disability level has currently been confirmed based on several studies (Klenerman et al. 1995; Vlaeyen et al. 1995; Fritz et al. 2001), its presumed negative influence on a patient's level of physical activity in daily life (PAL) is still inconclusive (Bousema et al. 2007). It can even be debated whether physical deconditioning in patients with CLBP really exists (Smeets et al. 2007; Smeets and Wittink 2007; Wittink et al. 2008).

In this chapter we will examine the deconditioning paradigm by summarizing the existing literature on this topic. We will start with a section on PALs in patients with CLBP. Next we will discuss studies describing the various aspects of health related fitness in patients with CLBP, followed by the latest theories regarding activity-related behaviour and the measurement problems in assessing physical fitness parameters in patients with CLBP. And finally, overall conclusions on the impact of deconditioning in CLBP will be provided.

## 10.2 The level of physical activity in patients with CLBP

Are patients with CLBP really inactive in comparison with healthy individuals? During recent years, several cross-sectional studies have been performed to identify inactivity in patients with CLBP. Whereas both Nielens and Plaghki (2001) and Berg-Emons et al. (2007) reported a significantly lower PAL in patients with CLBP, this finding was not confirmed by the studies of Protas (1999) and Verbunt et al. (2001) that reported a PAL in patients with CLBP that was comparable with the PAL of healthy individuals matched for age and gender. In 2007, a literature review on the presence of disuse in chronic pain was published, which again could not confirm the existence of disuse. Although a lower mean activity level in patients with pain could not be confirmed, it seems that in patients with pain activity-fluctuations during the day are more pronounced (van Weering et al. 2007).

One explanation for the diversity in findings between studies focussing on disuse in CLBP could be a variation in the percentage of study-participants with paid jobs. Persons with CLBP who are still working at least will have a PAL that is sufficient to meet the physical demands of their jobs. A hypothesis could therefore be that patients with CLBP who are working will have higher PALs than those who are not working. Studies that did not report a decrease in PAL in patients with CLBP indeed did include a higher percentage of participants who were still engaged in occupational activities. However, whether the patients having a paid job also performed their job with the normally required level of activity and effort was not studied.

A second explanation for the diversity of findings in studies on disuse in CLBP could be the use of different assessment instruments to measure physical activity. Studies in which activity assessment was based on self-report measures more frequently report a lower activity level for patients with musculoskeletal pain as compared to studies using accelerometry or activity monitoring (van Weering et al. 2007; Verbunt et al. 2008). Studies using an outcome measure on the basis of accelerometry (total counts of activity above a threshold) found no difference compared to healthy matched controls (Verbunt et al 2001; Van Weering et al. 2008), while a study using activity monitoring, including a set of three acclerometers which allows differentiating to types of activity, showed a reduced PAL in patients with CLBP (Van den Berg-Emons et al, 2007).

In 2007, Bousema et al. presented the first prospective cohort study on physical activity assessed by self-reported questionnaires as well as accelerometry in patients with low back pain (LBP). Patients were measured at 4–7 weeks after the onset of LBP until 1 year later (Bousema et al. 2007). In individuals who recovered as well as those who developed CLBP, the activity level during this year increased. In addition, changes in the level of physical activity and health-related fitness-parameters such as strength and lean body mass did not differ between both groups. Unexpectedly, the perceived level of disability of the individuals who developed CLBP was not associated with the level of registered activity, but was associated with the perceived decline in the level of activities after the onset of pain (Verbunt et al. 2005b). In summary, although hypothesized, the presence of physical inactivity in patients with chronic pain has still not been confirmed in the literature on physical activity in chronic musculoskeletal pain.

## 10.3 Health-related fitness in patients with CLBP

Are patients with musculoskeletal pain really deconditioned in comparison with healthy individuals? If they are, the components of health-related fitness defined as morphological (body composition, and bone strength), muscular (muscular strength, muscular endurance, and flexibility), motor (postural control), cardiorespiratory ($VO_{2max}$) and metabolic fitness (carbohydrate and lipid metabolism) (Bouchard and Shephard 1994; Skinner and Oja, 1994) should be different from healthy controls. And, are all components of health-related fitness equally effected in patients with pain? We will describe the current research on health related fitness in patients with CLBP next.

### 10.3.1 Body composition and bone strength

Reduced physical activity while maintaining the same caloric intake tends to lead to weight gain and changes in *body composition*. Based on studies using a cross-sectional design, patients with CLBP have a higher percentage of body fat as compared to age and gender matched individuals (Toda et al. 2000; Verbunt et al. 2005a). In addition, in chronic pain patients, a significant relationship between weight gain and decreased physical activity, increased emotional distress, and accident liability was found (Jamison et al. 1990).

Reduced physical activity can also result in a change in *bone strength*; the response of the human skeleton to unloading appears to be a rapid and sustained increase in bone resorption and a more subtle decrease in bone formation (Zerwekh et al. 1998). The greatest bone loss occurs at weight-bearing skeletal sites. Recovery of bone mass after immobilization is typically much slower than the rate at which it is lost. A recent review suggests that there is evidence that back pain and impaired bone health share common environmental (such as a lower activity level), but also genetic correlates, indicating that bone health ought to be considered in the context of longer lasting back pain in otherwise healthy individuals (Briggs et al. 2008). Bone responds to mechanical load and the response tends to be U-shaped, where both reduced physical activity and very high levels of physical activity are associated with bone loss (Briggs et al. 2008). Changes in bone strength can also be explained by changes in muscle reactivity due to pain. Individuals with severe back pain tend to stiffen the trunk and limit normal movement at the intervertebral joints (van Dieen et al. 2003a). Furthermore, in order to enhance the stability of the lumbar spine, patients with LBP show altered trunk muscle recruitment patterns (Mok et al. 2007). This altered neuromuscular strategy can decrease the opportunity for normal physiologic stresses, necessary for the maintenance of skeletal integrity, to be transferred through the vertebrae. This might explain why a history of back pain is reportedly associated with site-specific decreased bone mineral density in adults.

## 10.3.2 Muscle strength and endurance

In response to decreased usage (i.e. a decrease in daily activities), skeletal muscle undergoes an adaptive reductive remodelling. This adaptive response has been found in muscle disuse that occurs especially in a situation of immobility, such as in detraining, space flight, bed rest and in a lesser extent in situations of inactivity and ageing (Gogia et al. 1988). A decrease in muscle strength, or muscle weakening, during detraining or reduced activity is attributable to both a loss of muscle mass and changes in muscle composition. Muscle mass decreases due to both a general reduction in muscle cross-sectional fibre area as well as a reduction in the overall number of muscle fibres. These changes are associated with a decline in force production and decreased electromyographic (EMG) activity (Mujika and Padilla 2001).

Decreases of 6–40% in muscle strength have been observed within 4–6 weeks of bed rest (Bloomfield 1997). In micro-gravity simulation models, postural muscles that normally counteract the effects of gravity have been reported to become atrophic to a greater extent than fast contracting locomotor muscles (Convertino et al. 1997). This implies that especially muscles situated on the trunk and lower extremities are affected by physical deconditioning (Berry et al. 1993, Greenleaf 1997) with a consequence of early back muscle fatigue as presented in chapter 11. This assumption of physical deconditioning in trunk muscles was indeed shown in an eight-week bed rest study in 10 healthy males that indicated that bed rest resulted in selective atrophy of the multifidus muscles. An increased cross-sectional area (CSA) of the trunk flexor musculature (increases in psoas, anterolateral abdominal, and rectus abdominus muscles) is thought to reflect muscle shortening or possible overactivity during bed rest (Hides et al. 2007). According to some researchers, some of the changes resemble those seen in LBP and may partly explain the negative effects of bed rest seen in LBP sufferers.

Besides changes in muscle mass, physical deconditioning can also result in changes in muscle composition. As presented in Chapter 9, the human muscles are composed of different muscle fibres. Muscle disuse is often accompanied by increased fatigability of the muscle because of the reduced oxidative capacity of disused muscles. Muscle capillary density decreases within 2–3 weeks of disuse (Greenleaf 1997). Furthermore, capillary loss and reductions in blood flow at rest and arteriolar responsiveness may contribute to this increased fatigability through the resulting impairment of the supply of energy substrates and oxygen to the muscle (Degens and Alway 2006).

If patients with CLBP are really deconditioned, it would be reasonable to assume that they have measurable muscle atrophy, and reduced muscle strength and endurance. Over the last two decades much research has been done on the specific role of changes in muscle strength of the low back muscles, especially the paraspinal and in particular the multifidus muscles, in the segmental stability of the lower spine. It is hypothesized that segmental instability is an important contributing factor in the persistence of low back pain; when the stability at the segmental level is not sufficient, even little disturbances at this level might result in high forces at the region of the intervertebral disc and surrounding tissues. This could result in repetitive high strains and possibly re-injury of these tissues and eventually causing pain (Panjabi 1992a, 1992b; Danneels et al. 2001). It has been suggested that specific training of these paraspinal, and more specifically the lumbar multifidus muscles, is effective in non-specific CLBP (O'Sullivan et al. 1997; Hides et al. 2007) although the evidence is inconclusive (Macedo et al. 2009).

*Muscle atrophy in CLBP* has been studied based on a number of imaging studies. Several magnetic resonance imaging (MRI) or computed tomography (CT) studies showed a smaller CSA of the paraspinal muscles, psoas and multifidus (Gibbons et al. 1997a; Parkkola et al. 1993).

Danneels et al. studied the total paraspinal muscle mass, the isolated multifidus, and the psoas at three different levels using CT. The results showed that only the CSA of the multifidus and only at the lowest level (lower end-plate of L4) was found to be statistically smaller in patients with CLBP (Danneels et al. 2000). Others confirmed these findings of a localized rather than generalized pattern of multifidus and psoas muscle atrophy in patients with CLBP (Mayer et al. 1989; Kader et al. 2000; Barker et al. 2004; Hides et al. 2007).

The greatest asymmetry between sides was seen at the L5 vertebral level in patients with unilateral pain presentations. This asymmetry might be caused, at least partly, by inactivity/disuse and ageing. One study on patients with unilateral back pain shows clear atrophy of both the multifidus and psoas muscle at the symptomatic side suggesting that not only disuse but also neuromuscular changes play a role (Barker et al. 2004). However, there are inconsistencies between studies. When one corrects for age, gender, body mass index and activity level there is limited evidence that once LBP originates, atrophy of the multifidus muscles might play a role in the complex of CLBP and its resulting disability.

The overall results of studies reporting on changes in *muscle composition in CLBP* based on biopsy findings are inconclusive; several studies suggest the existence of type II fibres atrophy in CLBP (Matilla et al. 1986; Zhu et al. 1989; Weber et al. 1997), but others state that type IIX fibres are generally smaller even in healthy back muscles and decrease with advancing age. Several studies show that the longer the duration of LBP the more fibre-type transformation seems to occur (increased IIX:IIA ratio and decreased I:IIX ratio) (Zhu et al. 1989; Mannion et al. 2000). The observed atrophy may simply represent atrophy of this type IIX fibre (Rantanen et al. 1993; Mannion et al. 2000). One study with healthy controls matched for age and anthropometry does not show this transformation, although no further distinction in fibre type II was made (Crossman et al. 2004). No study has yet been able to convincingly show significant differences in the ratio of the size of the type I:IIX fibres between patients with CLBP and matched controls.

### 10.3.3 **Postural control**

Due to physical immobility or inactivity, changes in motor unit recruitment may occur that include an impairment of the ability to activate motor units (Sale et al. 1982). Immobility decreases coordination and balance (Haines 1974). Motor control is reported to be affected after a period of bed rest. Maintaining a high degree of coordination requires frequent performance of an activity under conditions in which the sensory perception of the motor performance can be checked for accuracy and errors may be corrected. Bed rest decreases the amount of proprioceptive stimuli, which are responsible for regulating neuromuscular performance.

Hides et al. studied the effect of bed rest on trunk muscle activation in 10 healthy males who underwent 8 weeks of bed rest with a 1-year follow-up (Hides et al. 2007). A repetitive knee movement model at four movement speeds in non-weight bearing was used to assess activity in five superficial lumbopelvic (LP) muscles and abdominal flexor-lumbar extensor co-contraction for lumbopelvic stabilization. Increased muscle activity and decreased co contraction during a repetitive-movement task were found. During bed rest, increased activity appeared at the highest movement speed and seemed generalized across all five superficial LP muscles up to 1 year after bed rest. The same subjects showed significant atrophy of the deep multifidus muscles, but not in the lumbar erector spinae or abdominal muscles (Hides et al. 2007) The authors suggest that due to this deep muscle atrophy, in order to maintain the necessary amount of LP stiffness for the knee movement task, the central nervous system increased the recruitment of the superficial LP muscle systems. However, research in patients with acute LBP is not available.

There is a wide variability in reported changes in sensorimotor control of the trunk muscles in low back and pelvic pain. Flexion-relaxation (FR) refers to a pattern of muscle activity during trunk flexion, in which the lumbar muscles initially contract, but ultimately relax, at what appears to be a distinct point in the flexion range of motion (ROM). ROM and FR are anatomically correlated, and hence, a large ROM will induce FR. The variables are not necessarily independent. Studies have shown FR of the lumbar muscles to be a consistent and predictable pattern in most normal subjects without back pain. As compared with normal subjects with no history of back pain, subjects with CLBP often show elevated muscle activity during full voluntary trunk flexion and fail to achieve FR (Watson et al. 1997; Neblett et al. 2003). However, it should be noted that patients with CLBP often fail to reach the ROM necessary for FR. Patients may be anatomically limited or have fear and/or pain during forward bending which will influence the results of the test.

During static tasks, such as standing, inconsistent levels of trunk muscle activation have been found in patients with CLBP. Patients with CLBP have been reported to have increased (Arena et al. 1989; Healey et al. 2005), decreased (Ahern et al. 1988; Cassisi et al. 1993) and similar surface electromyography (sEMG) (Kravitz et al. 1981) amplitudes compared with controls. Wong et al; reported, that workers with LBP spent a significantly higher percentage of time in static trunk posture when compared to normal (Wong et al; 2009). In a study investigating sEMG during unsupported 'usual' versus 'slumped' sitting no differences in trunk muscle activity between healthy controls and patients with CLBP were observed (Dankaerts et al. 2006). However, when these patients were subdivided into an active extension pattern group and a flexion pattern group, differences were identified. A study comparing patients with CLBP to healthy controls while performing slow trunk motions about the neutral posture and isometric ramp contractions while seated upright, showed greater ratios of EMG amplitudes of antagonists over agonists, and of lumbar over thoracic erector spinae muscles in patients (van Dieen et al. 2003a).

The recruitment of stabilizing trunk muscles during motion of the upper limbs appears to be different in persons with and without back pain (Hodges 2001). A number of studies have found increased superficial lumbar muscle activation in patients with LBP and increased coactivation of the abdominal muscles enhancing the stability of the lumbar spine. In addition activation of the deep lumbar muscles is impaired (Hodges et al. 2003; van Dieen et al. 2003b; Geisser et al. 2005). Several studies showed disturbances of propriosepsis in patients with CLBP (Brumagne et al. 2000; Leinonen et al. 2002; O'Sullivan et al. 2002), and some not (Asell et al. 2006). In most of these studies PAL of the subjects was not controlled for. It is therefore unclear if deconditioning influenced these results.

### 10.3.4 **Aerobic capacity**

Aerobic capacity is a measure of the ability and efficiency of the body to take up oxygen and use it to convert fat and carbohydrates into energy. It is an important index of cardiovascular fitness and increases with sustained rhythmic contractions of a large percentage of muscle mass. The oxygen uptake system has a central and a peripheral component. The central component is cardiac output (Q), which is equivalent to heart rate (HR) multiplied by stroke volume (SV). The peripheral component ($a\text{-}vO_2$) is the difference between arterial and mixed venous blood. Therefore, the level of $\dot{V}O_{2max}$ depends on both the heart's ability to pump blood as well as the capacity of the muscle tissues to extract oxygen from the blood. Aerobic capacity is expressed in litres/minute (l/min) and often adjusted for bodyweight millilitres/kilogram/minute ($ml \times kg^{-1} \times min^{-1}$). The magnitude of reduction in $\dot{V}O_{2max}$ $ml \times kg^{-1} \times min^{-1}$ varies according to the duration of inactivity and the initial level of aerobic capacity, but appears to be independent of age or gender. In general, fitter people appear to experience relatively greater losses in $\dot{V}O_{2max}$, but retain a more efficient oxygen uptake system than people who are sedentary or who have not exercised for prolonged periods (Saltin et al. 1968; Coyle et al. 1984). The decline in $\dot{V}O_{2max}$ is the result of a combination of central (cardiac output) and peripheral factors (arterio-venous difference). The rate at which $\dot{V}O_{2max}$ changes is determined by two factors: one fast-related to cardiac output, one slow-related to decrease in muscle oxidative potential (see also 'Muscle strength and endurance' section).

Most physical activities are described in terms of their energy or metabolic cost (Ainsworth et al. 2000). Physical activities are coded in metabolic equivalent (MET) intensity levels. One MET is considered a resting metabolic rate obtained during quiet sitting and equals an oxygen uptake of 3.5ml/kg/min. The oxygen cost for physical activities ranges from 0.9MET for sleeping to 18MET for running at 10.9mph (Ainsworth et al. 2000). For occupational activities energy cost ranges from about 1.5MET for sitting in a meeting to 17MET for fast axe chopping in forestry. The higher a person's $\dot{V}O_{2max}$, the more energy is available to perform physical activities. For an individual with a good aerobic exercise capacity, physical activity generates less fatigue, which means that he or she is capable of performing at a higher level of energy demand (i.e. 'do more').

The $\dot{V}O_{2peak}$[1] attained during a graded maximal exercise to volitional exhaustion is considered as the single best indicator of aerobic exercise capacity by the World Health Organization (Shephard et al. 1968). The gold standard for determining $\dot{V}O_{2peak}$ in an individual is by metabolic measurement system analysis of $O_2$ and $CO_2$ gas in expired air at regular intervals and a plateauing of $VO_2$ during increasing workloads (Oddsson et al. 1997). However, in many subjects including children, patients, and athletes a plateau in $\dot{V}O_2$ is not observed (Rowland 1993; Wassermen et al. 1999; Lucia et al. 2006). Several secondary parameters have therefore been established to determine $\dot{V}O_{2max}$ without a $\dot{V}O_2$ plateau. These parameters includes a failure of HR to increase with further increases in exercise intensity, a respiratory exchange ratio (RER) >1.15 and a rating of perceived exertion of more than 17 (Borg 6–20 scale) (Howley et al. 1995).

The mode of exercise testing and the age and gender of the subject determine oxygen uptake with exercise testing. In general, the highest oxygen uptake is achieved with the type of exercise that uses the greatest amount of muscle mass. In normal subjects, the highest $\dot{V}O_{2max}$ is obtained with treadmill testing due to the quantity of the muscle mass involved, followed by bicycle testing. $\dot{V}O_{2max}$ achieved by bicycle testing is reported to be 5–15% lower than with treadmill testing in normal subjects (Hermansen and Saltin 1969; Hermansen et al. 1970). A variety of (submaximal) tests have been developed estimating aerobic capacity, when direct measurement is not possible (See, for review, Noonan and Dean 2000.) These tests usually involve running/walking for a given time or distance, such as the 12min walk/run test (Cooper 1968), the shuttle test (Leger and Lambert 1982), various step tests (Siconolfi et al. 1985; Francis, 1987) and the 2km walk test (Oja et al. 1991). Longer distances and shorter test times are associated with higher levels of aerobic fitness.

Other tests estimate $\dot{V}O_{2max}$ by submaximal testing and extrapolation to maximal heart rate by treadmill walking or bicycling against a predetermined load with measurement of heart rates (Astrand and Ryhming 1954). These tests were mostly developed for testing aerobic capacity in healthy people and were validated by comparing actual measured $\dot{V}O_{2max}$ to predicted $\dot{V}O_{2max}$ or to the test performance. Nomograms and prediction equations, derived from exercise testing

---

[1] Maximal exercise tests in patients are usually terminated when the subject despite strong verbal encouragement from the experimenters, is unwilling or unable to continue. The appropriate term to use is therefore peak oxygen consumption ($\dot{V}O_{2peak}$), which represents the highest oxygen uptake during an exercise test to volitional exhaustion. Both terms will be used interchanged throughout this chapter.

large samples of subjects, were developed to estimate $\dot{V}O_{2max}$ in healthy populations. Even as they include age and gender corrections, they reflect a *mean* aerobic capacity level for a particular gender at a particular age and can therefore never be as precise as direct measurement of oxygen uptake. Maximal heart rate may be predicted from age using any of several published equations, such as 220 minus age, however interindividual variability is quite high (standard deviation is 10–12 beats/min) (Oddsson et al. 1997). As a result, there is potential for considerable error in the use of methods that extrapolate submaximal test data to an age-predicted HRmax (ACSM, 2000).

Whether patients with CLBP have a lower level of aerobic capacity as compared to healthy controls was a subject of various studies. In a systematic review, nine studies in which at least 50% of the patients had CLBP were assessed with a submaximal testing procedure to calculate the $\dot{V}O_{2max}$ were identified (Smeets et al. 2006). The studies are difficult to compare due to the heterogeneity of protocols, populations and controls used. These studies used different testing procedures and methods to calculate $\dot{V}O_{2max}$, sometimes even without adjustments for gender. Most studies used submaximal exercise-testing. Those studies that attempted maximal testing found that most patients were not able to reach the criteria for VO$_2$max (Wittink et al. 2000b). Furthermore, most studies used inappropriate healthy controls (no matching for age and gender) or used normative data of insufficiently relevant healthy population. Populations differed between studies in, for example, work status and diagnosis (herniated disc versus non-specific CLBP).

Despite the long existence of the deconditioning theory, this review concluded that it still is not clear whether symptoms of physical deconditioning, especially a reduced level of aerobic capacity, develop or even exist in patients with CLBP. However, authors have been consistent in suggesting that differences in levels of physical activity may contribute to their discrepant findings. For instance, Nielens and Plaghki (2001) and Wittink et al. (2000a) found male–female differences in $\dot{V}O_{2max}$ and suggested that these differences are attributable to different levels of physical activity, especially regarding work, household, sport, and leisure time. More recently, Brox et al. reported a lower aerobic capacity in patients with low back pain who were sick-listed for 8–12 weeks, but not in patients with CLBP waiting for lumbar instrumented fusion, compared with healthy persons matched for gender and age (Brox et al. 2005). Unfortunately, they only used four age cohorts, which limits its generalizability. Rasmussen-Barr et al. showed that male but not female patients with recurrent low back pain who were still at work have a similar aerobic capacity level as age- and gender matched controls, indicating that staying active at work might indeed be an important factor in the prevention of aerobic deconditioning (Rasmussen-Barr et al. 2008).

More recently, Smeets et al. reported that patients with moderately to severely disabling CLBP had a significantly lower level of aerobic capacity compared to healthy subjects matched for age, gender, and sport activity (Smeets et al. 2009). Men with CLPB even had a significantly lower level of $\dot{V}O_{2max}$ than women with CLBP. It appeared that the level of physical activity during leisure time as well as work including household work were significantly associated with this lower level of aerobic capacity. A possible explanation for the significantly lower level in aerobic capacity for men compared to women with CLBP (20% lower versus 13% lower than normative population) may be the significantly higher level of household activities performed by women, confirming the hypothesis of Nielens and Plaghki (2001) that women with chronic pain are generally more active once they are at home because they are still engaged in childcare and various household duties. Since this loss of aerobic capacity might also be caused by variables of the fear-avoidance model, Smeets et al. also investigated the role of these factors, and their results clearly showed that pain intensity, pain-catastrophizing, fear of movement and depression were not significantly associated with the loss of aerobic capacity (Smeets et al. 2009).

Since all above mentioned studies are based on cross-sectional designs, the possibility that deconditioning was already present before patients developed back pain cannot be ruled out. This explanation might by supported by the finding that almost 40% of the level of $VO_2$max can be explained by genetic factors (McArdle et al. 2001). Nevertheless, prospective research in healthy subjects has not identified low aerobic capacity levels or physical inactivity as a risk factor for developing CLBP (Battie et al. 1989; Picavet and Schuit 2003). To further investigate the development and impact of loss of aerobic capacity levels, longitudinal studies should be performed in patients with acute LBP, while monitoring all putative influential factors.

### 10.3.5 Metabolic factors

Insulin is the major hormonal regulator of energy storage and release. It stimulates glycogen synthesis, aerobic and anaerobic glycolysis and the synthesis of proteins and fatty acids in the liver. In numerous bed rest studies, it has been shown that bed rest reduces sensitivity to insulin (Pavy-Le Traon et al. 2007). Five days of bed rest only, was already associated with the development of insulin resistance, dyslipidaemia, increased blood pressure, and impaired microvascular function in 20 healthy volunteers (Hamburg et al. 2007). In a recent preliminary study, 18 non-exercising healthy volunteers in their twenties decreased their daily walking for 2–3 weeks to 1500 pedometer-recorded steps from a mean value of more than 6000 steps. During this period they developed metabolic changes that suggested a decrease in insulin sensitivity and an attenuation of post-prandial lipid metabolism, and physical changes that suggested that calories used to maintain muscle mass with greater stepping may have been partitioned to visceral fat (Olsen et al. 2008). Extrapolating from these data it would seem evident that patients with CLBP would show metabolic changes as a result from inactivity. To date, there are however no studies that have investigated metabolic changes in patients with CLBP.

### 10.3.6 Conclusion on health-related fitness in patients with CLBP

Currently, no consistent evidence could be found in the literature that the spectrum of changes in morphological, muscular, motor (postural control), cardiorespiratory ($VO_2$max) or metabolic factors (carbohydrate and lipid metabolism) in patients with CLBP are due to physical deconditioning.

## 10.4 Future research

### 10.4.1 Future research on physical activity in CLBP

What could explain why not all patients with musculoskeletal pain who feel highly disabled eventually become inactive? In recent years, several explanatory models (Vlaeyen and Morley 2004; Hasenbring and Verbunt 2010) have been introduced to explain differences in activity related behaviour in chronic pain. In addition to the fear avoidance model that introduced fear of movement/re-injury as the explaining factor for a disabling decrease in physical activity, alternative models have been proposed to explain other strategies concerning activity related behaviour in chronic pain. Hasenbring and colleagues hypothesized that, in addition to patients using avoidance strategies as a coping mechanism, other patients with pain will have the tendency to cope with pain by using persistent strategies (Hasenbring et al. 1994). These patients persist in the performance of activities and appear to ignore their pain and overload their muscles (overuse), resulting in muscular hyperactivity (further information is presented in Chapter 15). Long-term muscular hyperactivity and long term false straining of the muscles eventually can result in chronification of pain.

In accordance with the hypothesis of Hasenbring, Van Houdenhove suggested that, especially in patients with fibromyalgia and chronic fatigue syndrome, a high level of 'action proneness', promoting an overactive lifestyle, may play a predisposing, initiating and perpetuating role in the level of disability (Van Houdenhove et al. 1995). People who have an overactive lifestyle may be at a higher risk of overburdening. If these persons are deprived of overactivity as their favourite coping strategy, for example due to pain or functional limitations, the level of psychological distress can increase. An alternative explanation for differences in activity related behaviour in pain has been introduced by Vlaeyen and Morley in their Mood-as-Input Model (Vlaeyen and Morley 2004). This model explains why some patients will stop, whereas others will continue performing their activities when confronted by pain. According to the Mood-as-Input Model, the informational value of the mood in a certain context, rather than the mood itself, determines whether participants persist at a certain task. For some individuals a negative mood will facilitate task persistence; whereas for others it will lead to disengagement. Mood can result in different motivational effects leading to inactivity or persistence in activities regardless the level of pain. The hypothesis of Hasenbring and Vlaeyen and Morley could explain the coexistence of high levels of physical activity and high levels of disability. Research to confirm different activity related strategies in chronic pain has to be performed.

For future research on activity assessment in pain we urge the incorporation of monitoring of activities in daily life, preferably combined with methods to measure the total energy consumption (Westerterp 1999; Philippaerts et al. 2001; van den Berg-Emons et al. 2007; Verbunt et al. 2008). And we do need more cohort studies of patients with acute LBP in order to determine whether changes in the level of activities, and even more important the type of activities, occur, and whether deconditioning symptoms appear in case the pain persists.

## 10.4.2 Future research on health related fitness in CLBP

Two important topics have to be addressed in order to be able to answer the question whether physical deconditioning has a perpetuating role in CLBP. The first, major issue is to agree upon or develop valid and reliable measurement tools for the assessment of physical fitness parameters in people who experience pain. Assessment of fitness related parameters most often requires functional testing, in which patients with pain have to perform an exercise test. To obtain valid and reliable measurements of aerobic capacity, muscle strength and endurance, maximal effort is needed. Researchers warn that submaximal performance may play a role in the outcome of fitness testing in patients with pain and that influences such as motivation, fear that the action will cause pain or damage and the emotional state of a patient, level of pain, avoidance of pain, self-efficacy and deconditioning, need to be considered when the results are assessed (Keller et al. 1999; Watson 1999; Oddsson and De Luca 2003; Crossman et al. 2004; Kramer et al. 2005; Verbunt et al. 2005a; Smeets et al. 2007). Since voluntary muscle strength is influenced by many of the above mentioned factors strength and endurance testing is regarded as a invalid method to assess whether muscular deconditioning is present in patients with low back pain. Also the use of EMG-studies as a valid and reliable of back muscle weakness and muscle composition based on EMG-assessment is still controversial (Lariviere et al. 2002; Crossman et al. 2004). More research on influencing factors during performance testing in chronic pain is needed to be able to improve assessment of physical fitness related parameters in pain.

Second, current evidence on deconditioning related parameters in pain is especially based on cross-sectional research. To further investigate the development and impact of loss of the level of aerobic capacity, longitudinal studies should be performed in patients with acute LBP, while monitoring all putative influential factors.

## 10.5 **General conclusion**

The general assumption that patients with CLBP suffer from disuse and physical deconditioning still lacks empirical ground. The level of physical activity and fitness-related health of patients with CLBP seems less or equal as compared to healthy individuals. However, results of functional testing in patients with pain are often influenced by submaximal during performance testing of patients as compared to healthy individuals. Further longitudinal research especially is therefore needed to improve assessment of both physical activity and fitness-related health parameters in patients with pain, to distinguish different styles of activity-related behaviour in pain, and to identify and control for factors influencing performance testing in CLBP.

## **References**

ACSM (2000) *American College of Sports Medicine: Guideline for exercise testing and prescription,* Philadelphia, PA: Lippincott, Williams and Wilkins.

Ahern, D. K., Follick, M. J., Council, J. R., Laser-Wolston, N. & Litchman, H. (1988) Comparison of lumbar paravertebral EMG patterns in chronic low back pain patients and non-patient controls. *Pain,* **34**, 153–60.

Ainsworth, B. E., Haskell, W. L., Whitt, M. C., *et al.* (2000) Compendium of physical activities: an update of activity codes and MET intensities. *Med Sci Sports Exerc,* **32**, S498–504.

Arena, J. G., Sherman, R. A., Bruno, G. M. & Young, T. R. (1989) Electromyographic recordings of 5 types of low back pain subjects and non-pain controls in different positions. *Pain,* **37**, 57–65.

Asell, M., Sjolander, P., Kerschbaumer, H. & Djupsjobacka, M. (2006) Are lumbar repositioning errors larger among patients with chronic low back pain compared with asymptomatic subjects? *Arch Phys Med Rehabil,* **87**, 1170–6.

Astrand, P. O. & Ryhming, I. (1954) A nomogram for calculation of aerobic capacity (physical fitness) from pulse rate during sub-maximal work. *J Appl Physiol,* **7**, 218–21.

Barker, K. L., Shamley, D. R. & Jackson, D. (2004) Changes in the cross-sectional area of multifidus and psoas in patients with unilateral back pain: the relationship to pain and disability. *Spine,* **29**, E515–9.

Battie, M. C., Bigos, S. J., Fisher, L. D., *et al.* (1989) A prospective study of the role of cardiovascular risk factors and fitness in industrial back pain complaints. *Spine,* **14**, 141–7.

Berry, P., Berry, I. & Manelfe, C. (1993) Magnetic resonance imaging evaluation of lower limb muscles during bed rest—a microgravity simulation model. *Aviat Space Environ Med,* **64**, 212–8.

Bloomfield, S. A. (1997) Changes in musculoskeletal structure and function with prolonged bed rest. *Med Sci Sports Exerc,* **29**, 197–206.

Bouchard, C. & Shephard, R. J. (1994) Physical activity, fitness and health: the model and key concepts. *Physical activity, fitness and health. International Proceedings and consensus statement.* Champaign, IL: Kuman Kinetics.

Bousema, E. J., Verbunt, J. A., Seelen, H. A., Vlaeyen, J. W. & Knottnerus, J. A. (2007) Disuse and physical deconditioning in the first year after the onset of back pain. *Pain,* **130**, 279–86.

Briggs, A. M., Straker, L. M. & Wark, J. D. (2008) Bone health and back pain: What do we know and where should we go? *Osteoporos Int.,* 2009, 209–19.

Brox, J. I., Storheim, K., Holm, I., Friis, A. & Reikeras, O. (2005) Disability, pain, psychological factors and physical performance in healthy controls, patients with sub-acute and chronic low back pain: a case-control study. *J Rehabil Med,* **37**, 95–9.

Brumagne, S., Cordo, P., Lysens, R., Verschueren, S. & Swinnen, S. (2000) The role of paraspinal muscle spindles in lumbosacral position sense in individuals with and without low back pain. *Spine,* **25**, 989–94.

Cassisi, J. E., Robinson, M. E., O'Conner, P. & MacMillan, M. (1993) Trunk strength and lumbar paraspinal muscle activity during isometric exercise in chronic low-back pain patients and controls. *Spine,* **18**, 245–51.

Convertino, V. A., Bloomfield, S. A. & Greenleaf, J. E. (1997) An overview of the issues: physiological effects of bed rest and restricted physical activity. *Med Sci Sports Exerc,* **29,** 187–90.

Cooper, K.H. (1968) A means of assessing maximal oxygen intake. *JAMA,* **203,** 201–4.

Coyle, E. F., Martin, W. H., 3rd, Sinacore, D. R., Joyner, M. J., Hagberg, J. M. & Holloszy, J. O. (1984) Time course of loss of adaptations after stopping prolonged intense endurance training. *J Appl Physiol,* **57,** 1857–64.

Crossman, K. B. M., Mahon, M. M., Watson, P. J. P. M., *et al.* (2004) Chronic low back pain-associated paraspinal muscle dysfunction is not the result of a constitutionally determined 'adverse' fiber-type composition. *Spine,* **29,** 628–34.

Dankaerts, W., O'Sullivan, P., Burnett, A. & Straker, L. (2006) Altered patterns of superficial trunk muscle activation during sitting in nonspecific chronic low back pain patients: importance of subclassification. *Spine,* **31,** 2017–23.

Danneels, L. A., Vanderstraeten, G. G., Cambier, D. C., Witvrouw, E. E. & De Cuyper, H. J. (2000) CT imaging of trunk muscles in chronic low back pain patients and healthy control subjects. *Eur Spine J,* **9,** 266–72.

Danneels, L. A., Cools, A. M., Vanderstraeten, G. G., *et al.* (2001) The effects of three different training modalities on the cross-sectional area of the paravertebral muscles. *Scan J Med Sci Sports,* **11,** 335–41.

Danneels, L. A., Vanderstraeten, G. G., Cambier, D. C., Witvrouw, E. E. & De Cuyper, H. J. (2000) CT imaging of trunk muscles in chronic low back pain patients and healthy control subjects. *Eur Spine J,* **9,** 266–72.

Degens, H. & Alway, S. E. (2006) Control of muscle size during disuse, disease, and aging. *Int J Sports Med,* **27,** 94–9.

Francis, K. T. (1987) Fitness assessment using step tests. *Compr Ther,* **13,** 36–41.

Fritz, J. M., George, S. Z. & Delitto, A. (2001) The role of fear-avoidance beliefs in acute low back pain: relationships with current and future disability and work status. *Pain,* **94,** 7–15.

Geisser, M. E., Ranavaya, M., Haig, A. J., *et al.* (2005) A meta-analytic review of surface electromyography among persons with low back pain and normal, healthy controls. *J Pain,* **6,** 711–26.

Gibbons, L. E., Videman, T. & Battie, M. C. (1997a) Isokinetic and psychophysical lifting strength, static back muscle endurance, and magnetic resonance imaging of the paraspinal muscles as predictors of low back pain in men. *Scan J Rehab Med,* **29,** 187–91.

Gibbons, L. E., Videman, T. & Crites Battié, M. (1997b) Determinants of isokinetic and psychophysical lifting strength and static back muscle endurance: A study of male monozygotic twins. *Spine,* **23,** 2412–21.

Gogia, P., Schneider, V. S., Leblanc, A. D., Krebs, J., Kasson, C. & Pientok, C. (1988) Bed rest effect on extremity muscle torque in healthy men. *Arch Phys Med Rehabil,* **69,** 1030–2.

Greenleaf, J. (2004) *Deconditioning and Reconditioning.* Boca Baton, FL: CRC Press LLC.

Greenleaf, J. E. (1997) Intensive exercise training during bed rest attenuates deconditioning. *Med Sci Sports Exerc,* **29,** 207–15.

Haines, R. F. (1974) Effect of bed rest and exercise on body balance. *J Appl Physiol,* **36,** 323–7.

Hamburg, N. M., McMackin, C. J., Huang, A. L., *et al* (2007) Physical inactivity rapidly induces insulin resistance and microvascular dysfunction in healthy volunteers. *Arterioscler Thromb Vasc Biol,* **27,** 2650–6.

Hasenbring, M. & Verbunt, J. (2010). Fear-avoidance and endurance-related responses to pain: new models of behaviour and their consequences for clinical practice. *Clin J Pain,* **26**(9), 747–53.

Hasenbring, M., Marienfeld, G., Kuhlendahl, D. & Soyka, D. (1994) Risk factors of chronicity in lumbar disc patients. A prospective investigation of biologic, psychologic, and social predictors of therapy outcome. *Spine,* **19,** 2759–65.

Healey, E. L., Fowler, N. E., Burden, A. M. & Mcewan, I. M. (2005) The influence of different unloading positions upon stature recovery and paraspinal muscle activity. *Clin Biomech,* **20,** 365–71.

Hermansen, L. & Saltin, B. (1969) Oxygen uptake during maximal treadmill and bicycle exercise. *J Appl Physiol*, **26**, 31–7.

Hermansen, L., Ekblom, B. & Saltin, B. (1970) Cardiac output during submaximal and maximal treadmill and bicycle exercise. *J Appl Physiol*, **29**, 82–6.

Hides, J. A., Belavy, D. L., Stanton, W., *et al.* (2007) Magnetic resonance imaging assessment of trunk muscles during prolonged bed rest. *Spine*, **32**, 1687–92.

Hodges, P. W. (2001) Changes in motor planning of feedforward postural responses of the trunk muscles in low back pain. *Exp Brain Res*, **141**, 261–6.

Hodges, P. W., Moseley, G. L., Gabrielsson, A. & Gandevia, S. C. (2003) Experimental muscle pain changes feedforward postural responses of the trunk muscles. *Exp Brain Res*, **151**, 262–71.

Howley, E. T., Bassett, D. R., JR. & Welch, H. G. (1995) Criteria for maximal oxygen uptake: review and commentary. *Med Sci Sports Exerc*, **27**, 1292–301.

Jamison, R. N., Stetson, B., Sbrocco, T. & Parris, W. C. (1990) Effects of significant weight gain on chronic pain patients. *Clin J Pain*, **6**, 47–50.

Kader, D. F., Wardlaw, D. & Smith, F. W. (2000) Correlation between the MRI changes in the lumbar multifidus muscles and leg pain. *Clin Radiol*, **55**, 145–9.

Keller, A., Johansen, J. G., Hellesnes, J. & Brox, J. I. (1999) Predictors of isokinetic back muscle strength in patients with low back pain. *Spine*, **24**, 275–80.

Klenerman, L., Slade, P. D., Stanley, I. M., *et al.* (1995) The prediction of chronicity in patients with an acute attack of low back pain in a general practice setting. *Spine*, **20**, 478–84.

Kramer, M., Ebert, V., Kinzl, L., Dehner, C., Elbel, M. & Hartwig, E. (2005) Surface electromyography of the paravertebral muscles in patients with chronic low back pain. *Arch Phys Med Rehabil*, **86**, 31–6.

Kravitz, E., Moore, M. E. & Glaros, A. (1981) Paralumbar muscle activity in chronic low back pain. *Arch Phys Med Rehabil*, **62**, 172–6.

Lariviere, C., Arsenault, B., Gravel, D., Gagnon, D., Loisel, P. & Vadeboncoeur, R. (2002) Electromyographic assessment of back muscle weakness and muscle composition: reliability and validity issues. *Arch Phys Med Rehabil*, **83**, 1206–14.

Leger, L. A. & Lambert, J. (1982) A maximal multistage 20-m shuttle run test to predict VO2 max. *Eur J Appl Physiol Occup Physiol*, **49**, 1–12.

Leinonen, V., Maatta, S., Taimela, S., *et al.* (2002) Impaired lumbar movement perception in association with postural stability and motor- and somatosensory-evoked potentials in lumbar spinal stenosis. *Spine*, **27**, 975–83.

Lucia, A., Rabadan, M., Hoyos, J., *et al.* (2006) Frequency of the VO2max plateau phenomenon in world-class cyclists. *Int J Sports Med*, **27**, 984–92.

Macedo, L. G., Maher, C. G., Latimer, J. & McAuley, J. H. (2009) Motor control exercise for persistent, nonspecific low back pain: a systematic review. *Phys Ther*, **89**(1), 9–25.

Mannion, A. F., Kaser, L., Weber, E., Rhyner, A., Dvorak, J. & Muntener, M. (2000) Influence of age and duration of symptoms on fibre type distribution and size of the back muscles in chronic low back pain patients. *Eur Spine J*, **9**, 273–81.

Mattila, M., Hurme, M., Alaranta, H., *et al* (1986) The multifidus muscle in patients with lumbar disc herniation. A histochemical and morphometric analysis of intraoperative biopsies. *Spine*, **11**, 732–8.

Mayer, T. G., Gatchel, R. J., Kishino, N., *et al.* (1985) Objective assessment of spine function following industrial injury. A prospective study with comparison group and one-year follow-up. *Spine*, **10**, 482–93.

Mayer, T. G., Gatchel, R. J., Kishino, N., *et al.* (1986) A prospective short-term study of chronic low back pain patients utilizing novel objective functional measurement. *Pain*, **25**, 53–68.

Mayer, T. G., Vanharanta, H., Gatchel, R. J., *et al.* (1989) Comparison of CT scan muscle measurements and isokinetic trunk strength in postoperative patients. *Spine*, **14**, 33–6.

McArdle, W., Katch, F.I. & Katch, V.L. (2001) *Exercise Physiology: energy, nutrition, and human performance*. Baltimore, MD: Lippincott Wiliams & Wilkins.

Mok, N. W., Brauer, S. G. & Hodges, P. W. (2007) Failure to use movement in postural strategies leads to increased spinal displacement in low back pain. *Spine,* **32,** E537–43.

Mujika, I. & Padilla, S. (2001) Cardiorespiratory and metabolic characteristics of detraining in humans. *Med Sci Sports Exerc,* **33,** 413–21.

Neblett, R., Mayer, T. G., Gatchel, R. J., Keeley, J., Proctor, T. & Anagnostis, C. (2003) Quantifying the lumbar flexion-relaxation phenomenon: theory, normative data, and clinical applications. *Spine,* **28,** 1435–46.

Nielens, H. & Plaghki, L. (2001) Cardiorespiratory fitness, physical activity level, and chronic pain: are men more affected than women? *Clin J Pain,* **17,** 129–37.

Noonan, V. & Dean, E. (2000) Submaximal exercise testing: clinical application and interpretation. *Phys Ther,* **80,** 782–807.

O'Sullivan, P. B., Grahamslaw, K. M., Kendell, M., Lapenskie, S. C., Moller, N. E. & Richards, K. V. (2002) The effect of different standing and sitting postures on trunk muscle activity in a pain-free population. *Spine,* **27,** 1238–44.

O'Sullivan, P. B., Phyty, G. D., Twomey, L. T. & Allison, G. T. (1997) Evaluation of specific stabilizing exercise in the treatment of chronic low back pain with radiologic diagnosis of spondylolysis or spondylolisthesis. *Spine,* **22,** 2959–67.

Oddsson, L. I. & De Luca, C. J. (2003) Activation imbalances in lumbar spine muscles in the presence of chronic low back pain. *J Appl Physiol,* **94,** 1410–20.

Oddsson, L. I., Giphart, J. E., Buijs, R. J., Roy, S. H., Taylor, H. P. & De Luca, C. J. (1997) Development of new protocols and analysis procedures for the assessment of LBP by surface EMG techniques. *J Rehabil Res Dev,* **34,** 415–26.

Oja, P., Laukkanen, R., Pasanen, M., Tyry, T. & Vuori, I. (1991) A 2-km walking test for assessing the cardiorespiratory fitness of healthy adults. *Int J Sports Med,* **12,** 356–62.

Oldridge, N. B. (2008) Economic burden of physical inactivity: healthcare costs associated with cardiovascular disease. *Eur J Cardiovasc Prev Rehabil,* **15,** 130–9.

Olsen, R. H., Krogh-Madsen, R., Thomsen, C., Booth, F. W. & Pedersen, B. K. (2008) Metabolic responses to reduced daily steps in healthy nonexercising men. *JAMA,* **299,** 1261–3.

Panjabi, M. M. (1992a) The stabilizing system of the spine. Part I. Function, dysfunction, adaptation, and enhancement. *J Spinal Disord,* **5,** 383–9.

Panjabi, M. M. (1992b) The stabilizing system of the spine. Part II. Neutral zone and instability hypothesis. *J Spinal Disord,* **5,** 390–6.

Parkkola, R., Rytokoski, U. & Kormano, M. (1993) Magnetic resonance imaging of the discs and trunk muscles in patients with chronic low back pain and healthy control subjects. *Spine,* **18,** 830–6.

Pavy-Le Traon, A., Heer, M., Narici, M. V., Rittweger, J. & Vernikos, J. (2007) From space to Earth: advances in human physiology from 20 years of bed rest studies (1986–2006). *Eur J Appl Physiol,* **101,** 143–94.

Philippaerts, R. M., Westerterp, K. R. & Lefevre, J. (2001) Comparison of two questionnaires with a tri-axial accelerometer to assess physical activity patterns. *Int J Sports Med,* **22,** 34–9.

Picavet, H. S. & Schuit, A. J. (2003) Physical inactivity: a risk factor for low back pain in the general population? *J Epidemiol Community Health,* **57,** 517–8.

Protas, E. J. (1999) Physical activity and low back pain. In Mitchell, M. (Ed.) *An updated review; refresher course syllabus 9th World Congress on pain.* Seattle, WA: IASP Press.

Rantanen, J., Hurme, M., Falck, B., *et al.* (1993) The lumbar multifidus muscle five years after surgery for a lumbar intervertebral disc herniation. *Spine,* **18,** 568–74.

Rasmussen-Barr, E., Lundqvist, L., Nilsson-Wikmar, L. & Ljungquist, T. (2008) Aerobic fitness in patients at work despite recurrent low back pain: a cross-sectional study with healthy age- and gender-matched controls. *J Rehabil Med,* **40,** 359–65.

Rowland, T. W. (1993) Does peak VO2 reflect VO2max in children?: evidence from supramaximal testing. *Med Sci Sports Exerc,* **25,** 689–93.

Sale, D. G., Mccomas, A. J., Macdougall, J. D. & Upton, A. R. (1982) Neuromuscular adaptation in human thenar muscles following strength training and immobilization. *J Appl Physiol*, **53**, 419–24.

Saltin, B., Blomqvist, G., Mitchell, J. H., Johnson, R. L., JR., Wildenthal, K. & Chapman, C. B. (1968) Response to exercise after bed rest and after training. *Circulation*, **38**, VII1–78.

Shephard, R. J., Allen, C., Benade, A. J., *et al.* (1968) The maximum oxygen uptake. An international reference standard of cardiorespiratory fitness. *Bulletin of the World Health Organization*, **38**, 757–64.

Siconolfi, S. F., Garber, C. E., Lasater, T. M. & Carleton, R. A. (1985) A simple, valid step test for estimating maximal oxygen uptake in epidemiologic studies. *Am J Epidemiol*, **121**, 382–90.

Skinner, J. & Oja, P. (1994) Laboratory and field tests for assessing health-related fitness. *Physical activity, fitness and health*. Champaign, IL: Human Kinetics.

Smeets, R. J. & Wittink, H. (2007) The deconditioning paradigm for chronic low back pain unmasked? *Pain*, **130**, 201–2.

Smeets, R. J., Wittink, H., Hidding, A. & Knottnerus, J. A. (2006) Do patients with chronic low back pain have a lower level of aerobic fitness than healthy controls?: are pain, disability, fear of injury, working status, or level of leisure time activity associated with the difference in aerobic fitness level? *Spine*, **31**, 90–7; discussion 98.

Smeets, R. J., Van Geel, A. C., Kester, A. D. & Knottnerus, J. A. (2007) Physical capacity tasks in chronic low back pain: what is the contributing role of cardiovascular capacity, pain and psychological factors? *Disabil Rehabil*, **29**, 577–86.

Smeets, R. J., Geel, K. V. & Verbunt, J. A. (2009) Is the fear avoidance model associated with the reduced level of aerobic fitness in patients with chronic low back pain? *Arch Phys Med Rehabil*, **90**, 109–17.

Toda, Y., Segal, N., Toda, T., Morimoto, T. & Ogawa, R. (2000) Lean body mass and body fat distribution in participants with chronic low back pain. *Arch Intern Med*, **160**, 3265–9.

Van Den Berg-Emons, R. J., Schasfoort, F. C., De Vos, L. A., Bussmann, J. B. & Stam, H. J. (2007) Impact of chronic pain on everyday physical activity. *Eur J Pain*, **11**, 587–93.

Van Dieen, J. H., Cholewicki, J. & Radebold, A. (2003a) Trunk muscle recruitment patterns in patients with low back pain enhance the stability of the lumbar spine. *Spine*, **28**, 834–41.

Van Dieen, J. H., Selen, L. P. & Cholewicki, J. (2003b) Trunk muscle activation in low-back pain patients, an analysis of the literature. *J Electromyogr Kinesiol*, **13**, 333–51.

Van Houdenhove, B., Onghena, P., Neerinckx, E. & Hellin, J. (1995) Does high 'action-proneness' make people more vulnerable to chronic fatigue syndrome? A controlled psychometric study. *J Psychosom Res*, **39**, 633–40.

Van Weering, M., Vollenbroek-Hutten, M. M., Kotte, E. M. & Hermens, H. J. (2007) Daily physical activities of patients with chronic pain or fatigue versus asymptomatic controls. A systematic review. *Clin Rehabil*, **21**, 1007–23.

Van Weering, M.G., Vollenbroek-Hutten, M.M., Tönis, T.M., & Hermens, H.J. (2009) Daily physical activities in chronic lower back pain patients assessed with accelerometry. *Eur J Pain*, **13**(6): 649–54.

Verbunt, J. A., Westerterp, K. R., Van Der Heijden, G. J., Seelen, H. A., Vlaeyen, J. W. & Knottnerus, J. A. (2001) Physical activity in daily life in patients with chronic low back pain. *Arch Phys Med Rehabil*, **82**, 726–30.

Verbunt, J. A., Seelen, H. A., Vlaeyen, J. W., *et al* (2003) Disuse and deconditioning in chronic low back pain: concepts and hypotheses on contributing mechanisms. *Eur J Pain*, **7**, 9–21.

Verbunt, J. A., Seelen, H. A., Vlaeyen, J. W., *et al* (2005a) Pain-related factors contributing to muscle inhibition in patients with chronic low back pain: an experimental investigation based on superimposed electrical stimulation. *Clin J Pain*, **21**, 232–40.

Verbunt, J. A., Sieben, J. M., Seelen, H. A., *et al.* (2005b) Decline in physical activity, disability and pain-related fear in sub-acute low back pain. *Eur J Pain*, **9**, 417–25.

Verbunt, J. A., Huijnen, I. P. & Koke, A. (2008) Assessment of physical activity in daily life in patients with musculoskeletal pain. *Eur J Pain*, **13**, 231–42.

Vlaeyen, J. W. & Linton, S. J. (2000) Fear-avoidance and its consequences in chronic musculoskeletal pain: a state of the art. *Pain, 85*, 317–32.

Vlaeyen, J. W. & Morley, S. (2004) Active despite pain: the putative role of stop-rules and current mood. *Pain, 110*, 512–6.

Vlaeyen, J. W., Kole-Snijders, A. M., Boeren, R. G. & Van Eek, H. (1995) Fear of movement/(re)injury in chronic low back pain and its relation to behavioral performance. *Pain, 62*, 363–72.

Wasserman, K., Hansen, J. E., Sue, D. Y., Casaburi, R. & Whipp, B. J. (1999) *Principles of Exercise Testing and Interpretation*. Baltimore, MD: Williams and Wilkins.

Watson, P. J. (1999) Non-psychological determinants of physical performance in musculoskeletal pain. In Mitchell, M. (Ed.) *Pain 1999- an updated review: Refresher course syllabus 9th World Congress on Pain*, pp. 153–8. Seattle, WA: IASP Press.

Watson, P. J., Booker, C. K., Main, C. J. & Chen, A. C. (1997) Surface electromyography in the identification of chronic low back pain patients: the development of the flexion relaxation ratio. *Clin Biomech, 12*, 165–171.

Weber, B. R., Grob, D., Dvorak, J. & Muntener, M. (1997) Posterior surgical approach to the lumbar spine and its effect on the multifidus muscle. *Spine, 22*, 1765–72.

Westerterp, K. R. (1999) Assessment of physical activity level in relation to obesity: current evidence and research issues. *Med Sci Sports Exerc, 31*, S522–5.

Wittink, H., Hoskins Michel, T., Wagner, A., Sukiennik, A. & Rogers, W. (2000a) Deconditioning in patients with chronic low back pain: fact or fiction? *Spine, 25*, 2221–8.

Wittink, H., Michel, T. H., Kulich, R., Wagner, A., Sukiennik, A., Maciewicz, R. & Rogers, W. (2000b) Aerobic fitness testing in patients with chronic low back pain: which test is best? *Spine, 25*, 1704–10.

Wittink, H., Nicholas, M., Kralik, D. & Verbunt, J. (2008) Are we measuring what we need to measure? *Clin J Pain, 24*, 316–24.

Wong, K., Lee, R., Yeung, S. (2009) The association between back pain and trunk posture of workers in a special school for the severe handicaps. *BMC Musculoskeletal Dis, 10*, 43.

Zerwekh, J. E., Ruml, L. A., Gottschalk, F. & Pak, C. Y. (1998) The effects of twelve weeks of bed rest on bone histology, biochemical markers of bone turnover, and calcium homeostasis in eleven normal subjects. *J Bone Miner Res, 13*, 1594–601.

Zhu, X. Z., Parnianpour, M., Nordin, M. & Kahanovitz, N. (1989) Histochemistry and morphology of erector spinae muscle in lumbar disc herniation. *Spine, 14*, 391–7.

# Part 4

# Risk Factors of Chronic Back Pain and Disability: Sociodemographic and Psychosocial Mechanisms

Part II

# Risk Factors of Chronic Back Pain and Disability: Sociodemographic and Psychosocial Mechanisms

# Chapter 11

# Screening of Psychosocial Risk Factors (Yellow Flags) for Chronic Back Pain and Disability

Chris J. Main, Nicholas A.S. Kendall, and Monika I. Hasenbring

## 11.1 Introduction

There is a wide range of pain conditions in which there is evidence of significant dysfunction but little or no evidence of disease or nerve damage. The impact of non-specific pain conditions on suffering is considerable, as is the cost in terms of healthcare provision and work compromise. When a clearly identifiable 'pain generator' is not apparent, as is often the case, then promise of a complete cure seems improbable. What then can be done? Two major strategies have emerged:

◆ Prevention of chronic pain becoming unnecessarily disabling.

◆ Prevention of the development of chronic pain/disability in patients with acute/subacute pain.

Health and safety legislation has improved the safety of the workplace but population surveys and consultation rates still indicate a high prevalence of back pain in the community. Differences in methodology have made it difficult to compare directly the results from different studies, e.g. differing criteria for the identification of 'new episodes' lead to different estimates. Waddell (2004) in a further analysis of the data from the South Manchester population study (Thomas et al. 1999), found that 38% had had back pain in the previous year and of those who had been pain-free, 19% reported new episodes in the following year. Furthermore, of the 32% of those who had had intermittent or less disabling pain in the previous year, almost half would have further episodes during the following year and of the 6% with longstanding or seriously disabling back pain, one-third would improve to some extent. There is thus a significant minority of people experiencing pain who go on to develop persistent pain, and may develop long-lasting disability, in terms of reduced participation in usual activity and work, and the concomitant psychological impact on their mood, self-confidence, and personal identity (Pincus and Morley 2001). The goal of completely preventing the onset of all musculoskeletal pain is simply not achievable and attempts to clinically alleviate pain, or reduce its severity are often less effective than hoped. However, reducing the impact of pain by preventing it becoming unnecessary disabling and enhancing the back sufferer's quality of life, do appear to be worthwhile endeavours.

There is some evidence for the effectiveness of intervention strategies for people with chronic musculoskeletal pain problems, and the potential for secondary prevention, has now been recognized for more than a decade (Linton and Anderson 2000). In fact clear guidelines have been developed for the management of acute non-specific low back pain (LBP; Box 11.1).

> ## Box 11.1 Recommendations for treatment of acute non-specific low-back pain
>
> ◆ Give adequate information and reassure the patient.
>
> ◆ Do not describe bed rest as a treatment.
>
> ◆ Advise patients to stay active and continue normal daily activities including work if possible.
>
> ◆ Prescribe medication, if necessary for pain relief; preferably to be taken at regular intervals; first choice paracetamol, second choice NSAIDs.
>
> ◆ Consider adding a short course of muscle relaxants on its own or added to NSAIDs, if paracetamol or NSAIDs have failed to reduce pain.
>
> ◆ Consider (referral for) spinal manipulation for patients who are failing to return to normal activities.
>
> ◆ Multidisciplinary treatment programmes in occupational settings may be an option for workers with subacute low back pain and sick leave for more than 4–8 weeks.
>
> Adapted from Van Tulder et al. (2005).

Although psychosocial factors seem to be stronger predictors of outcome than biomedical/ biomechanical factors (Burton et al. 1999; Crombez et al. 1999), and several randomized controlled trials (RCTs) in early intervention (Hay et al. 2005; Jellema et al. 2005) have demonstrated the feasibility of early intervention tackling these risk factors, there is not clear evidence of superiority of clinical outcomes for biopsychosocial approaches over usual care, either because they don't work or because of methodological limitations in the design of the research. Van der Windt et al. (2008) have identified a number of methodological limitations such as insufficient statistical power or adoption of a 'one size fits all approach' to the intervention, the relative lack of therapeutic power in the treatments offered, or the inability to match the right treatment to the right patient at the right time (see for more detail Chapter 27). A possible solution in terms of an approach combining screening and targeting approach is described and discussed later in this chapter.

Estimation of risk is at the core of screening but the literature contains a number of overlapping and similar terms such as 'risk factors', 'predictive factors', and 'prognostic factors' that at times are used interchangeably. As a precursor to considering the nature and efficacy of risk factor identification and screening for improved outcome, we offer our understanding of these terms.

## 11.2 Terminology

### 11.2.1 Risk factors, predictive factors, and prognostic factors

*Risk factors* are usually taken to refer to features associated with the future development or occurrence of an event such as a disease of some sort. They may or may not be implicated causally in the development of the disease, but the disease is not present at the time of risk estimation. Further investigations may be able to demonstrate a direct causal relationship, but the relationship may be indirect (possibly mediated by other factors) or, in so far as can be investigated, may turn out to be a chance association.

*Predictive factors* refer to those that are associated statistically with some sort of future outcome. Whether or not they are predictive therefore is a matter of statistical association, using whatever criteria are appropriate. There is no assumption required about the relationship, or lack of, between the two sets of events. In practice, they can be divided into risk factors and prognostic factors.

*Prognostic factors* refer to factors predictive of outcome of a disease or condition already in progress. In terms of potential interventions however, the distinction between moderators and mediators is particularly important.

*Moderators (or treatment effect modifiers)* are baseline characteristics which influence the outcome of treatment. Thus people with leg pain as well as back pain might improve less with a particular type of therapy

*Mediators* are factors which change during or as a consequence of treatment and thereby influence outcome. Thus, for example, it might be hypothesized that increase in exercise tolerance in physiotherapy might be mediated by reduction in fear of movement

However, two caveats are in order. Firstly, it should be noted that in understanding the development of pain, chronic pain, and pain-associated disability, predictors may act as both risk factors and prognostic factors. For example, psychological distress may be a risk factor for the development of pain, a prognostic factor in terms of the development of chronic pain, a risk factor for the development of disability, and a prognostic factor for further change in disability. Similarly, pain severity may be both a risk factor for sickness absence and a prognostic factor for recovery. Secondly, the distinction between modifiable and unmodifiable predictive factors (whether risk factors or prognostic factors) although perhaps less important from a conceptual point of view is fundamental to the design (and implementation) of interventions.

### 11.2.2 **Flags as a method of risk identification**

The term 'yellow flags' has become a familiar term used to describe psychosocial risk factors for chronicity. The original flag system (Kendall et al. 1997), and its later developments (Main et al. 2005; Kendall et al. 2009) is one such approach to risk identification. It has been described as a methodological compromise between the inflexibilities of a purely actuarial model and a purely subjective approach based on clinical judgement (Linton et al. 2005). In this context it has three important features. Firstly, it offers a 'systems perspective' and assumes that an adequate understanding of the problem requires consideration of both the injured worker and the individual's social and occupational context. Secondly, it contains both clinical and occupational elements. Thirdly, it makes an important distinction between the individual's perception of the situation and the objective features.

The flags approach can be viewed as a conceptual framework potentially capable of including both actuarial data and individually-assessed risk factors informing different types of specifically targeted interventions based on modifiable risk. An attempted mapping of the flags onto the individual predictors of chronic pain and disability is illustrated in Table 11.1. Different flags, and combinations of flags, require different types on interventions, and a multiflag approach appears to lend itself flexibly to both individual clinical decision-making and widescale system applications (Main et al. 2005; Kendall et al. 2009). However, its predictive accuracy in administrative applications will likely be lower than one arising from a purely statistical or 'actuarial' approach and will likely result in over-identification of individuals at risk. Further reflections on the linking of screening with targeting are offered below.

As far as individual risk factors for long-term work disability are concerned, Sullivan et al. (2005) in their review found evidence for fear, beliefs in severity of health conditions, and catastrophizing (yellow flags). Nicholas et al. (2011) having reviewed the evidence both for the influence of yellow flags on outcomes in people with acute/subacute LBP, and of yellow flag targeting on outcomes, concluded:

> Overall, from the evidence gathered here the studies that target interventions on known psychological risk factors for disability do seem to be reporting more consistently positive results relative to those interventions that either ignore these risk factors or provide omnibus interventions to people regardless of psychological risk factors. It seems that the identification of those with these risk factors is an important precursor to psychological interventions.

Predictors of occupational outcomes have also been investigated. Shaw et al. (2009) in addition to pain severity and level of depressive symptoms also identified workplace factors such as job stress, co-worker support, job dissatisfaction, employer attitudes, job autonomy, and availability of modified work as influences on duration of work disability and return-to-work (RTW) outcomes. Their findings are consistent with an earlier more widespread review of predictors of chronic pain and disability (Waddell et al, 2003). It is sometimes difficult, however, to distinguish clinical outcomes such as increase in activity or postural tolerance from occupational variables such as RTW rates or indices of work capability.

In fact, the COST B13 prevention guidelines (Burton et al. 2004a) offered a distinction between the general population and workers. Despite some variation in the level of evidence available, the similarity among the recommendations is striking.

The guidelines for workers obviously contain a number of recommendations specific to work settings, but otherwise, in terms of the usefulness of information or educational approaches, the lack of support for traditional biomechanical and biomedical approaches, and for traditional clinical interventions is similar. In fact, over the last decade, with the exception of a series of reviews in the Cochrane Library (http://www2.cochrane.org/reviews/) synthesizing the findings of earlier conservative management, and studies of outcome of surgery (which are beyond the remit of this chapter), there appears to have been relatively little new research with clinical outcomes as a primary focus.

Waddell et al. (2003) appraised the evidence for different sorts of predictors of chronic pain and disability. In their first set of evidence tables they summarize the findings from published studies of clinical and psychosocial predictors (Table 11.1) where the strength of evidence and strength of predictors are shown along with a tentative flag assignment in the right-hand column.

Aggregation of such a large set of data, with such a wide variety of specific variables is by nature imprecise, as are the 27 variables under which the predictors have been gathered. Accepting these strictures, it can be seen that there is evidence for an influence of both sociodemographic and personal history variables, but the strongest influences appear to be from yellow or blue flags (most of which are potentially modifiable) and black flags (which are more immutable, although may present opportunities for a 'systems solution'; equivalent to Sullivan et al.'s (2005) Type-I (individually centred) and Type-II (workplace or system-based) solutions.

## 11.3 The nature and focus of risk identification

The identification of predictors of outcome may enable us to select subgroups, whether in terms of possible benefit from treatment ('screening in') or failure to benefit from treatment ('screening out') (Foster et al. 2011). Furthermore, identification of predictors may lead to the identification of new and different approaches to treatment for patients with differing presenting characteristics, as in the screening/targeting approach developed by Hay and colleagues (Hay et al. 2008), or at different stages of pain chronicity.

**Table 11.1** Individual clinical and psychosocial predictors of chronic pain and disability

| | Strength of evidence | Strength of predictor | Type of variable | Flag assignment |
|---|---|---|---|---|
| Age | ∗∗∗ | ∗∗∗ | Demog. | |
| Gender | ∗ | Variable | Demog. | |
| Ethnicity | ∗∗ | Not signif. | | |
| Marital status | ∗ | Variable | Demog. | |
| Education | ∗ | ∗ | Demog. | |
| Clin. history | ∗∗∗ (LBP) | ∗∗∗ | Clinical | ?Red ?Yellow |
| Clin. exam | ∗ | ∗ | Clinical | ?Red |
| Comorbidity | ∗∗∗ | ∗ | Clinical | ?Red |
| Alc./sub. abuse | ∗ | ∗ | Clinical | Orange |
| Personality | ∗ | ∗ | | Orange |
| Psychol. hist. | ∗ | ∗ | | ?Orange |
| Anxiety | ∗ | ∗ | | ?Orange |
| Stressful life events | ∗ | ∗ | | ?Orange |
| Pain intensity, functional disability | ∗∗∗ | ∗∗ | Clinical | ? |
| Poor perceptions of general health | ∗∗∗ | ∗∗ | Clinical | Yellow |
| Psychological distress | ∗∗∗ | ∗∗∗ | Clinical | Yellow/orange |
| Depression | ∗∗∗ | ∗∗ | Clinical | Orange/yellow |
| Fear avoidance | ∗∗ | ∗∗ | Clinical | Yellow |
| Maladaptive coping (catastrophizing) | ∗∗∗ | ∗∗ | Clinical | Yellow |
| Pain behaviour | ∗∗∗ | ∗∗ | Clinical | Yellow |
| Duration sickness absence | ∗∗∗ | ∗∗∗ | Clin./Occ. | Yellow/blue ?Black |
| Employment status | ∗∗∗ | ∗∗∗ | Occ. | Blue/black |
| Job dissatisfaction | ∗∗∗ | ∗∗∗ | Occ. | Blue |
| Expectations re: RTW | ∗∗∗ | ∗∗∗ | | Blue |
| Physical demands of work | ∗∗∗ | ∗ | Occ. | Black |
| Financial incentives | ∗∗∗ | ∗∗∗ | Occ. | Black |
| Unemployment rates | ∗∗ | ∗∗∗ | Occ. | Black |

∗∗∗ Strong; ∗∗ Moderate; ∗ Weak.

## 11.3.1 Understanding the natural history of chronic low back pain (CLBP)

For many purposes it is convenient to assume that either acute pain resolves, or it does not, and in the latter event there is a smooth and clearly identifiable trajectory into chronic pain. This assumption, however, would appear to be unsafe. Burton et al. (2004b), in a prospective cohort study of 252 LBP patients attending for manipulative care, were able to follow up 60% of the sample 4 years later. Of those attending initially with *acute* LBP, 60.9% had further episodes, with 50% identifying between one and five episodes over the ensuing 4 years, and 10.9% identifying more than six episodes of persistent pain. The comparable figures for the *subacute* group were

70.6%, 32.3%, and 38.2%. For the *chronic* group, the comparable figures are 88.9%, 33.3%, and 55.6%. Admittedly the actual numbers in this study are relatively small, but they suggest firstly that most back pain is recurrent and secondly that the future course is influenced by the clinical history at the time of initial consultation.

Conventionally, the development of chronicity is viewed along a continuous timeline, with pragmatic cut-off points devised primarily as a way of deciding about resource allocation. As can be inferred from some of the previous discussion, however, there is significant variation in the clinical course of back pain. Von Korff and Miglioretti (2006, see also Chapter 2 in this volume) have suggested a new approach to the definition of pain, by classifying it in terms of the probability of significant pain being present 1 or more years in the future; making a further distinction between possible chronic back pain (with a likelihood of occurrence of 50%) and probable chronic back pain (with a likelihood of occurrence of 80%). They based their estimation on three variables. Using a baseline score, with cut-offs as a basis for risk estimation, they found that 58.7% of possible and 82.1% of probable chronic back pain patients had a Chronic Pain Grade of 2–4 1 year later, and the classification also strongly predicted the presence of clinically significant back pain at years 2 and 5. Furthermore, of those with probable chronic back pain at year 1, 90.9% and 76.5% had clinically significant back pain at years 2 and 5 respectively. This prognostic approach would seem to merit further investigation since potentially it offers an opportunity for screening and targeting.

### 11.3.2 Defining the outcome

In the development of CLBP, the most common outcome variables of interest are pain intensity, pain-related disability, and pain-related work compromise. Unfortunately in many studies only a single outcome measure is employed and it is difficult therefore to differentiate between persistence of pain and pain-associated disability. Furthermore, since arguably one of the most appealing, and to some extent effective, ways of controlling pain is to diminish activities, the variables are not independent; and there are some patients who suffer from intense pain yet do not manifest significant levels of disability (see Chapter 15). It might be argued further that while an exclusive focus on pain, although consistent with a specific biomedical focus on pain nociception, may be important particularly in the management of neoplastic and neuropathic pain, it is more problematic in the management of 'non-specific' musculoskeletal pain, since the 'pain generator' cannot be clearly identified and targeted. Most evidence for the efficacy of treatment for acute pain problems lies in pharmacological trials, but there have recently been a number of trials published on the Cochrane website (http://www.cochrane.org) of a range of other sorts of treatment. The need for a broader view was recognized by the European Commission which, under the COST B13 funding initiative, established three working groups charged with developing LBP guidelines for acute pain, chronic pain and prevention, respectively. The acute non-specific LBP guidelines (van Tulder et al. 2005) described in Box 11.1, are targeted primarily on the management of pain, although there is recognition that with the passage of time a broader approach might be considered. A parallel working group (Burton et al. 2004a) considered prevention. It has extensive specific evidence-based recommendations which can be found on the website but it also offers a summary of the concepts of prevention accompanied by some overarching comments (see Box 11.2).

### Risk identification in population studies

The linking of harm with exposures is at the heart of population and clinical epidemiology. By their nature such investigations are descriptive rather than explanatory, and while statistically significant associations may serve as a foundation for major clinical initiatives (such as immunization) or

## Box 11.2 Concepts of prevention and overarching comments (extracts)

- There is limited scope for preventing its incidence (first-time onset).
- Prevention in the context of this guideline is focused primarily on reduction of the impact and consequences of LBP.
- There is considerable scope, in principle, for prevention of the consequences of LBP.
- Different interventions and outcomes will be appropriate for different populations.
- The most promising approaches seem to involve physical activity/exercise and appropriate biopsychosocial education, at least for adults.
- But, no single intervention is likely to be effective to prevent the overall problem of LBP, owing to its multidimensional nature.
- Optimal progress on prevention in LBP will likely require a cultural shift in the way LBP is viewed, its relation with activity and work, how it may best be tackled and just what is reasonable to expect from preventative strategies.
- It is important to get all the players onside, but innovative studies are required to understand better the mechanisms and delivery of prevention in LBP.

Reprinted from *Manual Therapy*, **9**(1), A. Kim Burton, Timothy D. McClune, Robert D. Clarke, and Chris J. Main, Long-term follow-up of patients with low back pain attending for manipulative care: outcomes and predictors, pp. 30–5, Copyright (2004), with permission from Elsevier.

social policy decisions involving the redirection of resources, such risk factors are usually not sufficiently powerful to inform decision-making on an individual basis.

Epidemiological studies can inform us of the prevalence of pain and other symptoms among the general (non-clinical) population, using a variety of prevalence estimates. It is possible to determine the incidence of new pain episodes, and longitudinal studies begin to inform us about the various (risk) factors that are associated with persistent pain. We can construct a map of the context of pain and its future development, enabling identification of predictors of chronicity as well as recovery at a population level. In this manner, demographic and ethnicity variables may lead to public health initiatives focused on particular subgroups or delivered in a variety of ways. At a population level even relatively weak levels of prediction may be of considerable importance in terms of informing public health policy, in terms of prioritizing initiatives or in optimizing use of resources.

However, population predictors are usually unhelpful in the management of individual patients since: (1) population predictors are insufficiently robust in terms of sensitivity and specificity for use in the individual patient; and (2) individual management needs to tackle modifiable risk factors, and many population factors are difficult to modify or unmodifiable.

### Risk identification in clinical epidemiology

Clinical studies are often more narrowly focused, typically on healthcare outcomes, than epidemiological investigations, and therefore potentially provide a better basis for clinical intervention in suggesting particular therapeutic targets or in assisting the design of preventative intervention. However, there are important issues of sensitivity and specificity that need to be evaluated prior to use in clinical decision-making for individuals. These are discussed below.

Epidemiological data from population studies have provided useful sign-posting for clinical epidemiology, and studies of pain patients in which much stronger predictors of the natural history and treatment outcome have been identified. There have been many studies of treatment outcome for specific neuropathic, neuroplastic and non-cancer pain conditions. Given the importance of abolishing pain, wherever possible, there has been a major emphasis on the biomedical parameters associated with outcome of acute pain conditions. Unfortunately, initial biomedical parameters seem to be relatively weak predictors in contrast with the relative strength of psychosocial predictors. The potential for screening for these psychosocial factors appears to merit attention.

### Conceptualizing risk identification for individuals

We believe we have made a strong case in principle for secondary prevention, but is there any way in which we can capitalize on what we have learned from population and clinical epidemiology? Can we link our knowledge of populations, and understanding of sub-populations (such as consulters), in an effort to improve our management of the individual?

There are two further important considerations. Firstly, in considering management of an individual patient in a clinical setting it is clear not only that there is a wide range of potentially relevant risk factors to consider, but furthermore, these may differ according to the outcome of interest. Secondly, not all risk factors are modifiable and so it would seem appropriate, as in the flags initiative, to narrow the focus to risk factors which are potential obstacles to recovery (Shaw et al. 2009; Nicholas et al. 2011) as a way of identifying opportunities for change which could be targeted.

## 11.4 **From risk identification to screening**

### 11.4.1 **Principles of screening**

The concept of risk factors has entered common parlance, although there is frequent confusion between the concepts of absolute and relative risk, with incorrect usage in media reports sometimes leading to unnecessary levels of concern and anxiety. Screening was developed initially in the context of the development of screening programmes for particular diseases and Muir Gray (2004) emphasizes particularly the need for careful evaluation of both the benefits and harm of screening as well as quality assurance, in an economically constrained healthcare system.

A number of approaches to screening, however, have been developed on a variety of clinical populations and it is important to appraise their utility as a part of overall clinical management. Prior to examining their utility specifically for the identification of risk and prognostic factors for pain and pain-associated limitations (disability), the nature of screening will be addressed.

The WHO criteria are shown in Box 11.3.

### 11.4.2 **Purposes of screening**

The importance of clarifying the purpose of screening, emphasized by Waddell et al. (2003, p. 5) in consideration of screening for long-term incapacity, identified a number of different purposes for screening.

*Some examples*

◆ Identifying people at higher risk of:
  • Long-term pain.
  • Long-term self-reported disability.
  • Long-term sickness absence and early retirement.

---

**Box 11.3 WHO screening criteria (adapted from Wilson and Junger 1968)**

1 Important health problem

2 Accepted treatment for recognized disease.

3 Facilities for diagnosis and treatment.

4 Suitable latent and symptomatic stage.

5 Suitable test or examination.

6 Test acceptable to population.

7 Natural history of condition understood.

8 Agreed on policy on whom to treat.

9 Cost of finding economically balanced with overall health.

10 Case finding should be continuous process.

---

◆ Identifying people who need:

 • Extra educational advice.

 • Extra therapeutic or rehabilitation help.

◆ Informing:

 • A rehabilitation programme or other work-focused intervention.

 • The decision-making processes and case management.

In the case of psychosocial risk factors indicating a high probability of the development of chronic pain and disability, the offer of an individually targeted intervention focusing on a modification of these psychosocial factors as early as possible but also as cost-effective as possible is one of the primary challenges of a yellow-flag screening programme. Turk (1990) has long been an advocate of customizing patients for treatment on the basis of their initial presenting characteristics. Screening has to be understood in context, not only in terms of the specific purposes of screening and the stage in illness, but also in terms of the base rates of the characteristic of interest in the particular group being screened. Most screening, however, can be described in terms of 'screening in', 'screening out', and 'screening with targeting', and the sensitivities/specificities need to be examined in relationship to the specific purpose of screening. However there is an important caveat which should be borne in mind: screening out from one treatment does not necessary imply screening in for another sort of treatment.

Since all screening measures are in effect proxies (i.e. short-cuts) for a full appraisal, the value of a screening procedure is dependent not only on its *accuracy* (in terms of the predictive value), but its *cost*, and of course increased accuracy usually comes at increased cost, but the worth of screening is also related to its *importance*. In clinical practice, screening for a potentially fatal disease such as cancer, lack of specificity (and therefore increased cost) may be considered a price worth paying for a higher degree of accuracy in identifying those at risk. The consequences of risk identification may be costly in terms of resources so decisions are made in terms of the probable additional benefit likely to accrue from various degrees of effort in improving overall accuracy. In back pain research, appraisal of cost of treatment has become an important consideration in healthcare funding and metrics such as the QALY (quality-adjusted life year) are now frequently employed as a measure of cost-effectiveness (Ratcliffe et al. 2006) In extreme cases, such as screening for potential terrorists, it may be decided politically that since the cost of failure is so catastrophic, that almost limitless resources are assigned to identify extremely rare events, but usually cost is a factor. For example, in screening for clinical depression it would seem reasonable to consider whether the increased cost of a clinical interview over a simple screening question-naire, as might be used in a population survey, is justified by the increased accuracy in case iden-tification. In considering the identification of individuals at risk of a particular clinical or occupational outcome, it is indeed relevant therefore to make use of all available information and to consider how much can be learned from population and clinical epidemiology.

### 11.4.3 Methods of screening

The value of screening depends not only on the content of the items, but the manner in which the information is collected and the way the information is integrated. Different methods may be required to elicit different sorts of information. Routinely available administrative data may be useful at a population, insurance system or organizational level, but usually it has been designed for different purposes such as audit or population risk estimates. More individualized and clini-cally relevant information may be collected using questionnaire, telephone or face-to-face inter-view. The additional potential value has to be offset against much greater cost and practical difficulties in eliciting and interpreting the information obtained.

Accepting the reality of financially constrained healthcare, insurance, and social security systems, a comprehensive evaluation on an individual basis, however desirable, is never likely to be funda-ble, or even acceptable. It is likely that there will always be a need for some sort of filtering or screen-ing as a precursor to intervention, but before considering screening per se, it is appropriate to reflect upon the process of clinical decision-making, We offer the view that at the heart of the proc-ess of clinical decision-making are probabilistic judgements and in this respect, arrival at a decision involves risk estimation in the context of risk of good and poor outcome (and by implication, whether to offer pain management, and what to offer). A number of core functions for a system of screening have been identified. They comprise: (1) identification of items of information that pre-dict the outcome of interest; (2) development of a practical and usable method of collecting the information; (3) development of a method of combining the information or scoring the instru-ment; and (4) measurement of the accuracy of prediction (adapted from Waddell et al. 2003, p. 7).

### Actuarial versus clinical methods

**Actuarial methods** A central issue in screening is the accuracy of predicting future ill health or disability based on various initial data sets. In clinical practice, treatment recommendations are usually based on implicit outcome predictions made by a practitioner. An alternative is to adopt a statistical approach based on population statistics, such that each individual is compared with a wider group in terms of a number of characteristics and a risk profile thus obtained from data often gathered for administrative rather than clinical purposes. This empirical approach has been called *actuarial* and lends itself to wide administrative applications (Dawes et al. 1989). The exact nature of the predictors is relatively unimportant, but their strength in terms of accuracy of pre-diction is critical. There is no inherent ordering of variables in terms of the significance and many different types of predictors may end up as part of the optimal algorithm, as the selection is based on each variable's contribution to the prediction of outcomes, such as duration of disability, RTW, or costs.

**Strengths and limitations of the actuarial model** Although there are a number of strengths of the actuarial model, such as accuracy of data, and maximization of use of the available data, with the promise of accurate quantification of the relationship between risk factors and future status and the potential for the construction of algorithms and prediction rules applicable to large purposes, there are also a number of limitations. Linton et al. (2005) have identified some inherent limitations of the actuarial model:

> First, it assumes that the variables are stable and static. Second, there is no room for individual differences as the same statistical formula is always used, leading to misclassifications. Third, the actuarial approach is problematic when critically important salient data are not collected. Fourth, the utility of a strictly actuarial model is limited when the ceiling for predictive accuracy is relatively low and when the underlying evidence is weak. In addition, the generalizability of such statistical prediction models to other populations and contexts is often unknown. Lastly, since prediction is the driving factor, the modifiability of the risk factors may be of secondary importance. Therefore, actuarial models may not be easily translated into secondary prevention (Linton et al. 2005, p. 462).

In summary, actuarial models as a basis from which to develop secondary prevention applications are inherently limited.

**Clinical methods: the role of clinical decision-making** Giving the striking variability in clinical presentation, an alternative and somewhat more intuitive strategy is to use incorporate clinical information about the condition or the particular individual into the clinical decision-making process. At the heart of clinical decision-making is a judgement matching the needs of the patient with the possible benefits from our intervention and known prognostic factors for a particular condition seem obvious contenders as a starting point from which to identify factors likely be of relevance to management of the individual.

Clinical decision-making can be a complex task. We know in clinical practice that there are at times different opinions expressed, both in terms of clinical formulation (and diagnosis) and about what treatment is appropriate for a particular patient. However a number of researchers have advocated the use of *clinical prediction* rules as an aid to clinical decision-making. These tools are designed to assist medical decision-making in the management of low back pain, by combining information from a number of variables, usually from the history, diagnostic tests and/or physical examination. Typically they quantify the probability of an outcome, e.g. the persistence/recurrence of LBP after a time period of 1 year as an indicator of the development of chronic pain and suggest a diagnostic or therapeutic course of action. The use of clinical or disability prediction rules has intuitive appeal and perhaps some utility as a 'middle-way' but is extremely context dependent, is based on an averaging of scores across individuals and in assuming a fixed relationship amongst the items effectively is restricted to a 'snap-shot' derived at a particular point in time.

Wasson et al. (1985) have specified a number of standards against which such rules should be appraised. They state inter alia that the outcome being predicted by a rule:

(1) *Should be clearly defined and clinically important.*
   When predicting chronicity of pain the most important outcomes considered should include pain intensity, pain-related disability, and work absenteeism

(2) *Assessed in a blinded manner.*
   Thus the presence versus absence or the degree of an outcome should ideally be assessed without knowledge of the status of the predictor variables, especially, when the outcome is determined by self-reported data or subject to interpretation;

(3) *The process of identification and definition of the predictor variables should be reported.*
   Multivariate predictive models (such as multiple regression) depend on the variables included in a model. In order to develop reproducible prediction rules, all variables need to be taken into account otherwise clinicians in daily practice will not be able to confidently apply the rule with their patients.

(4) *Predictor variables as well as the outcomes must be assessed in a standardized format.*

(5) *Patient characteristics that might have an impact on the predictive value of a prediction rule should be assessed and reported.*
e.g. gender, age, duration of pain.

(6) *Aspects of the site where the study was done should be described.*
e.g. the type of the institution (primary, secondary, or tertiary care), the setting (office, clinic, outpatient setting of general practitioners, orthopaedics or physiotherapists.

(7) *Mathematical procedures must be described in detail.*
e.g. logistic regression, discriminant function analysis used to create the prediction rule, and

(8) *Methods of testing the accuracy and prospective validity must be reported.*

Further extensions of these standards for prognostic studies reported by Linton et al. (2005) are shown in Table 11.2.

The identification of predictors, however, is only a first step. For risk assessment in the context of clinical application, it is necessary to be able to apply the model on an individual level with a view on utilizing the screening technique to improve the results of interventions.

**Table 11.2** Methodological issues isolated in the prognosis research field

| Issue | Recommendation |
| --- | --- |
| Design | Prospective, inception cohorts required |
| Sampling | Strictly outline inclusion/exclusion criteria |
| | State enrolment time point clearly |
| | For many questions, clear, early enrolment is necessary (< 3 weeks following onset) |
| | Representative sampling techniques (random selection or consecutive cases) |
| Prognostic indicators | Strictly define constructs of measure |
| | Selection should flow from conceptual framework, recognizing the multifactorial nature of the problem |
| | Use standardized, psychometrically sound instruments |
| Analysis | Multivariable techniques to adjust for all potential confounders |
| | Avoid over-fitting the data (too many covariates for sample size) |
| | Prospective validation in homogenous cohorts required |
| Follow-up | Strictly define outcome(s) of interest |
| | Adequate duration of follow-up (years) |
| | Strive for >80% follow-up rate |
| | Patterns of attrition should be investigated to determine if is random or systematic |
| | Blinded outcome measurement with standardized, psychometrically sound instruments |
| Conceptual framework | Strictly define the construct of the problem being studied |
| | Account for the recurrent and multifactorial nature of back pain disability |
| | Overarching theory needed identifying specific hypothesized relationships between variables |
| | Broaden the view to include factors over the usual professional/discipline boundaries |

With kind permission from Springer Science+Business Media: *Journal of Occupational Rehabilitation*, Prognosis and the identification of workers risking disability: Research issues and directions for future research, **15**(4), 2005, Steven J. Linton.

## Accuracy of screening

In addition to general requirements of reliability and content validity for all measurements, in consideration of screening, there are a number of key parameters by which accuracy should be appraised. These are: sensitivity, specificity, and positive and negative predictive value. In practice, patient screening methods often necessitate a compromise between reliability and predictive validity on the one hand, and practical utility (in terms of length and ease of administration) on the other. Reliability may be demonstrated in terms of interobserver agreement, internal consistency, and/or test-retest-reliability. Although reliability does not guarantee high predictive power, an unreliable test will probably not be sufficiently valid to be useful.

The accuracy of a clinical prediction rule or a simple screening test in identifying people with subacute back pain who go on to develop a negative outcome is referred to as the sensitivity of the test. The *sensitivity* of the test thus is defined as the percentage of cases with a positive screening score (derived from prospective longitudinal studies) at baseline, who in fact go on to develop the adverse outcome (whether persistent/recurrent pain, disability and/or work absenteeism) at follow-up. In contrast, *specificity* is a measure of the proportion of patients who are classified as probable cases of good outcome, who do not in fact go on to develop a poor outcome. Ideally a test will have both a very high sensitivity (accuracy in identifying those who go on to have a poor outcome) and high specificity (a low rate of 'false positives'). There often has to be a 'trade-off' in terms of false negatives (missed cases) and false positives (incorrectly identified cases) and the worth of the test will be determined by the value which is placed on the accuracy of identification, e.g. a high proportion of false negatives may be considered an acceptable price to pay for a high level of identification of those at risk of a potentially fatal disease.

The number of false positives of a test is known as its *positive predictive value* of a test (PPV) and false negatives termed as the *negative predictive value* of a test (NPV).

These estimates are also affected by the prevalence of the risk at early stages of the disease. For example, in case of a very low prevalence of psychosocial risk factors (5%), the PPV of a test, showing sensitivity of 70% and a specificity of 96%, will yield a PPV of about 48% (and a NPV of nearly 98%). However with a prevalence of 35% and same sensitivity and specificity, the PNV will be about 90% and the NPV 86% (Lund et al. 1995). In the case of a yellow flag screening, it is therefore important to consider both prevalence and length of follow-up (to outcome) in considering the utility of screening methods. As a number of epidemiological studies, including clinical studies, have shown, psychosocial risk factors will be of low prevalence during the first 2–4 weeks of duration of non-specific low back pain, while the prevalence will increase up to 30–40%, 6–12 weeks later (during the subacute phase). Although a precise demarcation between acute and a subacute phases is probably not merited, recent flag guidelines (Kendall et al. 2009), have recommended screening optimally should be conducted at the subacute stage of the disease.

## The importance of timing (lead time of screening)

A further difficulty for screening in addition to method and accuracy is the issue of *timing* since different predictors emerge at different stages of illness or disability. When the screening is undertaken has a major influence on the accuracy of the screening and there may be different challenges facing screening at different times. Waddell et al. (2003) illustrate this in consideration of the prediction of incapacity whereby, at the time of initial presentation, the task for a screening tool may be to identify the 1–2% of individuals who will go on to develop long-term incapacity from amongst the 98–99% with relatively simple problems, most of whom are likely to return to work quite rapidly, more or less irrespective of any intervention. However, with benefit claimants identified only at 26% the task may be to identify the 40% likely to continue on long-term benefit from those who might (or could) be returned to work.

The interval from screening detection of risk factors (yellow flags) to the time of clinical diagnosis, or, in the case of LBP, to the time of development of chronic pain, disability, prolonged work absenteeism and early retirement is defined as 'lead time', a term borrowed from early studies in cancer screening (Hutchison and Shapiro 1968), while the time from disease onset to clinical diagnosis is labelled a 'sojourn time' (Draisma et al. 2009). The advantage gained by screening of yellow flags as risk factors for the development of chronic pain and disability depends on the extent to which diagnosis can be advanced by this procedure. The key challenge for screening is to identify cases before they have become chronic and therefore open the possibility of interrupting the path to chronicity.

Consider a hypothetical case of the development of chronic low back pain, as shown in Figure 11.1 which begins with an episode of acute non-specific LBP that leads someone to visiting a primary care physician.

An acute episode of pain is commonly defined by a new onset of pain following a pain-free interval of at least 6 months (Von Korff et al. 1992). However, as Von Korff and Miglioretti (2006, see also Chapter 2 by Dunn et al. in this volume) have shown, a number of patients are characterized by a high variability of pain episodes of different intensity, a different degree of disabling character and with different duration of pain-free phases. In the single case it is therefore difficult to reliably detect the point of an acute episode of pain that fits into the definition proposed by Von Korff et al. (1992).

It is important to note that there is a relation between the duration of lead time and the probability of overdiagnosis (false positives). As Draisma and colleagues have shown convincingly for the screening of prostate cancer, the longer the duration of lead time, the higher was the probability of false positive predictions (Draisma et al. 2009). It therefore depends on the utility of risk-factor based interventions (e.g. the efficacy of treatment psychosocial risk factors) on the one hand and the costs of these interventions on the other, which of defined lead times or screening time points might show an optimal cost-effectiveness.

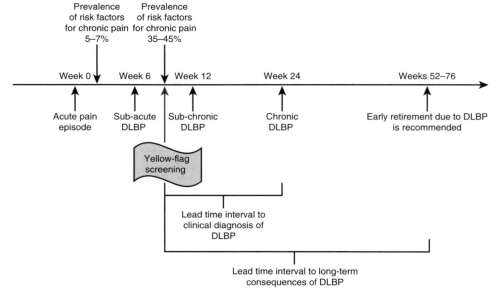

**Fig. 11.1** (See also Colour Plate 8) Phases in the development of chronic disabling low back pain (DLBP): hypothetical case.

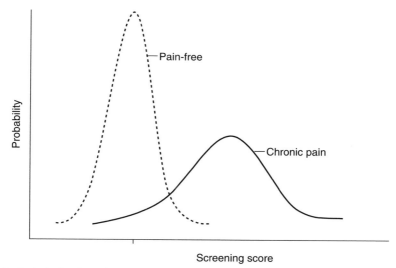

**Fig. 11.2** Typical distribution of screening scores in chronic pain and healthy samples.

## The determination of optimal cut-off points

A screening test provides clinicians with a defined cut-off point enabling them to predict positive (e.g. ongoing moderate or severe pain at the follow-up) or negative (e.g. pain-free) cases. Depending of the accuracy of a screening test, both populations will overlap to a specific degree. Patients who develop persistent/recurrent pain at the follow-up will mostly show a greater variability in the screening scores than the patients developed free of pain (Schwarzer et al. 2002, see also Figure 11.2).

All patients, who develop persistent pain at the follow-up, but with a screening score below this cut-off score will be incorrectly classified as free of risk of future pain (false negative). All patients who become pain-free, but with a screening score above the cut-off will be incorrectly classified as positive (false positive). With a low cut-off point, the probability of a false negative prediction is much less than a false positive (as shown in Figure 11.3).

Results from a hypothetical prospective study are shown in Table 11.3 where 94 out of 500 patients with subacute LBP (18.8%) are found to have developed persistent pain at follow-up. In this example, the low cut-off point for the yellow-flag screening yields three false negative prediction (3.2%) and 91 correct predictions (i.e. an overall sensitivity 96.8%). However, 139 out of 406 patients who did not show a persistent pain at follow-up (34.3%) and were therefore incorrectly classified as high risk patients (false positive), leading to a specificity of 65.7%.

In contrast, with a high cut-off point, the probability of false negative predictions will increase and the false positive will decrease (see Figure 11.4).

Thus in the example in Table 11.4, seven out of 94 patients developing chronic pain (7.4%) had a negative test result (sensitivity 92.5%), while only six out of 406 patients, who did not develop persistent pain, were false positive tests (1.5%), and with this high cut-off point, the specificity was 98.5%.

Ultimately, the choice of the cut-off point is a clinical one (Schwarzer et al. 2002). It is determined, as reasoned above, by the utility and the costs of the consequences of a positive screening result. Using the procedure of receiver operating characteristic (ROC) curves finding an optimal

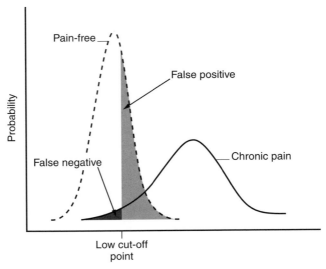

**Fig. 11.3** False positive and false negative predictions in the case of a low cut-off point. Reproduced from Schwarzer, G., Türp, J.C., Antes, G., EbM-Splitter: Die Vierfeldertafel (in Diagnosestudien): Sensitivität und Spezifität, *Deutsche Zahnärztliche Zeitschrift* 2002;**57**:446–447, Figures 2 and 3, © with permission from Deutscher Ärzte-Verlag.

cut-off point is a method becoming increasingly popular in judging the discriminative power of new screening measures (Hanley and McNeil, 1982; Hill et al. 2008).

## Combining different screening tools to improve prediction

As it is shown in the later section 'Methods for screening yellow flags', currently available screening tools differ in their ability to predict different outcomes such as future pain or pain-related disability and days off work due to back pain. Furthermore, single risk factors are of limited predictive value (McIntosh and Pepe 2002; Wald et al. 2005). A potential solution might be to combine multiple markers in some way to increase the predictive power of both outcomes, pain intensity and also disability, but this possibility for yellow flags has not as yet been explored and accuracy of prediction will have to be considered in terms of feasibility in clinical practice, since if the system of screening is too long or complex it will simply not be used.

**Table 11.3** Prediction in the case of a low cut-off point

|  |  | Persistent pain at the follow-up | | |
|---|---|---|---|---|
|  |  | Yes | No | |
| Screening | Positive | 91 | 139 | 230 |
|  | Negative | 3 | 267 | 270 |
|  |  | 94 | 406 | 500 |

Reprinted from *Manual Therapy*, **9** (1), A. Kim Burton, Timothy D. McClune, Robert D. Clarke, and Chris J. Main, Long-term follow-up of patients with low back pain attending for manipulative care: outcomes and predictors, pp. 30-5, Copyright (2004), with permission from Elsevier.

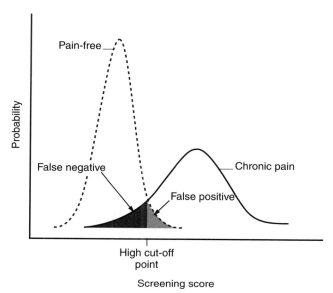

**Fig. 11.4** False positive and false negative predictions in the case of a high cut-off point. Reproduced from Schwarzer, G., Türp, J.C., Antes, G., EbM-Splitter: Die Vierfeldertafel (in Diagnosestudien): Sensitivität und Spezifität, *Deutsche Zahnärztliche Zeitschrift* 2002;**57**:446–447, Figures 2 and 3, © with permission from Deutscher Ärzte-Verlag.

## Feasibility of screening

Ideally, screening procedures must be acceptable in terms of content not only to the population which are being screened but, in the case of LBP, to healthcare providers as well as to the purchasers of healthcare, whether insurance companies or government departments. However if they are actually to be used in practice, yellow-flag screening should be *convenient* to physicians and patients and thus be easy and economical to administer. Finally of course, perhaps hardest of all, if it cannot contribute to the development of treatments effective in *preventing* chronic phases of disease, then the initiative will be valueless

How then do we decide whether a proposed method of screening is actually worthwhile? High economic or emotional costs of screening can only be justified if a high level of prediction (i.e. high predictive value, PV) is achieved, but a somewhat lower level of prediction might be considered acceptable with a relatively inexpensive screening which is easily tolerated by patients. In conclusion therefore, optimal yellow flag screening should be easy to administer and acceptable to patients, offer a high level of detection of those likely to become chronic and in addition facilitate effective physician-patient communication in the context of secondary prevention.

**Table 11.4** Results for screening using a high cut-off point

|  |  | Persistent pain at the follow-up | | |
|---|---|---|---|---|
|  |  | Yes | No | |
| Screening | Positive | 87 | 6 | 230 |
|  | Negative | 7 | 400 | 270 |
|  |  | 94 | 406 | 500 |

## 11.5 **Methods for screening yellow flags**

During the past two decades, a number of screening measures for the assessment of psychosocial risk factors, indicating a high probability of chronic pain and disability development, have been published. For example, Dionne (2005) predicted the level of disability 2 years later with 82% accuracy from the patients' initial level of distress.

Studies however differ with respect to the healthcare setting in which they have been validated (occupational versus clinical setting, primary-care versus specialized care settings), in the degree of specificity of screening and in the extent to which they have been empirically or theoretically underpinned.

While approaches to occupational screening are described in more detail in Chapter 19 of this volume, there are several examples of clinical screening which merit attention in this chapter. Turk (1990, 2005) has been a long advocate of customizing patients for treatment on the basis of their initial presenting characteristics. Most screening, can be described in terms of 'screening in', 'screening out' or 'screening with targeting'. However, the sensitivities/specificities need to be examined in relationship to the specific purpose of screening, and it should be emphasized that screening out from one treatment does not necessary imply screening in for another sort of treatment.

We have, for purposes of illustration, described four different assessment tools, which differ in their construction, validation and range of utility. The first tool, the Distress Risk Assessment Method or DRAM (Main et al. 1992) is a symptom-based measure designed for use in orthopaedic clinics (or similar musculoskeletal services). It was developed in response to a specific challenge, that of incorporating a measure of distress in patients under consideration for orthopaedic treatment. At the time of its development it was not considered feasible to incorporate a complex psychological tool within the context of time-constrained orthopaedic clinics, and so it was developed specifically as a first-stage screener. The STarT Back Decision Tool or SBDT (Hill et al. 2008), is also a first-stage screener, but developed for primary care. Although in a shorter dichotomous format, it captures a wider range of information (using psychosocial and biomedical predictors of chronicity). The Örebro Musculoskeletal Pain Screening Questionnaire or ÖMPSQ (Linton and Halden 1998; Boersma and Linton 2002) has a much stronger psychosocial focus and since its incorporation into the original yellow flag assessment system (Kendall et al.1997) has come to be widely used in physiotherapy clinics as a secondary prevention screener in patients already referred from primary care. Although relatively little information has been provided on its structural properties in terms of construct validity, it has proved to be clinically robust, is widely used and now available in a shorter form. Finally we appraise the The RIsk SCreening of Back Pain or RISC-BP (Hallner and Hasenbring 2004), an instrument with a complex aetiology, explicitly derived from research into the psychological processes underpinning pain coping strategies, and which includes a focus on cognitive, behavioural, and emotional factors and was developed specifically for the prediction of persistent or recurrent pain.

### 11.5.1 **Distress Risk Assessment Method (DRAM)**

DRAM (Main et al. 1992) was developed specifically as a screening tool for the identification of distress in LBP patients. It comprises a somatic awareness scale (The MSPQ and the Modified Zung Depression Inventory). DRAM offers a simple classification of patients into those showing no psychological distress, those at risk of developing major psychological overlay, and those clearly distressed. Four patient types were identified on the basis of scores on the two short questionnaires.

## Classification

N: Modified Zung score 17.

R: Modified Zung score 17–33 and MSPQ score LE 12.

DD: Modified Zung score GE 34.

DS: Modified Zung score 17–33 and MSPQ score GE 13.

In the original validation study, the authors found increased risk of poor outcome across the distress categories for *no improvement of pain* (N vs. Type R: odds ratio (OR) 2.0; N vs. DD/DS: OR 3.5), *higher levels of disability* (N vs. R: OR 1.9; N vs. DD/DS: OR 5.2), and for *not working* (N vs. R: OR 1.5; N vs. DD/DS: OR 2.5). In a study of outcome of osteopathic treatment, Burton et al. (2004b) found that a higher level of somatic symptoms (MSPQ) inter alia was associated with poorer outcome. Trief et al. (2000), in a prospective study of psychological predictors of lumbar surgery found the DRAM classification to be a strong predictor of outcome.

However, a caveat is in order, in patients with significantly troublesome pain problems, a patient-centred approach to evaluation is always appropriate and it is certainly not appropriate to view distress as a contraindication to treatment with good surgical indications (Hobby et al. 2001).

## Recommendations for use

- ◆ Recommended in secondary and tertiary care clinics as a screening tool to aid clinical appraisal of the patient.
- ◆ Particularly recommended in problem back clinics and pain clinics.
- ◆ Should be viewed as a first-stage screener, not as a complete psychological assessment or as a test of malingering.
- ◆ Distress and its management should always be considered as part of decisions about surgery.
- ◆ Distress patients not requiring surgery require pain management.

Adapted from Main et al. (1992, p. 52).

Although based on a restricted domain (somatic and depressive symptoms only), this short screening test has been validated specifically for patients consulting with LBP and does seem to have predictive validity for a range of outcomes

## 11.5.2 **The STarT Back Decision Tool (SBDT)**

Hill et al. (2008), have developed a screening tool, SBDT, as the basis of a system of triaging and targeting LBP patients presenting with modifiable physical and psychosocial prognostic indicators for persistent pain at the time of consultation to their GP in primary care. An initial set of items was selected on the basis of secondary analysis of pre-existing data on 1200 LBP consulters to primary care, an extensive literature review and input from an expert panel of clinicians. All items for the tool were developed from validated primary-care measurement tools. For prognostic indicators measured using composite instruments, individual questions were chosen using ROCs with high sensitivity and at least moderate specificity for identifying patients above the median on full scores of their composite measures. The clinical validity of the items was confirmed following appraisal by a consensus group of some 40 GPs and clinical physiotherapists, and blinded ratings of 12 videotaped 20-minute interviews of patients who had independently completed the SBDT (Hill et al. 2010).The tool was then tested for feasibility, repeatability and validity on a consecutive series of 244 patients consulting with LBP in eight GP practices.

Following examination of the distribution of SBDT scores, optimal cut-offs, based on the prognostic indicators included were derived, to allocate patients into one of three groups. An SBDT score of 0–3 was determined to be low risk; a score of four or more of the five psychosocial items (items 1, 4, 7, 8 and 9), allocates patients to the high-risk group. The remainder (SBDT score of more than 3, but less than four of the five psychosocial items) allocates patients to the medium-risk group. This procedure led to an allocation of 40% into the low-risk group, with 35% into the medium-risk group, with predominantly physical indicators, and 25% into the high-risk group with a higher proportion of psychological indicators.

The external validity of the tool was examined in an independent observational sample of 500 LBP primary-care consulters. SBDT scores were similar and recommended cut-offs for allocation to the three subgroups validated. The SBDT also demonstrated high predictive abilities with medium- and high-risk groups having relative risks of 3.0 and 4.5 respectively, compared to the low-risk group for high disability (RMDQ 7) at 6-month follow-up. It forms the basis for the STarT Back screening and targeted approach (Hay et al. 2008) in which clinicians have been trained in delivery of interventions on patients identified according to their risk profile. Preliminary analyses suggest that the screening and targeting approach has proved superior, particularly in the more complex patients to a non-screening or targeting approach at 4 months after treatment, and to be more cost-effective in the management of low risk patients.

### 11.5.3 Örebro Musculoskeletal Pain Screening Questionnaire (ÖMPSQ)

Linton and Hallden (1998)[1] developed a screening tool, primarily for psychosocial risk factors for chronic pain and chronicity. Although not offering clustering as such, the widespread clinical use of cut-off scores to identify the presence of significant psychosocial risk factors enable patient screening. It was included in the New Zealand Screening Instrument (Kendall et al. 1997) and was published later in a slightly modified form as the Örebro Screening Questionnaire for Pain (Boersma and Linton 2002). The final version comprises 25 items, of which six deal with background factors, and 19 deal with a variety of background factors. There are extremely minor differences in the precise descriptors between the New Zealand and Swedish versions and the way in which employment status is coded (featuring as an additional numbered item) but in all important respects the versions seem to be equivalent. The authors state that in order to give all items equal weight, they were scaled from 0 to 10 (with some items reversed) and the scores summated to form a total score. Since the background items (1–4) were not found to contribute statistically, they were not included in the calculation of the total score. A scoring system was provided such that a total score could be obtained.

In the earlier publication (Linton and Hallden 1998), it was stated that a cut-off of 105 enabled 75% correct identification of those not requiring alteration to ongoing management, 86% correct identification of those who would have between 1 and 30 days off work in the next year and 83% correct identification of those who would have more than 30 days off work.

Hurley et al. (2000), in an investigation of the instrument's utility in predicting RTW after physical therapy, found that a cut-off of 112 correctly identified 80% of patients failing to RTW at the end of treatment (sensitivity) and 59% of those who did RTW (specificity). In further analysis of the same cohort of patients (Hurley et al. 2001) they found that scores on the instrument (labelled the ALBPSQ) were correlated with the patients' level of pain and reported

---

[1] The original Linton and Hallden Questionnaire appeared originally in the first yellow flags monograph (Kendall et al. 1997); and thereffer has appeared in various publications in very slightly modified forms as the ÖMPQ, the ÖMPSQ and the ALBPSQ; and there is now a short-form (Linton et al. 2010).

disability at 1-year follow-up and 'correctly identified all patients reporting some degree of work loss but had minimal predictive strength for the other patient-centred variables evaluated'.

In the more recent publication (Boersma and Linton 2002), the authors report satisfactory test–retest reliability (0.83), using a cut-off of 105 (the maximum is 210), and a specificity of 0.75 with a sensitivity of 0.88 in the prediction of future absenteeism, and examine the utility of various cut-off scores in the prediction of sick listing (ranging from 90–120) and for functional ability (ranging from 80–110) in terms of sensitivity and specificity. As they point out, decisions about the trade-off between sensitivity and specificity may be different in relation to differing goals among healthcare professionals.

The questionnaire has considerable appeal as a general psychosocial screener, and is now fairly widely used in clinical practice. It has both strengths and limitations. The questionnaire targets important predictors of long-term pain-associated functional limitations and also occupational outcomes such as duration of sick leave and RTW, but on the evidence currently available would seem to function best in relation to occupational outcomes. As a screener therefore it is to be recommended.

It is clear that very different clinical and occupational profiles can yield similar scores on the questionnaire. This may not be critical in terms of first-level screening, but, as mentioned earlier in this chapter, screening should only be undertaken with specific purposes in mind. As the properties of the questionnaire become clearer with its use in a range of settings, it will be possible hopefully to examine its utility as a stand-alone screener, and also, possibly linking with more detailed and specific evaluations, to identify individuals likely to benefit from targeted interventions of various types.

It is to be hoped that as part of its further development, there will be further appraisal of its structural properties with the development of more sensitive scoring systems. As things stand it represents an extremely worthwhile addition to the psychometric validation.

### 11.5.4 **The Risk Screening of Back Pain (RISC-BP)**

Hasenbring and colleagues developed a screening tool, RISC-BP, to identify LBP patients with and without radiating pain during a subacute phase, who would develop persistent or recurrent pain in a primary care or a specialized care setting (Hallner and Hasenbring, 2004).

The RISC-BP is part of a large-scale assessment of potential psychosocial risk factors that have been investigated in different prospective longitudinal studies in patients with subacute low back and leg pain (Hasenbring et al. 1994; Grebner et al. 1999; Hallner and Hasenbring, 2004). These studies originally started with a large pool of standardized scales, such as the BDI, a measure of health-related locus of control, a measure of daily stress in 15 life areas, and the Kiel Pain Inventory or KPI, Hasenbring 1994), the latter consisting of 18 subscales of pain-related emotional, cognitive, and behavioural responses. The construction of the KPI was theory driven, based on the behavioural theory of operant conditioning (Fordyce 1976), blended with the cognitive stress and coping theory of Lazarus (1993), and the integrated cognitive-behavioural model of pain (Turk et al. 1983). The full assessment battery (excluding pain variables) comprised 162 items. The predictive power of these scales has been investigated using several statistical prediction rules and a variety of statistical methods (multiple regression analyses, discriminant analyses, neuronal network). In the initial study with 111 patients with subacute back and leg pain prior to an inpatient conservative medical treatment, Hasenbring et al. (1994) demonstrated that, after control for depression, the contrasting behavioural pain responses of high avoidance behaviour and endurance despite severe pain revealed significant and important predictive power. The psychosocial predictor variables yielded a sensitivity of 79% and specificity of 81% predicting pain at the 6-months follow-up. Whereas different pain responses were highly predictive of future pain intensity in this study, application for early retirement due to work absenteeism (the second out-come of interest) was predicted only by depression and distress at work with sensitivity of 75%, a specificity of 86% (Hasenbring et al. 1994).

The classification of three high-risk groups focuses explicitly on cognitive, behavioural, and emotional factors. Specific subgroup analyses based on pain-related avoidance versus endurance and depression, using both a clinical cut-off procedure (Hasenbring 1993) and an empirical approach of cluster analysis (Grebner et al. 1999) created the basis for the formulation of a first version of the avoidance-endurance model (AEM) (Hasenbring 2000). The clinical cut-offs used in the Hasenbring (1993) study were based on a BDI score of 9, which was published as a highly reliable and valid cut-off in low back pain patients (Geisser et al. 1997). Using the Thought Suppression Scale (TSS) and the Behavioural Endurance Scale (BES) of the KPI as further marker variables, mean scores of '3' ('this happens to me sometimes') on a scale ranging from '0' (never) to '6' (always) were taken as a cut-off score. Patients are characterized in terms of distress endur-ance responses (DER) if the BDI sum score was equal or above 9 and if the TSS and/or the BES was above or equal the cut-off score of 3 and as eustress endurance responses (EER) if the BDI was below 9. When the BDI was above/equal 9 and both, TSS and BES were below 3, patients were considered to show fear-avoidance pain responses (FARs). Patients whose scores were below the cut-offs on all three variables were considered to show adaptive responses (ARs). This AEM-based classification of psychosocial risk for chronic back pain is indicating targeted cognitive-behavioural interventions, described in more detail in Chapter 27 of this volume.

The current measure of the RISC-BP includes a measure of depression (using the Beck Depression Inventory (Beck et al. 1961), and measures of both thought suppression and behav-ioural endurance, derived from the avoidance-endurance model of pain (as described in Chapter 15) and identified by the Avoidance-Endurance Questionnaire or AEQ (Hasenbring et al. 2009. All three scales demonstrate sufficient to high internal consistency and are widely validated in pain patients (Hasenbring 1993; Hasenbring et al. 1994, 2009; Geisser et al. 1997).

The accuracy of the RISC-BP has been shown as to be sufficient or high in two independent prospective trials. Using an artificial neural network analysis, Hallner and Hasenbring (2004) calculated the predictive power of the three subscales BDI, TSS, and BES, later named as RISC-BP, in a sample of 90 subacute back and leg pain patients before and 6 months after an inpatient medical treatment. In this cross-validated study, persistent/recurrent pain at the 6-months fol-low-up was correctly classified in 83% of the patients with a sensitivity of 73% and a specificity of 97%. In a recent prospective study in patients with non-specific subacute low back pain (pain duration <90 days), who underwent an outpatient medical treatment in primary care, the RISC-BP demonstrated a sensitivity of 80%, specificity of 62% and a positive predictive value (PPV) of 77.9%, a prevalence (pre-test probability) of 57% presupposed (Hasenbring et al. in prep).

There is preliminary evidence that avoidance-endurance model based subgroups showing a pattern of cognitions of thought suppression, anxious/depressive mood and task/pain persistence behaviour (distress endurance responses) or a pattern of cognitions of ignoring/minimizing pain, positive mood despite pain and task/pain persistence behaviour (eustress endurance responses) will develop more pain prospectively and show higher levels of specific strain postures, measured by accelerometer, than patients showing adaptive pain responses (Hasenbring et al. 2006). Interestingly, the eustress endurance subgroup has been shown to develop rather low scores of disability despite severe pain intensity (see Chapter 15).

Finally, the RISC-BP is available both in a paper–pencil version as well as in a computer-based version (Hasenbring and Hallner, 1999) and therefore is easy to administer and interpret. The test duration, investigated in a number of primary care practices (GPs as well as orthopaedic practitioners), on average was about 10 minutes, and found to be both feasible and acceptable by patients attending a 1-day education programme for primary care providers.

## 11.6 **Summary and conclusion**

Based on a huge number of methodically well-controlled prospective longitudinal studies in subacute LBP patients, conducted during the past two decades, psychosocial factors have been shown as important predictive or prognostic factors indicating the high risk for developing chronic pain and pain-related disability in the long term. While high inter-correlations among some of these variables clearly are of methodological concern (Foster et al. 2010) in terms of conceptual overlap, and of practical concern in terms of the pragmatics of screening, there is convincing evidence that variables such as depression, distress in daily life, and maladaptive modes of cognitive/affective and behavioural pain responses play a significant role as so-called yellow flags. (Blue and black flags, both relevant within occupational settings, are reviewed in Chapter 19 of this volume).

In the assessment of yellow flags and appraising their utility, we have identified a number of important influences on their validity and utility (such as accuracy, time and context of identification, and the determination of optimal cut-off scores) and more practical issues such as feasibility. We have specifically examined four different measures which have been used for psychosocial screening, have been validated on clinical samples and for which some predictive validity has been demonstrated. Thus while three of these screening tools (DRAM, SBDT, and Örebro) are highly predictive of pain-related disability (and the ÖMPSQ also for occupational outcomes), the RISC-BP shows high predictive validity particularly for future pain intensity, perhaps as a consequence of its specific focus on endurance-related pain-responses, as it has been shown in several well controlled studies, that pain-related disability is more related to distress and pain-related fear than to pain intensity itself (Crombez et al. 1999). However, while consistent evidence has confirmed the role of fear-avoidance responses to pain and pain-related disability measured via self-report, the influence of fear-avoidance responses on objectively assessed physical activity is less clear.

In considering screening from a public health perspective, it is important to identify all potential risk factors that may be of relevance. We have drawn a distinction between actuarial screening, based principally on administrative data, and individual screening in the context of consideration for pain management. We have emphasized the need for clarity in terms of purpose for screening, since predictors are, to an extent, outcome specific, and may highlight the potential value of different types of interventions.

Most screening, however, can be described in terms of 'screening in', 'screening out' with consideration of the sensitivities/specificities in relationship to the specific purpose of screening. As aforementioned, screening out from one treatment does not necessary imply screening in for another sort of treatment.

The attempted link of screening with targeting in the case of yellow flags is found both in with more general targeted cognitive-behavioural interventions (e.g. Linton and Anderson 2000; Gatchel et al. 2003; Hill et al. 2008) and also with more specifically targeted interventions, such as high fears of (re)injury (Vlaeyen et al. 2002), catastrophizing (Sullivan et al. 2006), or fear-avoidance versus pain-related endurance (Hasenbring et al. 1999). These early interventions are described in more detail in Chapter 27.

Risk identification and screening has a long tradition in public health, and with the advent of evidence-based medicine the focus and 'outcome' has required a new way of thinking about the possibilities for pain management. The biomedical and biomechanical models of pain and function to an extent have served us well, but newer understandings of the influences on and effects of pain have required a broader perspective, and the biopsychosocial model has served as a vehicle for this. We have, however, moved beyond descriptions, classifications, and model building to a focus not only on treatment but towards prevention. In our view we now need a conceptual framework that allows us to understand the pain patient in context.

In our view, screening has to be linked with appraisal and management of the individual in pain and the main value of these tools may be in highlighting patients requiring a more comprehensive assessment or in further clinic assignment. With significant pain problems, this will need to include a clinical assessment by a competent healthcare professional and may require further expertise to evaluate and address specific occupational problems.

Although valuable, however, all screening tools are inherently limited in the context of decision-making at an individual level. Hill et al. (2010) directly compared the use of the StarTBack Tool with clinical decision-making and concluded:

> Clinicians are, therefore, advised to use the instrument as an adjunct to their own decision-making rather than a replacement to their considered clinical acumen. The strengths of the SBST are likely to be its systematic and consistent allocation of patients to subgroups, which contrasts with the experts' overwhelming inconsistencies in decision-making, and their lack of confidence in decision-making among more complex back pain cases.

The StarTBack initiative (Hay et al. 2008; Hill et al. submitted) in linking specifically tailored interventions to subgroups identified on the basis of screening, in offering a 'middle-way' between identifying risk factors at the level of clinical epidemiology and the delivery of treatment, is a model which would seem to merit further investigation in other groups of patients.

The review offered in this chapter clearly demonstrates the potential for yellow flag screening (discussed further in Nicholas et al. 2011) and we believe serves as an encouragement to strive to further improve the focus, nature, and quality of our interventions within an evidence-based framework and with a clear focus on a range of outcomes (as recommended in The Hopkinton Think Tank meeting in 2005) with its methodological recommendations for improvement in disability research (Linton et al. 2005).

## References

Beck, A.T., Ward, C.H., Mendelson, M., Mock, J., Erbaugh, J. (1961). An inventory for measuring depression. *Archives of General Psychiatry*, **4**, 561–71.

Boersma, K., Linton, S.J. (2002). Early assessment of psychological factors: the Örebro Screening Questionnaire for Pain. In Linton, S.J. (Ed.) *New avenues for the prevention of chronic musculoskeletal pain and disability. Pain research and clinical management, vol 12*, pp. 205–13. Amsterdam: Elsevier.

Burton, A.K., Battie, M.C., Main, C.J. (1999). The Relative Importance of Biomechanical and Psychosocial Factors in Low Back Injuries. In Karwoski W., Marras W.S. (Eds.) *The Handbook of Industrial Ergonomics*, pp. 1127–38. New York: CRC Press.

Burton, A.K., Balague, F., Cardon, G., *et al.* (2004a). European guidelines for prevention in low back pain. www.backpaineurope.org

Burton, A.K., McClune, T.D., Clarke, R.D., *et al.* (2004b). Long- term follow-up of patients with low back pain attending for manipulative care: outcomes and predictors. *Manual Therapy* **9**, 30–5.

Crombez, G., Vlaeyen, J.W.S., Heautz, P.H.T.G., Lysens, R. (1999). Pain-related fear is more disabling than pain itself: evidence on the role of pain-related fear in chronic back pain disability. *Pain* **80**, 329–39.

Dawes, R.M., Faust, D., Meehl, P.E. (1989). Clinical versus actuarial judgment. *Science* **243**, 1668–74.

Dionne, C. (2005). Psychological distress confirmed as predictor of long-term back-related functional limitations in primary care settings. *Journal of Clinical Epidemiology* **58**, 714–18.

Draisma, G., Etzioni, R., Tsodikov, A. *et al.* (2009). Lead time and overdiagnosis in prostate-specific antigen screening: importance of methods and context. *Journal of the National Cancer Institute* **101**, 374–83.

Fordyce, W.E. (1976). *Behavioural Methods for Chronic Pain and Illness*. St. Louis, MO: C.V. Mosby.

Foster, N.E., Thomas, E., Bishop, A., Dunn, K.M., Main, C.J. (2010). Distinctiveness of psychological obstacles to recovery in low back pain patients in primary care. *Pain,* **148**, 398–406.

Foster, N.E., Hill, J.C., Hay, E.M. (2011). Subgrouping patients with low back pain in primary care: Are we getting any better at it? *Manual Therapy* 16(1), 3–8.

Gatchel, R.J., Polatin, P.B., Noe, C.E., *et al.* (2003). Treatment- and cost-effectiveness of early intervention for acute low back pain patients: A one-year prospective study. *Journal of Occupational Rehabilitation* **13**, 1–9

Geisser, M.E., Roth, R.S., Robinson, M.E. (1997). Assessing depression among persons with chronic pain using the Center for Epidemiological Studies-Depression Scale and the Beck Depression Inventory: A comparative analysis. *Clinical Journal of Pain* **13**, 163–70.

Grebner, M., Breme, K., Rothoerl, R., Woertgen, C., Hartmann, A., Thomé, C. (1999). Coping and convalescence course after lumbar disk operations. *Der Schmerz* **13**, 19–30.

Hallner, D., Hasenbring, M. (2004). Classification of psychosocial risk factors (yellow flags) for the development of chronic low back and leg pain using artificial neural network. *Neuroscience Letters* **361**, 151–4.

Hanley, J.A., McNeil, B.J. (1982). The meaning and use of the area under a receiver operating characteristic (ROC) curve. *Radiology* **143**, 29–36

Hasenbring, M. (1993). Endurance strategies - a neglected phenomenon in the research and therapy of chronic pain? *Der Schmerz* **7**, 304–13.

Hasenbring, M. (1994). *Das Kieler Schmerzinventar. [The Kiel Pain Inventory-Manual. Three questionnaire scales for the assessment of pain-related cognitions, emotions and coping strategies]*. Bern: Huber.

Hasenbring, M. (2000). Attentional control of pain and the process of chronification. In: J. Sandkühler, B. Bromm, G.F. Gebhart (Eds.) *Progress in Pain Research Vol* 129, pp. 525–34. New York: Elsevier Science.

Hasenbring, M., Hallner, D. (1999). Telemedical system of patient diagnostics. *Deutsches Ärzteblatt, PC-Spektrum*, 49–50.

Hasenbring, M., Marienfeld, G., Kuhlendahl, D., Soyka, D. (1994). Risk factors of chronicity in lumbar disc patients. A prospective investigation of biologic, psychologic, and social predictors of therapy outcome. *Spine,* **19**, 2759–65.

Hasenbring, M., Ulrich, H.W., Hartmann, M., Soyka, D. (1999). The efficacy of a risk factor based cognitive behavioral intervention and EMG-biofeedback in patients with acute sciatic pain: an attempt to prevent chronicity. *Spine,* **24**, 2525–35.

Hasenbring, M. I., Plaas, H., Fischbein, B. and Willburger, R. (2006). The relationship between activity and pain in patients 6 months after lumbar disc surgery: do pain-related coping modes act as moderator variables? *European Journal of Pain,* **10**, 701–9.

Hasenbring, M.I., Hallner, D., Rusu, A.C. (2009). Fear-avoidance- and endurance-related responses to pain: development and validation of the Avoidance-Endurance Questionnaire (AEQ). *European Journal of Pain,* **13**, 620–8.

Hay, E.M., Mullis, R., Lewis, M., *et al.* (2005). Comparison of physical treatments versus a brief pain management programme for back pain in primary care: a randomised clinical trial in physiotherapy practice. *Lancet* **365**, 2024–30.

Hay, E.M., Dunn, K.M., Hill, J.C., *et al.* (2008). A randomised clinical trial of subgrouping and targeted treatment for low back pain compared with best current care. The STarT Back Trial Study Protocol *BMC Musculskeletal Disorders* **9**, 58.

Hill, J.C., Dunn, K.M., Lewis, M., *et al.* (2008). A Primary Care Back Pain Screening Tool: Identifying Patient Subgroups for Initial Treatment. *Arthritis and Rheumatism* **9**, 632–41.

Hill J.C., Vohora K., Dunn K.M., Main C.J, Hay E.M. (2010). Comparing the STarT Back screening tool's subgroup allocation of individual patients with that of independent clinical experts. *Clinical Journal of Pain* **26**(9), 783–7.

Hill, J.H., Dunn, K., Mason, L., *et al.* (2011). Comparison of stratified primary care management for low back pain with current best practice (STarT Back): a randomised controlled trial. *The Lancet* 29 September 2011 [Epub ahead of print].

Hobby. J.L., Lutchman. L.N., Powell. J.M., *et al.* (2001). The Distress Risk Assessment Method (DRAM): Failure to predict the outcome of lumbar discectomy. *Journal of Bone and Joint Surgery* **83B**(1), 19–21.

Hurley, D.A., Dusoir, T., McDonough, S., *et al.* (2000). Biopsychosocial screening questionnaire for patients with low back pain: Preliminary report of utility in physiotherapy practice in N Ireland. *Clinical Journal of Pain* **16**, 214–28.

Hurley, D.A., Dusoir, T., McDonough, S., *et al.* (2001). How effective is the Acute Low Back Screening Questionnaire for predicting one-year follow-up in patients with low back pain? *Clinical Journal of Pain* **17**, 256–63.

Hutchison, G.B., Shapiro, S. (1968). Lead time gained by diagnostic screening for breast cancer *Journal of the National Cancer Institute* **41**, 665–81.

Jellema, P., van der Windt, D.A.W., vander Horst, H.E., Twisk, J.W.R., Stalman, W.A.B, Bouter, L.M. (2005). Should treatment of (sub)acute low back pain be aimed at psychosocial prognostic factors? Cluster randomised clinical trial in general practice. *British Medical Journal* **331**, 84–8.

Kendall, N.A.S., Linton, S.L., Main, C.J. (1997). *Guide to assessing psychological yellow flags in acute low back pain: risk factors for long term disability and work loss.* Wellington: Accident Rehabilitation and Compensation Insurance Corporation of New Zealand and the National Health Committee. Wellington.

Kendall, N.A.S., Burton, A.K., Main, C.J., Watson, P.J. (2009). *Musculoskeletal Problems, A Guide For The Clinic and Workplace: Identifying Obstacles using the Psychosocial Flags framework.* London: The Stationery Office.

Lazarus, R.S. (1993). Coping theory and research: Past, present, and future. *Psychosomatic Medicine*, **55**, 234–47.

Linton, S.J., Andersson, T. (2000). Can chronic disability be prevented? A randomized trial of a cognitive-behavioural intervention and two forms of information for patients with spinal pain. *Spine* **25**, 2825–31.

Linton, S.J., Hallden, K. (1998). Can we screen for problematic back pain? A screening questionnaire for predicting out-come in acute and subacute back pain. *Clinical Journal of Pain* **14**, 209–15.

Linton, S.J., Gross, D., Schultz, I.Z., *et al.* (2005). Prognosis and the identification of workers risking disability: Research issues and directions for future research. *Journal of Occupational Rehabilitation* **15**, 459–74.

Linton, S.L., Nicholas, M.K., MacDonald, S. (2010). Development of a Short Form of the Örebro Musculoskeletal Pain Screening Questionnaire. *Spine* Dec 29. [Epub ahead of print].

Lund, J.P., Widmer, C.G., Feine, J.S. (1995). Validity of diagnostic and monitoring tests used for temperomandibular disorders. *Journal of Dental Research* **74**, 1133–43.

Main, C.J., Wood, P.L.R., Hollis, S., *et al.* (1992). The distress assessment method: A simple patient classification to identify distress and evaluate risk of poor outcome. *Spine* **17**, 42–50.

Main, C.J., Phillips, C.J., Watson, P.J. (2005). Secondary prevention in health care and occupational settings in musculoskeletal conditions focusing on low back pain. In: Schultz I Z, Gatchel R J (eds) *Handbook of complex occupational disability claims: Early risk identification, intervention and prevention,* pp. 387–404. New York: Springer.

McIntosh, M.W., Pepe, M.S. (2002). Combining several screening tests: optimality of the risk score. *Biometrics*, **58**, 657–64.

Muir Gray, J.A. (2004). New concepts of screening. *British Journal of General Practice* **54**, 292–8.

Nicholas, M.K., Watson, P.J., Linton, S.J., Main, C.J. (2011). The identification and management of psychosocial risk factors (Yellow Flags) in patients with low back pain. *Physical Therapy* **91**(5), 737–53.

Pincus, T., Morley, S.J. (2001). Cognitive-processing bias in chronic pain: a review and integration. *Psychological Bulletin* **127**, 599–617.

Ratcliffe, J., Thomas, K.J., MacPherson, H., Brazier, J. (2006). A randomized controlled trial of acupuncture care for persistent low back pain: cost effectiveness analysis. *British Medical Journal* **333**, 626.

Schwarzer, G., Türp, J.C., Antes, G. (2002). EbM-Splitter: Die Vierfeldertafel (in Diagnosestudien): Sensitivität und Spezifität. *Dtsch Zahnärztl Z,* **57**, 446–7.

Shaw, W.S., van der Windt, D.A., Main C.J., Loisel, P., Linton, S.J. (2009). Now tell me about your work: the feasibility of early screening and intervention to address occupational factors ("Blue Flags") in back disability. *Journal of Occupational Rehabilitation* **19**, 64–80.

Sullivan, M.J.L., Ward, L.C., Tripp, D., *et al.* (2005). Secondary prevention of work disability: Community-based psycho- social intervention for musculoskeletal disorders. *Journal of Occupational Rehabilitation* **15**, 377–92.

Sullivan, M.J.L., Adams, H., Rhodenizer, T., *et al.* (2006). A psycho- social risk factor targeted intervention for the prevention of chronic pain and disability following whiplash injury. *Physical Therapy* **86**, 8–18.

Thomas, E., Silman, A.J., Croft, P.R., Papageorgiou, A.C., Jayson, M.I.V., Macfarlane, G. (1999). Predicting who develops chronic back pain in primary care: a prospective study. *Britsh Medical Journal* **318**, 1662–7.

Trief, P., Grant, W., Fredrickson. B. (2000). A prospective study of psychological predictors of lumbar surgery outcome. *Spine* **25**, 2616–21.

Turk, D.C. (1990). Customising treatment for chronic pain patients; who, what, and why. *Clinical Journal of Pain* **6**, 255–70.

Turk, D.C. (2005). The potential of treatment matching for subgroups of patients with chronic pain: Lumping versus splitting. *Clinical Journal of Pain* **21**, 44–55.

Turk, D.C., Meichenbaum, D., Genest, D. (1983). *Pain and behavioral medicine: a cognitive-behavioural perspective.* New York: Guilford.

Van der Windt, D., Hay, E., Jellema, P., Main C.J. (2008). Psychosocial interventions for low back pain in Primary Care. *Spine,* **33**, 81–9.

Van Tulder, M., Becker, A., Bekkering, T. *et al.* on behalf of the COST B23 Working Group on Guidelines for the management of Acute Low Back pain in Primary Care (2005). www. backpaineurope.org

Vlaeyen, J.W., De Jong, J.R., Onghena, P., *et al.* (2002). Can pain-related fear be reduced? The application of cognitive-behavioral exposure in vivo. *Pain Research and Management* **7**, 144–53.

Von Korff, M., Miglioretti, D.L. (2006). A prospective approach to defining chronic pain. In: Flor, H., Kalso, E., Dostrovsky, J.O. (eds) *Proceedings of the 11th World Congress on Pain,* pp. 761–9. Seattle, WA: IASP Press.

Von Korff, M., Ormel, J., Keefe, F., *et al.* (1992). Grading the severity of chronic pain. *Pain* **50**, 133–49.

Waddell, G. (2004). *The back pain revolution* (2nd edn.). Edinburgh: Churchill Livingstone.

Waddell, G., Burton, A.K., Main, C.J. (2003). *Screening of DWP clients for risk of long-term incapacity: a conceptual and scientific review* (Royal Society of Medicine Monograph). London: Royal Society of Medicine Press.

Wald, N.J., Morris, J.K., Rish, S. (2005). The efficacy of combining several risk factors as a screening test. *Journal of Medical Screening,* **12**, 197–201.

Wasson, J.H., Sox, H.C., Neff, R.K., Golman, L. (1985). Clinical prediction rules–applications and methodological standards *New England Journal of Medicine* **313**, 793–9.

Wilson, J.M.G., Jungner, J.J. (1968). *Principles and practice of screening for disease.* World Health Organization, Geneva.

# Chapter 12

# Dispositional Fear, Anxiety Sensitivity, and Hypervigilance

R. Nicholas Carleton and Gordon J.G. Asmundson

## 12.1 Introduction

Diathesis–stress models are becoming popular and intuitive ways for researchers to describe the course of psychopathology (McKeever and Huff 2003). Predispositional traits align with specific environmental stressors resulting in pathological states. In the absence of either the precedent trait or the appropriate environmental state, psychopathology does not develop. Theorists have gone on to develop diathesis–stress models in which the stressor—and subsequent psychopathology—become diatheses for subsequent stressors (Asmundson et al. 2002; Sharp and Harvey 2001; Turk 2002; Vlaeyen and Linton 2000). The self-perpetuating cycles depicted by these models are understandably pernicious and difficult to break; however, identifying and ameliorating the fundamental predispositional trait(s) may be an effective way to provide treatment for diathesis–stress psychopathology (Carleton and Asmundson 2009; Taylor 1993).

Chronic musculoskeletal pain—pain persisting beyond the expected duration required for the healing of damaged tissue (International Association for the Study of Pain 1986)—is currently explained using diathesis–stress models. Most often, the stressor is an injurious event followed by persistent pain despite tissue repair. It is also possible, though presumably less common, for pain to begin without a definitive injurious event and persist or even worsen in the absence of definitive biological aetiology. Perhaps most importantly, the identification of a definitive injurious event appears to be a relatively small component of chronic musculoskeletal pain pathology. Indeed, tissue damage has now long been recognized as having relatively little association with pain (Beecher 1946, 1959; Melzack and Perry 1975). A similarly venerable notion is that chronic musculoskeletal pain symptoms can have a basis in organic pathology but nonetheless be maintained by psychological factors (Breuer and Freud 1974). Given the relatively small association between pain and tissue damage, it is reasonable to expect that the psychological factors will play a substantially greater role in chronic pain pathology. Accordingly, the psychological factors likely function as the key diatheses that are further mitigated by social factors (Fordyce 1976; Fordyce et al. 1982). It is within this context that researchers have investigated fundamental predispositional traits associated with psychopathology as potential diatheses for chronic musculoskeletal pain.

Anxiety sensitivity (AS), illness/injury sensitivity (IIS), and fear of negative evaluation (FNE) were among the first constructs suggested to be fundamental predispositional constructs associated with more common fearful reactions and psychopathology (Reiss 1991; Reiss and McNally 1985). The fundamental fears have been argued to be inherently noxious stimuli that represent fundamental predispositions not otherwise logically reducible to other fears (Reiss 1991; Taylor 1993). In contrast, the same investigators have argued that other fears (e.g. fear of snakes, fear of panic attacks) are common because those fears can be reduced to one or more of AS, FNE, and IIS. More recent research (Carleton and Asmundson 2009; Carleton et al. 2007b) has suggested that at least two other constructs—pain-related anxiety and intolerance of uncertainty (IU)—also meet the original requirements for inclusion as fundamental fears (Reiss 1991). Each of these predispositional psychological constructs has been identified as a potentially critical diathesis for the development and maintenance of chronic musculoskeletal pain (Asmundson and Carleton 2008; Asmundson et al. 2004a; Carleton et al. 2007b). Across all of these constructs, pain-related anxiety and fear may be among the most investigated and culpable constructs with regard to the development and maintenance of chronic musculoskeletal pain; pain-related anxiety and fear are generally thought to be key diathetic variables (Carleton and Asmundson 2009; Vlaeyen and Linton 2000) and may be more disabling than pain itself (Crombez et al. 1999).

Current fear-anxiety-avoidance models of chronic musculoskeletal pain (Asmundson et al. 2004b; Vlaeyen and Linton 2000) have been developed based on work conducted by several researchers (Asmundson et al. 1999a; McCracken et al. 1992; Vlaeyen et al. 1995; Waddell et al. 1993). Research on the fear-anxiety-avoidance models has resulted in considerable empirical support (Asmundson et al. 1999a; Asmundson et al. 2004b; Leeuw et al. 2008; Vlaeyen and Linton 2000). The models were generally intended to describe people with idiopathic chronic musculoskeletal pain, but they have also been found applicable to other pain conditions such as headache (Norton and Asmundson 2004), fibromyalgia (Goubert et al. 2004), and severe burns (Sgroi et al. 2005). These contemporary fear-anxiety-avoidance models of chronic musculoskeletal typically share similar basic elements (see also Chapter 14). These elements are as follows:

(1) Once the nociceptive stimulus is perceived, a judgement of the meaning or purpose of the pain is placed on the experience.

(2) For most people, the nociceptive stimulus is judged to be undesirable and unpleasant, but not catastrophic or suggestive of a major calamity. Accordingly, most people engage in appropriate behavioural restriction followed by graduated increases in activity until healing has occurred.

(3) For a significant minority of people, a catastrophic meaning (i.e. 'This pain means I'm never going to be able to do the things I like doing') is placed on the experience of pain. The quality and intensity of the catastrophizing is influenced by predispositional and current psychological factors, and results in pain-related anxiety and/or fear of (re)injury.

(4) Pain-related anxiety spirals into a vicious and self-perpetuating cycle that promotes and maintains avoidance, activity limitations, disability, pain, as well as additional catastrophizing.

Researchers and theorists continue to develop these models, with proposed modifications and additions based on evidence that the aforementioned predispositional traits can be associated with the development and maintenance of chronic musculoskeletal pain. Below we describe each of the posited predispositional traits–including pain-related anxiety and fear, AS, IU, IIS, and FNE–as depicted in some fear-avoidance models of chronic pain (see, for example, Figure 12.1– the predispositions listed below 'Pain catastrophizing').

## 12.2 **Pain-related anxiety and fear**

Pain-related fear and anxiety are typically referred to collectively as fear of pain (Carleton and Asmundson 2009); however, there is growing evidence that the difference may be far from semantic. The precedent distinction between present-tense fear and future-oriented anxiety has been recognized as important for years (Barlow 2000, 2002), providing theoretical and clinical utility; nevertheless, in models of chronic musculoskeletal pain the distinction remains somewhat novel.

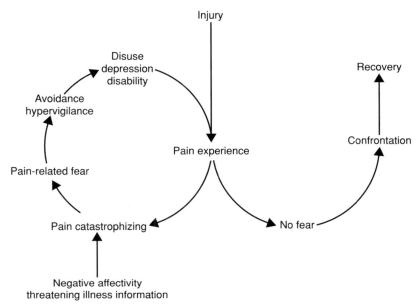

**Fig. 12.1** Fear-Avoidance Model of chronic pain. Adapted from Vlaeyen and Linton (2000). This figure has been reproduced with permission of the International Association for the Study of Pain® (IASP®). The figure may not be reproduced for any other purpose without permission.

The distinction between pain-related fear and anxiety has been suggested to parallel the distinction drawn in context of anxiety disorders; specifically, pain-related fear can be conceptualized as a present-oriented emotive state associated with nociceptive stimulation (e.g. pain from an injection), whereas pain-related anxiety can be conceptualized as a more general, future-oriented emotive state that does not require nociceptive stimulation, but occurs in anticipation of nociception (e.g. the possibility of pain from an injection). This formal distinction is relatively novel within the pain literature (Carleton and Asmundson 2009); however, earlier research identified distinctions between pain-related fear and anxiety responses within a chronic musculoskeletal pain sample (McCracken et al. 1996). In that initial study, self-reports of pain-related fear were found to be correlated primarily with pain complaints, whereas self-reports of pain-related anxiety were correlated primarily with pain severity and disability.

Subsequent research has supported the importance of the distinction, possibly extending it to a neuronal level. For example, hyperalgesia has been associated with anxiety-provoking unpredictable pain, while hypoalgesia has been associated with fear-provoking predictable pain (Ploghaus et al. 2003). There is also evidence that exposure-based therapies (e.g. graded activity, graded *in vivo* exposure) that reduce avoidance by confronting painful anxiety-provoking stimuli can reduce disabling chronic musculoskeletal pain in a fashion similar to exposure treatments for anxiety disorders (Bailey et al. 2010).

Despite the apparent association with the development of chronic musculoskeletal pain, pain-related anxiety plays an important protective role within injury-healing processes. Without some pain-related anxiety, people would be less motivated to engage in avoidance of behaviours expected to provoke pain, resulting in higher frequencies of tissue damage and reducing the evolutionary utility of pain. Accordingly, it makes intuitive sense that situationally-appropriate pain-related anxiety is beneficial; however, determining what is appropriate is likely to be a matter for debate. Research evidence suggests that there is substantial variation across the entire population and no readily apparent qualitative break that distinguishes between normal and pathological levels of the trait (Asmundson et al. 2007, 2009). Accordingly, nociceptive stimulation in people with increasing pain-related anxiety is likely to result in rumination, thereby further increasing pain-related anxiety, and potentially reinforcing unnecessary avoidance behaviours.

### 12.2.1 Assessment of pain-related fear and anxiety

Pain-related fear is commonly measured with the 30-item Fear of Pain Questionnaire-III (FPQ-III; McNeil and Rainwater 1998) and, more recently, the 20-item Fear of Pain Questionnaire-Short Form (FPQ-SF; Asmundson et al. 2008b). Items on both scales are responded to using a 5-point Likert scale ranging from 1 (not at all) to 5 (extreme). The short-form resulted from a factor-analytic investigation that removed unstable items and revised the originally proposed three-factor structure of the FPQ-III (i.e. minor pain, severe pain, medical pain) into a more robust four-factor structure. The four factorially distinct subscales of the FPQ-SF are each related to a specific type of pain: Minor Pain (e.g. biting your tongue while eating), Severe Pain (e.g. having someone slam a heavy car door on your hand), Injection Pain (e.g. having a blood sample drawn with a hypodermic needle), and Dental Pain (e.g. having one of your teeth drilled). There remain questions regarding the additive utility of the Injection Pain and Dental Pain factors, such that they have been argued to be optional (Asmundson et al. 2008b). Both measures have good internal consistency and there is evidence of good test-retest reliability for the FPQ-III (McNeil and Rainwater 1998; Osman et al. 2002).

Pain-related anxiety is most commonly measured with either the original 40-item Pain Anxiety Symptoms Scale (McCracken et al. 1993; McCracken et al. 1992) or the 20-item Pain Anxiety Symptoms Scale-20 (PASS-20; McCracken and Dhingra 2002). Items on both scales are responded to using a 6-point Likert scale anchored from 0 (never) to 5 (always). Both measures consist of four factorially distinct components of pain-related anxiety: (1) Cognitive Anxiety (e.g. I can't think straight when in pain), (2) Pain-related Fear, (e.g. Pain sensations are terrifying), (3) Escape and Avoidance (e.g. I try to avoid activities that cause pain), and (4) Physiological Anxiety (e.g. Pain makes me nauseous). The 40-item PASS has been used to assess pain-related anxiety in clinical (McCracken et al. 1992) and community (Larsen et al. 1997; Osman et al. 1994) samples. Factorial validity for both the total and subscale scores of the PASS-20 has been demonstrated for clinical (Coons et al. 2004) and non-clinical (Abrams et al. 2007) samples. Neither the instructions for the PASS or PASS-20, nor the items themselves, preclude the use of either measure with participants who do not have current pain.

### 12.2.2 Treatment of pain-related fear and anxiety

The apparent importance of pain-related fear and anxiety in the development and maintenance of chronic musculoskeletal pain has resulted in the derivation of at least two specific multidisciplinary treatment protocols. Graded *in vivo* exposure (GivE) is a cognitive-behavioural therapy that targets pain-related fear and anxiety (Vlaeyen et al. 2002). Proponents of GivE assert that pain-related fear and anxiety, as well as the associated disability, can be ameliorated by deliberating exposing people to activities previously avoided because of pain-related anxiety.

Acceptance and commitment therapy (ACT) and related approaches focus on concepts of mindfulness, acceptance, and values-based action (Hayes 2004; Hayes and Duckworth 2006; Hofmann and Asmundson 2008), with the ideal result being reduced pain-related anxiety, catastrophic beliefs, and fewer avoidance behaviours (Vowles et al. 2008). Proponents of ACT assert that patients with chronic pain need to shift the focus of their life from the pain and onto things of greater interest or importance. A recent comprehensive review of treatments for pain-related fear, anxiety, avoidance, and the associated disability suggested that GivE may function as a faster treatment protocol than ACT; however, ACT may have a lower dropout rate (Bailey et al. 2010).

## 12.3 **Anxiety sensitivity**

Paralleling more than a decade of research on pain-related fear and anxiety has been a growing interest in the relationship between AS and the development and maintenance of chronic musculoskeletal pain. The AS construct represents a heritable propensity (Stein et al. 1999) to appraise anxiety-related physiological sensations (e.g. increased heart rate, palpitations, trembling), cognitive changes (e.g. difficulty concentrating, racing thoughts), and social consequences (e.g. humiliation, rejection) based on the belief that these sensations have harmful consequences (Taylor 1999). The catastrophic appraisal of these sensations, changes, and consequences facilitates avoidance behaviours which, in turn, reinforce the fearful appraisals. AS is qualitatively different from trait anxiety (Reiss et al. 1986); specifically, AS focuses on fearing unknown or potential dangers associated with the sensations of anxiety rather than the anxiety-provoking stimulus itself (Taylor et al. 1992). In other words, AS focuses on identifiable stimuli—the object of fear is the anxiety-related sensations themselves. The catastrophic misappraisal of the stimuli associated with AS requires an anxiety-related sensation accompanied by uncertainty regarding the subsequent consequences of the sensation (Reiss et al. 1986). Accordingly, higher levels of AS can contribute to catastrophic misinterpretations of physical sensations related to pain or general arousal (Asmundson 1999; Asmundson and Norton 1995; Asmundson and Taylor 1996).

The 16-item Anxiety Sensitivity Index (ASI; Peterson and Reiss 1992) is the most commonly used measure of AS. Factor analytic investigations of the ASI indicate that it comprises three internally consistent lower-order factors—i.e. fear of somatic sensations; somatic (e.g. It scares me when my heart beats rapidly), fear of cognitive dyscontrol; cognitive (e.g. When I cannot keep my mind on a task, I worry that I may be going crazy), and fear of socially observable anxiety reactions; social (e.g. It is important to me not to appear nervous)—that load on to a single higher-order factor (Taylor et al. 1996; Zinbarg et al. 1997). The validity and reliability of using the ASI total or subscale scores have been well-documented (Peterson and Plehn 1999; Taylor 1999). Despite the relative popularity of the ASI, the measure is not without limitations. AS was not originally conceptualized as a multidimensional construct and, as such, the ASI was not created with multidimensional construct-driven factorial subscales in mind. Accordingly, the factor structure of the ASI is often found to be unstable. Subsequent research has led to the development of a new 18-item measure of AS—the ASI-3 (Taylor et al. 2007)—that appears to resolve the factorial difficulties related to measuring a multidimensional construct. Thus far, the ASI-3 has proven to be extremely robust, with a replicable factor structure, as well as good performance on indices of reliability and validity.

The relationships between pain, anxiety, and catastrophizing were established relatively early (Craig 1994; Rosenstiel and Keefe 1983; Sullivan and D'Eon 1990); however, the role of variant AS levels in pain was not explicitly investigated until Kuch and colleagues included the ASI in their investigation of phobias and pain (Kuch et al. 1994; Kuch et al. 1991). The importance of the relationship between AS and pain—in particular the physical concerns component of AS (Asmundson 1999)—was implied early by intuitive associations between pain-related anxiety and pain sensations (McCracken et al. 1993). Subsequent research further supported a relationship between AS and pain (Asmundson et al. 1999a), but primarily as an exacerbating construct influencing pain-related fear and avoidance (Asmundson 1999). Recent studies have demonstrated a relationship between AS and both laboratory-induced acute pain and chronic musculoskeletal pain (Keogh and Asmundson 2004).

People with heightened AS are prone to catastrophize about somatic sensations, which include pain sensations. Pain is naturally unpleasant, but not always interpreted catastrophically, unless the individual is predisposed to become anxious during the experience of somatic sensation. For such people, the pain is worse than unpleasant; instead, they are more likely to interpret pain as a harbinger of protracted physical, social, and financial hardship. The sensation and interpretation then function to initiate and maintain a spiralling cycle of sensations, catastrophic thoughts, and avoidance behaviours, which describe disabling chronic musculoskeletal pain.

AS is not consistently elevated in patients with chronic pain relative to non-clinical samples (Asmundson and Norton 1995; Asmundson and Taylor 1996). The results suggest that AS is critical for some, but not all, people with chronic pain (Asmundson et al. 2008a). In those with elevated AS, the fear of anxiety-related sensations, changes, and consequences may facilitate debilitating chronic pain. To illustrate, AS has been shown to increase the risk of pain-related avoidance and disability following physical injury (Asmundson and Norton 1995; Asmundson and Taylor 1996) and headache (Asmundson et al. 1999b). In a sample of patients with comparable injuries, patients reporting high levels of AS and chronic musculoskeletal pain were found to use more analgesic medication relative to patients with chronic musculoskeletal pain who reported low levels of AS (Asmundson and Norton 1995). Indeed, pain severity itself may be mediated by AS, given evidence that caffeine-related hypoalgesia (i.e. reduced pain) may occur specifically for women with low levels of AS (Keogh and Chaloner 2002). Women with high levels of AS also tend to demonstrate lower levels of pain tolerance relative to men (Thompson et al. 2008). In general, however, the evidence regarding whether the relationship between AS and pain is different for men relative to women is conflicting, with some data indicating differences (Keogh et al. 2006) and other data indicating no such differences (Conrod 2006; Tsao et al. 2006). In any case, contemporary fear-anxiety-avoidance models describe critical direct and indirect paths for AS in the development and maintenance of chronic musculoskeletal pain (Asmundson et al. 2004a).

## 12.4 Anxiety sensitivity and pain-related anxiety

Researchers have demonstrated that AS can directly and indirectly exacerbate pain-related fear, promoting avoidance behaviours even after controlling for differences in pain severity (Asmundson et al. 1999a; Asmundson and Taylor 1996; Zvolensky et al. 2001). The relationship between AS and pain-related anxiety is sufficiently interwoven that some researchers have suggested pain-related anxiety may be a manifestation of AS (Asmundson and Norton 1995; Asmundson and Taylor 1996). Pain-related anxiety is anxiety related to a somatic sensation and, therefore, arguably no different than anxiety related to other somatic sensations such as heart palpitations. In support of this argument, researchers have demonstrated that treatments for reducing AS (e.g. interoceptive exposure) may also reduce pain-related anxiety (Watt et al. 2006). Indeed, AS has been shown to account for most of the variance in pain-related anxiety (Greenberg and Burns 2003), even after controlling for other potential predictors of pain-related anxiety such as trait anxiety and pain intensity (Muris et al. 2001).

Pain-related anxiety can also be conceptualized as a fundamental fear (i.e. fears of inherently noxious stimuli that are not logically reducible to other fears; Reiss 1991; Taylor 1993) unto itself (Carleton and Asmundson 2009; Carleton et al. 2006b), rather than a manifestation of AS. In other words, nociceptive stimulation is inherently noxious and other more common fears can be logically reduced to a pain-related anxiety (e.g. fearing falling because it may cause pain). In this context pain-related anxiety and AS would be related but not necessarily dependent. The somatic sensations described in the AS construct can produce arousing and even fearful responses; however, those sensations are not inherently noxious. For example, a rapid heartbeat can be interpreted as exhilarating as easily as it can be interpreted as terrifying, depending on the context (e.g. lottery win vs. freefall off a building). In contrast, the somatic sensation associated with pain-related anxiety does not require contextual cues or a catastrophic misinterpretation for the sensation to be interpreted as noxious. Pain is almost always unpleasant, presumably by evolutionary design, and associated with specialized nociceptive pathways. Moreover, initial research evidence from clinical and non-clinical samples (Asmundson et al. 2007; Asmundson et al. 2009; McNeil and Rainwater 1998) suggests that pain-related anxiety is continuous in nature (i.e. occurring along a latent continuum ranging from low to high), whereas evidence to date suggests that AS is taxonic (i.e. having qualitatively distinct normative and pathological forms; Bernstein et al. 2006a; Bernstein et al. 2006b). Based on the available research to date, pain-related anxiety and AS appear to be related, but distinct (Carleton et al. 2011). Accordingly, it makes sense to continue to research the interdependent relationship of both constructs with pain.

## 12.5 **Intolerance of uncertainty**

Recent research has demonstrated a relationship between the AS and IU constructs, such that the two are interdependent because IU may be a necessary component of AS (Carleton et al. 2007b). Indeed, AS and IU appear to share a common basis in experiencing increased anxiety related to unknown, potentially harmful consequences. IU has been identified as a discriminating dispositional variable associated with worry (Laugesen et al. 2003) and state anxiety (Greco and Roger 2001). Moreover, IU is positively correlated with anxiety-related psychopathologies such as generalized anxiety disorder (GAD), obsessive–compulsive disorder (OCD), and panic disorder (Dugas et al. 1998; Dugas et al. 2001; Tolin et al. 2003). Given the established relationship between AS and pain, it makes sense that IU may play an important role in pain as well.

IU is the tendency for an individual to consider the possibility of a negative event occurring as unacceptable and threatening irrespective of the probability of its occurrence (Freeston et al. 1994; Holaway et al. 2006). Engaging in situations with uncertain outcomes (e.g. physical activity following an injury), is likely to induce and perpetuate a heightened level of anxiety in persons with heightened IU (Dugas et al. 2001). Moreover, people with high IU are likely to interpret ambiguous information (e.g. muscle tension) as threatening (Heydayati et al. 2003), contributing to increased arousal (e.g. increased heart rate and blood pressure; Greco and Roger 2001, 2003).

Despite the potential theoretical and clinical importance of understanding the role of IU in pain (Carleton et al. 2007a), there is a paucity of research exploring the relationship. IU has been suggested to be related to pain peripherally, as a function of GAD (Roemer and Orsillo 2007), OCD (Sookman and Pinard 2002), or health anxiety (Abramowitz et al. 2007). To date, there does not appear to be any research directly evaluating the relationship between IU and pain. The lack of research may be the result of historical difficulties measuring the construct in a psychometrically robust fashion. For example, the original Intolerance of Uncertainty Scale (IUS) was fairly long and the factor structures were not robust (Freeston et al. 1994); alterative measures were either longer than the IUS or had poor internal reliability and convergent validity (e.g. Intolerance of Ambiguity Scale: Budner 1962; Tolerance of Ambiguity Scale: Kirton 1981). A psychometrically stable 12-item version of the IUS, the IUS-12, has been proposed and has become increasingly popular (Carleton et al. 2007a); however, there have also been recent efforts to expand the scope of the construct using a newly proposed 30-item French measure (Gosselin et al. 2008). Given the current lack of general consensus and relatively rapid research developments regarding how to measure the IU construct, interested readers are encouraged to review the most current literature and evaluate how each measure might best fit with their research designs.

## 12.6 **Illness/injury sensitivity**

The relationship between IIS and pain—which has substantial intuitive face validity—remains relatively less explored than the relationship between pain and other predispositional variables. Indeed, most studies evaluate the construct either peripherally or split into fears of illness or fears of injury. The division makes sense, and the IIS construct does have explicit validity and is based on fears of becoming ill or injured; however, as a dispositional trait IIS is typically referred to as a unidimensional construct (Carleton et al. 2006b).

The original measure for IIS was open to confound with stimuli associated with common fears because the items were taken from the blood-injury items from the Fear Survey Schedule-II (FSS-II; Geer 1965). A second measure, the ISI, was created to overcome the confound (Taylor 1993). The measure included face-valid items for injury (e.g. I am frightened of being injured) and illness (e.g. I worry about becoming physically ill) evaluated on a 5-point Likert scale ranging from 0 (agree very little) to 4 (agree very much). The measure and its latent 2-factor structure was subsequently revised and confirmed (ISI-R; Carleton et al. 2005, 2006b), and is a common unitary measure of the IIS construct as a fundamental fear.

The ASI and ISI-R have recently been used to evaluate the predispositional development of AS and IIS (Watt et al. 2008). Development of AS and IIS both have been related to retrospective reports of learning through direct and vicarious experiences of chronic musculoskeletal pain. IIS has been shown to be a stronger predictor than AS of pain catastrophizing, pain-related fear, pain-related anxiety, and pain tolerance (Vancleef and Peters 2006b; Vancleef et al. 2006). In contrast, heightened AS appears related to learning to catastrophize about the meaning of somatic sensations, rather than catastrophizing about the sensations themselves (Stewart et al. 2001; Watt and Stewart 2000; Watt et al. 1998). In contrast, IIS appears linked to parental modelling and reinforcement of sick-role behaviour specifically related to aches and pains, which is in line with precedent research (Vancleef and Peters 2006b; Vancleef et al. 2006) that IIS may be subsumed within a more general fear of somatic sensations.

Reductions in fear of injury are generally considered to be important in pain management (Smeets et al. 2006), but whether they are as a result of an independent fear or because they function as a lower order construct of another fear remains to be determined. For example, pain-related fear has been proximally assessed using measures of fear of injury (Roelofs et al. 2006; Samwel et al. 2007), which implies that some researchers may believe either fear of pain or fear of injury could be derivatives or manifestations of one another. The notion of fear of re-injury continues to be a critical component of contemporary fear-anxiety-avoidance models (Leeuw et al. 2007a). Patients with chronic lower back pain report higher levels of fear of injury relative to healthy controls (Leeuw et al. 2007b); however, differences within chronic lower back pain groups based on fear of injury have ranged from being relatively small (Smeets et al. 2007) to being the best predictors of physical performance in people with this form of pain (Swinkels-Meewisse et al. 2006). Despite the lack of robust within-group differences, significant reductions in fear of injury have been recorded over the course of multidisciplinary treatments (van Wilgen et al. 2007). Moreover, movement-focused fear of (re)injury has been shown to be a sensitive measure of change associated with reports of pain severity (Ostelo et al. 2007). Finally, fear of injury has been related to lengthy bed rest immediately following an injury and increased levels of disability at 1 year post injury (Verbunt et al. 2008).

There is preliminary evidence that fear of illness is also higher in patients with chronic musculoskeletal pain that healthy controls (Carleton et al. 2006a); however, there is evidence that fear of illness may be heightened in persons with higher pain-related anxiety, while not being a specific predictor of pain or disability (Hadjistavropoulos et al. 2004). Furthermore, chronic pain patients with elevated health anxiety appear to be generally more susceptible to somatic sensations and catastrophic thoughts; but, this does not necessarily implicate fear of illness as a predictor for pain (Hadjistavropoulos et al. 2002). Additional hierarchical research is needed to determine what independent roll, if any, fear of illness plays in pain.

There are alternative measures that assess injury (e.g. the Tampa Scale for Kinesiophobia; [TSK] Kori et al. 1990; Miller et al. 1991) or illness (e.g. the Illness Attitudes Scale; [IAS] Kellner 1986) more broadly than the IIS. These alternative measures have been used in variety of pain-related investigations with varying results (see Smeets et al. 2006 and Crossmann and Pauli 2006, respectively). The items within each measure account for larger cognitive schemas than the items within the IIS. For example, the TSK measures fear of movement, with the implication being that such movement will result in re-injury. In other words, the respondent can state they are afraid to move because they are afraid to be re-injured, rather than having an option to state only that they are afraid to be injured. Similarly, the IAS measures broad health constructs, from specified diseases (e.g. cancer) to fears of death while simultaneously, but briefly, tapping concerns about somatic sensations similar to those assessed by the ASI. Researchers and clinicians are, of course, encouraged to select their illness- and injury-related measures based on intended use. The TSK and IAS may function better as symptom measures, whereas the IIS may function better as a measure of predispositional traits.

## 12.7 **Fear of negative evaluation**

The FNE construct focuses on fears of being judged disparagingly or hostilely by others (Leary 1983), and has been shown to be partially heritable (Stein et al. 1999). There is relatively solid support for the notion that social anxiety and Social Anxiety Disorder are driven in part or in whole by FNE (Rapee and Heimberg 1997). For people with pain, there are at least three major social foci affected by the pain experience. First, the possibility of chronic musculoskeletal pain has been suggested to be a significant threat to the person's sense of self (Morley and Eccleston 2004; Osborn and Smith 2006). Second, the legitimacy of the pain can be called into question, undermining the person's sense of self worth and perception of their own self (Aldrich et al. 2000; Eccleston et al. 1997). Third, either as a function of depression or due to inability to participate in social activities, chronic musculoskeletal pain serves to isolate people from their social support networks (Means-Christensen et al. 2008). There is also evidence that the development of pain-related anxiety may be affected by or partially dependent on social context (Chung 2005). Given the potentially pervasive relationship between FNE and chronic musculoskeletal pain, there is relatively little direct research. The research that is available suggests that, relative to the general population, patients with chronic musculoskeletal pain may be substantially more likely to experience clinically significant levels of social anxiety (Asmundson et al. 1996a, 1996b). There certainly appears to be evidence of social changes resulting from chronic pain, including social withdrawal (Gheldof et al. 2006); however, prospective studies are needed to delineate whether the increased social anxiety facilitates, or is the result of, chronic musculoskeletal pain.

The paucity of available research on FNE and pain may help to explain some of the conflicting findings currently available. For example, there are several researchers who have found no direct association between FNE and pain (Vancleef and Peters 2006a; Vancleef et al. 2007), reporting instead only peripheral or indirect relationships (Vancleef et al. 2006). In contrast, relatively higher levels of FNE and social anxiety have been found in samples of children with sickle cell anaemia (Wagner et al. 2004) and undergraduate adult samples with high levels of pain-related fear (Asmundson and Carleton 2005). The discrepant findings may also be the result of sampling differences, wherein some patient groups have come to expect negative evaluation as a result of their pain. Indeed, chronic disabling pain related to physiopathology has been associated with fears of negative evaluation, which were thought to drive symptoms of depression and anxiety (Richards et al. 2004). In any case, the interaction of FNE and pain is likely to be complex, refractory, and worth additional investigation within the context of psychosocial models of chronic musculoskeletal pain (Asmundson et al. 2004a).

## 12.8 **Hypervigilance**

Hypervigilance refers to a state of relatively heightened vigilance. With respect to pain, hypervigilance refers specifically to continuous scanning for somatic sensations that might be pain or preface pain (Van Damme et al. 2004). A person who is hypervigilant is not necessarily over-reporting symptoms. Instead, people who are hypervigilant are likely experiencing a relatively higher sensitivity to somatic sensations as well as an increased likelihood of catastrophic interpretations once somatic sensations are noticed. Hypervigilance is almost explicitly related to AS and catastrophizing (discussed in detail above); however, the focus here will be on the sensitivity and scanning aspects of hypervigilance.

Attending to pain requires at least some application of conscious attention (Eccleston 1995a, b; Miron et al. 1989); there is also perplexing evidence that attending to pain (Hadjistavropoulos et al. 2000; Keogh et al. 2000) or being distracted from pain (Villemure and Bushnell 2002) can both result in lower perceived pain intensities. Furthermore, growing evidence suggests that people with heightened pain-related fear or fear of re-injury are more likely to attend to pain sensations (Asmundson and Hadjistavropoulos 2007) without realizing the impact that fear may be having on their pain experience (LeDoux 1998). Evidence of this bias has been underscored in people who endure chronic musculoskeletal pain and have heightened pain-related fear or fear of re-injury (Khatibi et al. 2009). Evidence also exists that cognitively demanding tasks modulate neuronal activity in several regions involved in pain processing, including insular, cingulate, and premotor cortices, thalamus, and cerebellum (Bantick et al. 2002). In other words, pain is necessarily mediated by cognitive attentional biases that can result in hypervigilance.

The results of a recent review of attentional bias research were inconsistent (Pincus and Morley 2001). Only eight studies were available at time of review; nevertheless, the authors concluded that patients with chronic musculoskeletal pain do appear hypervigilant towards sensory pain-related stimuli. These results were further supported by a subsequent meta-analysis (Roelofs et al. 2002) that included five studies, all of which were included in the eight studies from the Pincus and Morley (2001) analysis. Despite general consensus for attentional biases towards threat stimuli relative to neutral stimuli (e.g. Andersson and Haldrup 2003; Asmundson et al. 2005; Duckworth et al. 1997; Roelofs et al. 2003), pain-related threat research is conflicting. Some research has resulted in differences (Beck et al. 2001; Boston and Sharpe 2005; Carleton et al. 2006a; Dehghani et al. 2004) and some has not (Asmundson et al. 2005; Petzke et al. 2003). The discrepant results may be explained by design differences surrounding the actual pain experienced during research efforts to assess hypervigilance (Vangronsveld et al. 2007). In addition, the different results are almost certainly due, in part, to the dispositional differences discussed in this chapter (e.g. pain-related fear and anxiety, AS, IIS, FNE). Such differences may function to mediate or moderate not only each pain experience, but also individual vigilance towards pain. There is also substantial evidence that individual differences in life events—particularly traumatic ones—can serve to maintain and exacerbate chronic pain (Sharp and Harvey 2001); however, a description of the mutual maintenance model of traumatic life events and pain is beyond the scope of this chapter.

## 12.9 **Conclusion**

Despite the growing body of research into the dynamic, complex, and individual experience of pain, a great deal remains to be learned. Researchers are continuing to explore the relationships between dispositional fears, hypervigilance, and chronic musculoskeletal pain. Treatment outcomes for chronic musculoskeletal pain are often less encouraging than hoped, due largely to a lack of data on, and understanding of, the mechanisms that underlie chronicity. Recent efforts to design treatment protocols that reduce pain-related disability by addressing pain-related fear and anxiety have been promising (Bailey et al. 2010) as have efforts to treat pain-related anxiety through interoceptive exposure protocols developed to address elevated AS (Watt et al. 2006). Future research should consider employing Watt and colleagues' interoceptive treatment example with people who have chronic musculoskeletal pain—the study would allow an evaluation of whether the promising results obtained in undergraduate students with elevated pain-related anxiety can be achieved in those disabled by their pain experiences. Given the relationship between AS and IU (Carleton et al. 2007b), researchers might also explore whether ambiguous pain (e.g. chronic non-specific back pain, chronic unexplained headache) is more threatening and therefore more disabling than other types of pain for which there is sometimes a reasonably clear medical explanation (e.g. arthritis). The AS and IU constructs, both of which drive catastrophizing, appear to offer promising avenues for future research into ameliorating chronic musculoskeletal pain. Alternatively, researchers might continue with efforts to clearly delineate the nature and magnitude of attentional biases associated with hypervigilance. If the biases are sufficiently specific, modifications such as those described in recent anxiety disorder research may provide additional relief for some patients (Amir et al. 2009a; Amir et al. 2009b). In any case, improving our understanding of each of the predispositional variables described in this chapter should lead to better a understanding and, thereby, potentially improved therapeutic interventions for people trying to cope with chronic musculoskeletal pain.

## References

Abramowitz, J. S., Olatunji, B. O. and Deacon, B. J. (2007). Health anxiety, hypochondriasis, and the anxiety disorders. *Behavior Therapy*, **38**, 86–94.

Abrams, M. P., Carleton, R. N. and Asmundson, G. J. G. (2007). An exploration of the psychometric properties of the PASS-20 with a nonclinical sample. *The Journal of Pain*, **8**, 879–86.

Aldrich, S., Eccleston, C. and Crombez, G. (2000). Worrying about chronic pain: vigilance to threat and misdirected problem solving. *Behaviour Research and Therapy*, **38**, 457–70.

Amir, N., Beard, C., Burns, M. and Bomyea, J. (2009a). Attention modification program in individuals with generalized anxiety disorder. *Journal of Abnormal Psychology*, **118**, 28–33.

Amir, N., Najmi, S. and Morrison, A. S. (2009b). Attenuation of attention bias in obsessive-compulsive disorder. *Behaviour Research and Therapy*, **47**, 153–7.

Andersson, G. and Haldrup, D. (2003). Personalized pain words and Stroop interference in chronic pain patients. *European Journal of Pain*, **7**, 431–8.

Asmundson, G. J. G. (1999). Anxiety sensitivity and chronic pain: Empirical findings, clinical implications, and future directions. In S. Taylor (ed.) *Anxiety sensitivity: theory, research and treatment of the fear of anxiety*, pp.269–85. New Jersey: Erlbaum.

Asmundson, G. J. G., Abrams, M. P. and Collimore, K. C. (2008a). Pain and anxiety disorders. In M. J. Zvolensky and J. A. J. Smits (eds.) *Health behaviors and physical illness in anxiety and its disorders: Contemporary theory and research*, pp.207–35. New York: Springer.

Asmundson, G. J. G., Bovell, C. V., Carleton, R. N. and McWilliams, L. A. (2008b). The Fear of Pain Questionnaire - Short Form (FPQ-SF): Factorial validity and psychometric properties. *Pain*, **134**, 51–8.

Asmundson, G. J. G. and Carleton, R. N. (2005). Fear of pain is elevated in adults with co-occurring trauma-related stress and social anxiety symptoms. *Cognitive Behaviour Therapy*, **34**, 248–55.

Asmundson, G. J. G. and Carleton, R. N. (2008). Fear of pain. In M. M. Antony and M. B. Stein (eds.) *Handbook of anxiety and the anxiety disorders*, pp. 551–61. New York: Oxford University Press.

Asmundson, G. J. G., Collimore, K. C., Bernstein, A., Zvolensky, M. J. and Hadjistavropoulos, H. D. (2007). Is the latent structure of fear of pain continuous or discontinuous among pain patients? Taxometric analysis of the pain anxiety symptoms scale. *The Journal of Pain*, **8**, 387–95.

Asmundson, G. J. G., Coons, M. J., Taylor, S. and Katz, J. (2002). PTSD and the experience of pain: research and clinical implications of shared vulnerability and mutual maintenance models. *Canadian Journal of Psychiatry*, **47**, 930–7.

Asmundson, G. J. G. and Hadjistavropoulos, H. D. (2007). Is high fear of pain associated with general hypervigilance? A categorical re-analysis. *The Journal of Pain*, **8**, 11–18.

Asmundson, G. J. G., Hadjistavropoulos, T., Bernstein, A. and Zvolensky, M. J. (2009). Latent structure of fear of pain: an empirical test among a sample of community dwelling older adults. *European Journal of Pain*, **13**, 419–25.

Asmundson, G. J. G., Jacobson, S. J., Allerdings, M. D. and Norton, G. R. (1996a). Social phobia in disabled workers with chronic musculoskeletal pain. *Behavior Research and Therapy*, **34**, 939–43.

Asmundson, G. J. G. and Norton, G. R. (1995). Anxiety sensitivity in patients with physically unexplained chronic back pain: a preliminary report. *Behaviour Research and Therapy*, **33**, 771–7

Asmundson, G. J. G., Norton, G. R. and Jacobson, S. J. (1996b). Social, blood/injury, and agoraphobic fears in patients with physically unexplained chronic pain: are they clinically significant? *Anxiety*, **2**, 28–33.

Asmundson, G. J. G., Norton, P. J. and Norton, G. R. (1999a). Beyond pain: the role of fear and avoidance in chronicity. *Clinical Psychology Review*, **19**, 97–119.

Asmundson, G. J. G., Norton, P. J. and Veloso, F. (1999b). Anxiety sensitivity and fear of pain in patients with recurring headaches. *Behaviour Research and Therapy*, **37**, 703–13.

Asmundson, G. J. G., Norton, P. J. and Vlaeyen, J. W. S. (2004a). Fear-avoidance models of chronic pain: An overview. In G. J. G. Asmundson, J. W. S. Vlaeyen and G. Crombez (eds.) *Understanding and Treating Fear of Pain*, pp.3–24. Oxford: Oxford University Press.

Asmundson, G. J. G. and Taylor, S. (1996). Role of anxiety sensitivity in pain-related fear and avoidance. *Journal of Behavioral Medicine*, **19**, 577–86.

Asmundson, G. J. G., Vlaeyen, J. W. S. and Crombez, G. eds. (2004b). *Understanding and treating fear of pain*. New York: Oxford.

Asmundson, G. J. G., Wright, K. D. and Hadjistavropoulos, H. D. (2005). Hypervigilance and attentional fixedness in chronic musculoskeletal pain: consistency of findings across modified stroop and dot-probe tasks. *The Journal of Pain*, **6**, 497–506.

Bailey, K. M., Carleton, R. N., Vlaeyen, J. W. and Asmundson, G. J. (2010). Treatments Addressing Pain-Related Fear and Anxiety in Patients with Chronic Musculoskeletal Pain: A Preliminary Review. *Cognitive Behaviour Therapy*, **39**, 46–63.

Bantick, S. J., Wise, R. G., Ploghaus, A., Clare, S., Smith, S. M. and Tracey, I. (2002). Imaging how attention modulates pain in humans using functional MRI. *Brain*, **125**, 310–19.

Barlow, D. H. (2000). Unraveling the mysteries of anxiety and its disorders from the perspective of emotion theory. *American Psychologist*, **55**, 1247–63.

Barlow, D. H. (2002). *Anxiety and Its Disorders*. 2nd Edition. New York, NY: Guilford Press.

Beck, J. G., Freeman, J. B., Shipherd, J. C., Hamblen, J. L. and Lackner, J. M. (2001). Specificity of Stroop interference in patients with pain and PTSD. *Journal of Abnormal Psychology*, **110**, 536–43.

Beecher, H. K. (1946). Pain in men wounded in battle. Bulletin. *United States Army Medical Department*, **5**, 445–54.

Beecher, H. K. (1959). Generalization from pain of various types and diverse origins. *Science*, **130**, 267–8.

Bernstein, A., Leen-Feldner, E. W., Kotov, R., Schmidt, N. B. and Zvolensky, M. J. (2006a). A test of a panicrelevant diathesis-stress model using a taxonic index of anxiety sensitivity. In A. J. Sanfelippo (ed.) *Panic Disorders: New Research*, pp.15–40. Hauppauge, NY: Nova Science Publishers Inc.

Bernstein, A., Zvolensky, M. J., Kotov, R., *et al.* (2006b). Taxonicity of anxiety sensitivity: a multi-national analysis. *Journal of Anxiety Disorders*, **20**, 1–22.

Boston, A. and Sharpe, L. (2005). The role of threat-expectancy in acute pain: effects on attentional bias, coping strategy effectiveness and response to pain. *Pain*, **119**, 168–75.

Breuer, J. and Freud, S. (1974). *Studies on hysteria*. New York: Basic Books.

Budner, S. (1962). Intolerance for ambiguity as a personal variable. *Journal of Personality*, **30**, 29–50.

Carleton, R. N. and Asmundson, G. J. G. (2009). The multidimensionality of fear of pain: Construct independence for the Fear of Pain Questionnaire-Short Form and the Pain Anxiety Symptoms Scale-20. *The Journal of Pain*, **10**, 29–37.

Carleton, R. N., Asmundson, G. J. G., Antony, M. M. and McCabe, R. (2011). Pain-related anxiety and anxiety sensitivity across anxiety and depressive disorders. *Journal of Anxiety Disorders*, **23**, 791–8.

Carleton, R. N., Adams, M. P., Asmundson, G. J. G., Collimore, K. C. and Ellwanger, J. (2006a). Strategic and automatic threat processing in chronic musculoskeletal pain: a startle probe investigation. *Cognitive Behaviour Therapy*, **35**, 236–47.

Carleton, R. N., Asmundson, G. J. G. and Taylor, S. (2005). Fear of Physical Harm: Factor Structure and Psychometric Properties of the Injury/Illness Sensitivity Index. *Journal of Psychopathology and Behavioral Assessment*, **27**, 235–41.

Carleton, R. N., Norton, M. A. and Asmundson, G. J. G. (2007a). Fearing the unknown: a short version of the Intolerance of Uncertainty Scale. *Journal of Anxiety Disorders*, **21**, 105–17.

Carleton, R. N., Park, I. and Asmundson, G. J. G. (2006b). The Illness/Injury Sensitivity Index: an examination of construct validity. *Depression and Anxiety*, **23**, 340–6.

Carleton, R. N., Sharpe, D. and Asmundson, G. J. G. (2007b). Anxiety sensitivity and intolerance of uncertainty: requisites of the fundamental fears? *Behaviour Research and Therapy*, **45**, 2307–16.

Chung, D. (2005). Something for nothing: understanding purchasing behaviors in social virtual environments. *Cyberpsychological Behavior*, **8**, 538–54.

Conrod, P. J. (2006). The role of anxiety sensitivity in subjective and physiologic responses to social and physical stressors. *Cognitive Behaviour Therapy*, **35**, 216–25.

Coons, M. J., Hadjistavropoulos, H. D. and Asmundson, G. J. G. (2004). Factor structure and psychometric properties of the Pain Anxiety Symptoms Scale-20 in a community physiotherapy clinic sample. *European Journal of Pain*, **8**, 511–16

Craig, K. D. (1994). Emotional aspects of pain. In P.D. Wall and R. Melzack (eds.) *The textbook of pain*, pp.261–74. Edinburgh: Churchill Livingstone.

Crombez, G., Vlaeyen, J. W. S., Heuts, P. H. T. G. and Lysens, R. (1999). Pain-related fear is more disabling than pain itself: Evidence on the role of pain-related fear in chronic back pain disability. *Pain*, **80**, 329–39.

Crossmann, A. and Pauli, P. (2006). The factor structure and reliability of the Illness Attitude Scales in a student and a patient sample. *BMC Psychiatry*, **6**, 46.

Dehghani, M., Sharpe, L. and Nicholas, M. K. (2004). Modification of attentional biases in chronic pain patients: a preliminary study. *European Journal of Pain*, **8**, 585–94.

Duckworth, M. P., Iezzi, A., Adams, H. E. and Hale, D. (1997). Information processing in chronic pain disorder: A preliminary analysis. *Journal of Psychopathology and Behavioral Assessment*, **19**, 239–55.

Dugas, M. J., Gagnon, F., Ladouceur, R. and Freeston, M. H. (1998). Generalized anxiety disorder: a preliminary test of a conceptual model. *Behavior Reseach and Therapy*, **36**, 215–26.

Dugas, M. J., Gosselin, P. and Landouceur, R. (2001). Intolerance of Uncertainty and Worry: Investigating Specificity in a Nonclinical Sample. *Cognitive Therapy and Research*, **25**, 551–8.

Eccleston, C. (1995a). The attentional control of pain: methodological and theoretical concerns. *Pain*, **63**, 3–10.

Eccleston, C. (1995b). Chronic pain and distraction: an experimental investigation into the role of sustained and shifting attention in the processing of chronic persistent pain. *Behavior Reseach and Therapy*, **33**, 391–405.

Eccleston, C., Williams, A. C. and Rogers, W. S. (1997). Patients' and professionals' understandings of the causes of chronic pain: blame, responsibility and identity protection. *Social Science Medicine*, **45**, 699–709.

Fordyce, W. E. (1976). *Behavioral methods for chronic pain and illness*. St. Louis: Mosby., MO

Fordyce, W. E., Shelton, J. L. and Dundore, D. E. (1982). The modification of avoidance learning pain behaviors. *Journal of Behavioral Medicine*, **5**, 405–14.

Freeston, M., Rhéaume, J., Letarte, H., Dugas, M. J. and Ladouceur, R. (1994). Why do people worry? *Personality and Individual Differences*, **17**, 791–802.

Geer, J. H. (1965). The development of a scale to measure fear. *Behaviour Reseach and Therapy*, **3**, 45–53.

Gheldof, E. L., Vinck, J., Van den Bussche, E., Vlaeyen, J. W., Hidding, A. and Crombez, G. (2006). Pain and pain-related fear are associated with functional and social disability in an occupational setting: evidence of mediation by pain-related fear. *European Journal of Pain*, **10**, 513–25.

Gosselin, P., Ladouceur, R., Evers, A., Laverdiere, A., Routhier, S. and Tremblay-Picard, M. (2008). Evaluation of intolerance of uncertainty: development and validation of a new self-report measure. *Journal of Anxiety Disorders*, **22**, 1427–39.

Goubert, L., Crombez, G., Van Damme, S., Vlaeyen, J. W. S., Bijttebier, P. and Roelofs, J. (2004). Confirmatory Factor Analysis of the Tampa Scale for Kinesiophobia: Invariant Two-Factor Model Across Low Back Pain Patients and Fibromyalgia Patients. *Clinical Journal of Pain*, **20**, 103–10.

Greco, V. and Roger, D. (2001). Coping with uncertainty: the construction and validation of a new measure. *Personality and Individual Differences*, **31**, 519–34.

Greco, V. and Roger, D. (2003). Uncertainty, stress and health. *Personality and Individual Differences*, **34**, 1057–68.

Greenberg, J. and Burns, J. W. (2003). Pain anxiety among chronic pain patients: specific phobia or manifestation of anxiety sensitivity? *Behaviour Research and Therapy*, **41**, 223–40.

Hadjistavropoulos, H. D., Asmundson, G. J. and Kowalyk, K. M. (2004). Measures of anxiety: is there a difference in their ability to predict functioning at three-month follow-up among pain patients? *European Journal of Pain*, **8**, 1–11.

Hadjistavropoulos, H. D., Asmundson, G. J., LaChapelle, D. L. and Quine, A. (2002). The role of health anxiety among patients with chronic pain in determining response to therapy. *Pain Research and Management*, **7**, 127–33.

Hadjistavropoulos, H. D., Hadjistavropoulos, T. and Quine, A. (2000). Health anxiety moderates the effects of distraction versus attention to pain. *Behavior Reseach and Therapy*, **38**, 425–38.

Hayes, S. C. (2004). Acceptance and Commitment Therapy, Relational Frame Theory, and the Third Wave of Behavioral and Cognitive Therapies. *Behavior Therapy*, **35**, 639–65.

Hayes, S. C. and Duckworth, M. P. (2006). Acceptance and Commitment Therapy and Traditional Cognitive Behavior Therapy Approaches to Pain. *Cognitive and Behavioral Practice*, **13**, 185–7.

Heydayati, M., Dugas, M. J., Buhr, K. and Francis, K. (2003). The relationship between intolerance of uncertainty and the interpretation of ambiguous and unambiguous information. In Annual Convention of the Association for Advancement of Behaviour Therapy, Boston, MA.

Hofmann, S. G. and Asmundson, G. J. G. (2008). Acceptance and mindfulness-based therapy: New wave or old hat? *Clinical Psychology Review*, **28**, 1–16.

Holaway, R. M., Heimberg, R. G. and Coles, M. E. (2006). A comparison of intolerance of uncertainty in analogue obsessive-compulsive disorder and generalized anxiety disorder. *Journal of Anxiety Disorders*, **20**, 158–74.

International Association for the Study of Pain Subcommittee on Taxonomy. (1986). Classification of chronic pain. Descriptions of chronic pain syndromes and definitions of pain terms. *Pain Suppl,* **3**, S1–226.

Kellner, R. (1986). *Somatization and Hypochondriasis.* New York: Praeger Publishers.

Keogh, E. and Asmundson, G. J. G. (2004). Negative affectivity, catastrophizing, and anxiety sensitivity. In G. J. G. Asmundson, J. W. S. Vlaeyen and G. Crombez (eds.) *Understanding and Treating Fear of Pain,* pp. 91–115. Oxford: Oxford University Press.

Keogh, E., Barlow, C., Mounce, C. and Bond, F. W. (2006). Assessing the relationship between cold pressor pain responses and dimensions of the anxiety sensitivity profile in healthy men and women. *Cognitive Behaviour Therapy,* **35**, 198–206.

Keogh, E. and Chaloner, N. (2002). The moderating effect of anxiety sensitivity on caffeine-induced hypoalgesia in healthy women. *Psychopharmacology (Berl),* **164**, 429–31.

Keogh, E., Hatton, K. and Ellery, D. (2000). Avoidance versus focused attention and the perception of pain: differential effects for men and women. *Pain,* **85**, 225–30.

Khatibi, A., Dehghani, M., Sharpe, L., Asmundson, G. J. and Pouretemad, H. (2009). Selective attention towards painful faces among chronic pain patients: evidence from a modified version of the dot-probe. *Pain,* **142**, 42–7.

Kirton, M. J. (1981). A reanalysis of two scales of tolerance of ambiguity. *Journal of Personality Assessment,* **45**, 407–14.

Kori, S. H., Miller, R. P. and Todd, D. D. (1990). Kinesiophobia: A new view of chronic pain behavior. *Pain Management,* **3**, 35–43.

Kuch, K., Cox, B. J., Evans, R. J. and Schulman, I. (1994). Phobias, panic, and pain in 55 survivors of road vehicle accidents. *Journal of Anxiety Disorders,* **8**, 181–7.

Kuch, K., Cox, B. J., Woszczyna, C. B., Swinson, R. P. and Shulman, I. (1991). Chronic pain in panic disorder. *Journal of Behavior Therapy and Experimental Psychiatry,* **22**, 255–9.

Larsen, D. K., Taylor, S. and Asmundson, G. J. G. (1997). Exploratory factor analysis of the Pain Anxiety Symptoms Scale in patients with chronic pain complaints. *Pain,* **69**, 27–34.

Laugesen, N., Dugas, M. J. and Bukowski, W. M. (2003). Understanding adolescent worry: the application of a cognitive model. *Journal of Abnormal Child Psychology,* **31**, 55–64.

Leary, M. R. (1983). A brief version of the Fear of Negative Evaluation Scale. *Personality and Social Psychology Bulletin,* **9**, 371–5.

LeDoux, J. (1998). *The emotional brain.* New York: Simon & Schuster.

Leeuw, M., Goossens, M. E., Linton, S. J., Crombez, G., Boersma, K. and Vlaeyen, J. W. (2007a). The fear-avoidance model of musculoskeletal pain: current state of scientific evidence. *Journal of Behavioral Medicine,* **30**, 77–94

Leeuw, M., Goossens, M. E., van Breukelen, G. J., de Jong, J. R., Heuts, P. H., Smeets, R. J., Koke, A. J. and Vlaeyen, J. W. (2008). Exposure in vivo versus operant graded activity in chronic low back pain patients: results of a randomized controlled trial. *Pain,* **138**, 192–207.

Leeuw, M., Peters, M. L., Wiers, R. W. and Vlaeyen, J. W. (2007b). Measuring fear of movement/(re)injury in chronic low back pain using implicit measures. *Cognitive Behaviour Therapy,* **36**, 52–64.

McCracken, L. M. and Dhingra, L. (2002). A short version of the Pain Anxiety Symptoms Scale (PASS-20): preliminary development and validity. *Pain Research and Management,* **7**, 45–50.

McCracken, L. M., Gross, R. T., Aikens, J. and Carnrike, C. L., Jr. (1996). The assessment of anxiety and fear in persons with chronic pain: a comparison of instruments. *Behaviour Research and Therapy,* **34**, 927–33.

McCracken, L. M., Gross, R. T., Sorg, P. J. and Edmands, T. A. (1993). Prediction of pain in patients with chronic low back pain: effects of inaccurate prediction and pain-related anxiety. *Behaviour Research and Therapy,* **31**, 647–52.

McCracken, L. M., Zayfert, C. and Gross, R. T. (1992). The Pain Anxiety Symptoms Scale: development and validation of a scale to measure fear of pain. *Pain,* **50**, 67–73.

McKeever, V. M. and Huff, M. E. (2003). A diathesis-stress model of posttraumatic stress disorder: Ecological, biological, and residual stress pathways. *Review of General Psychology*, **7**, 237–50.

McNeil, D. W. and Rainwater, A. J., 3rd. (1998). Development of the Fear of Pain Questionnaire—III. *Journal of Behavioral Medicine*, **21**, 389–410.

Means-Christensen, A. J., Roy-Byrne, P. P., Sherbourne, C. D., Craske, M. G. and Stein, M. B. (2008). Relationships among pain, anxiety, and depression in primary care. *Depression and Anxiety*, **25**, 593–600.

Melzack, R. and Perry, C. (1975). Self-regulation of pain: The use of alpha-feedback and hypnotic training for the control of chronic pain. *Experimental Neurology*, **46**, 452–69.

Miller, R. P., Kori, S. H. and Todd, D. D. (1991). '*The Tampa Scale for Kinesiophobia*.' Tampa, FL: Unpublished work.

Miron, D., Duncan, G. H. and Bushnell, M. C. (1989). Effects of attention on the intensity and unpleasantness of thermal pain. *Pain*, **39**, 345–52.

Morley, S. and Eccleston, C. (2004). The object of pain. In G. J. G. Asmundson, J. W. S. Vlaeyen and G. Crombez (eds.) *Understanding and Treating Fear of Pain* pp.163–88. Oxford: Oxford University Press.

Muris, P., Vlaeyen, J. and Meesters, C. (2001). The relationship between anxiety sensitivity and fear of pain in healthy adolescents. *Behavior Reseach and Therapy*, **39**, 1357–68.

Norton, P. J. and Asmundson, G. J. (2004). Anxiety sensitivity, fear, and avoidance behavior in headache pain. *Pain*, **111**, 218–23.

Osborn, M. and Smith, J. A. (2006). Living with a body separate from the self. The experience of the body in chronic benign low back pain: An interpretative phenomenological analysis. *Journal for Caring Sciences*, **20**, 216–22.

Osman, A., Barrios, F. X., Osman, J. R., Schneekloth, R. and Troutman, J. A. (1994). The Pain Anxiety Symptoms Scale: psychometric properties in a community sample. *Journal of Behavioral Medicine*, **17**, 511–22.

Osman, A., Breitenstein, J. L., Barrios, F. X., Gutierrez, P. M. and Kopper, B. A. (2002). The fear of pain questionnaire-III: Further reliability and validity with nonclinical samples. *Journal of Behavioral Medicine*, **25**, 155–73.

Ostelo, R. W., Swinkels-Meewisse, I. J., Knol, D. L., Vlaeyen, J. W. and de Vet, H. C. (2007). Assessing pain and pain-related fear in acute low back pain: what is the smallest detectable change? *Int J Behav Med*, **14**, 242–8.

Peterson, R. A. and Plehn, K. (1999). Measuring anxiety sensitivity. In S. Taylor (ed.) *Anxiety sensitivity: Theory, research, and treatment*, pp.61–81. Mahwah, NJ: Erlbaum.

Peterson, R. A. and Reiss, S. (1992). *Anxiety Sensitivity Index Manual*. 2nd Edition. Worthington, OH: International Diagnostic Systems

Petzke, F., Clauw, D. J., Ambrose, K., Khine, A. and Gracely, R. H. (2003). Increased pain sensitivity in fibromyalgia: effects of stimulus type and mode of presentation. *Pain*, **105**, 403–13.

Pincus, T. and Morley, S. (2001). Cognitive processing bias in chronic pain: A review and integration. *Psychological Bulletin*, **127**, 599–617.

Ploghaus, A., Becerra, L., Borras, C. and Borsook, D. (2003). Neural circuitry underlying pain modulation: expectation, hypnosis, placebo. *Trends Cogn Sci*, **7**, 197–200.

Rapee, R. M. and Heimberg, R. G. (1997). A cognitive-behavioral model of anxiety in social phobia. *Behaviour Research and Therapy*, **35**, 741–56.

Reiss, S. (1991). Expectancy model of fear, anxiety, and panic. *Clinical Psychology Review*, **11**, 141–53.

Reiss, S. and McNally, R. J. (1985). The expectancy model of fear. In S. Reiss and R. R. Bootzin (eds.) *Theoretical Issues in Behaviour Therapy*, pp.107–21. New York, NY: Academic Press.

Reiss, S., Peterson, R. A., Gursky, D. M. and McNally, R. J. (1986). Anxiety sensitivity, anxiety frequency and the predictions of fearfulness. *Behaviour Research and Therapy*, **24**, 1–8.

Richards, H. L., Herrick, A. L., Griffin, K., Gwilliam, P. D. H. and Fortune, D. G. (2004). Psychological adjustment to systemic sclerosis: Exploring the association of disease factors, functional ability, body related attitudes and fear of negative evaluation. *Psychology, Health & Medicine*, **9**, 29–39.

Roelofs, J., Peters, M. L., Patijn, J., Schouten, E. G. and Vlaeyen, J. W. (2006). An electronic diary assessment of the effects of distraction and attentional focusing on pain intensity in chronic low back pain patients. *Br J Health Psychol*, **11**, 595–606.

Roelofs, J., Peters, M. L. and Vlaeyen, J. W. (2003). The modified Stroop paradigm as a measure of selective attention towards pain-related information in patients with chronic low back pain. *Psycholoical Reports*, **92**, 707–15.

Roelofs, J., Peters, M. L., Zeegers, M. P. and Vlaeyen, J. W. (2002). The modified Stroop paradigm as a measure of selective attention towards pain-related stimuli among chronic pain patients: a meta-analysis. *European Journal of Pain*, **6**, 273–81.

Roemer, L. and Orsillo, S. M. (2007). An open trial of an acceptance-based behavior therapy for generalized anxiety disorder. *Behaviour Research and Therapy*, **38**, 72–85.

Rosenstiel, A. K. and Keefe, F. J. (1983). The use of coping strategies in chronic low back pain patients: relationship to patient characteristics and current adjustment. *Pain*, **17**, 33–44.

Samwel, H. J., Kraaimaat, F. W., Crul, B. J. and Evers, A. W. (2007). The role of fear-avoidance and helplessness in explaining functional disability in chronic pain: a prospective study. *Int J Behav Med*, **14**, 237–41.

Sgroi, M. I., Willebrand, M., Ekselius, L., Gerdin, B. and Andersson, G. (2005). Fear-avoidance in Recovered Burn Patients: Association with Psychological and Somatic Symptoms. *Journal of Health Psychology*, **10**, 491–502.

Sharp, T. J. and Harvey, A. G. (2001). Chronic pain and posttraumatic stress disorder: mutual maintenance? *Clinical Psychology Review*, **21**, 857–77.

Smeets, R. J., van Geel, A. C., Kester, A. D. and Knottnerus, J. A. (2007). Physical capacity tasks in chronic low back pain: what is the contributing role of cardiovascular capacity, pain and psychological factors? *Disability and Rehabilitation*, **29**, 577–86.

Smeets, R. J., Vlaeyen, J. W., Kester, A. D. and Knottnerus, J. A. (2006). Reduction of pain catastrophizing mediates the outcome of both physical and cognitive-behavioral treatment in chronic low back pain. *The Journal of Pain*, **7**, 261–71.

Sookman, D. and Pinard, G. (2002). Overestimation of threat and intolerance of uncertainty in obsessive compulsive disorder. In R. O. Frost and G. Steketee (eds.) *Cognitive Approaches to Obsessions and Compulsions: Theory, Assessment and Treatment*, pp.63–89. Oxford: Elsevier Press.

Stein, M. B., Jang, K. L. and Livesley, W. J. (1999). Heritability of anxiety sensitivity: a twin study. *Am J Psychiatry*, **156**, 246–51.

Stewart, S. H., Taylor, S., Jang, K. L., *et al.* (2001). Causal modeling of relations among learning history, anxiety sensitivity, and panic attacks. *Behavior Reseach and Therapy*, **39**, 443–56.

Sullivan, M. J. and D'Eon, J. L. (1990). Relation between catastrophizing and depression in chronic pain patients. *Journal of Abnormal Psychology*, **99**, 260–3.

Swinkels-Meewisse, I. E., Roelofs, J., Oostendorp, R. A., Verbeek, A. L. and Vlaeyen, J. W. (2006). Acute low back pain: pain-related fear and pain catastrophizing influence physical performance and perceived disability. *Pain*, **120**, 36–43.

Taylor, S. (1993). The structure of fundamental fears. *Journal of Behavior Therapy and Experimental Psychiatry*, **24**, 289–99.

Taylor, S. ed. (1999). *Anxiety sensitivity: Theory, research, and treatment of the fear of anxiety*. Mahwah, NJ: Erlbaum.

Taylor, S., Koch, W. J. and McNally, R. J. (1992). How does anxiety sensitivity vary across the anxiety disorders? . *Journal of Anxiety Disorders*, **6**, 249–59.

Taylor, S., Koch, W. J., Woody, S. and McLean, P. (1996). Anxiety sensitivity and depression: how are they related? *Journal of Abnormal Psychology*, **105**, 474–9.

Taylor, S., Zvolensky, M. J., Cox, B. J., *et al.* (2007). Robust dimensions of anxiety sensitivity: development and initial validation of the Anxiety Sensitivity Index-3. *Psychological Assessment*, **19**, 176–88

Thompson, T., Keogh, E., French, C. C. and Davis, R. (2008). Anxiety sensitivity and pain: generalisability across noxious stimuli. *Pain*, **134**, 187–96.

Tolin, D. F., Abramowitz, J. S., Brigidi, B. D. and Foa, E. B. (2003). Intolerance of uncertainty in obsessive-compulsive disorder. *Journal of Anxiety Disorders*, **17**, 233–42.

Tsao, J. C., Lu, Q., Kim, S. C. and Zeltzer, L. K. (2006). Relationships among anxious symptomatology, anxiety sensitivity and laboratory pain responsivity in children. *Cognitive Behaviour Therapy*, **35**, 207–15.

Turk, D. C. (2002). A diathesis-stress model of chronic pain and disability following traumatic injury. *Pain Research and Management*, **7**, 9–19.

Van Damme, S., Crombez, G., Eccleston, C. and Roelofs, J. (2004). The role of hypervigilance in the experience of pain. In G. J. G. Asmundson, J. W. S. Vlaeyen and G. Crombez (eds.) *Understanding and Treating Fear of Pain*, pp.71–90. Oxford: Oxford University Press.

van Wilgen, C. P., Bloten, H. and Oeseburg, B. (2007). Results of a multidisciplinary program for patients with fibromyalgia implemented in the primary care. *Disability & Rehabilitation*, **29**, 1207–13.

Vancleef, L. M. and Peters, M. L. (2006a). The interruptive effect of pain on attention. *The Journal of Pain*, **7**, 21–2.

Vancleef, L. M. and Peters, M. L. (2006b). Pain catastrophizing, but not injury/illness sensitivity or anxiety sensitivity, enhances attentional interference by pain. *The Journal of Pain*, **7**, 23–30.

Vancleef, L. M., Peters, M. L., Gilissen, S. M. and De Jong, P. J. (2007). Understanding the role of injury/illness sensitivity and anxiety sensitivity in (automatic) pain processing: an examination using the extrinsic affective simon task. *The Journal of Pain*, **8**, 563–72.

Vancleef, L. M., Peters, M. L., Roelofs, J. and Asmundson, G. J. G. (2006). Do fundamental fears differentially contribute to pain-related fear and pain catastrophizing? An evaluation of the sensitivity index. *European Journal of Pain*, **10**, 527–36.

Vangronsveld, K., Van Damme, S., Peters, M., Vlaeyen, J., Goossens, M. and Crombez, G. (2007). An experimental investigation on attentional interference by threatening fixations of the neck in patients with chronic whiplash syndrome. *Pain*, **127**, 121–8.

Verbunt, J. A., Sieben, J., Vlaeyen, J. W., Portegijs, P. and Andre Knottnerus, J. (2008). A new episode of low back pain: who relies on bed rest? *European Journal of Pain*, **12**, 508–16.

Villemure, C. and Bushnell, M. C. (2002). Cognitive modulation of pain: how do attention and emotion influence pain processing? *Pain*, **95**, 195–9.

Vlaeyen, J. W., de Jong, J., Geilen, M., Heuts, P. H. and van Breukelen, G. (2002). The treatment of fear of movement/(re)injury in chronic low back pain: further evidence on the effectiveness of exposure in vivo. *Clinical Journal of Pain*, **18**, 251–61.

Vlaeyen, J. W., Kole-Snijders, A. M., Boeren, R. G. and van Eek, H. (1995). Fear of movement/(re)injury in chronic low back pain and its relation to behavioral performance. *Pain*, **62**, 363–72.

Vlaeyen, J. W. and Linton, S. J. (2000). Fear-avoidance and its consequences in chronic musculoskeletal pain: a state of the art. *Pain*, **85**, 317–32.

Vowles, K. E., McCracken, L. M. and Eccleston, C. (2008). Patient functioning and catastrophizing in chronic pain: The mediating effects of acceptance. *Health Psychology*, **27**, S136–S43.

Waddell, G., Newton, M., Henderson, I., Somerville, D. and Main, C. J. (1993). A Fear-Avoidance Beliefs Questionnaire (FABQ) and the role of fear-avoidance beliefs in chronic low back pain and disability. *Pain*, **52**, 157–68.

Wagner, J. L., Connelly, M. A., Brown, R. T., Taylor, L., Rittle, C. and Cloues, B. (2004). Predictors of social anxiety in children and adolescents with sickle cell disease. *Journal of Clinical Psychology in Medical Settings*, **11**, 243–52.

Watt, M. C., O'Connor, R., Stewart, S., Moon, E. and Terry, L. (2008). Specificity of childhood learning experiences related to anxiety sensitivity and illness/injury sensitivity: implications for health anxiety and pain. *Journal of Cognitive Psychotherapy*, **22**, 128–42.

Watt, M. C. and Stewart, S. H. (2000). Anxiety sensitivity mediates the relationships between childhood learning experiences and elevated hypochondriacal concerns in young adulthood. *Journal of Psychosomatic Research*, **49**, 107–18.

Watt, M. C., Stewart, S. H. and Cox, B. J. (1998). A retrospective study of the learning history origins of anxiety sensitivity. *Behavior Reseach and Therapy*, **36**, 505–25.

Watt, M. C., Stewart, S. H., Lefaivre, M. J. and Uman, L. S. (2006). A brief cognitive-behavioral approach to reducing anxiety sensitivity decreases pain-related anxiety. *Cognitive Behaviour Therapy*, **35**, 248–56.

Zinbarg, R. E., Barlow, D. H. and Brown, T. A. (1997). Hierarchical structure and general factor saturation of the anxiety sensitivity index. *Psychological Assessment*, **9**, 277–84.

Zvolensky, M. J., Goodie, J. L., McNeil, D. W., Sperry, J. A. and Sorrell, J. T. (2001). Anxiety sensitivity in the prediction of pain-related fear and anxiety in a heterogeneous chronic pain population. *Behaviour Research and Therapy*, **39**, 683–96.

Chapter 13

# Processes Underlying the Relation between Catastrophizing and Chronic Pain: Implications for Intervention

Michael J.L. Sullivan and Marc O. Martel

## 13.1 Introduction

Over the past two decades, pain catastrophizing has emerged as one of the most robust psychological predictors of pain-related outcomes (Edwards et al. 2006a; Sullivan et al. 2001b; Turk et al. 1983; Weissman-Fogel et al. 2008). Hundreds of studies have documented associations between pain catastrophizing and adverse pain outcomes, including heightened pain intensity, emotional distress, and disability (Edwards et al. 2006a; Keefe et al. 2004; Sullivan et al. 2001b; Turk and Okifuji 2002).

Increasingly, researchers have turned their attention to questions concerning the mechanisms by which pain catastrophizing impacts on pain outcomes (Seminowicz and Davis 2006; Sullivan 2008; Turner and Aaron 2001). Research in this area has identified psychological, interpersonal (Cano 2004), physiological (Wolff et al. 2008), and neuroanatomical (Gracely et al. 2004) correlates of pain catastrophizing that might explain how pain catastrophizing impacts on pain experience. The identification of the mechanisms that link pain catastrophizing to pain outcomes has both clinical and theoretical implications. From a clinical perspective, understanding the processes by which pain catastrophizing influences the experience or expression of pain might point to new avenues for intervention that could reduce the suffering and burden of persistent pain conditions. From a theoretical perspective, understanding how pain catastrophizing influences pain might contribute to the elaboration or refinement of conceptual frameworks that address the linkages between psychology and physiology in the generation of pain experience.

This chapter summarizes research that has addressed the mechanisms implicated in the relation between pain catastrophizing and pain outcomes. Given the volume of research that has been conducted in this area, the review of the literature is intended to be illustrative as opposed to exhaustive. The chapter ends with a discussion of the clinical and theoretical implications of the research that has accumulated to date.

## 13.2 Catastrophizing: the construct

Pain catastrophizing has been broadly defined as an exaggerated negative orientation to actual or anticipated pain comprising elements of rumination, magnification and helplessness (Sullivan et al. 2001b). In 1995, Sullivan et al. (1995) suggested that different elements of catastrophizing might be related to primary and secondary appraisal processes (e.g. (Lazarus and Folkman 1984). At least at a descriptive level, magnification (e.g. exaggerating the threat value of pain) and rumination (e.g. excessive focus on pain-related stimuli) overlap with the defining features of primary

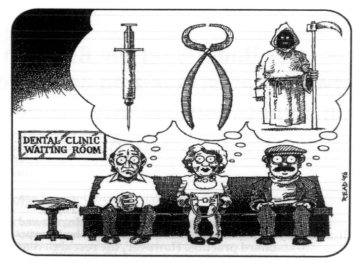

**Fig. 13.1** The mindset of catastrophizing. Original artwork produced by Stephen Read.

appraisals (e.g. evaluating the threat value of a stimulus) (Sullivan et al. 1995). The helplessness dimension of catastrophizing overlaps with the defining features of secondary appraisals (e.g. evaluation of one's ability to effectively deal with the stress situation).

Although the appraisal conceptualization of pain catastrophizing has been debated, it remains the view espoused by most researchers in this area of research (Jensen et al. 1991b; Keefe et al. 1999; Severeijns et al. 2004; Turner and Aaron 2001). The appraisal conceptualization of pain catastrophizing places the construct within a cognitive theory framework (Beck et al. 1978; Turk 1996). In its most general form, cognitive theory predicts that exaggerated threat appraisals will lead to emotional reactions such as anxiety or fear (Lazarus and Folkman 1984). Vlaeyen and his colleagues have elaborated a cognitive-behavioural model of pain-related disability where pain catastrophizing is viewed as a key factor in the development of problematic pain outcomes (Leeuw et al. 2007; Vlaeyen and Linton 2000). The model predicts that catastrophic thinking following the onset of pain will contribute to heightened fears of movement and increased hyper-vigilance to pain symptoms. In turn, fear is expected to lead to avoidance or escape of activity that might be associated with pain (Vlaeyen and Linton 2000). The model is recursive such that increased pain symptoms, distress and disability become the input for further catastrophic or alarmist thinking (Vlaeyen and Linton 2000).

It has also been suggested that pain catastrophizing might serve as an interpersonal coping function (Sullivan et al. 2000). The Communal Coping Model of pain catastrophizing draws on theoretical perspectives addressing the interpersonal objectives of coping (Coyne and Fiske 1992; Lackner and Gurtman 2004; Lyons et al. 1995; Taylor 2000). According to the Communal Coping Model, the pain expressions of high pain catastrophizers serve a social communicative function aimed at maximizing the probability that distress will be managed within a social/interpersonal context (Sullivan et al. 2000). Sullivan et al. (2001) suggested that high pain catastrophizers might engage in exaggerated pain expression in order to maximize proximity, or to solicit assistance or empathic responses from others. Pain catastrophizers' expressive pain displays might also be used to induce others to alter their expectations, reduce performance demands or as a means of managing interpersonal conflict.

Although the coping style of high pain catastrophizers might appear maladaptive, it is important to consider that a communal coping style might only become truly maladaptive under chronic pain or chronic illness conditions. In response to acute pain, exaggerated pain displays might result in a precarious, but sustainable, balance between satisfying support or affiliative needs, and increasing distress. Under acute pain conditions, overall benefits may outweigh costs, and reinforcement contingencies (e.g. increased support, attention, empathic responses) may actually serve to maintain the expressive style of high pain catastrophizers. When conditions become chronic, this balance may be disrupted such that costs begin to outweigh benefits. Others' responses may become increasingly negative when distress displays extend over time (Cano 2004). The disrupted balance may find expression as increased interpersonal conflict, social rejection and depression (Keefe et al. 2003).

## 13.3 Processes linking pain catastrophizing to adverse pain outcomes

An appraisal conceptualization of pain catastrophizing suggests several cognitive and emotional processes through which pain catastrophizing might impact on pain experience. These might include expectancies, attentional mechanisms, emotional distress states and the mobilization of distress reduction strategies (i.e. coping strategies). Research examining the role of these variables as determinants of the relation between pain catastrophizing and pain outcomes will be briefly reviewed.

### 13.3.1 Expectancies

Expectancies are essentially an individual's predictions about the future. In pain research, researchers have distinguished between 'response expectancies' and 'efficacy expectancies' (Bandura 1977; Kirsch 1985). Predictions about non-volitional responses to a particular stimulus are referred to as 'response expectancies'. Efficacy expectancies (e.g. self-efficacy) refer to the confidence individuals' have that they possess the ability to successfully execute the behaviour required to yield a desired outcome (Bandura 1977). Considerable research has shown that there is a high degree of concordance between pain expectancies and pain experience (Jensen et al. 1991a; Lacker et al. 1996).

Response expectancies for pain have been discussed as a significant determinant of actual pain experience (Crombez et al. 1996; Jensen et al. 1991a). For example, the powerful analgesic effects of placebos have been discussed in terms of expectancy manipulations (Pollo et al. 2001; Whalley et al. 2008). It has been suggested that many psychological interventions for pain management may exert their effects, at least in part, through their influence on pain expectancies (Milling et al. 2006; Milling et al. 2007).

Research has provided support for a relation between pain catastrophizing and response expectancies. In an experimental study, Sullivan et al (Sullivan et al. 2001a) reported that pain catastrophizing was associated with expectancies for heightened pain and emotional distress. Van Damme et al (Van Damme et al. 2002) also found a significant relation between pain catastrophizing and pain expectancies and suggested that the pain expectancies of high pain catastrophizers might promote hypervigilance to pain signals. Not only do high pain catastrophizers expect to experience more pain, but there are findings to suggest that high pain catastrophizers fail to correct their pain expectancies in the face of disconfirming evidence (Crombez et al. 2002; Van Damme et al. 2002).

A number of investigations have shown a close association between self-efficacy expectancies and pain catastrophizing (Keefe et al. 1997b; Thorn et al. 2007). For example, scale items that assess self-efficacy for coping with pain have frequently loaded on the same factor as scale items that assess catastrophic thinking (Sullivan et al. 2001b). Albeit a close association, the two constructs do not appear to be redundant. One investigation revealed that self-efficacy prospectively predicted pain behaviour and activity avoidance, even when controlling for pain catastrophizing (Asghari and Nicholas 2001). In a recent study of patients with osteoarthritis, Shelby et al. (2008) found that domain-specific self-efficacy mediated the relation between pain catastrophizing and pain intensity.

There are indications that the impact of expectancies on pain outcomes might be unmediated (at least with respect to psychological variables). Kirsch (1985) has proposed that response expectancies may represent one of the most basic psychological variables. This position has significant implications for explicating the underlying basis of several psychological determinants of pain experience. Expectancies may represent the final common pathway of several psychological influences on pain perception.

Research suggests that similar brain regions might modulate the effects of pain catastrophizing and pain expectancies (Gracely et al. 2004; Ploghaus et al. 2003; Ploghaus et al. 1999). In addition, there are indications that catastrophizing and expectancies might exert influence on endogenous opioid mechanisms (Peyron et al. 2000). For example, it has been shown that the analgesic effects of high self-efficacy can be blocked with naloxone (i.e. an opioid antagonist) (Bandura et al. 1987). High levels of pain catastrophizing have been associated with poorer response to opioids for both clinical and experimental pain (Fillingim et al. 2005; Haythornthwaite et al. 2003; Jacobsen and Butler 1996).

### 13.3.2 **Attention**

It has been suggested that pain catastrophizing might impact on pain experience by increasing attention to pain sensations. It has long been established that increased attention to pain sensations augments the intensity of perceived pain (Arntz et al. 1991; Bushnell et al. 2004; Eccleston and Crombez 1999; McCracken 1997). A number of early studies provided data indicating that attention diversion strategies such as distraction were less effective when used by individuals with high levels of pain catastrophizing (Heyneman et al. 1990; Spanos et al. 1979; Sullivan et al. 1995). Additionally, several studies have reported that among the three subscales of the Pain Catastrophizing Scale (i.e. rumination, magnification, helplessness), rumination was the best predictor of pain intensity and pain-related disability (Devoulyte and Sullivan 2003; Sullivan and Neish 1998; Sullivan et al. 1998).

One study showed that when individuals were asked to suppress thought about an upcoming pain procedure, individuals with high pain catastrophizing scores reported experiencing more pain-related thought intrusions than individuals with low pain catastrophizing scores (Sullivan et al. 1997). In an elegant series of studies, Van Damme et al (Van Damme et al. 2002; Van Damme et al. 2004) reported findings suggesting that pain catastrophizing might be associated with an attentional disengagement deficit. The results of the latter studies indicated that pain catastrophizing does not necessarily lead individuals to be more vigilant to pain, but once attention has been oriented to a pain stimulus, pain catastrophizing appears to interfere with disengagement from the pain stimulus.

Neuroimaging research has shown that focusing attention on pain may activate a distributed network of brain regions, including prefrontal and parietal areas, parts of the anterior cingulate cortex, and the thalamus (Bushnell et al. 2004; Derbyshire et al. 1997; Peyron et al. 2000). During painful stimulation, some regions of the 'attentional network' have been shown to be significantly more activated in high pain catastrophizers, particularly the dorsolateral prefrontal cortex, the anterior cingulate cortex, and the inferior parietal cortex (Gracely et al. 2004; Seminowicz and

Davis 2006). These findings provide neural evidence that attentional mechanisms might account, at least in part, for the relation between catastrophic thinking and pain experience (Seminowicz and Davis 2006; Sullivan et al. 2001b).

### 13.3.3 Emotion

A basic tenet of cognitive theories of emotion is that negative cognitions can lead to negative emotions (Banks and Kerns 1996; Beck et al. 1978; Lazarus and Folkman 1984). Researchers have appealed to variations of this general framework to understand the relation between catastrophic thinking and negative emotional reactions (Turner and Aaron 2001; Vlaeyen and Linton 2000). The relations among pain catastrophizing, fear, and depression have been the focus of numerous investigations (Keefe et al. 2005; Sullivan and D'Eon 1990). Research has been consistent in showing that measures of catastrophic thinking are significantly correlated with measures of depression, anxiety, and fear (Borsbo et al. 2008; Drahovzal et al. 2006; Edwards et al. 2006a; Edwards et al. 2006b; Leeuw et al. 2007). Keefe et al (Keefe et al. 1989) reported that pain catastrophizing prospectively predicted depressive symptoms in a sample of individuals with arthritis. The pattern of findings that has emerged suggests that catastrophic thinking might contribute to the development or maintenance of anxiety, fear or depression associated with pain.

The study of the relation between emotion and pain dates back several decades (Craig 1989; Schwarz 1962). There is a sizeable literature that has examined the relation between trait measures of emotional distress and pain outcomes. Numerous investigators have reported significant cross-sectional and prospective relations between trait measures of depression, anxiety, fear, anger, and heightened pain experience (Banks and Kerns 1996; Leeuw et al. 2007; Rudy et al. 1988; Sullivan and Neish 1998; Turk 1996; Turk and Okifuji 2002; Vlaeyen et al. 1995). For example, Smith and Zautra (2008) reported that anxiety was prospectively related to heightened pain intensity in a sample of women with arthritis (Smith and Zautra 2008). Carroll et al (2004) reported that depressive symptoms might increase susceptibility to exacerbation of musculoskeletal pain symptoms (Carroll et al. 2004).

Fewer studies have addressed the role of situation-specific or experimentally induced emotional distress on responses to painful stimulation. Findings from experimental studies are not entirely consistent with the pattern of findings using trait measures of emotional distress. For example, Meagher et al (Meagher et al. 2001) examined the effects of viewing emotional slides prior to participating in an experimental pain procedure. Their findings indicated that viewing slides of fear or disgust resulted in a decrease as opposed to an increase in pain intensity. However, consistent with the research using trait measures of emotional distress, Carter et al. (2002) reported that experimental induction of negative emotions (i.e. anxiety, depression) led to increased pain severity during a cold pressor task. Tang et al. (2008) reported that listening to sad music led to more intense pain experience and lower pain tolerance in chronic back pain patients. Thus, although the research on the effects of situation-specific negative mood on pain is not as consistent as the literature using trait measures of emotional distress, the findings point to a possible hyperalgesic effect of emotional distress in both healthy individuals and chronic pain patients.

Studies using functional brain imaging techniques have identified a number of brain areas responsible for producing emotional/affective responses associated with pain, including feelings of unpleasantness and distress. For example, studies have been consistent in showing that painful stimulation leads to increased neural activity in the anterior cingulate and insular cortices, both part of the limbic system (for a review, see Apkarian et al. 2005). It is generally assumed that neural activity in limbic areas contributes to heightened pain experience by increasing the emotional valence attributed to pain sensations.

Recent efforts have been made to examine the neural mechanisms underlying the effects of emotional states on pain processing. For example, Phillips et al (Phillips et al. 2003) have shown that experimentally induced negative mood can enhance neural activity in cingulate and insular cortices during visceral stimulation, leading to increased levels of pain-related discomfort. Similarly, Ploghaus et al (2001) have shown that experimentally induced anxiety can lead to hyperalgesic responses and increased neural activity in a number of brain areas associated with pain processing. Specifically, it has been shown that high levels of anxiety prior to painful heat stimulation can increase activity in the medial prefrontal cortex, the anterior cingulate cortex, and parts of the hippocampal formation. These areas are considered to be directly involved in the amplification of pain experience and provide a neural basis for the effects of emotion on pain (Schweinhardt et al. 2008; Tracey and Mantyh 2007).

There is reason to believe that pain catastrophizing might influence pain experience through similar neural mechanisms to those involved in the relationship between emotional distress and pain. During painful stimulation, Seminowicz and Davis (2006) found that pain catastrophizing was significantly associated with activity in the medial prefrontal cortex, the anterior cingulate cortex, the insula, and parts of the hippocampal formation. Pain-evoked neural activity in some of these regions has been associated with negative affect (Phillips et al. 2003; Ploghaus et al. 2001), suggesting that pain catastrophizing is likely to overlap with other emotional processes in modulating brain responses to pain. These neuroimaging findings also suggest that pain catastrophizing might increase emotional distress, facilitating nociceptive processing in cortico-cortical circuits and augmenting the overall pain experience.

### 13.3.4 **Coping**

Coping generally refers to the strategies that individuals use to minimize the impact of life stressors on their psychological well-being (Lazarus and Folkman 1984). In the area of pain, strategies such as distraction, positive self-statements and re-appraisal have been discussed as 'adaptive' coping strategies that might reduce the intensity of pain or the emotional distress associated with pain (Turk et al. 1983; Turk and Okifuji 2002). Early research on coping and pain catastrophizing led to the suggestion that pain catastrophizing might represent a 'maladaptive' coping strategy (Keefe et al. 1989). This view was challenged by researchers who argued that pain catastrophizing was neither strategic or goal directed, and should be considered distinct from coping efforts (Jensen et al. 1991b; Thorn et al. 2003). As noted earlier, the Communal Coping Model proposed that pain catastrophizing might indeed be strategic, but the goals of this coping orientation might be more socially relevant than pain relevant (Sullivan et al. 2001b).

Evidence suggests that pain catastrophizers do not differ from non-catastrophizers in the type or number of 'adaptive' pain coping strategies they use. In one of the earliest studies to address the relation between coping and pain catastrophizing, Spanos et al. (1979) reported that pain catastrophizers and non-catastrophizers did not differ in the number of coping strategies they reported using during a cold pressor procedure. Interestingly however, for non-catastrophizers, there was an association between number of coping strategies and degree of pain reduction. For pain catastrophizers, number of coping strategies reported was not associated with pain reduction. Similar findings were subsequently reported by other investigators suggesting that coping strategies are less effective when used by pain catastrophizers (Heyneman et al. 1990; Sullivan et al. 1995).

It is interesting to note that individuals with high pre-treatment scores on measures of pain catastrophizing are less likely to benefit from pain management or disability management interventions (Sullivan et al. 2005b). Findings such as these have led investigators to suggest that reductions in pain catastrophizing might be a pre-requisite to the effective use of pain coping strategies (Thorn et al. 2002, 2007). Consistent with this perspective, a number of studies have shown that reductions in catastrophizing mediate the outcomes of pain rehabilitation programmes (Smeets et al. 2006; Spinhoven et al. 2004; Sullivan et al. 2006b, 2005b).

The Communal Coping Model suggests that pain behaviour displays might be used strategically by high pain catastrophizers as a means of soliciting attention or support from their social environment (Sullivan et al. 2001b). Pain catastrophizers' expressive pain displays might also be used to induce others to alter their expectations, reduce performance demands or as a means of managing interpersonal conflict (Keefe et al. 1997a). From this perspective, the expressive pain displays of pain catastrophizers could be construed as a form of coping.

Support for the Communal Coping Model has come primarily from studies showing that the pain experience and pain expressions of pain catastrophizers are sensitive to social context (Giardino et al. 2003; Sullivan et al. 2004). The relation between pain catastrophizing and pain severity is higher when pain patients are living with a spouse or caregiver (Giardino et al. 2003), and higher levels of pain catastrophizing are associated with higher levels of short term spousal support (Cano 2004). Sullivan et al (Sullivan et al. 2006c) found that pain catastrophizers' expressive displays of pain led observers to infer more intense (but not more accurate) pain experience. Pain catastrophizing has also been associated with negative interpersonal outcomes where the emotional demands of high pain catastrophizers seem to tax the support resources of significant others (Boothy et al. 2004; Keefe et al. 2003; Lackner and Gurtman 2004).

Numerous investigations have shown that pain catastrophizing is associated with heightened expression of pain behaviour (Keefe et al. 2000; Sullivan et al. 2000; Thibault et al. 2008; Vervoort et al. 2008). The relation between pain catastrophizing and pain behaviour has been shown to remain significant even when controlling for pain intensity (Thibault et al. 2008). As such, the heightened pain expressions of pain catastrophizers cannot be explained as simply being the consequence of experiencing more intense pain. Although a relation between pain catastrophizing and pain behaviour does not confirm that pain behaviour is being used strategically as a form of coping, there are indirect indications that pain behaviour might serve such a function. In one study, the presence of an observer led to increases in pain behaviour for pain catastrophizers but not for non-catastrophizers participating in an experimental pain procedure (Sullivan et al. 2004). In the latter study, increases in pain behaviour were associated with decreases in the use of cognitive coping strategies. It has also been shown that emotional disclosure reduces the pain experience of pain catastrophizers but not that of non-catastrophizers (Sullivan and Neish 1999).

Thus, the literature in this area suggests that pain catastrophizers do not differ from non-catastrophizers in the types of coping strategies they report using. However, coping strategies seem to be less effective when used by pain catastrophizers, and pain catastrophizers appear to benefit less from interventions designed to foster successful adaptation to chronic pain. It is possible that pain catastrophizers might use pain behaviour as a means of soliciting support to deal with their distress. Unfortunately, in attaining these interpersonal objectives, pain catastrophizers may inadvertently make their pain experience more aversive. Exaggerated display of pain behaviour may become maladaptive by actually contributing to heightened pain experience, perhaps through increased attention to pain. In addition, others' solicitous or reinforcing responses may serve to trigger, maintain, or reinforce pain catastrophizers' exaggerated pain expression (Romano et al. 1995).

### 13.3.5 Endogenous pain modulation

There are some indications that pain catastrophizing might have a direct impact on endogenous pain modulation mechanisms. As noted above, research suggests that pain catastrophizers might benefit less from rehabilitation interventions for chronic pain. There is also research to suggest that pain catastrophizing might interfere with the effectiveness of pharmacological interventions for pain. Haythornthwaite et al (2003) reported the findings of a study assessing the efficacy of an opiate medication for post-herpetic neuralgia. Analyses revealed that initial pain catastrophizing scores predicted higher post-treatment pain ratings, even when controlling for baseline pain. Sullivan et al (2008b) reported that catastrophizing was associated with poor response to a topical analgesic for neuropathic pain. In an experimental study investigating psychological factors related to pain perception and analgesia, Fillingim et al. (2005) found that catastrophizing in men was associated with poor overall analgesic responses to intravenous pentazocine.

The mechanisms by which psychological factors interfere with response to analgesics remain unclear. It has been suggested that individuals high in catastrophizing might produce endogenous nocebo-like responses due to their negative cognitions (Fillingim et al. 2005). It has also been suggested that catastrophizing might compromise processes involved in descending pain inhibition (Edwards and Fillingim 2001). For example, in a temporal summation paradigm, Edwards et al. (2006c) found that individuals with high levels of catastrophizing reported significantly greater increases in pain ratings than individuals with low levels of catastrophizing during the application of repeated painful heat stimulations. Similarly, George et al (2006) found that pain catastrophizing was a significant predictor of increases in pain ratings across repeated noxious heat pulses, even when controlling for sex and pain-related fear. These findings suggest that pain catastrophizing may facilitate processes involved in temporal summation of pain or 'windup' (Price et al. 2002). The findings also suggest that pain catastrophizing might interfere with descending pain-inhibitory systems, facilitate neuroplastic changes in the spinal cord during repeated painful stimulation, subsequently promoting sensitization in the central nervous system.

Other studies have also established a link between pain catastrophizing and the operation of endogenous pain-modulatory systems. For example, two recently published papers have reported a negative association between pain catastrophizing and diffuse noxious inhibitory controls, a psychophysical measure of endogenous pain inhibition (Goodin et al. 2008; Weissman-Fogel et al. 2008). On the basis of findings such as these, it has been suggested that pain catastrophizing might directly interfere with the efficacy of endogenous pain-inhibitory mechanisms (Goodin et al. 2008).

## 13.4 Processes mediating the relation between pain catastrophizing and pain outcomes

The literature reviewed in this chapter points to several processes or mechanisms that might underlie the relation between pain catastrophizing and pain outcomes. Research suggests that pain catastrophizing is significantly associated with expectancies for heightened pain experience, increased attention to pain sensations and increased negative mood. In turn, expectancies, attention and negative mood have been shown to contribute to heightened pain experience. Research also suggests that pain catastrophizing might interfere with the effectiveness of certain coping strategies and might be associated with strategies (e.g. distress displays) that inadvertently contribute to increased pain.

It is important to caution that observed relations between pain catastrophizing and expectancies, attention, negative mood and coping cannot be taken as evidence that these are the processes by which pain catastrophizing impacts on pain experience. In order to determine which of these variables underlie the relation between pain catastrophizing and pain outcomes, it is necessary to examine the degree to which the catastrophizing-pain relation is diminished when controlling, experimentally or statistically, for potential determinants (or mediators).

Unfortunately, few studies have conducted mediational analyses for variables that might under-lie the relation between pain catastrophizing and pain outcomes. Still, the available research permits some speculation about potential mediational candidates. Research addressing the role of expectancies in mediating the relation between pain catastrophizing and pain has yielded mixed findings. Sullivan et al. (2001a) reported that expectancies for pain experience prior to an experi-mental pain procedure partially mediated the relation between catastrophizing and pain. In a recent study of patients with osteoarthritis, Shelby et al (2008) reported that self-efficacy fully mediated of the relation between catastrophizing and pain in patients with osteoarthritis.

The research on the relation between pain catastrophizing and attention to pain is strongly sug-gestive that attention might mediate the catastrophizing-pain relation. Catastrophizing appears to be associated with a propensity to focus excessively on pain, and might also be associated with a deficit in mental control over pain-related stimuli such that individuals high in catastrophizing will have more difficulty disengaging their attention from a pain stimulus. Although the bulk of this research has been conducted within experimental paradigms, there is little basis for arguing that different processes might operate in patients with chronic pain. In chronic pain patients, pain catastrophizing has been shown to correlate significantly with self-reported vigilance to pain symptoms (Crombez et al. 2004). Surprisingly, research suggests that pain catastrophizing might mediate the relation between vigilance and pain, as opposed to vigilance mediating the relation between pain catastrophizing and pain (Crombez et al. 2004).

Questions concerning the role of emotional distress as a mediator of the relationship between catastrophizing and pain have been addressed in several investigations. Overall, the findings of this research do not support the mediating role of emotional distress. Many investigations have reported findings suggesting that instead of emotional distress mediating the relation between pain catastrophizing and pain outcomes, pain catastrophizing might mediate the relation between emotional distress and pain. Geisser et al. (1995) found that pain catastrophizing mediated the relation between depression and pain. Lackner and Quigley (2005) reported that pain catastro-phizing mediated the relation between worry and pain in individuals with irritable bowel syndrome. In a study using experimental pain and mood induction, Bartley and Rhudy (2008) found no evidence that pain catastrophizing exerted its effects on pain indirectly through mood.

Thus, it appears that emotional distress might not be a promising candidate as a mediator of the relation between pain catastrophizing and pain outcomes. Although emotional distress co-varies with catastrophic thinking to a significant degree, the research does not support the view that emotional distress is the vehicle through which pain catastrophizing exerts its impact on pain outcomes.

The role of coping as a mediator of the relation between catastrophizing and pain outcomes has been more challenging to address. First, the use of 'adaptive' coping strategies does not appear to co-vary with level of pain catastrophizing, although the effectiveness of coping strategies might be influenced by level of pain catastrophizing. It is possible that pain catastrophizers might use mala-daptive strategies, such as the expression of pain behaviour, that inadvertently contribute to adverse interpersonal or pain outcomes. However, if the use of pain behaviour to solicit attention or support is not driven by conscious intent, it will be difficult to establish whether such coping efforts are the process by which pain catastrophizing impacts negatively on pain outcomes.

## 13.5 Treatment implications

Research examining potential mediators of the relation between catastrophizing and pain outcomes might have important implications for the development of targeted interventions aimed at reducing pain catastrophizing, or minimizing the negative impact of pain catastrophizing on pain outcomes. Although numerous treatment studies have been shown to have an effect on catastrophic thinking, the critical elements of effective treatments for yielding meaningful change have yet to be identified.

Considerable research supports the view that pain catastrophizing is a modifiable variable (Keefe et al. 2005; Sullivan et al. 2005a). In the absence of intervention, pain catastrophizing shows some degree of stability over time (Sullivan et al. 2001b). However, numerous intervention studies have shown that catastrophic thinking decreases as a result of participation in treatment aimed at facilitating recovery or adaptation to chronic pain (Jensen et al. 2001; Smeets et al. 2006; Spinhoven et al. 2004). Many of these studies have pointed to importance of reducing pain catastrophizing as a key factor in determining the success of interventions for chronic pain (Spinhoven et al. 2004; Sullivan et al. 2005b).

Jensen et al (2001) reported that participation in a 3-week (82 hours) multidisciplinary pain treatment programme led to a 40% reduction in scores on a measure of catastrophizing (Jensen et al. 2001). Treatment-related changes in pain catastrophizing rose significantly at 6-month follow-up, but remained below baseline levels. Sullivan et al. (2003) reported a 33% reduction in catastrophizing scores following participation in a 10-week (10 hours) psychological intervention (led by psychologists) designed to target psychosocial risk factors for pain and disability (Sullivan and Stanish 2003). Sullivan et al. (2006a) reported a 43% reduction in catastrophizing following participation in a 10-week programme (50 hours) consisting of exercise and a psychosocial intervention (led by occupational therapists and physiotherapists) targeting risk factors for pain and disability. Adams et al. (2007) reported that reductions in pain catastrophizing following a 10-week (50 hours) treatment programme consisting of exercise and a psychosocial intervention varied as a function of level of chronicity. For patients in the subacute (4 weeks to 3 months) and early chronic period (3–6 months) of recovery, pain catastrophizing scores showed a reduction of 39%. For patients whose condition had become chronic (+6 months), pain catastrophizing scores decreased by only 10%.

There are also indications that psychological intervention might not be essential to yield reductions in catastrophic thinking. Sullivan et al (2006a) reported a 24% reduction in pain catastrophizing scores following participation in a 10-week (45 hours) physical therapy intervention. Another study reported a 27% decrease in pain catastrophizing scores following a 4-week (100 hours) functional restoration exercise programme (Sullivan et al. 2008a). Smeets et al. (Smeets et al. 2006) reported no significant difference in the magnitude of reduction in pain catastrophizing scores for patients who participated in active physiotherapy (−12%), problem-solving therapy (−10%) or combined treatment (−10%). In the latter study, each treatment programme consisted of approximately 11 hours of intervention.

The research conducted to date suggests that catastrophic thinking associated with pain can be reduced through a variety of means. However, some degree of caution must be exercised in the interpretation of the results of the studies described above. Studies vary in terms of the nature of the population being treated (recent onset versus long term disability; low back pain versus whiplash), the intensity of treatment (10–100 hours), the insurance context within which clients are treated (no fault versus tort), and the objectives of the intervention (pain management, functional improvement, or return to work). Initial values (high versus low) on measures of pain catastrophizing will play a role in determining the magnitude of reductions that will be observed and the relation between reductions in pain catastrophizing and clinical outcomes. In a related manner, there is currently limited information about the magnitude of reduction in pain catastrophizing scores that is required to impact in a clinically meaningful manner on pain outcomes.

Education, activity resumption and instruction in self-management skills characterize the content of most multidisciplinary programmes for the management of chronic pain

(Gatchel et al. 2007). It is not unreasonable to assume that each of these elements might impact directly or indirectly on catastrophic thinking. As noted earlier, catastrophizing has been discussed as a multidimensional construct comprising rumination, magnification and helplessness. Intervention techniques that impact on any of these dimensions might yield therapeutic benefit. Education might permit individuals to re-evaluate or re-appraise the degree of threat they associate with their condition or their participation in activity (Moseley 2004; Turk 2004). Participation in exercise or other physical activity might yield benefit by reducing the cognitive resources that can be allocated to catastrophic thinking. Activity participation and instruction in self-management skills might increase self-efficacy and, in turn, reduce the helplessness dimension of catastrophizing.

In recent years, targeted treatments have been designed specifically to reduce catastrophic thinking (Sullivan et al. 2006a; Thorn et al. 2002). Some of these have taken the form of group interventions using cognitive-behavioural techniques such as thought monitoring, cognitive re-structuring and re-appraisal (Thorn et al. 2002). Other interventions have taken the form of individual treatment where behavioural activation and life role resumption are used to augment the impact of cognitive-behavioural techniques for pain-related disability (Sullivan et al. 2006a). To date, limited evidence is available to address whether these targeted interventions have added value for reducing levels of catastrophic thinking.

Research reviewed in this chapter suggests additional avenues that might be considered in efforts to reduce catastrophic thinking. The research suggests that intervention techniques specifically targeting expectancies and attention might augment the impact of treatment programmes for chronic pain. However, expectancies and attention are broad constructs and might represent the final common pathways of numerous psychological processes. Indeed, it is difficult to point to intervention dimensions that will not in some way influence expectancies or attention. The challenge for future research appears to be the development of interventions that will yield reductions in catastrophic thinking of sufficient magnitude to have a meaningful impact on pain and rehabilitation outcomes.

There is a basis for suggesting that activity-based interventions targeting catastrophic thinking might have advantages over strictly cognitive approaches to reducing catastrophic thinking. The literature on disengagement deficits suggests that high pain catastrophizers might be limited in their ability to make effective use of cognitive techniques that might require disengagement such as distraction or cognitive-restructuring. Activity-based interventions might be useful in reducing the frequency of catastrophic thinking without appealing to disengagement abilities. The impoverished stimulus environment that characterizes sedentary or passive activities might leave the cognitive content of the high catastrophizer saturated with negative or pessimistic thoughts. Since activity participation requires some degree of cognitive resource investment, activity participation might result in fewer attentional resources devoted to catastrophic thinking, without having to rely on attentional disengagement abilities.

The research that has been cited in support of the Communal Coping Model of pain catastrophizing suggests that including techniques designed to target interpersonal or communicative aspects of pain might hold promise. Disclosure interventions might play a role in reducing pain severity and as well as reducing pain behaviour (Keefe et al. 2008; Sullivan and Neish 1999). Increased awareness of emotional or attachment needs and the development of more effective communication strategies might reduce reliance on the display of pain behaviour to solicit attention, care or proximity (Cano 2004; Ciechanowski et al. 2003; Gauthier et al. 2008).

The development of more targeted interventions for the reduction of pain catastrophizing might also have implications for the effectiveness of pharmacotherapeutic interventions for pain. As discussed earlier, pain catastrophizing has been shown to interfere with the effectiveness of analgesics. Brief interventions aimed at reducing catastrophic thinking might improve responses to analgesic medication. Such interventions might be particularly important in domains associated with treatment resistance such as neuropathic pain or fibromyalgia. Interventions designed to reduce catastrophic thinking might also prevent the development of chronic pain following surgical interventions (Forsythe et al. 2008).

The research conducted on the neurophysiological correlates of pain catastrophizing raises interesting questions about the bi-directionality of relations between cognitive processes and central mechanisms involved in nociceptive processing. Psychological interventions that yield reductions in catastrophizing might also impact directly or indirectly on activation patterns of brain centres associated with pain perception, and might even modify the functioning of endogenous opioid mechanisms. It follows that interventions that target central mechanisms of pain control might also influence catastrophic thinking.

## 13.6 **Summary**

Over the past two decades pain catastrophizing has emerged as one of the most robust psychological predictors of adverse pain outcomes. Recent research has begun to address the psychological and neurophysiological mechanisms that might underlie the relation between catastrophizing and pain outcomes. There are indications that psychological variables related to expectancies and attention might account, at least in part, for the relation between catastrophizing and pain outcomes. Some research suggests that catastrophic thinking might also impact directly on central mechanisms of pain control. Challenges for the future include the development of more targeted interventions for reducing catastrophic thinking. Future research on the relations between catastrophizing and central mechanisms of pain control might have implications for theoretical models that address the linkages between psychology and physiology in the modulation of pain experience.

## References

Adams, H., Ellis, T., Stanish, W. D., *et al.* Psychosocial factors related to return to work following rehabilitation of whiplash injuries. *J Occup Rehabil* (2007) **17**(2):305–15.

Apkarian, A. V., Bushnell, M. C., Treede, R. D., *et al.* Human brain mechanisms of pain perception and regulation in health and disease. *Eur J Pain* (2005) **9**(4):463–84.

Arntz, A., Dreesen, L., and Merckelbach, H. Attention, not anxiety, influences pain. *Behav Res Ther* (1991) **29**:41–50.

Asghari, A., and Nicholas, M. K. Pain self-efficacy beliefs and pain behavior: A prospective study. *Pain* (2001) **94**:85–100.

Bandura, A. *Self-Efficacy: The Exercise of Control.* New York: W.H. Freeman, 1977.

Bandura, A., O'Leary, A., Taylor, C. B., *et al.* Perceived self-efficacy and pain control: Opioid and nonopioid mechanims. *Journal of Personality and Social Psychology* (1987) **53**:563–71.

Banks, S., and Kerns, R. Explaining high rates of depression in chronic pain: A diathesis-stress formulation. *Psychological Bulletin* (1996) **119**:95–110.

Bartley, E. J., and Rhudy, J. L. The influence of pain catastrophizing on experimentally induced emotion and emotional modulation of nociception. *J Pain* (2008) **9**(5):388–96.

Beck, A. T., Rush, A. J., Shaw, B. F., *et al. Cognitive Therapy for Depression.* New York: Guilford, 1978.

Boothy, J., Thorn, B., Overduin, L., *et al.* Catastrophizing and perceived partner responses to pain. *Pain* (2004) **109**:500–506.

Borsbo, B., Peolsson, M., and Gerdle, B. Catastrophizing, depression, and pain: correlation with and influence on quality of life and health - a study of chronic whiplash-associated disorders. *J Rehabil Med* (2008) **40**(7):562–9.

Bushnell, M. C., Villemure, C., and Duncan, G. H. Psychophysical and neurophysiological studies of pain modulation by attention. In D. D. P. a. M. C. Bushnell., ed., *Psychological methods of pain control: Basic science and clinical perspectives.* IASP Press., 2004.

Cano, A. Pain catastrophizing and social support in married individuals with chronic pain: The moderating role of pain duration. *Pain* (2004) **110**:656–64.

Carroll, L. J., Cassidy, J. D., and Cote, P. Depression as a risk factor for onset of an episode of troublesome neck and low back pain. *Pain* (2004) **107**(1–2):134–9.

Carter, L. E., McNeil, D. W., Vowles, K. E., *et al.* Effects of emotion of pain reprots, tolerance and physiology. *Pain Res Manag* (2002) **7**:21–30.

Ciechanowski, P., Sullivan, M., Jensen, M., *et al.* The relationship of attachment style to depression, catastrophizing and health care utilization in patients with chronic pain. *Pain* (2003) **104**(3):627–37.

Coyne, J., and Fiske, V. Couples coping with chronic illness. In T. Akamatsu, J. Crowther, S. Hobfoll, et al. (eds.), *Family Health Psychology*, pp. 129–49. Washington DC: Hemisphere, 1992.

Craig, K. Emotional aspects of pain. In R. Melzack and P. Wall (eds.), *Textbook of Pain*, pp. 220–30. Edinburgh: Churchill Livingstone, 1989.

Crombez, G., Eccleston, C., Van den Broeck, A., *et al.* Hypervigilance to pain in fibromyalgia: the mediating role of pain intensity and catastrophic thinking about pain. *Clin J Pain* (2004) **20**(2):98–102.

Crombez, G., Eccleston, C., Vlaeyen, J. W., *et al.* Exposure to physical movements in low back pain patients: restricted effects of generalization. *Health Psychol* (2002) **21**(6):573–8.

Crombez, G., Vervaet, L., Baeyens, F., *et al.* Do pain expectancies cause pain in chronic low back patients? A clinical investigation. *Behav Res Ther* (1996) **34**(11–12):919–25.

Derbyshire, S. W. G., Jones, A. K., Gyulai, F., *et al.* Pain processing during three levels of noxious stimulation produces differential patterns of central activity. *Pain* (1997) **73**:431–45.

Devoulyte, K., and Sullivan, M. J. Pain catastrophizing and symptom severity during upper respiratory tract illness. *Clinical Journal of Pain* (2003) **19**(2):125–33.

Drahovzal, D. N., Stewart, S. H., and Sullivan, M. J. Tendency to catastrophize somatic sensations: pain catastrophizing and anxiety sensitivity in predicting headache. *Cogn Behav Ther* (2006) **35**(4):226–35.

Eccleston, C., and Crombez, G. Pain demands attention: a cognitive-affective model of the interruptive function of pain. *Psychol Bull* (1999) **125**(3):356–66.

Edwards, R. R., Bingham, C. O., 3rd, Bathon, J., *et al.* Catastrophizing and pain in arthritis, fibromyalgia, and other rheumatic diseases. *Arthritis Rheum* (2006a) **55**(2):325–32.

Edwards, R. R., and Fillingim, R. B. Effects of age on temporal summation and habituation of thermal pain: clinical relevance in health older and yonger adults. *J Pain* (2001) **2**:307–317.

Edwards, R. R., Smith, M. T., Kudel, I., *et al.* Pain-related catastrophizing as a risk factor for suicidal ideation in chronic pain. *Pain* (2006b) **126**(1–3):272–9.

Edwards, R. R., Smith, M. T., Stonerock, G., *et al.* Pain-related catastrophizing in healthy women is associated with greater temporal summation of and reduced habituation to thermal pain. *Clin J Pain* (2006c) **22**(8):730–7.

Fillingim, R. B., Hastie, B. A., Ness, T. J., *et al.* Sex-related psychological predictors of baseline pain perception and analgesic responses to pentazocine. *Biol Psychol* (2005) **69**(1):97–112.

Forsythe, M. E., Dunbar, M. J., Hennigar, A. W., *et al.* Prospective relation between catastrophizing and residual pain following knee arthroplasty: two-year follow-up. *Pain Res Manag* (2008) **13**(4):335–41.

Gatchel, R., Peng, Y. B., Peters, M. L., *et al.* The biopsychosocial approach to chronic pain: Scientific advances and future directions. *Psychol Bull* (2007) **133**:581–624.

Gauthier, N., Thibault, P., and Sullivan, M. J. Individual and relational correlates of pain-related empathic accuracy in spouses of chronic pain patients. *Clin J Pain* (2008) **24**(8):669–77.

Geisser, M. E., Robinson, M. E., Keefe, F. J., *et al.* Catastrophizing, depression and the sensory, affective and evaluative aspects of chronic pain. *Pain* (1995) **59**:79–83.

George, S. Z., Wittmer, V. T., Fillingim, R. B., *et al*. Fear-avoidance beliefs and temporal summation of evoked thermal pain influence self-report of disability in patients with chronic low back pain. *J Occup Rehabil* (2006) **16**(1):95–108.

Giardino, N., Jensen, M., Turner, J., *et al*. Social environment moderates the association between catastrophizing and pain among persons with a spinal cord injury. *Pain* (2003) **106**:19–25.

Goodin, B. R., McGuire, L., Allshouse, M., *et al*. Associations between catastrophizing and endogenous pain-inhibitory processes: sex differences. *J Pain* (2008) **10**:180–90.

Gracely, R. H., Geisser, M. E., Giesecke, T., *et al*. Pain catastrophizing and neural responses to pain among persons with fibromyagia. *Brain* (2004) **127**:835–43.

Haythornthwaite, J., Clark, M., Pappagallo, M., *et al*. Pain coping strategies play a role in the persistence of pain in post-herpetic neuralgia. *Pain* (2003) **106**:453–60.

Heyneman, N. E., Fremouw, W. J., Gano, D., *et al*. Individual differences and the effectiveness of different coping strategies for pain. *Cog Ther Res* (1990) **14**:63–77.

Jacobsen, P. B., and Butler, R. W. Relation of cognitive coping and catastrophizing to acute pain and analgesic use following breast cancer surgery. *Journal of Behavioral Medicine* (1996) **19**(1):17–29.

Jensen, M. P., Turner, J. A., and Romano, J. M. Self-efficacy and outcome expectancies: relationship to chronic pain coping strategies and adjustment. *Pain* (1991a) **44**(3):263–9.

Jensen, M. P., Turner, J. A., and Romano, J. M. Changes in beliefs, catastrophizing, and coping are associated with improvement in multidisciplinary pain treatment. *Journal of Consulting and Clinical Psychology* (2001) **69**:655 662.

Jensen, M. P., Turner, J. A., Romano, J. M., *et al*. Coping with chronic pain: a critical review of the literature. *Pain* (1991b) **47**(3):249–83.

Keefe, F., Lefebvre, J., and Smith, S. Catastrophizing research: Avoiding conceptual errors and maintaining a balnaced perspective. *Pain Forum* (1999) **8**:176–80.

Keefe, F., Lipkus, I., Lefebvre, J., *et al*. The social contex of gastrointestinal cancer pain: A preliminary study examining the relation of patient pain catastrophizing to patient perceptions of social support and caregiver stress and negative responses. *Pain* (2003) **103**:151–56.

Keefe, F., Rumble, M., Scipio, C., *et al*. Psychological aspects of persistent pain: Current state of the science. *Journal of Pain* (2004) **5**:195–211.

Keefe, F. J., Abernethy, A. P., and Campbell, L. C. Psychological approaches to understanding and treating disease-related pain. . *Annual Review of Psychology* (2005) **56**:601–30.

Keefe, F. J., Anderson, T., Lumley, M., *et al*. A randomized, controlled trial of emotional disclosure in rheumatoid arthritis: can clinician assistance enhance the effects? *Pain* (2008) **137**(1):164–72.

Keefe, F. J., Brown, G. K., Wallston, K. A., *et al*. Coping with rheumatoid arthritis pain: catastrophizing as a maladaptive strategy. *Pain* (1989) **37**(1):51–6.

Keefe, F. J., Kashikar-Zuck, S., Robinson, E., *et al*. Pain coping strategies that predict patients' and spouses' ratings of patients' self-efficacy. *Pain* (1997a) **73**(2):191–9.

Keefe, F. J., Lefebvre, J. C., Egert, J. R., *et al*. The relationship of gender to pain, pain behavior, and disability in osteoarthritis patients: the role of catastrophizing. *Pain* (2000) **87**(3):325–34.

Keefe, F. J., Lefebvre, J. C., Maixner, W., *et al*. Self-efficacy for arthritis pain: relationship to perception of thermal laboratory pain stimuli. *Arth Care Res* (1997b) **10**(3):177–84.

Kirsch, I. Response expectancy as a determinant of experience and behavior. *Am Psychol* (1985) **40**:1189–1202.

Lacker, J. M., Carosella, A. M., and Feuerstein, M. Pain expectancies, pain, and functional self-efficacy expectancies as determinants of disability in patients with chronic low back disorders. *J Consult Clin Psychol* (1996) **64**(1):212–20.

Lackner, J., and Gurtman, M. Pain catastrophizing and interpersonal problems: A circumplex analysis of the communal coping model. *Pain* (2004) **110**:597–604.

Lackner, J. M., and Quigley, B. M. Pain catastrophizing mediates the relationship between worry and pain suffering in patients with irritable bowel syndrome. *Behav Res Ther* (2005) **43**:943–57.

Lazarus, R., **and** Folkman, S. *Stress, appraisal and coping.* New York: Springer, 1984.

Leeuw, M., Goossens, M. E., Linton, S. J., *et al.* The fear-avoidance model of musculoskeletal pain: current state of scientific evidence. *J Behav Med* (2007) **30**(1):77–94.

Lyons, R., Sullivan, M., Ritvo, P., *et al. Relationships in Illness and Disability.* Sage, 1995.

McCracken, L. M. 'Attention' to pain in persons with chronic pain: a behavioral approach. *Behav Ther* (1997) **28**:271–84.

Meagher, M. W., Arnau, R. C., and Rhudy, J. L. Pain and emotion: effects of affective picture modulation. *Psychosom Med* (2001) **63**:79–90.

Milling, L. S., Reardon, J. M., and Carosella, G. M. Mediation and moderation of psychological pain treatments: response expectancies and hypnotic suggestibility. *J Consult Clin Psychol* (2006) **74**(2):253–62.

Milling, L. S., Shores, J. S., Coursen, E. L., *et al.* Response expectancies, treatment credibility, and hypnotic suggestibility: mediator and moderator effects in hypnotic and cognitive-behavioral pain interventions. *Ann Behav Med* (2007) **33**(2):167–78.

Moseley, G. L. Evidence for a direct relationship between cognitive and physical change during an education intervention in people with chronic low back pain. *Eur J Pain* (2004) **8**:39–45.

Peyron, R., Laurent, B., and Garcia-Larrea, L. Functional imaging of brain responses to pain. A review and meta-analysis (2000). *Neurophysiol Clin* (2000) **30**(5):263–88.

Phillips, M. L., Gregory, L. J., Cullen, S., *et al.* The effect of negative emotional context on neural and behavioural responses to oesophageal stimulation. *Brain* (2003) **126**(Pt 3):669–84.

Ploghaus, A., Becerra, L., Borras, C., *et al.* Neural circuitry underlying pain modulation: expectation, hypnosis, placebo. *Trends in Cog Sci* (2003) **7**:197–200.

Ploghaus, A., Narain, C., Beckmann, C. F., *et al.* Exacerbation of pain by anxiety is associated with activity in a hippocampal network. *J Neurosci* (2001) **21**(24):9896–903.

Ploghaus, A., Tracey, I., Gati, S., *et al.* Dissociating pain from its anticipation in the human brain. *Science* (1999) **284**:1979–81.

Pollo, A., Amanzio, M., Arslanian, A., *et al.* Response expectancies in placebo analgesia and their clinical relevance. *Pain* (2001) **93**(1):77–84.

Price, D. D., Staud, R., Robinson, M. E., *et al.* Enhanced temporal summation of second pain and its central modulation in fibromyalgia patients. *Pain* (2002) **99**(1–2):49–59.

Romano, J., Turner, J., Jensen, M., *et al.* Chronic pain patient-spouse interactions predict patient disability. *Pain* (1995) **65**:353–60.

Rudy, T., Kerns, R., and Turk, D. Chronic pain and depression: Toward a cognitive-behavioral mediation model. *Pain* (1988) **35**:129–40.

Schwarz, B. E. Pain and emotion. *J Med Soc N J* (1962) **59**:517.

Schweinhardt, P., Kalk, N., Wartolowska, K., *et al.* Investigation into the neural correlates of emotional augmentation of clinical pain. *Neuroimage* (2008) **40**(2):759–66.

Seminowicz, D. A., and Davis, K. D. Cortical responses to pain in healthy individuals depends on pain catastrophizing. *Pain* (2006) **120**(3):297–306.

Severeijns, R., Vlaeyen, J., and van den Hout, M. Do we need a communal coping model of pain catastrophizing? An alternative explanation. *Pain* (2004) **111**:226–29.

Shelby, R. A., Somers, T. J., Keefe, F. J., *et al.* Domain specific self-efficacy mediates the impact of pain catastrophizing on pain and disability in overweight and obese osteoarthritis patients. *J Pain* (2008) **9**(10):912–19.

Smeets, R. J., Vlaeyen, J. W., Kester, A. D., *et al.* **Reduction** of pain catastrophizing mediates the outcome of both physical and cognitive-behavioral treatment in chronic low back pain. *J Pain* (2006) **7**(4):261–71.

Smith, B. W., and Zautra, A. J. The effects of anxiety and depression on weekly pain in women with arthritis. *Pain* (2008) **138**:354–61.

Spanos, N. P., Radtke-Bodorik, H. L., Ferguson, J. D., *et al.* The effects of hypnotic susceptibility, suggestions for analgesia, and utilization of cognitive strategies on the reduction of pain. *Journal of Abnormal Psychology* (1979) **88**:282–92.

Spinhoven, P., Ter Kuile, M., Kole-Snijders, A. M., *et al.* Catastrophizing and internal pain control as mediators of outcome in the multidisciplinary treatment of chronic low back pain. *European Journal of Pain* (2004) **8**(3):211–9.

Sullivan, M., Bishop, S., and Pivik, J. The Pain Catastrophizing Scale: Development and validation. *Psychological Assessment* (1995) **7**:524–32.

Sullivan, M., Feuerstein, M., Gatchel, R. J., *et al.* Integrating psychological and behavioral interventions to achieve optimal rehabilitation outcomes. *J Occ Rehab* (2005a) **15**:475–89.

Sullivan, M. J., and Neish, N. The effects of disclosure on pain during dental hygiene treatment: the moderating role of catastrophizing. *Pain* (1999) **79**(2–3):155–63.

Sullivan, M. J. L. Toward a biopsychomotor conceptualisation of pain. *Clin J Pain* (2008) **24**:281–90.

Sullivan, M. J. L., Adams, A., Horan, S., *et al.* The role of perceived injustice in the experience of chronic pain and disability: Scale development and validation. *J Occ Rehab* (2008a) **18**:249–61.

Sullivan, M. J. L., Adams, A., Rhodenizer, T., *et al.* A psychosocial risk factor targeted intervention for the prevention of chronic pain and disability following whiplash injury. *Phys Ther* (2006a) **86**:8–18.

Sullivan, M. J. L., Adams, H., Rhodenizer, T., *et al.* A psychosocial risk factor—targeted intervention for the prevention of chronic pain and disability following whiplash injury. *Phys Ther* (2006b) **86**(1):8–18.

Sullivan, M. J. L., Adams, H., and Sullivan, M. E. Communicative dimensions of pain catastrophizing: social cueing effects on pain behaviour and coping. *Pain* (2004) **107**(3):220–6.

Sullivan, M. J. L., and D'Eon, J. L. Relation between catastrophizing and depression in chronic pain patients. *Journal of Abnormal Psychology* (1990) **99**(3):260–3.

Sullivan, M. J. L., Lynch, M. E., Clark, A. J., *et al.* Catastrophizing and treatment outcome: Impact on response to placebo and active treatment outcome. . *Contemporary Hypnosis* (2008b) **29**:129–40.

Sullivan, M. J. L., Martel, M. O., Tripp, D., *et al.* The relation between catastrophizing and the communication of pain experience. *Pain* (2006c) **122**(3):282–8.

Sullivan, M. J. L., and Neish, N. R. Catastrophizing, anxiety and pain during dental hygiene treatment. *Community Dentistry and Oral Epidemiology* (1998) **26**(5):344–9.

Sullivan, M. J. L., Rodgers, W. M., and Kirsch, I. Catastrophizing, depression and expectancies for pain and emotional distress. *Pain* (2001a) **91**:147–54.

Sullivan, M. J. L., Rouse, D., Bishop, S. R., *et al.* Thought suppression, catastrophizing and pain. *Cog Ther Res* (1997) **21**:555–68.

Sullivan, M. J. L., Stanish, W., Waite, H., *et al.* Catastrophizing, pain, and disability in patients with soft-tissue injuries. *Pain* (1998) **77**(3):253–60.

Sullivan, M. J. L., and Stanish, W. D. Psychologically based occupational rehabilitation: the Pain-Disability Prevention Program. *Clin J Pain* (2003) **19**(2):97–104.

Sullivan, M. J. L., Thorn, B., Haythornthwaite, J. A., *et al.* Theoretical perspectives on the relation between catastrophizing and pain. *Clin J Pain* (2001b) **17**(1):52–64.

Sullivan, M. J. L., Tripp, D., and Santor, D. Gender differences in pain and pain behavior: The role of catastrophizing. *Cog Ther Res* (2000) **24**:121–34.

Sullivan, M. J. L., Ward, L. C., Tripp, D., *et al.* Secondary prevention of work disability: community-based psychosocial intervention for musculoskeletal disorders. *J Occup Rehabil* (2005b) **15**(3):377–92.

Tang, N. K., Salkovskis, P. M., Hodges, A., *et al.* Effects of mood on pain responses and pain tolerance: an experimental study in chronic back pain patients. *Pain* (2008) **138**(2):392–401.

Taylor, S. Biobehavioral responses to stress in females: Tend-and befriend, not fight-or-flight. *Psychological Review* (2000) **107**:411–29.

Thibault, P., Loisel, P., Durand, M. J., *et al.* Psychological predictors of pain expression and activity intolerance in chronic pain patients. . *Pain* (2008) **139**:47–54.

**Thorn, B., Boothy, J., and Sullivan, M.** Targeted treatment of catastrophizing for the management of chronic pain. *Cognitive Behavior Practice* (2002) **9**:127–38.

**Thorn, B. E., Pence, L. B., Ward, L. C.,** *et al.* A randomized clinical trial of targeted cognitive behavioral treatment to reduce catastrophizing in chronic headache sufferers. *J Pain* (2007) **8**(12):938–49.

**Thorn, B. E., Ward, L. C., Sullivan, M. J.,** *et al.* Communal coping model of catastrophizing: conceptual model building. *Pain* (2003) **106**(1–2):1–2.

**Tracey, I., and Mantyh, P. W.** The cerebral signature for pain perception and its modulation. *Neuron* (2007) **55**(3):377–91.

**Turk, D.** Biopsychosocial perspective on chronic pain. In R. Gatchel and D. Turk (eds.), *Psychological Approaches to Pain Management*, pp. 138–58. New York: Guilford, 1996.

**Turk, D., Meichenbaum, D., and Genest, M.** *Pain and Behavioral Medicine: A Cognitive-Behavioral Perspective.* New York: Guilford, 1983.

**Turk, D., and Okifuji, A.** Psychological factors in chronic pain: Evolution and revolution. *Journal of Consulting and Clinical Psychology* (2002) **70**:678–90.

**Turk, D. C.** Understanding pain sufferers: the role of cognitive processes. *The Spine J* (2004) **4**:1–7.

**Turner, J., and Aaron, L.** Pain-related catastrophizing: What is it? *Clinical Journal of Pain* (2001) **17**:65–71.

**Van Damme, S., Crombez, G., and Eccleston, C.** Retarded disengagement from pain cues: the effects of pain catastrophizing and pain expectancy. *Pain* (2002) **100**(1–2):111–18.

**Van Damme, S., Crombez, G., and Eccleston, C.** Disengagement from pain: the role of catastrophic thinking about pain. *Pain* (2004) **107**(1–2):70–6.

**Vervoort, T., Goubert, L., Eccleston, C.,** *et al.* The effects of parental presence upon the facial expression of pain: the moderating role of child pain catastrophizing. *Pain* (2008) **138**(2):277–85.

**Vlaeyen, J. W., Kole-Snijders, A. M., Boeren, R. G.,** *et al.* Fear of movement/(re)injury in chronic low back pain and its relation to behavioral performance. *Pain* (1995) **62**(3):363–72.

**Vlaeyen, J. W., and Linton, S. J.** Fear-avoidance and its consequences in chronic musculoskeletal pain: a state of the art. *Pain* (2000) **85**(3):317–32.

**Weissman-Fogel, I., Sprecher, E., and Pud, D.** Effects of catastrophizing on pain perception and pain modulation. *Exp Brain Res* (2008) **186**(1):79–85.

**Whalley, B., Hyland, M. E., and Kirsch, I.** Consistency of the placebo effect. *J Psychosom Res* (2008) **64**(5):537–41.

**Wolff, B., Burns, J. W., Quartana, P. J.,** *et al.* Pain catastrophizing, physiological indexes, and chronic pain severity: tests of mediation and moderation models. *J Behav Med* (2008) **31**(2):105–14.

# Chapter 14

# Fear-Avoidance as a Risk Factor for the Development of Chronic Back Pain and Disability

Linda Vancleef, Ida Flink, Steven J. Linton, and Johan Vlaeyen

## 14.1 Introduction

Chronic musculoskeletal pain syndromes are responsible for enormous costs for healthcare and society (Linton 1998; Phillips et al. 2008; Picavet and Schouten 2003; Verhaak et al. 1998). Nowadays, the biopsychosocial perspective on pain offers a good foundation for a better insight into how pain can become a persistent problem (Fordyce 1976; Turk and Flor 1999). In this perspective, pain and pain disability are influenced by the dynamic interaction among biological, psychological, and social factors.

The present chapter focuses on the role of fear and avoidance in the development and maintenance of chronic low back pain (CLBP). In the following paragraphs, an overview on the aetiology of low back pain (LBP), the conceptualization of fear and avoidance, and the development of fear-avoidance models will be provided. Furthermore, empirical evidence on the role of fear and avoidance behaviour in chronic pain, stemming from studies conducted in pain patients and in healthy volunteers, will be reviewed. This chapter will then continue with a discussion on how to assess fear of pain both at a direct and indirect level. Finally, this chapter will end with perspectives on the cognitive-behavioural management of chronic pain in patients who are characterized by increased pain-related fear and avoidance behaviour.

### 14.1.1 Chronic low back pain

LBP is one of the most prevalent complaints in the musculoskeletal apparatus. LBP refers to pain in the area of the lower back that often radiates to the buttocks or the legs. Recent reviews indicated that about 60–90% of the general population report to have experienced complaints in the lower back at some point throughout the course of their lives (Picavet and Schouten 2003). Population-based studies estimate the lifetime prevalence of LBP between 60–80% (Nachemson et al. 2000; Walker 2000). A study in the Belgian population showed that 41.8% of the respondents indicated to have experienced LBP for at least one day in the past period of 6 months. Moreover, 8.2% of this group reported that the pain in their lower back was seriously impeding daily functioning (Goubert et al. 2004a). These figures are comparable to other Western countries (e.g. Schmidt et al. 2007; Walker et al. 2004).

Only in a minority of people with LBP specific causes such as nerve injury, fractures, inflammation or malign disease are found to be responsible for the pain (Waddell 2004). In most cases the pain is denoted as non-specific, meaning that no specific biomedical cause can be found for LBP. For the majority of back pain patients who seek care and refrain from work, the problem of pain resolves within a few weeks. These patients return to work and resume their daily activities within 4–6 weeks after the onset of the complaints. However, there is a small subgroup of patients (5–10% of the total population), in whom back pain persists for longer than 3 months, and who develop a chronic pain problem (Waddell 2004). Ironically, this relatively small group of back pain patients is responsible for the largest amount of healthcare and societal costs of back problems (Phillips et al. 2008; Waddell 2004). In addition, chronic pain is known to have an enormous impact on the personal and social relations of these chronic back pain patients (Sullivan et al. 2004; Morley and Eccleston 2004).

### 14.1.2 **General explanatory models**

Throughout time, several explanatory models have been put forward to explain why a small group of back pain patients become chronic pain sufferers. Biomedically oriented specialists have suggested that these patients have more serious impairments than those who resume daily activities earlier. However, no research supports this assumption. On the contrary, numerous studies have shown that there is no perfect relationship between impairment, pain, and disability. Patients with back problems often show no physical injury, and conversely, it happens that persons who do show physical injury do not report pain or disability (e.g. Jensen et al. 1994). The biomedical perspective that any pain is the result of structural and biomechanical abnormalities can also not account for phantom limb pain, where pain is experienced in missing body parts (Giummarra et al. 2007) or for the large interindividual differences that exist in the way persons experience, respond to, and cope with pain.

A biopsychosocial approach offers a better insight into how pain can become a persistent problem (Turk and Flor 1999; Waddell 2004). According to this approach, pain and pain disability are not only influenced by organic pathology, if present, but also by psychological and social factors. The interrelationship between the biological, psychological, and social factors, as well as their influence on the pain experience can be complex. As such, small content overlap does exist between the various factors, but different processes are assumed in each individual component of the model (Turk and Gatchel 2002; Waddel 2004). For example, processes and factors that influence the biomedical aspects of pain, like an injury, are different from those that influence the daily functioning of individuals in pain, like the affective evaluation of the sensory experience. In this multidimensional approach to pain, pain is conceived as a unique experience that can have divergent outcomes in terms of illness, disability and suffering. The major benefit of the biopsychosocial model concerns its flexibility in allowing a broad variety of factors to influence and determine each individual pain experience. On the other hand, the biopsychosocial model is conceived as a theoretical conceptualization only and does not possess explanatory power for the way in which biological, psychological, and social processes exert their influence on chronic pain. Under the biopsychosocial umbrella, several specific explanatory models have been developed that aim to clarify the role of specific factors in pain. Explanatory models on fear of pain are rooted in one of the most robust explanatory models in psychology, namely conditioning theory. Fear conditioning theories possess the power to explain why fears can exist and become chronic, even when the source of threat is not apparent.

## 14.2 **Fear and avoidance**

Fear and avoidance are central concepts to contemporary views on pain development and treatment.

*Fear* is generally conceived as a basic or pure emotion that represents a present-oriented state, an emotional reaction that is directed at an identifiable, concrete stimulus (Izard 1992;

Rachmann 2004). From an evolutionary perspective, fear serves to protect the individual from immediate threat. However, because fears can be both rational and irrational, fear responses can occur for either accurately or inaccurately perceived dangers. It is important to note at this point that fear cannot be equated to anxiety, although both terms are often used interchangeably. In contrast to fear, anxiety is a future-oriented state that is more diffuse, unfocussed, and less controllable than fear.

What pain patients are afraid of and what is thus seen as the object of fear in pain has been divided into three areas; fear of pain sensations (i.e. the pain itself), fear of pain-causing activities and fear of movement and (re)injury (Vlaeyen and Linton 2000). Other authors have emphasized that also more general aspects, such as threats to life-goals and identity, might be objects of fear in pain patients (Morley and Eccleston 2004). Fear of pain encompasses cognitive, physiologic, as well as motor processes Studies have demonstrated correlations between fear of pain and measures of anxiety, cognitive errors, depression, and disability (McCracken et al. 1992, 1996). CLBP patients may fear not only pain, but also activities that are expected to cause pain. In this case, fear is hypothesized to generalize to other situations that are closely linked to the feared stimulus. A specific fear is fear of movement and physical activity that is (wrongfully) assumed to cause (re) injury. Kori et al. (1990) introduced the term 'kinesiophobia' (kinesis=movement) for the condition in which a patient has 'an excessive, irrational, and debilitating fear of physical movement and activity resulting from a feeling of vulnerability to painful injury or re-injury'.

*Avoidance* refers to the performance (or withdrawal) of a behaviour so that an undesirable experience or situation is delayed or put off. Although in the case of chronic pain it is not possible to avoid the pain itself, activities that might increase pain or cause (re)injury can be avoided. Therefore, the suboptimal performance of activities is often taken as an index of avoidance behaviour in pain patients.

### 14.2.1 **Fear-avoidance learning**

Relying on both *classical* and *operant* conditioning principles, the two-factor theory by Mowrer (1947) has been an influential theory in explaining fear-avoidance acquisition. According to this theory, classical conditioning accounts for the acquisition of fear responses to aversive stimuli through learning of associations between stimuli. Neutral stimuli that are associated with unconditioned aversive stimuli (US) develop fearful qualities and become conditioned fear stimuli (CS). The likelihood of fear development is increased by exposure to high-intensity pain and/or fear situations, and by frequent repetitions of the association between the new conditioned stimulus and the pain/fear. Once objects or situations have acquired fear provoking qualities, they develop motivating properties and elicit conditioned (defensive) responses, including escape, avoidance, and safety seeking behaviours. For example, using a differential classical conditioning paradigm with visual cues as CS and electric shock as the US, Bradley et al. (2008) found that individuals responded with greater defensive reactivity in the context of threat cues (CS+) as compared to safe cues (CS−) which were never associated with the US. The operant conditioning component of the two factor theory describes how defensive responses (e.g. avoidance) become persistent through learning of associations between behaviour and its consequences. The reduction of fear that is invoked by these responses serves as their negative reinforcement. Although Mowrer's two-factor theory has been very influential in the fear-avoidance literature, it is troubled by a number of shortcomings. For example, it can not explain the persistence of avoidance behaviour when the aversive stimulus has been withdrawn for a repeated number of times. Following conditioning principles, the absence of repeated unpleasant experiences should lead to the extinction of acquired avoidance behaviour. Furthermore, the basic premise of the theory that *all* fears are acquired by classical conditioning cannot be sustained, since several instances are known in which persons develop fears for stimuli they have never encountered before (e.g. fear of snakes).

Fordyce et al. (1982) described how pain behaviour might result from avoidance learning. In the case of pain, a patient may no longer perform certain activities because he or she anticipates that these activities will increase pain and suffering. In the acute phase, avoidance behaviours such as resting, limping, or the use of supportive equipment are effective in reducing suffering from nociception. Later on, these protective pain and illness behaviours may persist in anticipation of pain, instead as of a response to it. Long-lasting avoidance of motor activities may lead to detrimental consequences, both physically (loss of mobility, muscle strength, and fitness, possibly resulting in the 'disuse syndrome') (Bortz 1984), and psychologically (loss of self-esteem, depression, and somatic preoccupation).

Although classical and operant learning principles are important mechanisms in the development of fear and avoidance behaviour, it seems likely that besides learning principles, other processes are important in fear-avoidance acquisition as well. Favouring a cognitive theory of avoidance learning, Philips (1987) takes the view that avoidance is influenced by the *expectancy* that further exposure to certain stimuli will promote pain and suffering. This expectancy is assumed to be based on previous aversive experiences in the same or similar situations. Since the avoidance behaviour displayed by pain patients and by patients with phobias shows large similarities, Philips suggested that, 'chronic pain and chronic fear—both aversive experiences which result in avoidance behaviour—may share important characteristics' (Philips 1987, p. 277). Several studies have focussed on the relationship between fear/anxiety and chronic pain, of which the object of fear has been fear of pain (Lethem et al. 1983), fear of work-related activities (Waddell 1987), and fear of movement that is assumed to cause (re)injury (Vlaeyen et al. 1995a, 1995b).

Usually, extinction of fear takes place when exposure to the feared stimulus does not lead to the adverse consequences anymore. In the area of pain, Philips was one of the first to argue for the systematic application of graded exposure to produce disconfirmations between expected and the actually experienced pain and harm (Philips 1987). Experimental support for this novel idea was provided by Crombez et al. (1996) in a sample of CLBP patients who were requested to perform four exercises (two with each leg) at maximal force. During each exercise, baseline pain and expected pain before the performance of the movement were recorded as well as the experienced pain during the movement. As predicted, the CLBP patients initially overpredicted pain, but after repeated exposure to the movements the overprediction was readily corrected. These findings were replicated with other movements, including bending forward and straight leg raising (Crombez et al. 2002b; Goubert et al. 2002). However, the later data also showed that these disconfirmations were context dependent. Indeed, when patients were exposed to a different movement, again overpredictions were made as if no exposure to a previous movement had taken place. This restriction of generalization was particularly true for those patients who catastrophically (mis)interpreted the pain. Exposure to the physical activities did not result in a fundamental change in the belief that certain movements are harmful or painful, but rather that the movements involved in the exposure sessions are less harmful or painful than anticipated.

## 14.2.2 Fear-avoidance model of pain

With the introduction of a 'fear-avoidance model of exaggerated pain perception' in 1983, Lethem and colleagues reserved a critical role for fear of pain and avoidance behaviour in the explanation of perpetuating pain complaints in the absence of organic pathology (Lethem et al. 1983). In this model, 'confrontation' and 'avoidance' are postulated as two extreme responses to the fear of pain.

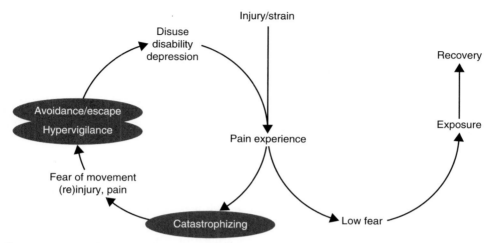

**Fig. 14.1** Fear avoidance model of chronic pain. This figure has been reproduced with permission of the International Association for the Study of Pain® (IASP®). The figure may not be reproduced for any other purpose without permission.

While confrontation will lead to the reduction of fear over time, avoidance leads to the maintenance or exacerbation of fear, possible developing into a phobic-like state. The avoidance results in the reduction of both social and physical activities, which in turn can lead to a number of physical and psychological consequences augmenting the disability.

After the introduction of the fear-avoidance model by Lethem and the emphasis on the role of cognitions in avoidance by Philips, various cognitive-behavioural models of chronic pain have been proposed. These models are commonly referred to as contemporary fear-avoidance models, in which pain disability is conceived as the result of a vicious process that is determined by the interaction between cognitions and behaviour (Asmundson et al. 1999; Vlaeyen et al. 1995b; Waddell et al. 1993). Subtle differences aside, contemporary fear-avoidance models all share the same basic tenets, which can be easily understood from the integrated model that is illustrated in Figure 14.1. Upon the initial perception of pain, individuals assign a certain meaning and purpose to the painful experience that is based upon current expectations regarding the pain and prior learning history. Although the majority of individuals will evaluate the pain experience as undesirable and unpleasant at this stage, most persons will not perceive it as an extreme threat or an insurmountable catastrophe. These individuals will proactively and gradually *confront* their pain, and resume their daily activities, promoting health behaviours and early recovery. However, for a minority of individuals, the painful experiences, which are intensified during movement, will elicit catastrophizing cognitions. These catastrophic cognitions can then lead to pain-related fear (fear of pain, fear of movement, fear of (re)injury), which in its turn initiates the *avoidance* of potential painful activities and hypervigilance for potential signals of additional pain and bodily harm. As such, a vicious and self-perpetuating spiral is activated with avoidance of more and more (daily) activities, leading to functional disability and possibly also to social isolation and depression. In addition, physical deconditioning and depression may fuel the fear-avoidance cycle by increasing pain intensity and increasing the fearful appraisal of and selective attention to pain. In addition to the avoidance of fearful activities, pain disability may also persist because of the immediate consequences to which it leads, such as diminished pain, increased attention from others, and the avoidance of social conflicts or responsibility.

### 14.2.3 Empirical support for the main components of the fear-avoidance model

The fear avoidance model has offered a fruitful framework within which the development and maintenance of persisting pain complaints can be understood. Empirical support for the model has been found within the area of CLBP, osteoarthritis, neck pain, and chronic headache (e.g. Fritz et al. 2001; Leeuw et al. 2007a; Vlaeyen and Linton 2000; Waddell et al. 1993). This paragraph reviews experimental evidence for the main components of the fear-avoidance model.

#### Pain catastrophizing

Pain catastrophizing is conceived as a cognitive construct that represents the tendency to make exaggerated negative or threatening interpretations of pain (Sullivan et al. 1995). Pain catastrophizing has often been found closely related to fear of pain. In addition, a few studies have reported about the predictive value of pain catastrophizing for pain-related fear (Leeuw et al. 2007c; Vlaeyen et al. 1995b; 2004b). Elevated levels of pain-catastrophizing have been consistently found related to pain disability in chronic pain samples, acute pain samples, and pain-free volunteers (Peters et al. 2005; Severeijns et al. 2005; Sullivan et al. 2005; Turner et al. 2004). Furthermore, persons who tend to catastrophize about pain are found to show more hypervigilance for pain-related information, less tolerance for pain, and to report increased pain intensity levels when experiencing pain (Crombez et al. 2002a; Haythornthwaite et al. 2003; Peters et al. 2005; Sullivan et al. 2005; Turner et al. 2002). In prospective studies, pain catastrophizing has been found predictive of elevated pain intensity levels during a painful procedure or after an operation (Edwards et al. 2004; Sullivan et al. 1995; Vlaeyen et al. 2004b). For more detailed information on pain catastrophizing see also Chapter 13.

#### Pain-related fear

The importance of pain-related fear has been demonstrated in chronic and acute pain samples as well as in healthy volunteers possessing elevated levels of pain-related fear (Crombez et al. 1999; Leeuw et al. 2007a; Swinkels-Meewisse et al. 2006; Vlaeyen and Linton 2000). As such, LBP patients who are high in pain-related fear perform less well on behavioural (physical) performance tasks, like a walking test or a lifting task (Al Obaidi et al. 2003; Vlaeyen et al. 1995a; Vlaeyen and Linton 2000; Vowles and Gross 2003). Fear of movement/(re)injury showed to be a stronger predictor for detrimental performance on physical tasks then biomedical symptoms or severity and duration of the pain experience (Vlaeyen and Linton 2000). Furthermore, pain-related fears about work have been found related to disability of daily living and work lost in the past year, more so than to biomedical variables such as the anatomic pattern, the time pattern, or the severity of pain (Fritz et al. 2001; Waddell et al. 1993). In pain-free individuals, elevated levels of pain-related fear have been found associated with increased pain intensity ratings for experimentally induced pain (George et al. 2006; Roelofs et al. 2004b; Hirsh et al. 2008). In a number of prospective studies, pain-related fear proved to be a powerful predictor of disability 6 months or 1 year after acute pain onset (Klenerman et al. 1995; Swinkels-Meewisse et al. 2006; Turner et al. 2006; Vlaeyen et al. 1995b).

#### Avoidance behaviour

In chronic pain research, avoidance behaviour is commonly derived from the suboptimal performance of activities. Several studies have demonstrated that pain patients perform less well on behavioural performance tasks like lifting or walking tasks (Vlaeyen and Linton 2000). In addition, Crombez and colleagues (1999) showed that pain-related fear was associated with escape/avoidance of physical activities, resulting in poor behavioural performance. More recently, a number of studies have provided support for the relation between pain-related fear and avoidance. Al Obaidi and colleagues (2003) demonstrated that pain-related fear was associated with decreased speed in preferred and fast walking. In addition, Geisser and colleagues (2000) and Vowles and Gross (2003) showed diminished performance on physical tasks in high pain-fearful individuals. Supporting the tenets of the fear-avoidance model, there is thus compelling evidence that pain-related fear underlies avoidance behaviours in chronic pain. Nevertheless, it should be noted that a number of studies failed to demonstrate a relationship between fear and avoidance (George et al. 2006; Huis in 't Veld et al. 2007, Michael and Burns 2004). For example, Reneman and colleagues found a weak to no relation at all between pain-related fear and performance of functional activities in a sample of CLBP patients (Reneman et al. 2003; Reneman et al. 2007). In addition, some studies showed conflicting results, in that pain-related fear was associated with task persistence rather than avoidance. Pain-related fear may elicit different behaviours depending on current goal context, and vice versa, outwardly similar behaviours may be driven by different motivational strategies. Such an affective-motivational perspective will probably initiate a next generation of studies addressing new questions including the following: (1) Can higher order goals inhibit the primary goal to protect the integrity of the body by hypervigilance, escape, and avoidance behaviour?; (2) What is the effect of life goal interference and goal conflict on pain-related fear (see e.g. Karsdorp et al. 2010; Van Damme et al. 2008; Vlaeyen and Morley 2004)?

## Hypervigilance and attention

Hypervigilance for pain is defined as the excessive orientation towards pain and pain-related stimuli in both the external and the internal environment. Using Stroop paradigms and dot-probe tasks, a number of studies have provided evidence that pain fearful individuals do show attentional bias towards pain-related information or bodily sensations (Asmundson and Hadjistavropoulos 2007; Keogh et al. 2001; Roelofs et al. 2002, 2003). Furthermore, a series of studies have shown that pain demands attention and disrupts ongoing activities (Crombez et al. 1998a, 2002a; Eccleston and Crombez 1999). This disruptive effect of pain on attention has been demonstrated in pain patients as well as in healthy controls, and is dependent upon the novelty, unpredictability, and intensity of pain (Crombez et al. 1998a). Furthermore, a series of studies showed that pain-fearful patients attend more to pain-threatening signals, are less able to ignore pain-related information, and perform worse on cognitive demanding tasks in comparison to non-fearful patients (Crombez et al. 1998b, 2002a; de Gier et al. 2003; Eccleston et al. 1997; Peters et al. 2002). Supporting the idea that pain vigilance is dependent on pain-related fear, Deghani and colleagues (2004) reported a study in which reductions in pain-related fear account for diminished attentional bias for pain after treatment. In addition, experimental laboratory studies have repeatedly demonstrated the association between elevated levels of pain catastrophizing and deteriorated cognitive task performance under conditions of pain (Crombez et al. 2002a; Van Damme et al. 2002; Vancleef and Peters 2006). Recent evidence has shown that the interruptive effect of pain on attention results from the difficulty to *disengage* attention from pain-related information, rather then from an attentional shift towards pain (Asmundson et al. 2005; Roelofs et al. 2005; Van Damme et al. 2002). This attentional disengagement has been proposed to be enhanced by the anticipation of pain (Van Damme et al. 2004).

## Depression

Although depressed mood is one of the presumed consequences of longstanding avoidance of daily activities, a small number of studies have actually examined depression in relation to pain-related fear. Grotle et al. (2004) found only modest associations between pain-related fear and a measure of distress, both in acute and CLBP patients. Sullivan et al. (2008) examined the effects of a pain rehabilitation program aimed at work resumption on changes in levels of pain and depression. This study revealed that changes in depression were mainly predicted by the level of chronicity, and that this relationship was mediated by pain reduction, and not by changes in pain catastrophizing or fear of movement/re-injury. There is a need for more systematic studies examining the association between pain-related fear and depression.

### Disuse

Frequent and enduring avoidance of daily activities may also result in gradual deterioration of a person's muscular system and fitness. The term 'disuse syndrome' refers to the physiological and psychological effects of a reduced level of physical activity in daily life (Bousema et al. 2007; Verbunt et al. 2003). Although often referred to in the literature, the disuse syndrome still is ill-defined (Wittink et al. 2000). Generally, two different aspects are distinguished: physical decon-ditioning, which can either be expressed in weakened muscle strength or reduced aerobic fitness, and disordered muscle coordination during physical activity (also called 'guarded movements'). Generally, the physical fitness levels of CLBP patients are found to be either lower or equal to that of healthy subjects (Verbunt et al. 2003). Only one current study succeeded in demonstrating that CLBP patients have lower aerobic fitness than matched healthy counterparts, while this could not be explained by pain-related fear or other relevant variables (Smeets et al. 2006). Evidence for disordered muscle coordination was found by Geisser and colleagues (2004), who showed that among CLBP patients pain-related fear was not only associated with reduced lumbar flexion and greater EMG in full flexion, but also to abnormalities in the muscle activity during flexion from the standing position. These changes in musculoskeletal functioning and flexion may be impor-tant for the understanding of how pain may interfere with daily life functioning. In sum, it still is unclear what the effects of pain-related fear are on physical functioning, both in terms of reduced aerobic fitness as disordered muscle coordination (see also Chapter 12).

### 14.2.4 **Vulnerabilities for fear of pain**

The foregoing paragraphs offer support for the importance of pain-related fear and associated avoidance behaviour in chronic pain. However, an interesting issue that presents itself concerns the aetiology of pain-related fear. Complementing fear-learning theories as described in earlier paragraphs, several factors have been proposed to constitute vulnerability for pain-related fear. As such, research has indicated that fear of pain is closely related to a number of negative emo-tional constructs, like negative affectivity, trait anxiety, anxiety sensitivity, and illness injury sen-sitivity (Keogh and Asmundson 2004; for more information see Chapter 12). Elevated levels of anxiety sensitivity and illness injury sensitivity have been frequently found related to maladaptive responses to pain in terms of reduced tolerance for pain, increased pain intensity levels, attention bias for pain etc (Stewart and Asmundson 2006; Vancleef and Peters 2006; Vancleef et al. 2006). In addition, trait anxiety and negative affectivity have been found related to increased pain inten-sity, increased discomfort and disability by the pain, hypervigilance for internal bodily sensations, and less adequate coping with and perceived control over pain (Keogh and Asmundson 2004; Stegen et al. 2001). One way to conceptualize the various constructs in relation to each other is by representing them in a hierarchical tree structure (Keogh and Asmundson 2004; Vancleef et al. 2006; Vancleef et al. 2009). In this hierarchical tree, fear of pain is conceived as the most *specific* construct that resides at the lowest level of the tree. Fear of pain is subordinated to anxiety sensi-tivity and illness injury sensitivity that in their turn subordinate to trait anxiety. One level above trait anxiety, negative affectivity represents the most *general* and stable negative emotional construct at the top of the tree. A hierarchical structure offers an elucidating framework for the conceptualization of pain-relevant negative emotional constructs. As such, content overlap between the constructs is accounted for by interrelations between constructs, while each individual construct possesses unique explanatory value for pain as well. According to the tree structure, pain-related fear will exert the most direct influence on pain, while influences of other constructs, like anxiety sensitivity for example, are understood to run through the specific fears that are found at the lower positioned levels. It is important to note that the hierarchical structure serves a mere theoretical conceptualization to date that serves to aid our understanding of the relative contribution of various negative emotional constructs to pain. Nevertheless, it seems obvious that general and stable anxiety related constructs entail vulnerability for pain-related fear and pain catastrophizing. Therefore, it is important that diagnostic and treatment approaches to pain keep these other pain anxiety constructs into account in understanding and treating individual pain problems.

## 14.3 Assessment of pain-related fear

Patients with fear of pain are at risk for developing persistent back pain and disability, which implies a need to make a thorough assessment of pain-related fear and avoidance. As pain-related fear involves cognitions, emotions, overt behaviour and physiological responses, several methods are needed to fully understand patients' reactions to pain. This section provides an overview of assessment tools that are frequently used in current research and clinical practice to assess pain-related fear. As such, both clinicians and researchers rely heavily on interviews and self-report measures to assess fear. Several widely used validated questionnaires are also useful tools in the  assessment of fear. Furthermore, another tool based on pictures of every day movements is helpful in determining fear and above all the avoidance of movements. In order to get a more complete picture and to be able to grasp different components of the object of pain-related fear, self-report measures are often combined with observational or physiological measures. A multimodal assessment presumably helps us to reach a better understanding of patients' fear of pain.

### 14.3.1 Self-report measures

The most common way to assess pain-related fear is through self-report measures which cover different aspects of fear. Most of these focus on cognitive and affective responsivity that may indicate fear. A challenge in developing self-report measures has been isolating the emotional response as opposed to measuring 'beliefs'. Indeed, many of the instruments available appear to tap into beliefs that the patient holds rather than things that actually provoke fear. Similarly, some instruments may measure affect but may be more oriented towards 'worry' rather than to actual fear. Although this may seem to some to be a mute point, the differences may be significant especially if the proposed treatment (see the section on exposure *in vivo*) focuses on fear. At present, a large number of self-report measures are available for the assessment of pain-related fear. The choice for one measure over the other mainly depends on the object of fear (e.g. fear of pain, fear of movement, fear of re-injury), and the fear specific concerns (e.g. cognitive concerns, physical concerns, emotional concerns) one aims to measure. Furthermore, whereas some measures are more generally applicable for assessing fear in both healthy and pain populations, others are more appropriate for assessment in specific pain patient groups only (e.g. cervical pain, back pain). Some of the most commonly used self-report measures of pain-related fear in the current assessment and treatment of pain-related fear are listed below. However, this list is not conclusive, and other measures, including modified versions of the questionnaires described below are eligible for use in pain research and clinical practice as well.

It should be noted that self-report instruments are subject to a number of drawbacks that have to be kept in mind when interpreting results of these measures. As such, respondents might not always report their genuine thoughts and feelings, because of social desirability, response bias, or simply because they are unable to access and grasp their real concerns. Furthermore, no one-to-one relationship between the measure and the latent construct it represents can be assumed. Nevertheless, keeping these drawbacks in mind, psychometric evaluated self-report measures are easy to administer, at low-cost, but still offer valuable information to researchers and clinicians.

## Fear of pain

The *Pain and Impairment Relationship Scale (PAIRS)* was an early attempt to capture chronic pain patients' beliefs and attitudes towards pain and ability to function despite pain (Riley et al. 1988). It consists of 15 statements about pain and activity (e.g. 'I can't go about my normal life activities when I am in pain', 'An increase in pain is an indication that I should stop what I am doing until the pain decreases') which are rated on a seven-point scale (0=completely disagree; 6=completely agree). The scale has been found to have good psychometric properties (DeGood and Shutty 1992) and may be used to assess beliefs about pain and activity. As this scale was a relatively early attempt to assess pain-related fear, it is not clear what processes it in fact captures. Indeed, it appears to assess a wide range of attitudes and beliefs concerning living with persistent pain that go beyond fear of pain.

The *Pain Anxiety Symptoms Scale (PASS)* was developed to measure general anxiety and fear in people with chronic pain (McCracken et al. 1992). The original scale consisted of 40 items intended to assess four aspects of pain-related anxiety: (1) fearful appraisal of pain (e.g. 'When I feel pain I am afraid something terrible will happen'): (2) cognitive anxiety (e.g. 'During painful episodes it is difficult for me to think of anything besides the pain'): (3) physiological anxiety (e.g. 'Pain seems to cause my heart to pound or race'): (4) escape and avoidance behaviour (e.g. 'I avoid important activities when I hurt'). Responders rate how often they have these thoughts or sensations on a six-point scale (0=never; 5=always). Later, a shortened version of the scale was developed and validated (PASS-20) (McCracken and Dhingra 2002). The short form version has 20 items and has been found to be a good reflection of the original PASS (Roelofs et al. 2004a). One of the advantages with this measure is that it includes bodily indicators of fear through questions about physiological arousal. However, as these reactions might appear as a direct consequence of pain, it is difficult to determine whether it actually captures indicators of fear. Furthermore, as bodily reactions are difficult to assess through self-report measures, physiological measures might be preferable if available. In addition, the questions in the PASS presume that the individual has an earlier or present experience of pain problems. This makes the PASS inappropriate for use with people who are not clinical pain patients.

The *Fear of Pain Questionnaire-III (FPQ-III)* (McNeil and Rainwater 1998) was developed to assess fear associated with both acute and chronic pain in healthy individuals. People are asked to rate their fear of pain in 30 situations, which are divided into: (1) severe pain (e.g. 'Breaking your leg'), (2) minor pain (e.g. 'Having a muscle cramp') and (3) medical pain (e.g. 'Having a tooth pulled'). Answers are given on a five-point scale (1=no fear at all; 5=extreme fear). Recently, a shortened version of the scale has been developed (FPQ-SF) (Asmundson et al. 2008). The authors suggest that the FPQ-SF is a more psychometrically sound alternative to the original scale. One advantage of the FPQ is that it is possible to use it both with pain and non-pain populations as the questions do not imply any earlier clinical experience of pain. However, the non-clinical focus of the scale might make it less relevant to use for clinical purposes as some of the items describe events that are far from clinical situations (e.g. having sand or dust blowing into your eyes; gulping a hot drink before it has cooled).

## Fear of pain-causing activities

The Fear-Avoidance Beliefs Questionnaire (FABQ) (Waddell et al. 1993) is used to assess pain patients' beliefs about possible harm from work and physical activities. It has 16 items which are divided into two subscales; (1) fear-avoidance beliefs about physical activity (e.g. 'Physical activity might harm my back') and (2) fear-avoidance beliefs about work ('My work aggravated my pain'). Answers are given on a seven-point scale (0=completely disagree; 6=completely agree). The scale has been found to have good psychometric properties in patients with both acute and long-term pain (Swinkels-Meewisse et al. 2003; Waddell et al. 1993), and may be used to identify beliefs that are related to pain-related disability and work loss. One of the disadvantages with this questionnaire might be in line with what the name of the scale indicates—that it assesses *beliefs* rather than fear per se. It might be possible that people hold such beliefs without being particularly fearful, which is important to take into account when using this scale in a clinical context.

## Fear of movement and (re)injury

The Tampa Scale for Kinesiophobia (TSK) (Kori et al. 1990) has been developed to assess patients' fear of (re)injury due to movement, and consists of 17 items (e.g. 'Pain always means I have injured my body' and 'If I try to overcome it, my pain would increase').

Later, a shorter version of the TSK has been developed and validated, containing only 13 items as it excludes the four items that are reverse scored. This version has greater internal consistency and is composed of two lower-order factors ('Activity Avoidance' and 'Somatic Focus') that also load on a single higher-order factor (Geisser et al. 2000). A number of studies have corroborated the two-factor structure of TSK, which also appeared invariant across pain diagnoses and Dutch, Swedish, and Canadian samples (Goubert et al. 2004b; Roelofs et al. 2007). One concern that has been highlighted about the TSK is that some items have troublesome wording (Pool et al. 2009). More specifically, some questions seem to be difficult to understand because they employ words such as 'dangerous' and 'injury' that may have different meanings for different patients. Some items also use negations which may be difficult for some patients to understand. These reflections might be important to take into consideration when using the TSK with patients.

## Perceived harmfulness of movements: the PHODA

When fear of movement is assessed in a clinical context, the Photograph Series of Daily Activities (PHODA) (Kugler et al. 1999) is a pictorial assessment tool which consists of 98 photographs of various daily-life activities (e.g. walking, lifting, bending, etc.). Patients are asked to rate how harmful they think each activity would be to their back by placing the photographs on a thermometer which ranges from 0 (=not at all harmful) to 100 (=extremely harmful). Although the PHODA mainly is used as a self-report measure, it also provides the clinician with an opportunity to observe and discuss the patient's fear when confronted with different activities. The PHODA is commonly used in the assessment phase of exposure *in vivo*, a treatment for pain-related fear that is described later in this chapter. Recently, an electronic and shortened version of the PHODA (PHODA-SeV) was developed and validated (Leeuw et al. 2007b). It showed excellent psychometric properties, which implies that it is a proper alternative to the original version. One limitation that has been raised is that the PHODA seems to be more appropriate for highly fearful pain patients and less applicable for those with low or mediate levels of fear (Trost et al. 2009). Nevertheless, because the PHODA consists of photographs of real activities, it may be a clinically useful tool for revealing the patients' beliefs and concerns about specific movements. This is an important basis for the exposure treatment and one which may be quite difficult without tools such as the PHODA.

An alternative measure to assess fear of movement is the Pictorial Fear of Activity Scale-Cervical (PFActS-C) (Turk et al. 2008). This instrument was recently developed to assess fear of movement that is specifically related to neck pain. The PFActS-C differs from the PHODA in its specific focus on neck pain and the varying degree of mechanical load that is incorporated in the photographs. The instrument consists of 77 photographs of movements with varying biomechanical stress. Respondents are asked, for each photograph, to rate on a scale from 0 (=no fear at all) to 10 (=extremely fearful) how worried or fearful they would be to perform the activity as shown in the picture. A first validation study in a group of neck pain patients indicated that the PFActS-C is a promising tool for assessing fear of movement in patients with cervical pain (Turk et al. 2008). However, since this tool is still rather new, more research is needed to examine its applicability.

### 14.3.2 Interview

Apart from questionnaires, every assessment of pain-related fear also involves a rigorous interview. The semi-structured interview is an important tool for collecting additional information about the patient's cognitions, emotions and overt behaviour (e.g. avoidance) in relation to pain. The clinician also may get a better picture of the role fear and avoidance may have played in the aetiology and maintenance of the pain and disability problem. However, as the interview provides a purely subjective picture of the pain problem, it should be complemented by other assessment tools. Some of the areas that are covered in the interview are listed in Table 14.1.

### 14.3.3 Self-assessment

Self-assessment is a useful supplement to the interview. Self-assessment is one of the most commonly used methods in psychological research and practice (Sigmon and LaMattina 2006). In self-assessment, the patients systematically observe and record their own behaviour. In pain

**Table 14.1** Interview in assessment of pain-related fear

| | |
|---|---|
| **Description of the pain** | Where do you have pain? |
| | What does the pain feel like? |
| | How intense is the pain? (0–10) |
| | When does it hurt more? |
| | When does it hurt less? |
| **Learning history** | When did the pain start? |
| | How did it develop? |
| | What do you think has made your pain problem worse? |
| **Cognitions** | What do you think causes your pain? |
| | When you do something that provokes the pain, what goes through your mind? |
| | What do you think it will lead to in the future? |
| | What is the worst thing that could happen? |
| **Emotions** | What emotions do you have in relation to the pain? |
| | Are there any activities that you are afraid of doing? |
| **Activities/ movements vs. avoidance** | What are you able to do despite the pain? |
| | What activities do you avoid because of the pain? |
| | How active are you in daily life? |
| **Coping vs. safety behaviours** | What do you do to stand the pain? |
| | What do you do when the pain gets worse? |
| | What do you do to be able to perform activities that are difficult because of pain? |

patients, diaries are used to keep record of situations that provoke fear and avoidance. Often, the patients also use the diary to register their daily activities, which may be an indirect measure of fear and avoidance. In the last years, research about the use of electronic diaries in pain assessment has increased (e.g. Jamison et al. 2001; Peters et al. 2000). Maybe this will become more common in clinical practice in the future. At the moment, however, paper-and-pencil diaries are still the most widely used tools in self-assessment of pain-related fear.

### 14.3.4 **Observational measures**

Even though it is well known that patients express fear of pain both verbally and non-verbally, there are few standardized tools to assess overt behaviour. Fear of pain has been associated with a number of overt behaviours, such as diminished physical performance and escape/avoidance behaviour (Leeuw et al. 2007a). In a clinical situation, clinicians may instinctively observe how the patient reacts to pain and movement, and use this information in the further assessment. Notwithstanding, a thorough observational assessment is seldom accomplished. There are observational measures which aim to assess pain behaviour (e.g. Weiner et al. 1996). However, these are not developed to capture fear. In verbal assessment of fear, we do not rely solely on one question or on what the patients tell us at first glance, but complement this with standardized questionnaires. A comparable scrupulous assessment of overt behaviour would help us to reach a better understanding of patients' pain-related fear.

Assessment of other overt behaviours may also help to reach a better understanding of pain-related fear. Facial expression has been suggested to be a potential target for assessment (McNeil and Vowles 2004). However, there is still a lack of appropriate assessment tools for facial expression as a non-verbal manifestation of pain-related fear.

### 14.3.5 **Physiological measures**

In the last decades, researchers have paid increasing attention to psychophysiological recordings as an assessment tool for pain-related fear and anxiety. In particular, Flor and her colleagues have contributed to the growing knowledge about how psychophysiological measures may be used in the area of pain (Flor et al. 2001), including as indicators of fear. Muscle tension, skin conductance, and heart rate are some of the targets for psychophysiological assessments in pain patients (Andrasik and Flor 2008). Also the startle reflex, an involuntary eye blink movement, has been used in experiments as an indicator of fear (e.g. Carleton et al. 2006; Naliboff et al. 2008). In clinical settings, however, it is still uncommon to include physiological measures when assessing fear. A challenge for the future is the development of sound psychophysiological measures that may be used in the clinical assessment of pain-related fear.

### 14.3.6 **Additional measures**

In addition to explicit and physiological measures of fear of pain, researchers have relied on *indirect* cognitive measures of indicators of fear and anxiety related to pain. In these measures, variables of interest (beliefs, attitudes, cognitive biases) are inferred from behavioural responses (e.g. reaction times, reading times) within a specific context. Characteristic to these measures is the fact that they assess cognitive processes, beliefs, and attitudes without the awareness or control of the participant. Experimental research often uses automatized cognitive processing tasks like the modified Stroop task and the dot probe paradigm to assess attention bias for pain. In the modified Stroop task, categories of sensory or affective pain words and neutral words are presented in different colours. Responders are asked to name the colour of each word and response times are compared. Typically, it takes longer to name the colour when the information is threatening; in this case when pain words are presented. In the dot probe paradigm, one neutral word and one pain-related word are presented simultaneously on a screen. Next, one of the words is replaced by a dot. Response times for when the dot replaces neutral and pain-related words are compared. In pain patients and pain-fearful individuals, reaction time is expected to be shorter when the dot replaces pain words, due to attentional biases. Both the modified Stroop task and the dot probe paradigm are tests of attentional bias which may presumably indicate fear. There are mixed results, however, concerning whether these tests are reliable indicators of fear (e.g. Asmundson et al. 2005; Pincus and Morley 2001; Roelofs et al. 2002).

Furthermore, a few studies have relied on *implicit association measures* to assess the attitudes and beliefs that pain-fearful individuals possess regarding pain and disability. These studies demonstrated that CLBP patient who are high in pain-related fear possess stronger associations between pain and threat than low-fearful patients do. Furthermore, Goubert et al. (2003) reported about a general implicit negative attitude towards back-stressing pictures in healthy individuals, using an affective priming task. Recently, Leeuw and colleagues (2007d) used two association tasks, the implicit association task and the go-no-go association task, to measure implicit fear of movement(re) injury in a group of CLBP patients and pain-free controls. Results did not indicate implicit fear of movement(re)injury in both groups, nor did the authors observe differences in the implicit attitudes between the patient and the control group. Nevertheless, the authors argued that psychometric and methodological difficulties of the paradigms might explain the lack of findings. In general implicit measures are promising techniques that might be able to reveal those aspects of pain-related fear that are inaccessible to explicit measures like self-report and interviews.

## 14.4 **Treating pain-related fear**

Exposure *in vivo* is a novel treatment approach which has been developed to target fear of pain. As seen earlier in this chapter, fear and avoidance may be essential factors that maintain pain and dysfunction in some patients. It has been stated that 'Fear of pain and what we do about it may be more disabling than pain itself' (Waddell et al. 1993, p. 164). Based on this, graded exposure *in vivo* recently was developed as a cognitive-behavioural treatment for patients with back pain and high levels of pain-related fear (Vlaeyen et al. 2004a). Today, it is the only standardized and evidence-based treatment which exclusively focuses on reducing pain-related fear and avoidance.

Because exposure *in vivo* is the 'treatment of choice' for patients suffering from excessive fears, e.g. phobias (Barlow 2000), it would also seem to be ideal for patients with pain-related fear. Accordingly, exposure *in vivo* for pain-related fear relies on the same principles as exposure therapy for phobia. In fact, Kori et al. (1990) went so far as to call pain-related fear a phobia, introducing the term 'kinesiophobia' as a description of 'an excessive, irrational, and debilitating fear of physical movement and activity resulting from a feeling of vulnerability to painful injury or reinjury'. Avoidance of the feared stimuli, which here refers to movements, maintains and exaggerates the fear. During exposure, phobic patients confront the feared stimuli until habituation, i.e. until the fear decreases and finally dissipates. The same principles may be transferred to pain patients. During exposure for pain-related fear, the patient is gradually exposed to movements following the hierarchy until extinction of defensive fear responses occur. Besides the effect of extinction there may also be benefits in terms of cognitions. As the fear and avoidance model underscores, performing a feared movement may be associated with catastrophic expectations which, during exposure *in vivo*, are challenged and disconfirmed (Vlaeyen et al. 2008). The main goal in exposure *in vivo* is hence that the patient confronts what (s)he is afraid of as a way to become less fearful. Recent evidence shows that learned associations between certain movements and pain are not abolished during exposure, but that inhibitory learning occurs. This means that the initial associations remain stored in memory, but that the individual has learned to inhibit the conditioned (defence) responses. Moreover, the inhibitory learning appears to be context dependent, thereby limiting generalization of extinction to other contexts (Craske et al. 2008; Crombez et al. 2002b).

## 14.4.1 Main components of exposure

### Assessment

The first step in graded exposure *in vivo* is to perform a thorough assessment of pain-related fear and avoidance. As assessment has been discussed earlier in this chapter, let us simply review this briefly here. A proper assessment is a prerequisite for the treatment as it serves to identify target movements for the exposure. The intention is to get a complete picture of how the patient's fear and avoidance maintain the pain problem. The PHODA (Leeuw et al. 2007b), an instrument with pictures of daily activities that patients rate for fear, is an especially important tool in the assessment. Thus, the PHODA provides information as to *which* movements the patient is fearful of and also *how* afraid they are of each movement. This information is employed to develop a hierarchy of feared movements. The PHODA may also be used to reveal catastrophic (mis)interpretations and irrational beliefs that patients have about movements and pain. At the end of assessment, the therapist should have a clear idea of what movements the patient avoids and what beliefs and catastrophic thoughts are linked to these movements; this will be the focus of the treatment.

### Defining goals

During the assessment phase, the patient and the therapist agree on a limited number of specific treatment goals. Goal setting serves a number of important functions. First, the goals serve as a clear statement of the aim of exposure. A primary aim in cognitive behavioural treatments for pain is to restore functional ability, and not simply to get rid of the pain. Therefore, goals should focus on activities and not on pain reduction. Second, when the patient has been involved in developing goals they view as quite valuable; they become more engaged in the treatment and naturally take a more active role in the treatment. Third, goals help to structure the treatment. By establishing goals the patient and the therapist share a picture of what they are striving towards. The goals also make it easier to establish a hierarchy which involves movements that are important for the patient to restore. Typically, a hierarchy includes daily activities that the patient desires to resume or develop such as hobbies, family life, or work. Fourth, goals are also used as an evaluation tool. With clear goals, both the patient and the therapist may evaluate treatment progress and see whether the exposure has succeeded or not. Typical example of treatment goals are shown in Table 14.2.

**Table 14.2** Typical examples of treatment goals

| Goal | Description |
| --- | --- |
| Play with my kids | Play actively with my kids 30 minutes in the garden twice a week, including lifting them, bending over etc. |
| Play soccer | Play soccer with my old team 1 hour once a week |
| Increase my work time | Increase my work time from 25% to 75% at my ordinary work place, including performing all duties. |
| Do the weekly shopping | Do the weekly shopping by myself, including carrying the bags to the car |

**Table 14.3** An example of a graded fear-hierarchy of pain-related fear stimuli

**Goal:** To play with my kids in the garden 30 minutes, twice a week

| Movement/activity | Pre-treatment PHODA score | Post-treatment PHODA score |
|---|---|---|
| Running while carrying a child on my shoulders | 100 | 20 |
| Riding off a pavement with a bicycle | 90 | 15 |
| Lifting a child from the floor | 80 | 0 |
| Bending forward to pick up tools from the floor | 70 | 0 |
| Jumping up and down | 50 | 0 |
| Walking up and down the stairs | 30 | 0 |

## Establishing hierarchies

Once treatment goals are identified, the therapist and the patient need to establish a fear hierarchy. The hierarchy consists of movements that provoke pain-related fear starting with those inducing only a little fear to those trigger a maximum of fear. It normally will include 5–10 steps or movements. An example of a graded fear-hierarchy is shown in Table 14.3. Exposure begins with a movement that provokes only a small amount of fear. When habituation occurs and the patient is able to perform the movement without provoking fear, then the next movement in the hierarchy is tackled. This procedure continues until the patient is able to perform all of the movements in the hierarchy, including the goal activity, without provoking very much fear. In this way, function is restored and the clear goals of the treatment are achieved.

## Education

Education is an important part of the treatment. The purpose of the psychoeducation is to provide a clear rational and to engage the patient. Before being exposed to any fear-provoking stimuli, the patient should understand how and why exposure should reduce fear, and how this will bring the patient closer to his or her goals. The therapist explains the fear-avoidance model, using the patient's own history and wording as much as possible. If the patient does not use the word 'fear', other words may be more suitable. An essential message in the education is that fear and avoidance are natural and normal responses to acute pain, but that they paradoxically maintain fear and pain in the long term. Another point is that long-term back, neck or shoulder pain typically signals that muscles are working too hard to protect the back (resulting in muscle pain) rather than from damage to the spine. There is some evidence that psychoeducation in itself may have some effect in reducing pain-related fear and disability (Burton et al. 1999; de Jong et al. 2005b; Moore et al. 2000). The psychoeducation aims to enhance the patient's understanding of how the exposure treatment will help them to deal with their fears and achieve their goals concerning function.

## Graded exposure

The keystone in exposure is, of course, when the patient actually exposes himself to previously avoided stimuli according to the fear hierarchy. The patient starts at lower level of the hierarchy, with a movement that provokes relatively less intense fear. First, the therapist serves as a role model and demonstrates the movement. Then, the patient performs the movement, with verbal support from the therapist. The general principles for exposure are followed: the patient is exposed to the feared stimuli for a prolonged time, until fear and anxiety decreases significantly. In exposure for pain-related fear, the patient consequently performs the movement several times.

The therapist encourages the patient to do the exposure without using safety behaviours, i.e. subtle strategies that patients use to 'protect' themselves (guarded walking, relaxation, seeking social support, etc.). Safety behaviours are subtle avoidance behaviours which may hinder the effect of exposure (Tang et al. 2007; Vlaeyen et al. 2004a). In between exposure sessions, the patient is told to continue the exposure at home by performing homework assignments. Besides reducing fear and re-establishing physical function, this helps the patient to generalize the effects and enhance self-efficacy. All treatment sessions follow the same structure, each time at a higher level in the hierarchy, to systematically decrease the patient's pain-related fear.

### Behavioural experiments

The graded exposure *in vivo* might be combined with behavioural experiments (Bennett-Levy et al. 2004; Vlaeyen et al. 2004a). Behavioural experiments have been developed from cognitive theory, to create a collaborative empiricism. The purpose is to challenge irrational beliefs and catastrophic (mis)interpretations about pain and movement. In a behavioural experiment, the patient first formulates the belief and rates its credibility. Then, an alternative belief is formulated and the patient rates its credibility. Next, the patient performs the movement and describes what happens. Finally, the outcome is compared to the expectation and conclusions are drawn. Table 14.4 displays an example of a behavioural experiment in a patient with pain-related fear. The main goal with behavioural experiments is to challenge and adjust irrational beliefs but may also be used as a way to encourage patients to view the exposure as an experiment in which new behaviours are tested.

### 14.4.2 **Evidence for exposure *in vivo***

Exposure *in vivo* is a promising treatment approach for patients with pain-related fear. Two recent reviews concluded that exposure *in vivo* is currently the treatment of choice for such patients (Bailey et al. 2010; Lohnberg 2007). The first research about the effect of exposure was a series of studies using a replicated single-case experimental design. These showed that graded exposure *in vivo* was effective in reducing pain-related fear, avoidance behaviour, and to some extent also pain intensity in patients with back pain (Boersma et al. 2004; Linton et al. 2002; Vlaeyen et al. 2001). Later, the same type of design was used to evaluate the effect in other groups of patients. These studies demonstrate the same basic results in patients with complex regional pain syndrome (de Jong et al. 2005a) and in patients with neck pain after a motor vehicle accident (de Jong et al. 2008). Further evidence was then provided in randomized control trials (RCTs). RCTs are generally seen as the most powerful way of demonstrating that an intervention is effective (Kazdin 2003). Recently, three RCTs have been published, evaluating the effect of exposure

**Table 14.4** An example of a behavioural experiment in a patient with pain-related fear

| Belief/thought | Rating of credibility before the experiment | Rating of credibility after the experiment |
|---|---|---|
| **Belief/catastrophic thought:** 'If I jump from the chair, I will get excruciating pain (10 on a scale 0–10)' | 85% | 20% |
| **Alternative belief:** 'If I jump from the chair, my pain will only increase slightly (2 on a scale 0–10)' | 15% | 80% |
| **What happened:** The pain increased slightly (from 2 to 3 on a scale 0–10) | | |
| **Conclusion:** The original thought was an overestimation of the harmfulness of the movement. The alternative belief is more realistic. | | |

in patients with long-term back pain (Leeuw et al. 2008; Linton et al. 2008; Woods and Asmundson 2008). Although the results are not as striking as in the single-subject studies, exposure was found to result in moderate to large effects for reducing pain-related fear, catastrophic thoughts, disability and pain. However, when compared to graded activity, a commonly used treatment in pain rehabilitation, the results were more modest (Leeuw et al. 2008; Woods and Asmundson 2008). The exposure groups showed larger improvements on measures of pain-related fear and anxiety, beliefs, and catastrophizing, but on measures of disability and pain both treatments appeared to be about equally effective. Overall, these studies show that exposure may be an important treatment, but that it cannot yet be recommended as a 'stand alone' treatment. As the authors of one of the studies suggest (Woods and Asmundson 2008), it is important to explore the use of exposure in applied multidisciplinary treatment settings. Given that patients with high levels of pain-related fear become noticeably less fearful and anxious through exposure, it has potential to be a successful addition to ordinary treatment packages for fearful patients suffering from long-term pain. Likewise, new advances in delivering exposure treatments may also improve its utility.

## 14.5 **Future directions**

This chapter shows that the literature on fear-avoidance has strong roots in the learning–conditioning theory. The classical conditioning account of fear development predicts that neutral stimuli can develop fearful qualities and become conditioned fear stimuli (CS) when they are associated with unconditioned aversive stimuli (US). Following this theory, the *nature* of the CS and the US determines the kind of fear. Future research should focus more on the nature of both types of stimuli in fear development. On a continuum from 'outside' to 'inside' the body—an exteroceptive-interoceptive continuum—three types of sensorial receptors can be distinguished. *Exteroceptors* are situated closely to the bodily surface and are sensitive to mechanical and electro-mechanical energetic fields surrounding the organism. *Proprioceptors* are sensitive to the orientation and the action of parts of the body in space. *Interoceptors* are located in the cavities of the body and form the basis for the neural representation of the viscera and the vascular system. Traditionally, human fear conditioning studies have used paradigms in which affectively neutral, exteroceptive stimuli (CSs, e.g. a picture or a tone) become predictors for an aversive physical event (e.g. pain). Pain research has focused more on proprioceptive stimuli (i.e. kinesiophobia). Certain movements may have acquired the features of a CS as they have been associated with a US (more pain), and create fear of movement. Strangely enough, there is much less information in the pain literature on interoceptive fear conditioning. Interoceptive cues (e.g. muscle spasms, mild pain, dizziness . . .) can also become CSs and this might be a particular form of fear conditioning differentiates the fear of 'pain' construct from the fear of 'movement' construct (De Peuter et al. 2010). The fear of pain construct might be more relevant in physical complaints where the musculoskeletal system is less involved. Besides the theoretical importance of examining this idea more into detail, findings may also lead to different therapeutic interventions. For example, interoceptive exposure has been reported as an effective treatment in patients with panic disorder, assumed to be mediated by interoceptive fear conditioning (Walker and Furer 2008). At this point, it is important to note that the term 'fear-avoidance' as introduced by Lethem et al. in 1983 might need reconsideration given the fact that it points only to one defensive mechanism: avoidance. It might be more appropriate to adopt the general term 'pain-related fear', which could be defined as the fear that originated in associations where pain is the US. Depending on the CS, this general term can then be subdivided in fear of movement (proprioceptive fear), fear of pain (interoceptive fear), fear of sounds (exteroceptieve fear, for example in headaches), etc . . . or more diffuse pain anxiety.

A second direction for further research on fear-avoidance stems from commonly observed and complex situations in which the individual cannot identify discrete cues that signal or predict the US. In that case the context in which the US occurs becomes the US, and theorists have introduced the term 'contextual' fear for this form of fear, which has a lot of resemblances with generalized anxiety disorder (Vansteenwegen et al. 2008). Some authors prefer the term 'anxiety' above fear. In the case of contextual fear with pain as the US, one could speak of 'pain anxiety'. The characteristics of pain anxiety are that the defensive responses last longer as contextual stimuli usually are temporally quite stable.

In sum, since the early writings in the 1980s we have made considerable progress in the understanding and management of pain-related fear and anxiety, and we look forward to further exploration and fine tuning of these processes in the near future.

## Acknowledgements

The contribution of Johan W. S. Vlaeyen was supported by the NWO Social Sciences Research Council of the Netherlands, Grant No. 453–04-003, and by an Odysseus Grant of the Research Foundation Flanders, Belgium (FWO).

## References

Al Obaidi, S. M., Al Zoabi, B., Al Shuwaie, N., Al Zaabie, N. and Nelson, R. M. (2003) The influence of pain and pain-related fear and disability beliefs on walking velocity in chronic low back pain. *International Journal of Rehabilitation Research*, **26**, 101–8.

Andrasik, F. and Flor, H. (2008) Biofeedback, in H. Breivik, W. Campbell and M.K. Nicholas (ed.) *Clinical Pain Management: Practice and procedures.* London: Hodder & Stoughton.

Asmundson, G. J. and Hadjistavropoulos, H. D. (2007) Is high fear of pain associated with attentional bias for pain-related or general threat? A categorical reanalysis. *Journal of Pain*, **8**, 11–18.

Asmundson, G. J. G., Bovell, C. V., Carleton, N. R. and McWilliams, L. A. (2008) The Fear of Pain Questionnnaire - Short Form (FPQ-SF): Factorial validity and psychometric properties. *Pain*, **134**, 51–58.

Asmundson, G. J. G., Carleton, N. R. and Ekong, J. (2005) Dot-probe evaluation of selective attentional processing of pain cues in patients with chronic headaches. *Pain*, **114**, 250–6.

Asmundson, G. J. G., Norton, P. J. and Norton, G. R. (1999) Beyond pain: The role of fear and avoidance in chronicity. *Clinical Psychology Review*, **19**, 97–119.

Bailey, K. M., Carleton, R. N., Vlaeyen, J. W., Asmundson, G. J. (2010) Treatments addressing pain-related fear and anxiety in patients with chronic musculoskeletal pain: A preliminary review. *Cognitive Behaviour Therapy*, **39**(1), 46–63.

Barlow, D. H. (2000) Unravelling the mysteries of anxiety and its disorders from the perspective of emotion theory. *American Psychologist*, **55**, 1247–63.

Bennett-Levy, J., Butler, G., Fennell, M., Hackmann, A., Mueller, M. and Westbrook, D. (2004) *Oxford Guide to Behavioral Experiments in Cognitive Psychology*, Oxford: Oxford University Press.

Boersma, K., Linton, S. J., Overmeer, T., Jansson, M., Vlaeyen, J. W. S. and de Jong, J. (2004) Lowering fear-avoidance and enhancing function through exposure in vivo. A multiple baseline study across six patients with back pain. *Pain*, **108**, 8–16.

Bortz, W. M. (1984) The disuse syndrome. *The Western Journal of Medicine*, **141**, 691–4.

Bousema, E. J., Verbunt, J. A., Seelen, H. A., Vlaeyen, J. W. and Knottnerus, J. A. (2007) Disuse and physical deconditioning in the first year after the onset of back pain. *Pain*, **130**, 279–86.

Bradley, M., Silakowski, T. and Lang, P. J. (2008) Fear of pain and defensive activation. *Pain*, **137**, 156–63.

Burton, A. K., Waddell, G., Tillotson, K. M. and Summerton, N. (1999) Information and advice to patients with back pain can have a positive effect. A randomized controlled trial of a novel educational booklet in primary care. *Spine*, **24**, 2484–91.

Carleton, N. R., Asmundson, G. J. G., Collimore, K. C. and Ellwanger, J. (2006) Strategic and automatic threat processing in chronic musculoskeletal pain: a startle probe investigation. *Cognitive Behaviour Therapy*, **35**, 236–47.

Craske, M. G., Kircanski, K., Zelikowsky, M., Mystkowski, J., Chowdhury, N. and Baker, A. (2008) Optimizing inhibitory learning during exposure therapy. *Behaviour Research and Therapy*, **46**, 5–27.

Crombez, G., Eccleston, C., Baeyens, F. and Eelen, P. (1998a) Attentional disruption is enhanced by the threat of pain. *Behaviour Research and Therapy*, **36**, 195–204.

Crombez, G., Eccleston, C., van den Broeck, A., van Houdenhove, B. and Goubert, L. (2002a) The effects of catastrophic thinking about pain on attentional interference by pain: No mediation of negative affectivity in healthy volunteers and in patients with low back pain. *Pain Research and Management*, **7**, 31–9.

Crombez, G., Eccleston, C., Vlaeyen, J. W. S., Vansteenwegen, D., Lysens, R. and Eelen, P. (2002b) Exposure to physical movements in low back pain patients: Restricted effects of generalization. *Health Psychology*, **21**, 573–78.

Crombez, G., Vervaet, L., Baeyens, F., Lysens, R. and Eelen, P. (1996) Do pain expectancies cause pain in chronic low back patients? A clinical investigation. *Behaviour Research and Therapy*, **34**, 919–25.

Crombez, G., Vervaet, L., Lysens, R., Baeyens, F. and Eelen, P. (1998b) Avoidance and confrontation of painful, back-straining movements in chronic back pain patients. *Behavior Modification*, **22**, 62–77.

Crombez, G., Vlaeyen, J. W. S., Heuts, P. H. T. G. and Lysens, R. (1999) Pain-related fear is more disabling than pain itself: evidence on the role of pain-related fear in chronic back pain disability. *Pain*, **80**, 329–39.

de Gier, M., Peters, M. L. and Vlaeyen, J. W. (2003) Fear of pain, physical performance, and attentional processes in patients with fibromyalgia. *Pain*, **104**, 121–30.

de Jong, J. R., Vangronsveld, K., Peters, M. L., et al. (2008) Reduction of pain-related fear and disability in post-traumatic neck pain: a replicated single-case experimental study of exposure in vivo. *Journal of Pain*, **9**, 1123–34.

de Jong, J. R., Vlaeyen, J. W. S., Onghena, P., Cuypers, C., den Hollander, M. and Ruijgrok, J. (2005a) Reduction of pain-related fear in complex regional pain syndrome type 1: the application of graded exposure in vivo. *Pain*, **116**, 264–75.

de Jong, J. R., Vlaeyen, J. W. S., Onghena, P., Goossens, M. E. J. B., Geilen, M. and Mulder, H. (2005b) Fear of Movement/(Re)injury in Chronic Low Back Pain: Education or Exposure In Vivo as Mediator to Fear Reduction? *Clinical Journal of Pain*, **21**, 9–17.

De Peuter, S., Van Diest, I., Vansteenwegen, D., Van den Bergh, O., Vlaeyen, J. W. S. Pain-related fear and chronic pain: Interoceptive fear conditioning as a novel approach. European Journal of Pain (submitted manuscript: accepted pending revision).

DeGood, D. E. and Shutty, M. S. (1992) Assessment of pain beliefs, coping and self-efficacy, in D. C.Turk and D.C. Melzack (ed.) *Handbook of pain assessment*. New York: Guilford.

Dehghani, M., Sharpe, L. and Nicholas, M. K. (2004) Modification of attentional biases in chronic pain patients: a preliminary study. *European Journal of Pain*, **8**, 585–94.

Eccleston, C. and Crombez, G. (1999) Pain demands attention: A cognitive-affective model of the interruptive function of pain. *Psychological Bulletin*, **125**, 356–66.

Eccleston, C., Crombez, G., Aldrich, S. and Stannard, C. (1997) Attention and somatic awareness in chronic pain. *Pain*, **72**, 209–15.

Edwards, R. R., Haythornthwaite, J. A., Sullivan, M. J. and Fillingim, R. B. (2004) Catastrophizing as a mediator of sex differences in pain: differential effects for daily pain versus laboratory-induced pain. *Pain*, **111**, 335–41.

Flor, H., Miltner, W. and Birbaumer, N. (2001) Psychophysiological recording methods. In D. C. T. Melzack (Ed.) *Handbook of Pain Assessment*. New York: Guilford.

Fordyce, W. E. (1976) *Behavioural methods for chronic pain and illness*, St. Louis, Mosby.

Fordyce, W. E., Shelton, J. L. and Dundore, D. E. (1982) The modification of avoidance learning in pain behaviors. *Journal of Behavioral Medicine,* 5, 405–14.

Fritz, J. M., George, S. Z. and Delitto, A. (2001) The role of fear-avoidance beliefs in acute low back pain: relationships with current and future disability and work status. *Pain,* 94, 7–15.

Geisser, M., Haig, A., Wallbom, A. and Wiggert, E. (2004) Pain-related fear, lumbar flexion, and dynamic EMG among persons with chronic musculoskeletal low back pain. *Clinical Journal of Pain* 20, 61–9.

Geisser, M. E., Haig, A. J. and Theisen, M. E. (2000) Activity avoidance and function in persons with chronic back pain. *Journal of Occupational Rehabilitation,* 10, 215–27.

George, S. Z., Dannecker, E. A. and Robinson, M. E. (2006) Fear of pain, not pain catastrophizing, predicts acute pain intensity, but neither factor predicts tolerance or blood pressure reactivity: An experimental investigation in pain-free individuals, 10, 457–65.

Giummarra, M. J., Gibson, S. J., Georgiou Karistianis, N. and Bradshaw, J. L. (2007) Central mechanisms in phantom limb perception: the past, present and future. *Brain Research Reviews,* 54, 219–32.

Goubert, L., Crombez, G. and De Bourdeaudhuij, I. (2004a) Low back pain, disability and back pain myths in a community sample: prevalence and interrelationships. *European Journal of Pain,* 8, 385–94.

Goubert, L., Crombez, G., Hermans, D. and Vanderstraeten, G. (2003) Implicit attitude towards pictures of back-stressing activities in pain-free subjects and patients with low back pain. *European Journal of Pain,* 7, 33–42.

Goubert, L., Crombez, G., Van Damme, S., Vlaeyen, J. W. S., Bijttebier, P. and Roelofs, J. (2004b) Confirmatory factor analysis of the Tampa Scale for Kinesiophobia: invariant two-factor model across low back pain patients and fibromyalgia patients. *Clinical Journal of Pain,* 20, 103–10.

Goubert, L., Francken, G., Crombez, G., Vansteenwegen, D. and Lysens, R. (2002) Exposure to physical movement in chronic back pain patients: No evidence for generalization across different movements. *Behaviour Research and Therapy,* 40, 415–29.

Grotle, M., Vollestad, N. K., Veierod, M. B. and Brox, J. I. (2004) Fear-avoidance beliefs and distress in relation to disability in acute and chronic low back pain. *Pain,* 112, 343–52.

Haythornthwaite, J. A., Clark, M. R., Pappagallo, M. and Raja, S. N. (2003) Pain coping strategies play a role in the persistence of pain in post-herpetic neuralgia. *Pain,* 106, 453–60.

Hirsh, A. T., George, S. Z., Bialosky, J. E. and Robinson, M. E. (2008) Fear of pain, pain catastrophizing, and acute pain perception: relative prediction and timing of assessment. *Journal of Pain,* 9, 806–12.

Huis in 't Veld, R. M. H. A., Vollenbroek-Hutten, M. M. R., Groothuis-Oudshoorn, K. C. G. M. and Hermenss H. J. (2007) The role of the fear-avoidance model in female workers with neck-shoulder pain related to computer work. *Clinical Journal of Pain,* 23, 28–34.

Izard, C. E. (1992) Basic emotions, relations among emotions, and emotion-cognition relations. *Psychological Review,* 99, 561–5.

Jamison, R. N., Raymond, S. A., Levine, J. G., Slawsby, E. A., Nedeljkovic, S. S. and Katz, N. P. (2001) Electronic diaries for monitoring chronic pain: 1-year validation study. *Pain,* 91, 277–85.

Jensen, M. P., Brant-Zawadzki, M., Obuchowski, N., Modic, M., Malkasian, D. and Ross, J. (1994) Magnetic resonance imaging of the lumbar spine in people without back pain. *New England Journal of Medicine,* 331, 69–73.

Karsdorp, P. A., Nijst, S. E., Goossens, M. E. and Vlaeyen, J. W. S. (2009) The role of current mood and stop rules on physical task performance: An experimental investigation in patients with work-related upper extremity pain. *European Journal of Pain,* 14(4), 434–40.

Kazdin, A. E. (2003) *Research design in clinical psychology.* Boston, MA: Allyn & Bacon.

Keogh, E. and Asmundson, G. J. G. (2004) Negative affectivity, catastrophizing, and anxiety sensitivity. In G. J. G.Asmundson, J. W. S.Vlaeyen and G. Crombez, G. (ed.) *Understanding and treating fear of pain.* New York: Oxford University Press.

Keogh, E., Ellery, D., Hunt, C. and Hannent, I. (2001) Selective attentional bias for pain-related stimuli amongst pain fearful individuals. *Pain,* 91, 91–100.

Klenerman, L., Slade, P. D., Stanley, I. M., et al. (1995) The prediction of chronicity in patients with an acute attack of low back pain in a general practice setting. *Spine*, **20**, 478–84.

Kori, S. H., Miller, R. and Todd, D. (1990) Kinesiophobia: a new view of chronic pain behavior. *Pain Management*, Jan/Feb, 35–43.

Kugler, K., Wijn, J., Geilen, M., de Jong, J. and Vlaeyen, J. W. S. (1999) *The photograph series of daily activities (PHODA). CD-rom version 1.0.*, Heerlen, The Netherlands: Institute for Rehabilitation Research and School for Physiotherapy.

Leeuw, M., Goossens, M. E., Linton, S. J., Crombez, G., Boersma, K. and Vlaeyen, J. W. (2007a) The fear-avoidance model of musculoskeletal pain: current state of scientific evidence. *Journal of Behavioral Medicine*, **30**, 77–94.

Leeuw, M., Goossens, M. E. J. B., van Breukelen, G. J. P., Boersma, K. and Vlaeyen, J. W. S. (2007b) Measuring perceived harmfulness of physical activities in patients with chronic low back pain: The photograph series of daily activities – Short electronic version. *Journal of Pain*, **8**, 840–49.

Leeuw, M., Goossens, M. E. J. B., van Breukelen, G. J. P., et al. (2008) Exposure in vivo versus operant graded activity in chronic low back pain patients: Results of a randomized controlled trial. *Pain*, **138**, 192–207.

Leeuw, M., Houben, R. M., Severeijns, R., Picavet, H. S., Schouten, E. G. and Vlaeyen, J. W. (2007c) Pain-related fear in low back pain: a prospective study in the general population. *European Journal of Pain*, **11**, 256–66.

Leeuw, M., Peters, M. L., Wiers, R. W. and Vlaeyen, J. W. (2007d) Measuring Fear of Movement/(Re) injury in Chronic Low Back Pain Using Implicit Measures. *Cognitive Behaviour Therapy*, **36**, 52–64.

Lethem, J., Slade, P. D., Troup, J. D. and Bentley, G. (1983) Outline of a Fear-Avoidance Model of exaggerated pain perception—I. *Behaviour Research and Therapy*, **21**, 401–8.

Linton, S. J. (1998) The socioeconomic impact of chronic back pain: is anyone benefiting? *Pain*, **75**, 163–68.

Linton, S. J., Boersma, K., Jansson, M., Overmeer, T., Lindblom, K. and Vlaeyen, J. W. S. (2008) A randomized controlled trial of exposure in vivo for patients with spinal pain reporting fear of work-related activities. *European Journal of Pain*, **12**, 722–30.

Linton, S. J., Overmeer, T., Janson, M., Vlaeyen, J. W. S. and de Jong, J. R. (2002) Graded in-vivo exposure treatment for fear-avoidant pain patients with functional disability: A case study. *Cognitive Behaviour Therapy*, **31**, 49–58.

Lohnberg, J. (2007) A Review of Outcome Studies on Cognitive-Behavioral Therapy for Reducing Fear-Avoidance Beliefs Among Individuals With Chronic Pain. *Journal of Clinical Psychology in Medical Settings*, **14**, 113–22.

McCracken, L. M. and Dhingra, L. (2002) A short version of the Pain Anxiety Symptoms Scale (PASS—20): Preliminary development and validity. *Pain Research and Management*, **7**, 45–50.

McCracken, L. M., Gross, R. T., Aikens, J. and Carnrike, C. L. M., Jr. (1996) The assessment of anxiety and fear in persons with chronic pain: A comparison of instruments. *Behaviour Research and Therapy*, **34**, 927–33.

McCracken, L. M., Zayfert, C. and Gross, R. T. (1992) The pain anxiety symptoms scale: development and validation of a scale to measure fear of pain. *Pain*, **50**, 67–73.

McNeil, D. W. and Rainwater, A. J. (1998) Development of the Fear of Pain Questionnaire—III. *Journal of Behavioral Medicine*, **21**, 389–410.

McNeil, D. W. and Vowles, K. E. (2004) Assessment of fear and anxiety associated with pain: Conceptualization, methods, and measures, in G. J. G.Asmundson, J. W. S. Vlaeyen, and G. Crombez (ed) *Understanding and treating fear of pain*. New York: Oxford University Press.

Michael, E. S. and Bruns, J. W. (2004). Catastrophizing and pain sensitivity among chronic pain patients: moderating effects of sensory and affect focus. *Annals of Behavioral Medicine*, **27**, 185–94.

Moore, J. E., Von Korff, M., Cherkin, D., Saunders, K. and Lorig, K. (2000) A randomized trial of cognitive-behavioral program for enhancing back pain self care in a primary care setting. *Pain*, **88**, 145–53.

Morley, S. and Eccleston, C. (2004) The object of fear in pain, in G. J. G. Asmundson, J. W. S. Vlaeyen, and G. Crombez (ed.) *Understanding and treating fear of pain.* New York: Oxford University Press.

Mowrer, O. H. (1947) On the dual nature of learning: a reinterpretation of 'conditioning' an 'problem-solving'. *Harvard Educational Review,* **17,** 102–50.

Nachemson, A. L., Waddell, G. and Norlund, A. L. (2000) Epidemiology of neck and low back pain, in A. L. Nachemson and E. Johnsson (ed.) *Neck and back pain: the scientific evidence of causes, diagnosis, and treatment.* Philadelphia, PA: Lippincott, Williams, and Wilkins.

Naliboff, B. D., Waters, A. M., Labus, J. S., et al. (2008) Increased acoustic startle responses in ibs patients during abdominal and nonabdominal threat. *Psychosomatic Medicine,* **70,** 920–27.

Peters, M. L., Sorbi, M. J., Kruise, D. A., Kerssens, J. J., Veerhak, P. F. M. and Bensing, J. M. (2000) Electronic diary assessment of pain, disability and psychological adaptation in patients differing in duration of pain. *Pain,* **84,** 181–92.

Peters, M. L., Vlaeyen, J. W. and Weber, W. E. (2005) The joint contribution of physical pathology, pain-related fear and catastrophizing to chronic back pain disability. *Pain,* **113,** 45–50.

Peters, M. L., Vlaeyen, J. W. S. and Kunnen, A. M. W. (2002) Is pain-related fear a predictor of somatosensory hypervigilance in chronic low back pain patients? *Behaviour Research and Therapy,* **40,** 85–103.

Philips, H. C. (1987) Avoidance behaviour and its role in sustaining chronic pain. *Behaviour Research and Therapy,* **25,** 273–9.

Phillips, C., Main, C. J., Buck, R., Aylward, M., Wynne-Jones, G. and Farr, A. (2008) Prioristising pain in policy making: The need for a whole systems perspective. *Health Policy,* **88,** 166–75.

Picavet, H. S. and Schouten, J. S. (2003) Musculoskeletal pain in the Netherlands: prevalences, consequences and risk groups, the DMC(3)-study. *Pain,* **102,** 167–78.

Pincus, T. and Morley, S. (2001) Cognitive-processing bias in chronic pain: A review and integration. *Psychological Bulletin,* **127,** 599–617.

Pool, J. J. M., Hiralal, S., Ostelo, R. W. J. G., et al. (2009). The applicability of the Tampa Scale of Kinesiophobia for patients with sub-acute neck pain. *Quality and Quantity,* **43,** 773–80.

Rachmann, S. (2004) *Anxiety.* Hove: Psychological Press.

Reneman, M. F., Jorritsma, W., Dijkstra, S. J. and Dijkstra, P. U. (2003) Relationship between kinesiophobia and performance in a functional capacity evaluation. *Journal of Occupational Rehabilitation,* **13,** 277–85.

Reneman, M. F., Schiphorst Preuper, H. R., Kleen, M., Geertzen, J. H. B. and Dijkstra, P.U. (2007) Are pain intensity and pain related fear related to functional capacity evaluation performances of patients with chronic low back pain? *Journal of Occupational Rehabilitation,* **17,** 247–58.

Riley, J. F., Ahern, D. K. and Follnik, M. J. (1988) Chronic Pain and Functional Impairment: Assessing Beliefs About Their Relationship. *Archives of Physical Medicine and Rehabilitation,* **69,** 579–82.

Roelofs, J., McCracken, L. M., Peters, M. L., Crombez, G., van Breukelen, G. and Vlaeyen, J. W. S. (2004a) Psychometric evaluation of the Pain Anxiety Symptoms Scale (PASS) in chronic pain patients. *Journal of Behavioral Medicine,* **27,** 167–83.

Roelofs, J., Peters, M. L., Fassaert, T. and Vlaeyen, J. W. (2005) The role of fear of movement and injury in selective attentional processing in patients with chronic low back pain: a dot-probe evaluation. *Journal of Pain,* **6,** 294–300.

Roelofs, J., Peters, M. L., van der Zijden, M. and Vlaeyen, J. W. (2004b) Does fear of pain moderate the effects of sensory focusing and distraction on cold pressor pain in pain-free individuals? *Journal of Pain,* **5,** 250–6.

Roelofs, J., Peters, M. L. and Vlaeyen, J. W. S. (2003) The modified Stroop paradigm as a measure of selective attention towards pain-related information in patients with chronic low back pain. *Psychological Reports,* **92,** 707–15.

Roelofs, J., Peters, M. L., Zeegers, M. P. A. and Vlaeyen, J. W. S. (2002) The modified stroop paradigm as a measure of selective attention towards pain-related stimuli among chronic pain patients: a meta-analysis. *European Journal of Pain,* **6,** 273–81.

Roelofs, J., Sluiter, J. K., Frings-Dresen, M. H. W., et al. (2007) Fear of movement and (re)injury in chronis musculoskeletal pain: Evidence for an invariant two-factor model of the Tampa Scale for Kinesiophobia across pain diagnoses and Dutch, Swedish, and Canadian samples. *Pain,* **131,** 181–90.

Schmidt, C. O., Raspe, H., Pfingsten, M., et al. (2007) Back pain in the german adult population: Prevalence, severity, and sociodemographic correlates in a multiregional survey. *Spine,* **32,** 2005–11.

Severeijns, R., van den Hout, M. A. and Vlaeyen, J. W. S. (2005) The causal status of pain catastrophizing: An experimental test with healthy participants. *European Journal of Pain,* **9,** 257–65.

Sigmon, S. T. and LaMattina, S. M. (2006) Self-assessment, in M.Hersen (ed.) *Clinician's Handbook of Adult Behavioral Assessment.* Oxford: Academic Press.

Smeets, R. J. E. M., Wittink, H., Hidding, A. and Knottnerus, J. A. (2006) Do patients with chronic low back pain have a lower level of aerobic fitness than healthy controls? : Are pain, disability, fear of injury, working status, or level of leisure time activity associated with the difference in aerobic fitness level? *Spine,* **31,** 90–8.

Stegen, K., Van Diest, I., Van de Woestijne, K. P. and Van den Bergh, O. (2001) Do persons with negative affect have an attentional bias to bodily sensations? *Cognition and Emotion,* **15,** 813–29.

Stewart, S. H. and Asmundson, G. J. G. (2006) Anxiety sensitivity and its impact on pain experiences and conditions: a state of the art. *Cognitive Behaviour Therapy,* **35,** 185–8.

Sullivan, M. J., Adams, H. and Sullivan, M. E. (2004) Communicative dimensions of pain catastrophizing: social cueing effects on pain behaviour and coping. *Pain,* **107,** 220–6.

Sullivan, M. J., Adams, H., Tripp, D. A. and Stanish, W. (2008) Stage of chronicity and treatment response in patients with musculoskeletal injuries and concurrent symptoms of depression. *Pain,* **135,** 151–9.

Sullivan, M. J. L., Bishop, S. R. and Pivik, J. (1995) The Pain Catastrophizing Scale: Development and validation. *Psychological Assessment,* **7,** 524–32.

Sullivan, M. J. L., Lynch, M. E. and Clark, A. J. (2005) Dimensions of catastrophic thinking associated with pain experience and disability in patients with neuropathic pain conditions. *Pain,* **113,** 310–15.

Swinkels-Meewisse, E. J. C. M., Swinkels, R. A. H. M., Verbeek, A. L. M., Vlaeyen, J. W. S. and Oostendorp, R. A. B. (2003) Psychometric properties of the Tampa Scale for kinesiophobia and the fear-avoidance beliefs questionnaire in acute low back pain. *Manual Therapy,* **8,** 29–36.

Swinkels-Meewisse, I. E., Roelofs, J., Schouten, E. G., Verbeek, A. L., Oostendorp, R. A. and Vlaeyen, J. W. (2006) Fear of movement/(re)injury predicting chronic disabling low back pain: a prospective inception cohort study. *Spine,* **31,** 658–64.

Tang, N. K., Salkovskis, P. M., Poplavskaya, E., Wright, K. J., Hanna, M. and Hester, J. (2007) Increased use of safety-seeking behaviors in chronic back pain patients with high health anxiety. *Behaviour Research and Therapy,* **45,** 2821–35.

Trost, Z., France, C. R. and Thomas, J. S. (2009) Examination of the photograph series of daily activities (PHODA) scale in chronic low back pain patients with high and low kinesiophobia. *Pain,* **141,** 276–82.

Turk, D. C. and Flor, H. (1999) Chronic pain: A biobehavioral perspective. *Psychosocial factors in pain: Critical perspectives.* New York: Guilford Press.

Turk, D. C. and Gatchel, R. J. (2002) *Psychological approaches to pain management: A practitioner's handbook.* New York: Guildford.

Turk, D. C., Robinson, J. P., Sherman, J. J., Burwinkle, T. and Swanson, K. (2008) Assessing fear in patients with cervical pain: development and validation of the Pictorial Fear of Activity Scale-Cervical (PFActS-C). *Pain,* **139,** 55–62.

Turner, J. A., Franklin, G., Fulton-Kehoe, D., et al. (2006) Worker recovery expectations and fear-avoidance predict work disability in a population-based workers' compensation back pain sample. *Spine,* **31** 682–9.

Turner, J. A., Jensen, M. P., Warms, C. A. and Cardenas, D. D. (2002) Catastrophizing is associated with pain intensity, psychological distress, and pain-related disability among individuals with chronic pain after spinal cord injury. *Pain,* **98,** 127–34.

Turner, J. A., Mancl, L. and Aaron, L. A. (2004) Pain-related catastrophizing: a daily process study. *Pain,* **110**, 103–11.

Van Damme, S., Crombez, G. and Eccleston, C. (2002) Retarded disengagement from pain cues: the effects of pain catastrophizing and pain expectancy. *Pain,* **100**, 111–18.

Van Damme, S., Crombez, G., Eccleston, C. and Roelofs, J. (2004) The role of hypervigilance in the experience of pain, in G. J. G.Asmundson, J. W. S. Vlaeyen, and G. Crombez (ed.) *Understanding and treating fear of pain.* New York: Oxford University Press.

Van Damme, S, Crombez, G. and Eccleston, C. (2008) Coping with pain: A motivational perspective. *Pain,* **139**, 1–4.

Vancleef, L. M. G. and Peters, M. L. (2006) The interruptive effect of pain on attention. *Journal of Pain,* **7**, 21–2.

Vancleef, L. M. G., Peters, M. L., Roelofs, J. and Asmundson, G. J. G. (2006) Do fundamental fears differentially contribute to pain-related fear and pain catastrophizing? An evaluation of the sensitivity index. *European Journal of Pain,* **10**, 527–36.

Vancleef, L. M. G., Vlaeyen, J. W. and Peters, M. L. (2009) Dimensional and Componential Structure of a Hierarchical Organisation of Pain-related Anxiety Constructs. *Psychological Assessment,* **23**, 340–51.

Vansteenwegen, D., Iberico, C., Vervliet, B., Marescau, V. and Hermans, D. (2008) Contextual fear induced by unpredictability in a human fear conditioning preparation is related to the chronic expectation of a threatening US. *Biological Psychology,* **77**, 39–46.

Verbunt, J., Seelen, H., Vlaeyen, J., et al. (2003) Disuse and deconditioning in chronic low back pain: Concepts and hypotheses on contributing mechanisms. *European Journal of Pain,* **7**, 9–21.

Verhaak, P. F., Kerssens, J. J., Dekker, J., Sorbi, M. J. and Bensing, J. M. (1998) Prevalence of chronic benign pain disorder among adults: a review of the literature. *Pain,* **77**, 231–9.

Vlaeyen, J. W., De Jong, J., Leeuw, M. and Crombez, G. (2004a) Fear reduction in chronic pain: graded exposure in vivo with behavioural experiments, in G. J. G.Asmundson, J. W. S. Vlaeyen, and G. Crombez (ed.) *Understanding and treating fear of pain.* New York: Oxford University Press.

Vlaeyen, J. W., Kole-Snijders, A. M. J., Boeren, A. M. and Van Eek, H. (1995a) Fear of movemement/(re) injury in chronic low back pain and its relation to behavioral performance. *Pain,* **62**, 363–72.

Vlaeyen, J. W., Timmermans, C., Rodriguez, L. M., et al. (2004b) Catastrophic thinking about pain increases discomfort during internal atrial cardioversion. *Journal of Psychosomatic Research,* **56**, 139–44.

Vlaeyen, J. W. S., de Jong, J., Heuts, P. H. T. G. and Crombez, G. (2008) Graded exposure in vivo for pain-related fear, in H. Breivik, W. Campbell and M. K. Nicholas (ed.) *Clinical Pain Management: Practice and procedures.* 2nd edn. London, Hodder & Stoughton.

Vlaeyen, J. W. S., de Jong, J. R., Geilen, M., Heuts, P. and van Breukelen, G. (2001) Graded exposure in vivo in the treatment of pain-related fear: a replicated single-case experimental design in four patients with low back pain.. *Behaviour Research and Therapy,* **39**, 151–66.

Vlaeyen, J. W. S., Kole-Snijders, A. M. J., Rotteveel, A. M., Ruesink, R. et al. (1995b) The role of fear of movement/(re)injury in pain disability. *Journal of Occupational Rehabilitation,* **5**, 235–52.

Vlaeyen, J. W. S. and Linton, S. J. (2000) Fear-avoidance and its consequences in chronic musculoskeletal pain: A state of the art. *Pain,* **85**, 317–32.

Vlaeyen, J. W. and Morley, S. (2004). Active despite pain: The putative role of stop-rules and current mood. *Pain,* **110**, 512–16.

Vowles, K. E. and Gross, R. T. (2003) Work-related beliefs about injury and physical capability for work in individuals with chronic pain. *Pain,* **101**, 291–8.

Waddel, G. (2004) The biopsychosocial model, in G. Waddel (ed.) *The back pain revolution.* Edinburgh: Churchill Livingstone.

Waddell, G. (1987) Volvo award in clinical sciences. A new clinical model for the treatment of low back pain. *Spine,* **12**, 632–44.

Waddell, G. (2004) The epidemiology of back pain, in G. Waddel (ed.) *The back pain revolution.* Edinburgh: Churchill Livingstone.

Waddell, G., Newton, M., Henderson, I., et al. (1993) A Fear-Avoidance Beliefs Questionnaire (FABQ) and the role of fear-avoidance beliefs in chronic low back pain and disability. *Pain,* **52,** 157–68.

Walker, B. F. (2000) The prevalence of low back pain: a systematic review of the literature from 1966 to 1998. *Journal of Spinal Disorders,* **13,** 205–17.

Walker, B. F., Muller, R. and Grant, W. D. (2004) Low back pain in Australian adults. Prevalence and associated disability. *Journal of Manipulative Physiology and Therapy,* **27,** 238–44.

Walker, J. R. and Furer, P. (2008) Interoceptive exposure in the treatment of health anxiety and hypochondriasis. *Journal of Cognitive Psychotherapy,* **22,** 366–78.

Weiner, D., Pieper, C., McConnell, E., Martinez, S. and Keefe, F. (1996) Pain measurement in elders with chronic low back pain: traditional and alternative approaches. *Pain,* **67,** 461–7.

Wittink, H., Hoskins Michel, T. H., Wagner, A., Sukiennik, A. and Rogers, W. (2000) Deconditioning in patients with chronic low back pain: fact or fiction? *Spine,* **25,** 2221–8.

Woods, M. P. and Asmundson, G. J. G. (2008) Evaluating the efficacy of graded in vivo exposure for the treatment of fear in patients with chronic back pain: A randomized controlled trial. *Pain,* **136,** 271–80.

# Chapter 15

# Endurance-Related Pain Responses in the Development of Chronic Back Pain

Monika I. Hasenbring, Dirk Hallner, and
Adina C. Rusu

## 15.1 Introduction

During the past two decades, a significant amount of evidence has supported the impact of pain-related cognitive, affective, and behavioural responses on the development and mainte-nance of chronic musculoskeletal pain (Turk and Rudy 1992; Waddel 2004; Gatchel et al. 2007). For example, catastrophizing and pain-related fear were identified as important mediators of pain and disability (Linton 2000; Sullivan et al. 2001; Turner and Aaron 2001). The fear-avoidance model (FAM; Vlaeyen and Linton 2000) is a stimulating approach, postulating a pathway between these pain responses, physical disuse and chronic pain (Verbunt et al. 2003, see detailed discus-sion of the FAM in Chapter 14). However, recently, there is growing evidence that a second, potentially opposite pathway will also lead to the development and maintenance of chronic pain. This alternative pathway is based upon endurance-related responses and includes physical over-use or overload instead of physical disuse as main mediators (Bousema et al. 2007; Hasenbring et al. 2006; Smeets et al. 2007). The avoidance-endurance model (AEM) proposes several path-ways for chronicity of pain based on either endurance- or fear avoidance-related responses. The following review will at first focus on research concerning the frequency of self-reported endur-ance-related responses to pain, as a complement to the well-known fear-avoidance responses. Second, basic assumptions underlying the conceptualization of the AEM will be outlined. This will be followed by a review of existing empirical evidence supporting hypotheses related to the AEM and its consequences for the performance of daily activities will be presented. Finally, clini-cal implications, such as proposed modifications for behavioural interventions will be described.

## 15.2 The occurrence of endurance-related pain responses

Pain demands attention, specifically when it occurs suddenly. In an acute pain situation this symptom could be an indicator of a potential medical problem that has to be solved. Pain how-ever, often occurs in situations where people are engaged in several competing occupational, house work, and leisure activities. Therefore, at least two goals may be activated simultaneously—finding an explanation and solution for the pain problem on the one hand and to maintain cur-rent activities on the other. Due to the model of limited mental resources in goal-directed behaviour (Norman and Bobrow 1975), these competing goals may result in a goal-conflict trig-gering a goal-shielding mechanism, in which commitment to a focal goal inhibits the availability of alternative goals and distracting information (Fishbach and Fergusan 2007; Goschke and Dreisbach 2008). For example, suddenly occurring, intensive pain that occurs during house-work may become pre-potent leading to an interruption of ongoing activities and result in calling a doctor. In contrast, when several weeks later such an acute pain episode is resolving, recurrent episodes of milder pain may not have this interruptive quality. It more and more depends on the resulting individual goal interference, potential habitual mechanisms resolving these conflicts, as well as on situational demands, as to whether attention will be directed to this pain stimulus or to alternative activities.

Only recently, evidence has been acquired related to the frequency of attentional responses to pain symptoms, when these occur during other activities. When people are asked to evaluate coping strategies, distraction is rated as highly effective and is preferred over alternative techniques (McCaul and Haugtvedt 1982; Ahles et al. 1983). In a laboratory experiment, McCaul and Haugvedt (1982) reported that 80% of their subjects preferred distraction over attending sensations for coping with cold pressor pain, whereas 92% of subjects who were instructed to attend to the concrete sensations of the pain stimulus, reported less distress than subjects in the distraction condition. That means, distraction was preferred by most of the people although it was not an effective coping strategy, especially for severe pain (McCaul and Mallot 1984). The question arises, how people behave in their daily life, when confronted with pain? Do they divide their attention between the pain stimulus and their current activity? How does emotional arousal impact on the perception of pain, and what do individuals do in order to reduce pain?

Twenty-five years ago, Philips and Jahanshahi (1986) proposed avoidance as the most frequent and prominent behavioural response to pain. Their evaluation was based on a systematic comparison of three different pain related responses (avoidance, complaint, and help-seeking behaviour) in patients with chronic headache and low back pain (LBP). This study established the focus on an important maladaptive pattern of pain responses that was further conceptualized within several FAMs of pain (Lethem et al. 1983; Philips 1987; Asmundson et al. 1999; Vlaeyen and Linton 2000). Within this context, fear-avoidance responses (FAR) consist of avoidance of pain-associated activities on the behavioural level, elicited by fear (e.g. fear of pain-related movements) on the affective level and automatic thoughts, such as catastrophizing or more generalized appraisals (e.g. fear-avoidance beliefs) on the cognitive level.

However, focusing on coping responses, which encompasses both pain-related thoughts and behaviour, several studies have shown that task persistent behaviour despite pain and thought suppression seem to be as frequent as catastrophizing and avoidance. Using the Coping Strategies Questionnaire (CSQ), Rosenstiel and Keefe (1983) found that patients with chronic pain reported that they were active despite pain or ignored pain in the same frequency as they reported catastrophizing about pain. This finding was confirmed by others (Turner and Clancy 1986; Haythornetwaite et al 1998; Garcia-Campayo et al. 2007). Within the AEM of pain (described below), cognitions involving thought suppression, distraction or minimization, task persistence behaviour in spite of severe pain and potentially positive mood despite pain represent central aspects of pain-related endurance responses (ERs). Pain-related endurance is motivated by the goal of maintaining current activities despite feeling pain, either by struggling against the potentially alarming character of pain (thought suppression) or by successfully distracting from pain (Hasenbring 2000).

Hasenbring (1993) and Grebner et al. (1999) investigated the occurrence of fear-avoidance-versus endurance-related responses in samples of acute and subacute back and leg pain prior to lumbar disc surgery. Using the Kiel Pain Inventory (Hasenbring 1994), both research groups reported cognitions of thought suppression with at least the same frequency as helplessness, hopelessness, and catastrophizing. An identical finding was found for the relation of avoidance behaviour compared to endurance behaviour despite severe pain. Recently, in a sample of chronic back pain patients, using a Chinese version of the Chronic Pain Coping Inventory (CPCI, Jensen et al. 1995), Wong et al. (2010) found different coping strategies, such as guarding, resting, asking for assistance, relaxation and task persistence, were rated concerning the number of days over the past weeks that have been used for each of these strategies at least once. The authors reported the highest frequency scores for task persistence behaviour (mean 4.32, SD 1.75) compared to typical FA responses such as guarding (mean 3.06, SD 1.84) or resting (mean 3.64, SD 1.93). Pain responses that are to be seen as adaptive, such as relaxation (mean 1.94, SD 1.70) and exercise (mean 2.52, SD 1.89) were rated much lower. Concerning mood, in acute and subacute as well as in chronic LBP, positive mood despite pain was rated with higher frequency than anxiety and depressive mood (Hasenbring et al. 1994; Hasenbring et al. 2009).

Taken together, when confronted with acute, subacute, or chronic LBP in daily life, endurance responses such as positive mood despite pain, cognitions of distraction and thought suppression as well as task persistence behaviour seem to be more often occurring than FAR with anxious and depressive mood, cognitions of catastrophizing, helplessness/hopelessness, and avoidance behaviour. Whereas there is substantial evidence that FAR leads to increased pain-related disability and depression over time, the question arises as to the consequences following endurance responses.

## 15.3 Theoretical considerations: the Avoidance-Endurance Model (AEM) of pain

The AEM of pain was developed in order to address FAR as well as ER as important mediators in the development and maintenance of chronic pain and disability (Hasenbring 2000). While earlier formulations of this model primarily focused on potential maladaptive consequences of these different pain responses, the current version of the AEM also hypothesizes adaptive short-term consequences (positive or negative reinforcement) that may be responsible for the maintenance of these reactions.

### 15.3.1 Basic assumptions

Basic assumptions underlying the AEM are as follows. In accordance with the psychophysiological model of anxiety (Lang 1970) loose relations are hypothesized for the cognitive, affective, and behavioural responses to pain. Further, comparable to the Dynamic Model of Affect (DMA, Davis and Zautra 2004), an opposite pattern of FAR and ER are expected to exist on distinct dimensions, implying that opposite features can be activated independently. This assumption is supported by evidence of distinct neural systems for opposite affects and cognitions (e.g. Hass and Canli, 2008). We hypothesize that each individual will show a specific pattern of cognitive, affective, and behavioural pain responses when confronted with pain and that only specific, highly rigid and time-stable pattern of cognitive, affective, and behavioural pain responses will contribute to the maintenance of pain in the long-term run. We suggest that FAR represent a specific and highly rigid pattern of pain-related fear, cognitions of catastrophizing and helplessness, hopelessness, and behavioural avoidance (*FAR pattern*). In contrast, the AEM suggests that due to ER at least two different response pattern can be described influencing the maintenance of pain and disability. The distress-endurance pattern (DER) refers to marked thought suppression, emotions of anxiety and depression and to task persistence in spite of pain on the behavioural level. The eustress-endurance pattern (EER) refers to ignoring pain sensations and minimizing the meaning of pain experiences and marked task persistence behaviour, often accompanied by high scores on positive mood despite pain. Furthermore, an adaptive response (AR) pattern is suggested to be characterized by cognitions of sensory monitoring without ongoing negative affects, by a high degree of flexibility between avoidance and endurance responses to pain, supporting the effect of biomedical treatments. Finally, we suggest that there are a number of psychoneurobiological pathways from acute to chronic pain for FAR and ER that can be explained via learning conditioning theory in the long-term as well as maintaining mechanisms in the short-term.

### 15.3.2 **Fear-avoidance responses and physical disuse**

The pathway between catastrophizing, fear of pain, avoidance behaviour, and physical disuse is conceptualized within several FAMs in the literature (see for more detail Chapter 14). Patients, that will exclusively show FAR, will tend to avoid all physical and social activities that could elicit pain. Within this pattern, avoidance behaviour is assumed to be guided by conditioned stimuli (e.g. the imagination of a painful lifting activity elicits fear), shown preventively in order to avoid experience of pain (active avoidance). People will avoid physical activities that they believe will lead to increased back pain (e.g. heavy lifting, walking) as well as social events that are potentially pain provoking (e.g. sitting in a film theatre, having guests for dinner, playing tennis). In the short-term, preventive avoidance behaviour will lead to negative reinforcement, when pain is diminishing or when an increase of pain is lacking. As indicated in Figure 15.1, over time, decreasing physical activity will cause physical deconditioning including negative changes in muscular, motor, cardiorespiratory and metabolic aspects of physical fitness (Verbunt et al. 2003). Due to neurobiological processes of central sensitization, physical structures respond with pain during normal activities (Bortz 1984; see also Chapter 4 in this volume). The AEM assumes a further pathway between avoidance of social activities and the development of chronic pain via an increase in depression, mediated by a loss of social reinforcement and increased social isolation (Lewinsohn and Libet, 1972). These differential hypotheses concerning avoidance of physical versus social activities were supported by evidence of positive associations between the subscale Avoidance of Social Activities of the Avoidance-Endurance Questionnaire (AEQ; Hasenbring et al. 2009) and BDI depression and between the Avoidance of Physical Activities subscale and fear-avoidance beliefs concerning physical activities, measured with the Fear-Avoidance-Beliefs Questionnaire (FABQ), Waddell Physical Activity (Hasenbring et al. 2009).

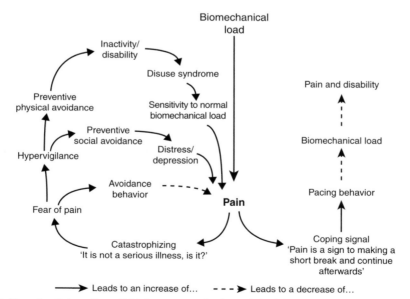

**Fig. 15.1** (See also Colour Plate 9) Maintenance of pain and disability by fear-avoidance responses to pain.

### 15.3.3 Endurance-response pattern and physical overuse/overload

Patients that will exclusively show an ER pattern with high scores on endurance behaviour despite severe pain (irrespective of the distress or eustress version) will have a high risk for physical over-activity leading to overuse or overload of physical structures. In a situation, in which a pain-related interruption of daily activities, normally taken into account, will be disdained or disregarded, overuse (based on repetitive movements) or overload (based on ongoing static strain postures) will result in a number of damages of muscle fibres, nerves, bones, and ligaments. These behaviour-related damages as well as the repetitive experience of pain will maintain pain and contribute to neurobiological mechanisms of peripheral and central sensitization. In the post-injury acute or subacute phase of pain, an ER pattern will disturb the normal recovery period, and can consequently result in a higher risk for developing chronic pain problems.

DER and EER patterns differ mainly in their cognitive and affective responses. Patients with a DER pattern tend to show thought suppression combined with an increased depressive mood. Thought suppression represents a cognitive response that blocks the perception of pain or the interruption of daily activities normally demanded by pain (Eccleston and Crombez 1999). Thought suppression attempts are often disorganized, non-focused, effortful, and at risk for fail-ure. It may be reasonable, that thought suppression is followed by processes of intermittent rein-forcement in the short term. Sometimes a successful suppression of a pain experience and concentration on concurrent daily activities may be possible whereas at other times pain will repeatedly come into one's focus of attention. Frequent failure of thought suppression, however, may lead to a decreased perception of self-efficacy and to an increased emotional distress. Moreover, a rebound phenomenon was suggested (Wegner et al. 1987) leading to more fre-quently occurring pain-related thoughts accompanied by the perception of additional failure, feelings of helplessness-, hopelessness, and depressive mood (see Figure 15.2).

In contrast, patients with an EER pattern tend to pain-related cognitive responses of distraction from pain or minimizing the meaning of pain experience and marked positive mood despite severe pain. Distraction from pain might be more successful than thought suppression as it rep-resents a more organized and focused way of attention diversion (Cioffi and Holloway 1993).

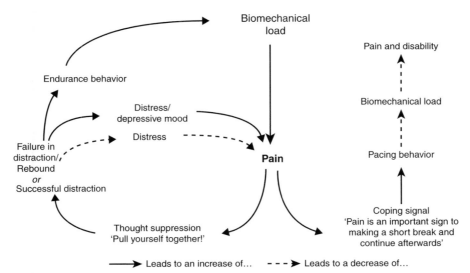

**Fig. 15.2** (See also Colour Plate 10) Maintenance of pain by distress-endurance responses to pain.

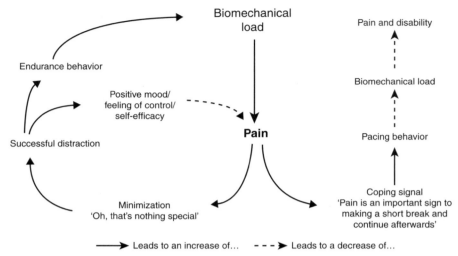

Fig. 15.3 (See also Colour Plate 11) Maintenance of pain by eustress-endurance responses (EER) to pain.

Successful distraction and maintaining concentration towards concurrent daily activities may lead to feelings of high self-control, high self-efficacy, and positive mood in the short term (see Figure 15.3). A rebound effect will occur less often or never. However, due to ongoing task persistence behaviour, these patients also tend to overlook pain experiences caused by strain-induced small and repetitive damages of soft tissues, such as muscles, ligaments and tendons and reveal overuse and overload in the long-term.

### 15.3.4 Adaptive pain responses and balancing of physical/mental load

The AEM assumes that there is an adaptive way to respond to back pain sensations that leads to a health-promoting balancing of activities including physical, mental, and social activities. In the phase of acute/subacute pain, when pain still has the function of a signal indicating some kind of physical damage, cognitions labelled as coping signal lead to a conscious awareness of individual needs. In the case, one has sat a long time, pain may be attributed as a signal to making a short break standing up and move a little. Lingering upon a static strain position, back pain normally increases over time. The earlier the break is realized, the less time is needed to reach a sensible relief in pain.

Imagine different people suffering from back pain who are invited to a champagne reception of a friend where all guests will stay the whole time. Normally, no seats will be available at this sort of party. All these individuals had experienced a heavy increase of pain in such a situation some time before. The AEM suggests that a man showing a pattern of FAR will be afraid of this pain increase and therefore decline this invitation. Another man showing a pattern of DER will visit this party despite this pain experience. When during standing and talking with friends pain will increase (for instance from a level of '3' at the beginning of the party up to a level of '5') his automatic thoughts may be as follows: 'Don't make such a fuss, an Indian does not know pain. You cannot interrupt this talk at this moment!'. He will continue to stay at this party for 2 or more hours and having a pain intensity level of '8' when he is leaving. He will be angry and depressed about the weakness of his body, and when pain has the level of '8', he tends to thoughts of catastrophizing: 'What will happen when this pain does not decrease today?' A third man showing a pattern of EER will also visit this party and will reach complete cognitive distraction by animated talking with his friends. At the end of the party he suddenly will sense pain of high intensity (for instance of level '8') and will wonder why he was not aware of an increase of pain during the time before. The AEM assumes that a man showing a pattern of adaptive pain responses will know that a party where all guests will stay a long time will lead to an unnecessary increase of back pain. He decides not to decline this party visit knowing that meeting his friends will increase positive mood. He decides to phone to his friend asking him to prepare some chairs giving him the chance of sitting for a while. During this party, he decides to make short breaks latest at an increase of pain from '3' to '5'.

What ingredients belong to this kind of adaptive pain response? First, the awareness of a slight pain increase at low levels of pain intensity. Second, the acceptance that standing for a long time represents a kind of biomechanical load leading to a delay of the recovery of back pain. Third, the acceptance of individual needs making a short break changing the bodily position. Fourth, the behavioural competence that enables him, asking his friend providing a chair.

Patients with elevated FAR or ER pattern report a great number of external obstacles (for instance, high social pressure, specific circumstances), internal cognitive/affective barriers (e.g. dysfunctional thoughts 'what will my friends think of me?') or behavioural deficits regarding social competence that makes it difficult to realize the above mentioned adaptive responding to pain. To our best knowledge, there is no empirical evidence concerning a systematic classification of external and internal obstacles until now. In Chapter 27 of this volume, we will describe different obstacles based on extensive clinical work as well as specific cognitive-behavioural treatment strategies aiming at overcoming individual barriers and promoting adaptive pain responses.

## 15.4 Evidence for endurance-related components of AEM

The degree to which single affective, cognitive and behavioural responses, described in the AEM as well as the more complex response pattern, will be adaptive is a matter of some debate. Whether single responses or a full pattern will be effective and adaptive or not depends on the outcome criterion used and on the different time-lags used to measure pain responses and the outcomes. For example, active avoidance behaviour may lead, in the short term, to a reduction or prevention of pain. However, in the long term, it may lead to physical disuse and an increase of disability. On the other hand, task persistence behaviour may lead to a feeling of control and short-term distress reduction, but in the long term, it can result in physical overuse and overload including pain increase, a consequence of repetitive micro-damaging of physical structures. Task persistence behaviour that is part of an exclusive DER is associated with cognitions of thought suppression. Due to the lack of success of these cognitions within this pattern, patients may even experience a rapid change between feelings of control and feelings of loss of control. With these considerations in mind, it is obvious that an evaluation of the effect of pain-related responses based on associations found in cross-sectional study designs will only deliver vague information that must interpreted cautiously. The evaluation of both short-term as well as long-term consequences of different response patterns need to be performed in prospective study designs. To identify short-term consequences, experimental trials and process-oriented correlation approaches have to be included. In addition, for identifying long-term consequences prospective cohort studies are necessary.

### 15.4.1 Measurement of endurance-related pain responses

While measurements of pain-related fear and fear-related beliefs are presented in Chapter 14 of this volume, the present chapter will mainly focus on measurements of pain-related endurance with its behavioural feature of task persistence, with the cognitive aspects of thought suppression and distraction and with the affective feature of positive mood despite pain.

## Measurement of behavioural responses

Task persistence behaviour is captured by the CPCI (Jensen et al. 1995), the Kiel Pain Inventory (KPI, Hasenbring 1994), and the KPI-derived Avoidance-Endurance Questionnaire (AEQ, Hasenbring et al. 2009). The scale Task Persistence is a subscale of the CPCI-42 (Jensen et al. 1995; Romano et al. 2003) consists of 42 items assessing coping strategies that patients might use to cope with chronic pain, for instance Guarding, Resting, Asking for Assistance, Relaxation, Task Persistence, Exercise/Stretch, Seeking Social Support, and Coping Self-Statements. Patients are asked to rate the number of days (0–7 days) over the past week that they used each of the strategies at least once. The subscale Task Persistence (TP) consists of 6 items (e.g. 'I kept on doing what I was doing' or 'I didn't let the pain interfere with my activities') and showed sufficient internal consistence (Cronbach's alpha between 0.85 and 0.74) but low re-test reliability ($r=0.66$). Results concerning validity seem to be inconclusive until now: low to moderate negative cross-sectional correlations were reported for task persistence and disability, pain intensity and depression in samples including back pain or mixed pain diagnoses (Jensen et al. 1995; Tan et al. 2001; Romano et al. 2003). No correlation was found for self-reported activity. Truchon and Coté (2005), however, did not find cross-sectional or prospective associations between CPCI-TP and the outcomes pain, disability or return to work, and Garcia-Campayo et al. (2007) reported positive correlations between TP and other so-called illness-focused subscales (e.g. Guarding and Resting) and also positive correlations with the outcome disability, fatigue and depression in a sample of 402 fibromyalgia patients.

The Behavioural Endurance Scale (BES) of the KPI consists of 11 items that focus on coping efforts to finish all activities just started in spite of severe pain (e.g. 'I keep all appointments even though I don't feel well'). Patients indicate on a 7-point scale (0 'never', 6 'always') how often they have acted in such a way in the past 14 days when they experienced pain. Higher scores indicate a higher number of self-reported endurance cognitions and behaviours. Cronbach's alpha for BES was $r=0.81$ (Hasenbring, 1994) in a sample of acute and chronic pain patients with different diagnoses. In a sample of 111 sciatic pain patients, no correlation with pain intensity was found cross-sectional, but positive associations pain intensity prospectively ($r=0.25$, $p <0.01$). Patients high on BES further showed a lower return-to-work rate at the six months follow-up ($p <0.05$). The original BES subscale from the KPI was included to the KPI-derived AEQ (Hasenbring et al. 2009) that was developed in order to measure typical fear-avoidance- as well as endurance-related features of pain responses. In a sample of 191 LBP patients, factorial structure indicated that the two subscales Pain Persistence (PPS, 7 items) and Distraction/Humour (HDS, 5 items) revealed sufficient internal consistency (0.78 and 0.76). The total BES score can be using additionally. Within this sample, there were positive but low correlations between BES, PPS and HDS and pain intensity and negative associations with self-reported disability, depression, fear of pain and days of sick listing (Hasenbring et al. 2009). BES is one of the three marker variables used for building the AEM-based subgroups (see 'AEM-based subgroups').

## Measurement of cognitive responses

The Thought Suppression Scale (TSS) is a subscale of the KPI as well as of the KPI-derived AEQ. The TSS consists of 4 items ('Pull yourself together!'), yielding an internal consistency of 0.78 (Cronbach's alpha) in the original sample of 405 pain patients with different diagnoses (Hasenbring 1994) and 0.80 in LBP patients (Hasenbring et al. 2009). TSS scores were unrelated to pain intensity in a cross-sectional study of acute sciatic pain patients, but positively related to pain as well to depression prospectively at a 6-month follow-up (Hasenbring et al. 1994, Klasen et al. 2006). TSS was more elevated in a dysfunctional subgroup of CLBP patients compared to adaptive copers (Rusu et al. 2008) using the Multidimensional Pain Inventory (MPI; Kerns et al. (1985) -derived subgroup analysis (Turk and Rudy 1988)). TSS is further one of the three marker variables used for building the AEM-based subgroups (see section 'AEM-based subgroups').

Cognitive distraction is captured at least by three measurements, the Humour/Distraction subscale of the AEQ (Hasenbring et al. 2009), the Coping Strategies Questionnaire (CSQ; Rosenstiel and Keefe, 1983) and the Pain-Coping Inventory (PCI; Kraimaat et al. 2003). The Diverting Attention subscale of the CSQ consists of 6 items and reveals sufficient internal consistency (e.g. Cronbach's alpha 0.80 in Hill et al. 1995). Based on exploratory or confirmatory components analyses, the Diverting Attention scale is one of 3–4 features summarized as coping attempts (Hill et al. 1995) or part of so-called active coping (Riley and Robinson, 1997). The same was seeing for the Distraction subscale of the PCI that consists of five items. Internal consistency, however, was rather low in different samples (Alpha <0.70; Kraimaat et al. 2003). It is important to note, that the distraction scale of the PCI contains items that serves to relaxation ('I distract myself by reading, listening to music') on the one hand, and to kinds of endurance behaviour on the other ('I distract myself by undertaking a physical activity'). The Humour/Distraction subscale of the AEQ consists of five items ('I take it with a laugh', 'I distract doing little jobs at home'), yielding an internal consistency of Alpha=0.78. Preliminary validation indicated a positive relationship with pain intensity but a negative one with self-reported disability, depression and fear of pain (Hasenbring et al. 2009).

## Measurement of endurance-related affective responses

The Positive Mood Scale (PMS) is a subscale of the KPI as well as of the KPI-derived AEQ. The KPI-PMS consists of 4 items ('I feel happy, anyway') yielding an internal consistency of .85 (Cronbach's alpha) in the original sample of 513 pain patients with different diagnoses (Hasenbring 1994) and 0.90 for the PMS scale of the AEQ (consisting of 3 items) in a LBP study (Hasenbring et al. 2009). The AEQ-PMS scores were cross-sectional unrelated to pain intensity but negatively correlated with disability, depression, and fear of pain measures (Hasenbring et al. 2009). As described above, the KPI-PMS scores were positively related to pain intensity prospectively, contributing to the prediction of pain condition at the time of discharge from a hospital stay due to sciatic pain (Hasenbring et al. 1994).

## 15.4.2 **AEM-based subgroups**

Research in FAR and ER pattern delivers preliminary support for the fact that subgroups of pain patients are to be identified by specific AEM-based pattern on the affective, cognitive, and behavioural level. Hasenbring (1993) compared for the first time patients with a DER or EER pattern with patients showing an adaptive response (AR) pattern. In this study, using the Beck Depression Inventory (BDI; Beck et al. 1961) and the KPI (Hasenbring, 1994), a cut-off for depression was defined as BDI >9 and the KPI subscales thought suppression and endurance behaviour (mean scale scores) were used in a sample of subacute sciatic pain patients. DER patients differed from AR with respect to higher thought suppression and depression (marker variables), higher pain-related helplessness, hopelessness, higher nonverbal pain behaviour and a higher degree of chronic distress in daily life. EER patients differed from AR showing significantly higher positive mood despite pain, less catastrophizing, less avoidance of physical as well as of social activities and less nonverbal pain behaviour, besides the higher scores in the marker variable endurance behaviour. Data concerning the four AEM-based subgroups had been also reported by Grebner and co-workers (1999). The authors investigated 82 patients prior to a lumbar disc surgery, using a cluster analysis procedure. DER patients revealed more thought suppression as well as more pain-related anxiety and less positive mood compared to EER patients, more thought suppression and pain-related anxiety than FAR and less positive mood compared to AR patients. FAR patients differed from AR showing less positive mood. With respect to avoidance behaviour, there was only a significant difference between EER patients and all other subgroups with lower avoidance in EER. Further data on content validity of AEM-based subgroups have been reporting in a recent study in patients suffering from subacute non-specific low back pain (Hasenbring et al. under review). Besides the marker variables depression, thought suppression and behavioural endurance, DER patients reveal significant higher scores in pain-related anxiety and helplessness/hopelessness as well as in work-related fear-avoidance beliefs. EER patients differ from AR in less avoidance and less work-related fear-avoidance beliefs. FAR patients differed from AR with respect to less behavioural endurance, and with higher avoidance due to mild pain from both ER subgroups.

Thus far, there are preliminary data supporting the content validity of the four subgroups suggested by the AEM, two times using clinical cut-off scores and one study using cluster analysis. Further results on criterion related and prospective validity will be reported in the subsections that follow.

### 15.4.3 **Endurance and pain-related outcomes**

#### Endurance and pain intensity

With regard to single endurance responses, *task persistence behaviour* seems to be the most often investigated feature in clinical research. There is first evidence from several prospective studies concerning short-term as well as long-term effects on the maintenance of pain, mediated by endurance behaviour. In a prospective study of acute and subacute sciatica patients, who underwent an inpatient medical treatment, Hasenbring et al. (1994) reported endurance behaviour as a unique, significant predictor of higher pain intensity at the time of discharge from the hospital as well as at the 6-month follow-up besides other psychological and biomedical predictor variables. In a recent prospective study of subacute non-specific back pain patients in an outpatient setting, endurance behaviour was the main predictor of pain intensity at the 6-month follow-up, after control for baseline pain variables and depression (Hasenbring et al. under review). Additionally, Turner and Clancy (1986) found that diverting attention combined with increasing behavioural activity was predictive of higher pain intensity after a cognitive-behavioural treatment in chronic back pain patients, using a former version of the CSQ. These first data concerning ER pain behaviour provide preliminary support for the AEM-based hypothesis of a link between endurance-related behaviour and the development of higher levels of future pain intensity.

Cross-sectional there is more inconsistent evidence for the relation between task persistence behaviour and pain intensity variables. Some studies reported absent or low positive correlations with pain (Rosenstiel and Keefe 1983; Hadjistavropoulos et al. 1999; Tan et al. 2001; Truchon and Coté 2005; Hasenbring et al. 2009), whereas others reported moderate positive associations with pain intensity (Osborne et al. 2007; Hasenbring et al. under review).

Thought suppression as a cognitive aspect of ER pain responses had been exploring within laboratory experimental studies comparing the effect of different cognitive coping strategies on pain intensity in healthy individuals as well as in clinical studies. Cioffi and Holloway (1993) investigated the effect of thought suppression in comparison to distraction and sensory monitoring. While participants in the distraction condition were told to form a vivid mental picture of their rooms at home, participants in the suppression condition were only told to not think about their hand sensations, to eliminate awareness of them. Furthermore, the authors studied

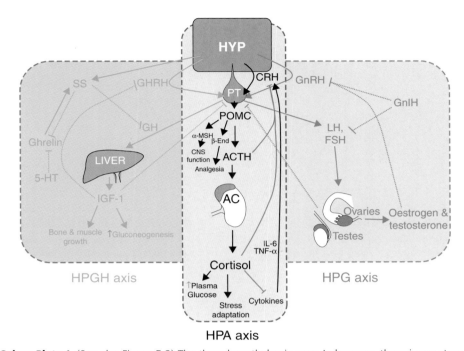

HPA axis

**Colour Plate 1** (See also Figure 5.2) The three hypothalamic axes. In humans, the primary stress response system, the hypothalamic pituitary adrenal (HPA) axis (grey), interacts with two other related neuroendocrine pathways, the hypothalamic pituitary growth hormone (HPGH, green) and hypothalamic pituitary gonadal (HPG, blue) axes. Under normal, stress-free conditions, these three hypothalamic pathways function independently and maintain homeostasis through positive (arrows) and negative (bars) regulation. Each axis is driven by hormonal secretion from the pituitary gland (PT). Corticotropin releasing hormone (CRH) released from the hypothalamus (HYP) initiates HPA activity, by stimulating pro-opiomelanocortin (POMC) production from the PT POMC is sequentially cleaved into a number of active components such as adrenocorticotropin hormone (ACTH) β-endorphin (β-E) and α-melanocyte-stimulating hormone (α-MSH). ACTH is responsible for activating the release of downstream element, cortisol, from the adrenal cortex (AC). Cortisol then suppresses HPA function at various levels as well as inhibiting the production of immune system components, such as interleukin-6 (IL-6) and tumour necrosis factor alpha (TNF-α). In comparison, HPGH activity is instigated by the release of gonadotrophin releasing hormone (GnRH) and the subsequent secretion of growth hormone (GH) by the PT Circulating GH then induces the liver to secrete insulin-like growth factor 1 (IGF-1) resulting in bone and muscle growth and gluconeogenesis. HPG activity is prompted by the hypothalamic release of gonadotrophin releasing hormone (GnRH) which stimulates luteinizing hormone (LH) and follicle stimulating hormone (FSH) secretion from the PT This results in the downstream release of oestrogen and testosterone and sequential inhibition of GnRH. Further, control of the HPG pathway is elicited by gonadotrophin inhibitory hormone (GnIH) which inhibits GnRH, LH and FSH secretion.

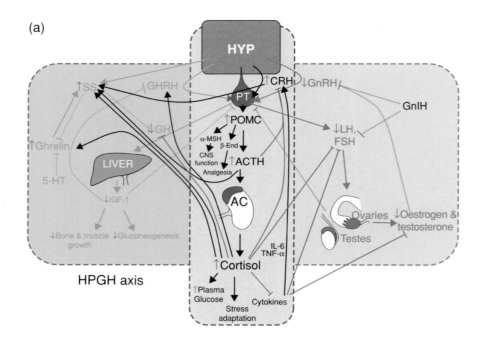

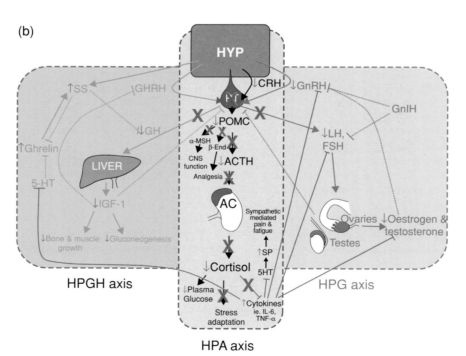

**Colour Plate 2** (See also Figure 5.3) The HPA dampens HPGH and HPG activity during acute stress (a), while chronic stress leads to HPA hypoactivity, excessive cytokine production and further down-regulation of the HPGH and HPG axes (b). HYP, hypothalamus; CRH, corticotropin releasing hormone; ACTH, adrenocorticotropin hormone; AC, adrenal cortex; POMC, pro-opiomelanocortin; β-End, β-endorphin; α-MSH, α-melanocyte-stimulating hormones; SS, somatostatin; GnRH, gonadotrophin releasing hormone; LH, luteinizing hormone; FSH, follicle stimulating hormone; GnIH, gonadotrophin inhibitory hormone.

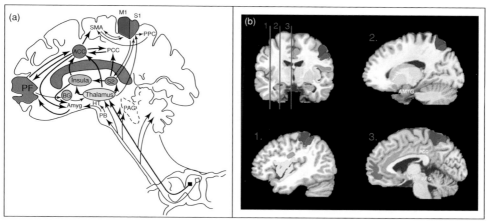

**Colour Plate 3** (See also Figure 6.1) Cortical and subcortical regions involved in pain perception. The locations of the regions are superimposed onto an example MRI. The areas primarily involved in pain perception are the primary somatosensory cortex (S1, red), the secondary somatosensory cortex (S2, orange), the anterior cingulate cortex (ACC, green), the insula (light blue), the thalamus (yellow), as well as the basal ganglia (BG, pink), the prefrontal cortex (PF; purple) and the primary motor cortex (M1, blue). Other regions are the supplementary motor area (SMA), the posterior cingulate cortex (PCC), the amygdale (AMYG), the parabrachial nuclei (PB) and the periaqueductal grey (PAG). Reprinted from *Progress in Neurobiology*, **87**(2), A. V. Apkarian, M. N. Baliki, and P. Y. Geha, Towards a theory of chronic pain, pp. 81–97, Copyright (2009), with permission from Elsevier.

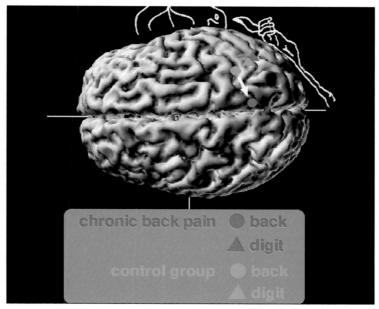

**Colour Plate 4** (See also Figure 6.2) Localization of the representation of the digits and the back in primary somatosensory cortex in back pain patients and healthy controls. Stimulation was on the left side of the body, the representations are on the hemisphere contralateral to the stimulation side. Please note the shift of the back representation of the back pain patients into a more medial position (i.e. towards the leg representation). The shift amounted to about 2–3 cm. Reprinted from *Neuroscience Letters*, **224**(1), H. Flor, C. Braun, T. Elbert, and N. Birbaumer, Extensive reorganization of primary somatosensory cortex in chronic back pain patients, pp. 5–8, Copyright (1997), with permission from Elsevier.

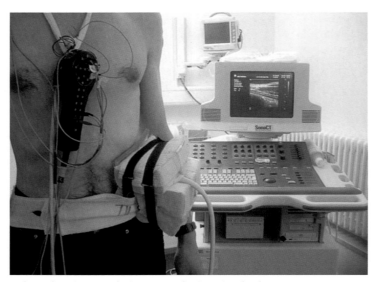

**Colour Plate 5** (See also Figure 8.1) Tissue Doppler imaging (TDI).

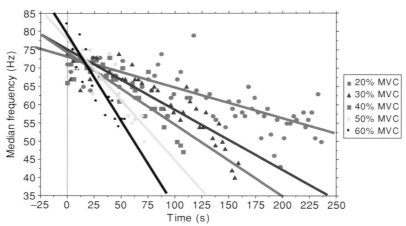

**Colour Plate 6** (See also Figure 9.5) Rate of decline in median frequency at differing submaximal contraction force outputs (% MVC) for the quadriceps femoris muscle. See Mannion and Dolan (1996b) for details. With kind permission from Springer Science+Business Media: *European Journal of Applied Physiology and Occupational Physiology*, Relationship between myoelectric and mechanical manifestations of fatigue in the quadriceps femoris muscle group, **74**(5), 1996, A. F. Mannion.

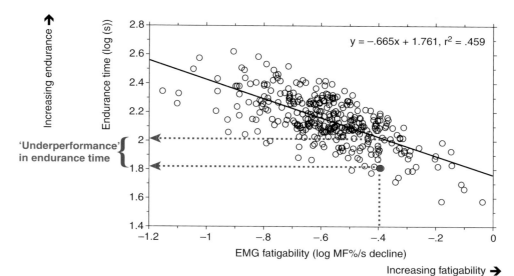

**Colour Plate 7** (See also Figure 9.7) Plot of the endurance time versus EMG-MF slope for individuals participating in a study of risk factors for LBP (for details, see Mannion et al. 1996). Using the slope of the relationship between these two measures, it was possible to predict the endurance time associated with a given EMG fatigability. The subject's actual performance (e.g. filled circle at approx. −0.4%/s below) could then be calculated in relation to his predicted endurance time (using the regression equation) and expressed as the number of seconds of either 'under-performance' or 'over-performance' compared with his/her peers.

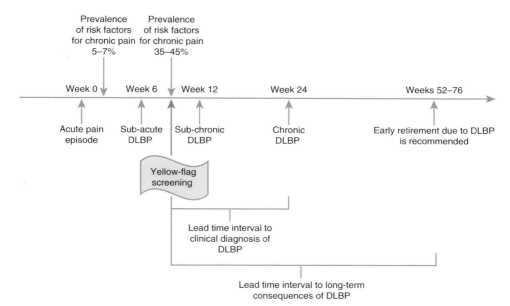

**Colour Plate 8** (See also Figure 11.1) Phases in the development of chronic disabling low back pain (DLBP): hypothetical case.

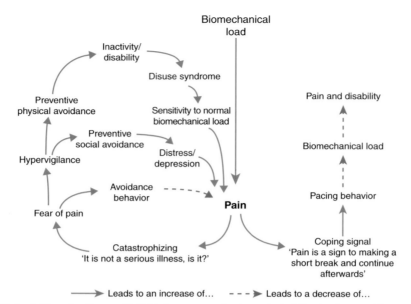

**Colour Plate 9** (See also Figure 15.1) Maintenance of pain and disability by fear-avoidance responses to pain.

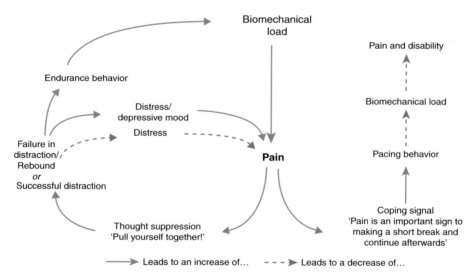

**Colour Plate 10** (See also Figure 15.2) Maintenance of pain by distress-endurance responses to pain.

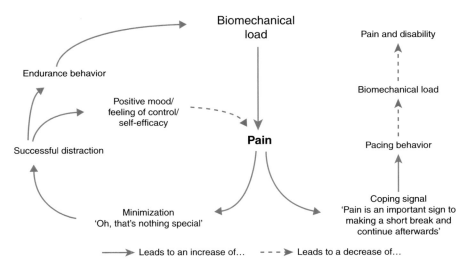

Biomechanical load

Endurance behavior

Pain and disability

Positive mood/
feeling of control/
self-efficacy

Biomechanical load

Successful distraction

**Pain**

Pacing behavior

Minimization
'Oh, that's nothing special'

Coping signal
'Pain is an important sign to
making a short break and
continue afterwards'

Leads to an increase of...    - - - ▶ Leads to a decrease of...

**Colour Plate 11** (See also Figure 15.3) Maintenance of pain by eustress-endurance responses (EER) to pain.

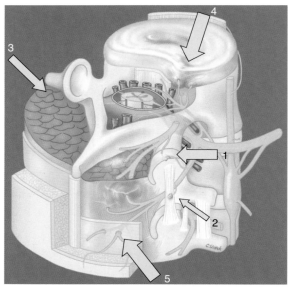

**Colour Plate 12** (See also Figure 25.1) Schematic drawing of the lumbar intervertebral joints (zygapophysial joints), indicating the site of increased nociception in LBP (1–5). Note (outlined in light blue) cartilage and synovialis of the intervertebral joints, painful when irritated and inflamed; (red) intervertebral musculature which may—in order to immobilize the joint—become painfully spastic; the lumbar nerves (yellow) squeezing through the narrow intervertebral foramen, nerve damage and irritation of the meninges, causing nociceptor activation; the intervertebral disc—when damaged—leads to invasion of nerves and activation of nociception. (pink in the (blue) intervertebral disk). Pathophysiological "sources" of low back pain: (1) Arthrosis of the vertebral joints (2) Damaged (extended) intervertebral ligaments (3) Spasticity of the deep intervertebral muscles (4) Raptured disc with secondary capillarisation and innervation (5) Damaged (irritated) neuronal fibers and sheaths due to degeneration and deformation of the lumbar spine and inflammatory processes in the meninges. Image by Christiane Wittek. Reproduced from Kubik, S.: FortbildK. Rheumatol., Bd.6, pp. 1-29 © Karger, Basel, 1981, with permission.

short- and mid-term outcomes in the laboratory by assessing pain intensity every 20s after pain stimulation over a period of 2min and by conducting a further experimental task. Thirty minutes after pain stimulation a mild vibration stimulus was applied at the participant's neck which was experienced as relatively neutral as assessed by a pre-test sample. Results indicated that participants in the suppression condition initially showed less intense pain but later during the 2-min interval showed more intense pain compared to the distractors or monitorers. They also rated the vibration stimulus as less pleasant compared to the distraction and sensory monitoring group. This differential short- and mid-term effect of suppression on pain intensity mirrors potentially different operant mechanisms in the maintenance of this cognitive pain response, as suggested in the AEM above (see Figure 15.2).

As noted previously, Cioffi and Holloway (1993) assumed that especially the instruction to suppression produces a rebound effect, which is well investigated in research on cognition and mental control (e.g. Wegner et al. 1987). This research has shown that when people were asked to suppress awareness of a thought they were, in fact, able to do it but this suppression produced a rebound effect—with the consequence that this thought occurred subsequently more often than if it has not been initially suppressed. Wegner and colleagues attributed this phenomenon to the different goal structures of distraction, sensory monitoring, and suppression. Whereas the goal of distraction is to replace one thought with another, therefore distraction specifies what to do, the goal of suppression is to remove a thought from the mind or it specifies what not to do. If people try to obtain goal-relevant feedback about the success of their mental strategy, in the case of suppression they ask themselves repeatedly how empty their mind will be of the thought X. As a consequence, in the case of pain stimulation, they focus to this pain stimulus again and again. In contrast, distraction and also sensory monitoring instructions give a concrete and vivid mental event, success is evaluated by an awareness of sensations irrelevant of unpleasant features of the pain stimulus. Furthermore, Wegner and colleagues have found that the instruction to suppress often induces a search for distractors that was disorganized, non-focused and which has often failed (Wegner et al. 1991). This search for distractors is more effortful than having a specific distractor given by the experimenter. Support for the assumption of a mid-term pain-increasing effect of thought suppression came also from an experimental study conducted by Masedo and Esteve (2007), comparing suppression, spontaneous coping and instructed acceptance of a cold-pressor stimulus.

In clinical pain patients, there is preliminary evidence for a pain-increasing or pain-maintaining effect of thought suppression as a single response. In a cross-sectional study including 191 subacute LBP and chronic LBP (CLBP) patients, a weak but positive correlation was found between thought suppression and pain intensity (Hasenbring et al. 2009). In another recent study, Rusu and Hasenbring (2008) found TSS scores significantly more elevated in a dysfunctional subgroup of CLBP patients compared to adaptive copers, using the MPI clustering methodology (Turk and Rudy, 1988).

In patient subgroups showing a DER pain response pattern, thought suppression goes along with enhanced depressive mood as well as with high pain-related task persistence behaviour. In a sample of acute/subacute sciatic pain patients prior to an inpatient treatment, DER patients revealed a significant decrease in pain intensity until the discharge from the hospital but they had shown a new increase at the 1-week and at the 6-month follow-up. At this last follow-up, 53% of this subgroup had not been return to work compared to 6% in the AR subgroup and 18% in the EER patients. Despite high positive mood and no depression, the EER patients also had a new increase in pain intensity at both follow-ups. Furthermore, both ER subgroups revealed significantly more often an application for early retirement due to pain (25% in EER, 31% in DER) compared to AR patients with 3% (Hasenbring 1993). These prospective data regarding pain intensity and pain-related work absenteeism was supported by the Grebner et al. subgroups study (Grebner et al. 1999).

### Endurance and pain-related disability

Past research has shown that pain intensity and disability are only marginally associated, while pain-related disability is highly linked with cognitive and affective aspects of pain-related fear, such as catastrophizing or fear-avoidance beliefs (see Chapter 14). However, the relationship between self-reported disability and pain-related endurance, such as thought suppression and task persistence behaviour, remains open. The AEM suggests that a person, who reports high pain-related endurance, will feel less disabled at that time. This hypothesis is to be investigating within cross-sectional designs. Reviewing the body of research using cross-sectional designs, this hypothesis is supported for task persistence behaviour but not for thought suppression. A majority of studies reported significant negative associations between pain-related task persistence behaviour as a single response and disability (Rosenstiel and Keefe 1983; Hadjistavropoulos et al. 1999; Tan et al. 2001; Truchon and Coté 2005; Hasenbring et al. 2009). First data reveal a significant negative association between positive mood as an endurance-related emotional response to pain and disability (Hasenbring et al. 2009). In contrast, only a few data published data concerning thought suppression as a single response and disability. In a cross-sectional study in non-specific back pain patients, Hasenbring et al. (2009) reported zero-correlations between thought suppression, assessed with the AEQ, and pain-related disability, measured with the Pain Disability Index (PDI; Tait et al. 1990).

As the AEM assumes that thought suppression effectively reduces pain only intermittently (see Figure 15.2), it may be linking with task persistence as well as with avoidance behaviour, specifically in the long-term run (Hasenbring and Verbunt, 2010). Future studies investigating bivariate the relation between thought suppression and disability should control for both behavioural features, for instance, using partial regression analysis.

### 15.4.4 **Endurance and overt physical activity**

A few studies that assess physical activity not only by self-report measures but also by overt behavioural methods found no difference in actual physical activity between CLBP patients and healthy controls, neither in adults (Verbunt et al. 2001) nor in children (Wedderkopp et al. 2003). They found also no correlation between self-ratings of pain intensity and the actual physical activity level (PAL) in CLBP patients (Sanders, 1983; Linton 1985; Vendrig and Lousberg 1997; Verbunt et al. 2001; Wedderkopp et al. 2003; Wittink et al. 2003). Wittink et al. (2003) had been discussing the possibility of a subgroup of CLBP patients that will under-report or underestimate their actual ability to function physically.

Subgroups of LBP patients showing self-reported disability despite a high level of overt physical activity have been published by Bousema and co-workers (2007). In this study, patients with subacute back pain were investigated over 1 year. The authors described a subgroup that developed an increase of back pain despite a significant increase of accelerometer-assessed physical activity, which was an unexpected finding. Interestingly, these patients with an increase in PAL, however, suffered of more disability.

As the AEM postulates that patients with high ER pain responses will tend to withstand pain-related interruptions of daily activities in order to pursuit current work-related goals, it is therefore suggested that ER patients will show signs of physical overuse and overload in their daily life. A first accelerometer study delivered preliminary evidence for this assumption (Hasenbring et al. 2006). A combined subgroup of ER patients revealed a trend to higher PAL compared to adaptive patients and a significantly higher number of constant strain positions (CP, sitting or standing upright or bending forward) during an 8-hour assessment period of a working day. It was a striking finding, that this ER subgroup revealed a higher overt activity level despite higher pain intensity, and, against expectations also despite higher self-reported disability. Due to small sample sizes, DER and EER patients could not be distinguished. It remains therefore open whether the high disability score comes more from DER as to be expected and not from EER patients. Furthermore, a high level of fatigue has been seen in the ER subgroup. Fatigue had been discussed as a response to repeating, often unsuccessful trials to distract from pain or to suppress pain experiences from consciousness (Eccleston and Crombez 1999). It can be hypothesized that not only unsuccessful mental trials to suppress pain but also the behavioural components of persisting daily activities in spite of pain may lead to increased fatigue, mentally and physically.

The prominent role of static physical strain positions in the maintenance of back pain was also captured by a recent cross-sectional study in teachers in schools for people with severe handicaps. Using accelerometer data, Wong et al. (2009) have shown that teachers with LBP showed significantly more static trunk postures during working days than pain-free colleagues.

Static strain positions have been shown to cause high loads to the spine inducing creep in the various viscoelastic tissues, such as ligament, discs and fascia (Solomonow et al. 2003a, 2003b). Sbriccoli et al (2004) have shown that the number of repetitions of a static load on the lumbar spine is a risk factor in the development of cumulative trauma disorder. The creep developed becomes more intense as the number of repetitions increases. Furthermore, the authors argue, if the creep does not fully recover, for instance overnight, people start a new workday with a residual creep from the previous day. As time goes on, the residual creep may accumulate from day to day, inducing micro-damages in the lumbar spinal tissues associated with acute inflammation as an attempt of healing of the damage. Further consequences of repetitive static load positions are the reduction of oxygenation of lumbar extensors due to the constant isometric contraction (McGill et al. 2000) as well as an increase of intradiscal pressure (Stokes and Iatridis 2004).

## 15.4.5 **Endurance and neurocognitive functions**

Within a recent neurocognitive model of pain (Legrain et al. 2009), attention to pain or to pain-irrelevant behavioural goals is conceptualized through involuntary (bottom-up) and intentional (top-down) processes, given the limited processing capacity of the brain. Among top-down processes, attention may be directed away from nociceptive stimuli in order to fulfil a concurrent cognitive task, leading to a specific effort due to the primary goal (attentional load hypothesis) or attention may be facilitated towards stimuli that are associated with defined goal-relevant stimuli, for instance, towards pain stimuli, when these are experienced as highly threatening (attentional set hypothesis).

The attentional load hypothesis was investigated in a number of laboratory experiments in healthy individuals using nociceptive stimulation while instructed to attend to a specific cognitive task. This kind of distraction seems able to reduce the intensity of experienced pain (Bingel et al. 2007) as well as to reduce brain activity, specifically in areas that are usually involved in the processing of pain perception and attentional control (Seminowicz and Davis 2006; Bingel et al. 2007; Seminowicz and Davis 2007). Within the context of the AEM model, the question arises whether people, who usually respond to pain with cognitive distraction, thought suppression, and task persistence behaviour (ER pattern), will show higher cognitive performance than individuals low in ERs. In a recent laboratory study, Held et al. (in prep.) instructed healthy volunteers to attend to a mental arithmetic task while pain was induced by a cold pressor stimulation. Using median split procedure, the participants high in task persistence behaviour, measured with the AEQ (Hasenbring et al. 2009) modified for healthy individuals (AEQ-H), revealed shorter response times in the mental task as well as a lower number of cognitive errors.

Furthermore, participants with high endurance revealed less pain intensity scores and significantly higher pain tolerance time than low endurance participants. These preliminary findings indicate that pain persistence behaviour enables a person to direct attention towards pain-irrelevant goals, which may in the short term be followed by a reduction of pain (negative reinforcement) and a better cognitive performance representing a kind of positive reinforcement.

### 15.4.6 Endurance and feelings of self-control and self-efficacy

The ability to respond with endurance behaviour in unpleasant or difficult situations is undoubtedly an important ability and may lead to an increase of feelings of self-control and high self-efficacy. In pain research, self-efficacy represents a set of cognitions predicting positive outcomes of medical as well as of psychological treatments (Nicholas 2007). In models of stress and coping (Zautra et al. 1995), pain is conceptualized as a stressor to which individuals show diverse adaptation patterns. Whereas cognitive responses to pain such as help-hopelessness are important precursors of feelings of loss of control and depression, several coping responses were positively associated with self-reported control. Based on a cross-sectional correlation study in 195 chronic pain patients, positive relations between the CSQ-factors ignoring pain sensations, increasing behavioural activity, diverting attention as well as for coping self-statements and reinterpreting pain sensations and feelings of control were reported (Haythornethwaite et al. 1998). Individual differences in pain coping, predicted the effects of experimentally induced controllability during heat pain stimulation in healthy individuals and indicate the critical role of prefrontal cortex areas (Salomons et al. 2004). More recently, two studies investigated the association between pain-related task persistence behaviour and basal adrenocortical activity represented by a neuroendocrinological stress parameter, such as level of salivary cortisol after awakening (Sudhaus et al. 2007, Sudhaus et al. 2009), both supporting the stress-reducing character of behavioural endurance. These data concerning the relation between endurance behaviour, pain-related stress and control provide preliminary support for the assumption of the AEM that behavioural endurance associated with effective distraction away from pain may have a stress-reducing short-term effect, potentially mediated by an increased sense of control and self-efficacy.

### 15.4.7 Endurance and affective responses

#### Positive mood despite pain

One of the most surprising and counterintuitive results in psychological pain research refer to the finding that patients with LBP, irrespective of the duration of pain, report feelings of positive mood despite pain, besides anxiety, depression, or irritated mood (Hasenbring et al. 1994; Hasenbring et al. 2009). Positive mood despite pain and endurance behaviour, both assessed with the KPI or with the AEQ were significantly positively correlated in a sample of 305 pain patients of different diagnoses (r=0.41; Hasenbring 1994) as well as in a recent studied sample of 191 LBP patients (r=0.46; Hasenbring et al. 2009). In contrast, PMS was unrelated to thought suppression in these both validation studies. In a former prospective study in acute or subacute sciatic pain patients, both, endurance behaviour and positive mood despite pain were positively correlated with pain intensity prospectively, to a lesser degree but in the same direction as for depression and avoidance behaviour (Hasenbring et al. 1994). Positive mood despite pain and endurance behaviour are the two marker variables representing the EER pattern, seen in a subgroup of patients who also tend to minimize pain experiences and to cognitive distraction. It remains to be determined whether attentional distraction in EER patients is more effective in reducing pain experiences and in enhancing the ability to continue with current daily activities and whether this is the main origin of positive mood. Habitual as well as situational characteristics are also potential precursors of the ability to maintain positive mood despite pain.

## Endurance and pain-related fear and depression

At a first glance, it seems plausible to suggest pain-related helplessness, hopelessness and beliefs that daily work will lead to an increase of pain as parts of a FAR pattern. It has been shown, however, that the DER subgroup of LBP patients, revealed even higher scores in pain anxiety, helplessness, hopelessness, and the belief that work will cause pain as well as in the belief of a poor work prognosis, compared to AR patients (Grebner et al. 1999; Hasenbring et al. under review). In a recent study in 146 patients with exercise induced leg pain (overuse group) and 154 CLBP patients, the overuse group revealed as high fear of re-injury pain (measured with the TSK) as the CLBP group (Lundberg and Styf 2009). These findings are in line with the assumption of the AEM, that pain-related fear and dysfunctional beliefs may not only be associated with avoidance behaviour but also with the opposite tendency of task persistence behaviour. Within this context, the question arises, whether the beliefs in DER patients that work will cause or increase pain, are really dysfunctional or alternatively whether these beliefs are based on real experiences and represent consequences of individual coping by dealing with daily work requirements in these patients.

A positive association between high fear and persistence behaviour has been also reported in other fields of research, for instance, in military psychology (Rachman 2004). Rachman describes soldiers trained to realize persistence behaviour in dangerous situations despite subjective feelings of fear or anxiety, labelling this pattern 'courageous behaviour'. Comprehensive training programmes, for instance in parachutists (Walk, 1956), led to a reduction of fear after a few jumps, representing learning principles of negative reinforcement. Within this context, it is important to note, that behavioural training programmes in patients suffering from anxiety of pain-related fear, using the principle of confrontation, also increase the ability of a patient to reveal courageous behaviour, namely persistence despite fear. While this procedure seems to be successful in FAR patients (see also Chapter 14), it can be questioned whether it would be also effective and indicated in patients showing a DER pattern, where we assume that high task persistence behaviour will lead to overuse and physical injury in the long term.

Increased depressive mood is an often seen and theoretically reasoned consequence of pain-related FAR pattern (see Chapter 14). Moreover, the AEM suggests a link between high thought suppression and increased depressive mood, due to the often experienced failure of attentional distraction and the rebound phenomenon reviewed previously. Preliminary, but conclusive evidence came from a multivariate study in chronic LBP patients, investigating the role of pain intensity, catastrophizing, helplessness, hopelessness, as well as thought suppression in the prediction of depression (Klasen et al. 2006). Using path analysis, the authors found a direct relationship between thought suppression and depressive mood, whereas catastrophizing revealed only an indirect association via cognitions of helplessness and hopelessness. In this study, pain intensity by itself had no direct association to depression.

## 15.4.8 Stability versus variability of pain-related endurance responses and AEM pattern

Knowledge of stability versus variability over time of response patterns is rare. In addition, no information is currently available indicating which situational demands, specific motivational factors and/or aspects of learning history will lead to an individual FAR or ER pattern. The AEM suggests that exclusive FAR or ER pattern are relatively stable in time unless modification is based on well-directed behavioural interventions. On the other hand, changes in response pattern may naturally occur during the long-term process of pain chronification. For example, the experience of long-term pain, which does not respond adequately to medical therapy, may lead to a change from an exclusive EER into a DER or even FAR pattern. Longitudinally, ER patients might be at risk for a decrease of task persistence and an increase of avoidance behaviour. In this situation, avoidance is assumed as a kind of passive avoidance behaviour, which may have several deteriorated consequences: First, patients postpone the interruption of painful daily activities for a long time. Consequently, when they eventually do interrupt (e.g. a short pause for relaxation) their activities, this will not lead to a regeneration of damaged physical structures and pain will not diminish. Therefore, patients will experience such an interruption as unsuccessful. Second, short pauses that will not result in a pain decrease, will lead to an increase of thought suppression with the consequences of rebound, feelings of failure, low self-esteem and depression. Third, when ER patients will only decide to interrupt their daily activities due to very severe pain, eventually, pain will guide these interruptions consciously or unconsciously. Therefore, although task persistence behaviour may first lead to feelings of control, in the long-term it can result in feelings of loss of control.

## 15.5 Consequences for clinical practice: implication for differentially targeted approaches

Preliminary clinical consequences for patients with both acute and chronic pain are considered in the following. Diverse national LBP guidelines advise, in a situation of acute non-specific LBP (excluding severe structural causes of pain (red flags)), to quickly return to a normal level of daily activity (Arnau et al. 2006). On a conceptual level, the avoidance and endurance-based research reported previously in this chapter suggest the need for a definition of the term 'normal' activity, as it is assumed that FAR patients would subjectively define their normal activity level differently compared to ER patients. Adding to the complexity, patients tend to evaluate their activity-related problem due to pain by comparing their current activity level in reference to their habitual activity level before pain-onset. Their perceived decline of activities since pain-onset appeared to be more disabling as their actual activity level (Verbunt et al 2001; Bousema et al. 2007).

Based on these considerations, the AEM suggests differential interventions for patient education, physical therapy, and cognitive-behavioural treatment approaches. Based on a preceding screening of AEM-derived pain response pattern, multimodal treatment strategies should be individually targeted dependant on FAR, DER, or EER pattern. For patients with FAR and related physical disuse, the approach of increasing one's activity level, based on graded activity and exposure *in vivo* (a behavioural approach in which fear of movement is the focus of treatment) seemed both effective, specifically in reducing pain-related disability (Vlaeyen at al. 2002; Leeuw et al. 2008). In contrast, patients showing an endurance-related response pattern should be encouraged to accept pain experience as a signal that has to be taken seriously in order to prepare short breaks in their daily activities and to reduce physical postures that cause high load on muscles and the spine. The general aim of an AEM-based CBT approach is to enable both, FAR and ER patients to a more flexible response pattern that is comparable to the AR patients.

A first randomized controlled intervention trial in patients suffering from subacute sciatic pain revealed preliminary evidence that an AEM-scheduled, risk-factor based CBT, offered besides conservative medical interventions, is significantly more effective in preventing future pain compared to a standardized psychological programme or to a control group receiving only medical treatment as usual (Hasenbring et al. 1999). Results from an additional randomized trial in subacute non-specific back pain patients provided further evidence concerning the efficacy of an individually scheduled, AEM-based short physician counselling with a 3-month follow-up (Hasenbring et al. under review, for more information see also Chapter 27 in this volume).

## 15.6 **Summary and conclusion**

Firm evidence identified FAR as an important mediator for the development and maintenance of chronic pain and disability. In addition, we found increasing evidence for the presence of a second and opposite pathway for chronicity in pain based on endurance-related responses. The impact of these opposite pathways on daily activities and their implication for clinical practice still need further research, but seem promising in the determination of more individualized treatment programmes for patients with chronic pain syndromes.

In conclusion, the AEM provides testable hypotheses concerning the development of pain-related disability and affective distress, such as increased depressed mood. Most of these hypotheses will require prospective study designs including diary studies exploring short-term relationships as well as longitudinal designs for the investigation of long-term processes, such as the recurrence of pain months or years following an acute episode. More research is required to understand the underlying mechanisms of endurance-related responses and several potential avenues for future research have been identified including, for instance, activity monitoring, neuroendocrinological and neurocognitive functions. Future research should also focus on the motivational mechanisms, situational demands, learning history and the potential impact of personality features on the development of rigid fear-avoidance and endurance pattern.

## References

Ahles, T., Blanchard, E. and Leventhal, H. (1983). Cognitive control of pain: attention to the sensory aspects of the cold pressor stimulus. *Cognitive Therapy and Research, 7*, 159–77.

Arnau, J.M., Vallano A, Lopez A, *et al.* (2006). A critical review of guidelines for low back pain treatment. *European Spine Journal*, **15**, 543–53.

Asmundson, G.J.G., Norton and P.J., Norton, G.R. (1999). Beyond pain: the role of fear and avoidance in chronicity. *Clinical Psychology Review*, **19**, 97–119.

Beck, A.T., Ward, C.H., Mendelson, M., Mock, J., Erbaugh, J. (1961). An inventory for measuring depression. *Archives of General Psychiatry*, **4**, 561–71.

Bingel, U., Rose, M., Gläscher, J. and Büchel, C. (2007). fMRI reveals how pain modulates visual object processing in the ventral visual stream. *Neuron*, **55**, 157–67.

Bortz, W.M. (1984). The disuse syndrome. *Western Journal of Medicine, 141*, 691–94.

Bousema, E.J., Verbunt, J.A., Seelen, H.A.M., Vlaeyen, J.W.S., Knottnerus, J.A. (2007). Disuse and physical deconditioning in the first year after the onset of back pain. *Pain*, **130**, 279–86.

Cioffy, D. and Holloway, J. (1993). Delayed costs of suppressed pain, *Journal of Personality and Clinical Psychology*, **64**, 274–82.

Commission on Behavioral and Social Sciences and Education, National Research Council and Institute of Medicine. (2001). *Musculosceletal disorders and the workplace: low back and upper extremities.* Washington, DC: National Academy Press.

Davis, M.C., Zautra, A.J. and Smith, B.W. (2004). Chronic pain, stress, and the dynamics of affective differentiation. *Journal of Personality, 72*, 1133–59.

Eccleston, C. and Crombez, G. (1999). Pain demands attention: a cognitive-affective model of the interruptive function of pain. *Psychological Bulletin*, **125**, 356–66.

Fishbach, A. and Ferguson, M.F. (2007). The goal construct in social psychology. In: A.W. Kruglanski and E.T. Higgins (Eds.) *Social Psychology: Handbook of basic principles*, pp. 490–515. New York: Guilford.

Garcia-Campayo, J.G., Pascual, A., Alda, M. and Ramirez, M.T.G. (2007). Coping with fibromyalgia: usefulness of the chronic pain coping inventory-42. *Pain, 132*, 68–76.

Gatchel, R.J., Peng, Y.B., Peters, M.L., Fuchs, P.N., Turk, D.D. (2007). The biopsychosocial approach to chronic pain: schientific advances and future directions. *Psychological Bulletin*, **133**, 581–624.

Goschke, T. and Dreisbach, G. (2008). Conflict-triggered goal-shielding: response conflicts attenuate background monitoring for prospective memory cues. *Psychological Science*, **19**, 25–32.

Grebner, M., Breme, K., Rothoerl, R., Woertgen, C., Hartmann, A. and Thomé, C. (1999). Coping and convalescence course after lumbar disk operations. *Der Schmerz,* **13**, 19–30.

Hadjistavropoulos HD, Frombach IK, Asmundson GJG. (1999). Exploratory and confirmatory factor analytic investigations of the Illness Attitudes Scale in a nonclinical sample. *Behaviour Research and Therapy*, **37**, 671–84.

Hasenbring, M. (1993). Endurance strategies - a neglected phenomenon in the research and therapy of chronic pain? *Der Schmerz,* **7**, 304–13.

Hasenbring, M. (1994). *Das Kieler Schmerzinventar.* [The Kiel Pain Inventory-Manual. Three questionnaire scales for the assessment of pain-related cognitions, emotions and coping strategies]. Bern: Huber.

Hasenbring, M. (2000). Attentional control of pain and the process of chronification. In: J. Sandkühler, B. Bromm and G.F. Gebhart (Eds.) *Progress in Pain Research Vol* 129, pp. 525–34. New York: Elsevier Science.

Hasenbring, M., Marienfeld, G., Kuhlendahl, D. and Soyka, D. (1994). Risk factors of chronicity in lumbar disc patients. A prospective investigation of biologic, psychologic, and social predictors of therapy outcome. *Spine,* **19**, 2759–65.

Hasenbring, M., Ulrich, H.W., Hartmann, M. and Soyka, D. (1999). The efficacy of a risk factor based cognitive behavioral intervention and EMG-biofeedback in patients with acute sciatic pain: an attempt to prevent chronicity. *Spine,* **24**, 2525–35.

Hasenbring, M.I., Plaas, H., Fischbein, B. and Willburger, R. (2006). The relationship between activity and pain in patients 6 months after lumbar disc surgery: do pain-related coping modes act as moderator variables? *European Journal of Pain,* **10**, 701–9.

Hasenbring, M.I., Hallner, D. and Rusu, A.C. (2009). Fear-avoidance- and endurance-related responses to pain: development and validation of the Avoidance-Endurance Questionnaire (AEQ). *European Journal of Pain,* **13**, 620–8.

Hasenbring, M.I., Verbunt, J.A. (2010). Fear-Avoidance and endurance-related responses to pain: new models of behavior and their consequences for clinical practice. *Clin J Pain,* **26**, 747–53.

Hass, B.W. and Canli, T. (2008). Emotional memory function, personality structure and psychopathology: a neural system approach to the identification of vulnerability markers. *Brain Research Review,* **58**, 71–84.

Haythornthwaite, J.A., Menefee, L.A., Heinberg, L.J. and Clark, M.R. (1998). Pain coping strategies predict perceived control over pain. *Pain,* **77**, 33–9.

Hill, A., Niven, C.A. and Knussen, C. (1995). The role of coping in adjustment to phantom limb pain. *Pain,* **62**, 79–86.

Jensen, M.P., Turner, J.A., Romano, J.M. and Strom, S.E. (1995). The Chronic Pain Coping Inventory: Development and preliminary validation. *Pain,* **60**, 203–16.

Kerns, R.D., Turk, D.C. and Rudy, T.E. (1985). The West Haven-Yale Multidimensional Pain Inventory (WHYMPI). *Pain,* **23**, 345–56.

Klasen, B.W., Bruggert, J., Hasenbring, M. (2006). The role of cognitive pain coping strategies for depression in chronic back pain path analysis of patients in primary care. *Der Schmerz,* **5**, 398–410.

Kraimaat, F.W. and Evers, A.W.M. (2003). Pain-coping strategies in chronic pain patients: psychometric characteristics of the pain-coping inventory (PCI). *International Journal of Behavioral Medicine,* **10**, 343–63.

Lang, P.J. (1970). Stimulus control, response control, and the desensitization of fear. In: D.J. Levis (Ed.) *Learning approaches to therapeutic behavior change*, pp. 148–73. Chicago, IL: Aldine Press.

Leeuw, M., Goossens, M.E., van Breukelen, G.J., *et al.* (2008). Exposure in vivo versus operant graded activity in chronic low back pain patients: results of a randomized controlled trial. *Pain,* **138**, 192–207.

Legrain, V., VanDamme, S., Eccleston, C., Davis, K.D., Seminowicz, D.A. and Crombez, G. (2009). A neurocognitive model of attention to pain: behavioral and neuroimaging evidence. *Pain,* **144**, 230–2.

Lethem, J., Slade, P.D., Troup, J.D.G. and Bentley, G. (1983). Outline of a fear-avoidance model of exaggerated pain perception. *Behavior Research and Therapy,* **21**, 401–8.

Lewinsohn, P.M., Libet, J.M. (1972). Pleasant events, activity schedules and depression. *Journal of Abnormal Psychology,* **79**, 291–5.

Linton, S. (1985). The relationship between activity and chronic back pain. *Pain*, **21**, 289–94.

Lundberg, M. and Styf, J. (2009). Kinesophobia among physiological overusers with musculoskeletal pain. *European Journal of Pain*, **13**, 655–9.

Masedo, A.I. and Esteve, R. (2007). Effects of suppression, acceptance and spontaneous coping on pain tolerance, pain intensity and distress. *Behaviour Research and Therapy*, **45**, 199–209.

McCaul, K.D. and Haugtvedt, C. (1982). Attention, distraction, and cold pressor pain. *Journal of Personality and Social Psychology*, **43**, 154–62.

McCaul, K.D., and Mallot, J.M. (1984). Distraction and coping with pain. *Psychological Bulletin*, **95**, 516–33.

McGill, S.M., Hughson, R.L. and Parks, K. (2000). Lumbar erector spinae oxygenation during prolonged contractions: implications for prolonged work. *Ergonomics*, **43**, 486–93.

Nicholas, M.K. (2007). The pain self-efficacy questionnaire: taking pain into account. *European Journal of Pain*, **11**, 153–63.

Norman, D.A. and Bobrow, D.G. (1975). On data-limited and resource-limited processes. *Cognitive Psychology*, **7**, 44–64.

Osborne, T.L., Jensen, M.P., Ehde, D.M., Hanley, M.A. and Kraft, G. (2007). Psychosocial factors associated with pain intensity, pain-related interference, and psychological functioning in persons with multiple sclerosis and pain. *Pain*, **127**, 52–62.

Philips, H. (1987). Avoidance behavior and its role in sustaining chronic pain. *Behavior Research and Therapy*, **25**, 273–9.

Philips, H.C. and Jahanshahi, M. (1986). The components of pain behavior report. *Behavior Research and Therapy*, **24**, 117–25.

Rachman, S.J. (2004). Fear and courage: a psychological perspective. *Social Research*, **71**, 149–76.

Riley, J.L. and Robinson, M.E. (1997). CSQ: Five factors or fiction? *The Clinical Journal of Pain*, **13**, 156–62.

Romano, J.M., Jensen, M.P.,and Turner, J.A. (2003). The Chronic Pain Coping Inventory-42: Reliability and validity. *Pain*, **104**, 65–73.

Rosenstiel, A.K. and Keefe, F.J. (1983). The use of coping strategies in chronic low back pain patients: relationship to patient characteristics and current adjustment. *Pain*, **17**, 33–44.

Rusu, A.C. and Hasenbring, M. (2008). Multidimensional pain inventory derived classifications of chronic pain: evidence for maladaptive pain-related coping within the dysfunctional group. *Pain*, **134**, 80–90

Salomons, T.V., Johnstone, T., Backonja, M. and Davidson, R.J. (2004). Perceived controllability modulates the neural response to pain. *Journal of Neuroscience*, **24**, 7199–203.

Sanders, S. (1983). Automated versus self-monitoring of up-time in chronic low-back pain patients: a comparative study. *Pain*, **15**, 399–405.

Sbriccoli, P., Yousuf, K., Kupershtein, I., Solomonow, M., Zhou, B.H., Zhu, M.P. *et al.* (2004). Static load repetition is a risk factor in the development of lumbar cumulative musculoskeletal disorder. *Spine*, **29**, 2643–53.

Seminowicz, D.A. and Davis, K.D. (2006). Cortical responses to pain in healthy individuals depends on pain catastrophizing. *Pain*, **120**, 297–306.

Seminowicz, D.A. and Davis, K.D. (2007). Interactions of pain intensity and cognitive load: the brain stays on task. *Cerebral Cortex*, **17**, 1412–22.

Solomonow, M., Hatipkarasulu, S., Zhou, B.H. *et al.* (2003a). Biomechanics and electromyography of a common idiopathic low back disorder. *Spine*, **28**, 1235–48.

Solomonow, M., Baratta, R.V., Zhou, B.H. *et al.* (2003b). Muscular dysfunction elicited by creep of lumbar viscoelastic tissues. *J Electromyogr Kinesiol*, **13**, 381–93.

Stokes, I.A.F. and Iatridis, J.C. (2004). Mechanical conditions that accelerate intervertebral disc degeneration: overload versus immobilization. *Spine*, **29**, 2724–32.

Sudhaus, S., Fricke, B., Schneider, S., Stachon, A., Klein, H., vonDüring, M. and Hasenbring, M. (2007). The cortisol awakening response in patients with acute and chronic low back pain. Relations with psychological risk factors of pain chronicity. *Schmerz*, **21**, 202–11.

Sudhaus, S., Fricke, B., Stachon, A., Schneider, S., Klein, H., vonDüring, M. and Hasenbring, M. (2009). Salivary cortisol and psychological mechanisms in patients with acute versus chronic low back pain. *PNEC*, **34**, 513–22.

Sullivan, M.J.L., Thorn, B., Haythornthwaite, J.A., et al. (2001). Theoretical perspectives on the relation between catastrophizing and pain. *Clin J Pain*, **17**, 52–64.

Tait, R.C., Chibnall, J.T., & Krause, S. (1990). The Pain Disbility Index: psychometric properties. *Pain*, **40**, 171–82.

Tan, G., Jensen, M.P., Robinson-Whelen, S., Thornby, J.I. and Monga, T.N. (2001). Coping with chronic pain: A comparison of two measures. *Pain*, **90**, 127–33.

Truchon, M. and Coté, D. (2005). Predictive validity of the chronic pain coping inventory in subacute low back pain. *Pain*, **116**, 205–212.

Turk, D.C. and Rudy, T.E. (1988). Toward an empirically derived taxonomy of chronic pain patients: integration of psychological assessment data. *Journal of Consulting and Clinical Psychology*, **56**, 233–8.

Turner, J.A. and Clancy, S. (1986). Strategies for coping with chronic low back pain: relationship to pain and disability. *Pain*, **24**, 355–64.

Turner, J.A. and Aaron, L.A. (2001). Pain-related catastrophizing: what is it? *Clin J Pain*, **17**, 65–71.

VanDamme, S., Crombez, G., Eccleston, C. and Roelofs, J. (2004). Impaired disengagement from threatening cues of impending pain in a crossmodal cueing paradigm. *European Journal of Pain*, **8**, 227–36.

Vendrig, A.A., Lousberg, R. (1997). Within-person relationships among pain intensity, mood and physical activity in chronic pain: a naturalistic approach. *Pain*, **73**, 71–6.

Verbunt, J., Westerterp, K., Van der Heijden, G.J., Seelen, H.A., Vlaeyen, J.W.S., Knottnerus, J.A. (2001). Physical activity in daily life in patients with chronic low back pain. *Arch Phys Med Rehabil*, **82**, 726–30.

Verbunt, J.A., Seelen, H.A., Vlaeyen, J.W., *et al.* (2003). Disuse and deconditioning in chronic low back pain: concepts and hypotheses on contributing mechanisms. *European Journal of Pain*, **7**, 9–21.

Vlaeyen, J.W. and Linton, S.J. (2000). Fear-avoidance and its consequences in chronic musculoskeletal pain: a state of the art. *Pain*, **85**, 317–32.

Vlaeyen, J.W.S., de Jong, J., Geilen, M., *et al.* (2002). The treatment of fear of movement/(re)injury in chronic low back pain: further evidence on the effectiveness of exposure in vivo. *Clinical Journal of Pain*, **18**, 251–61.

Waddel, G., Newton, M., Henderson, I., Somerville, D., Main, C.J. (1993). A fear-avoidance beliefs questionnaire (FABQ) and the role of fear-avoidance beliefs in chronic low back pain and disability. *Pain*, **52**, 157–68.

Waddell, G. (2004). The Back pain revolution. London: Churchill Livingston.

Walk, R. (1956). Self-ratings of fear in a fear-avoking situation. *Journal of Social and Abnormal Psychology*, **52**, 171–8.

Wedderkopp, N., Leboeuf-Yde, D.C., Andersen, L.B., Froberg, K., Hansen, H.S. (2003). Back pain in children. *Spine*, **17**, 2019–24.

Wegner, D.M., Schneider, D., Carter, S.R. and White, T.L. (1987). Paradoxical effects of thought suppression. *Journal of Personaliyt and Social Psychology*, **53**, 5–13.

Wittink, H., Rogers, W., Sukiennik, A., Carr, D.B. (2003). Physical functioning: self-report and performance measures are related but distinct. *Spine*, **20**, 2407–13.

Wong, K.C.H., Lee, R.Y.W. and Yeung, S.S. (2009). The association between back pain and trunk posture of workers in a special school for the severe handicaps. *BMC Musculoskeletal Disorders*, **10**, 43.

Wong, W.S., Jensen, M.P., Mak, K.H., Tam, B.K.H. and Fielding, R. (2010). Preliminary Psychometric Properties of the Chinese Version of the Chronic Pain Coping Inventory (ChCPCI) in a Hong Kong Chinese Population. *The Journal of Pain*, **11**, 672–80.

Zautra, A.J., Burleson, M.H., Smith, C.A. *et al.* (1995). Arthritis and perceptions of quality of life: an examination of positive and negative affects in rheumatoid arthritis patients. *Health Psychology*, **14**, 399–408.

Chapter 16

# Cognitive Processing and Self-Pain Enmeshment in Chronic Back Pain

Adina C. Rusu and Tamar Pincus

## 16.1 Introduction

Given the detrimental effect of chronic pain on the individual and his or her surrounding environment, research into the factors and mechanisms that contribute to the aetiology, persistence, and effective management of chronic pain has increased significantly in the last decades (Morley et al. 1999; McCracken and Turk 2002; Turk and Okifuji 2002). This growing research interest has (amongst other outcomes) resulted in the identification of a number of psychological factors and mechanisms that may predispose persons toward, or conversely protect them against the development of persistent pain. This chapter contributes to this line of research by focusing on the specific contribution of some of these proposed vulnerability factors. The present chapter focuses on cognitive mechanisms and processes occurring at strategic and automatic levels that constitute a mediating or moderating role in pain and pain-related disability. Before introducing the precise research questions that have been explored in this context, in the following paragraphs a brief overview of cognitive processing theories will be provided. The main part of this chapter will focus on the theoretical background against which the current research was conducted. Furthermore, empirical evidence on cognitive processing biases in chronic pain will be reviewed. Finally, this chapter will end with perspectives on the main clinical implications of this line of research and future research directions.

## 16.2 Cognitive processing and schemas

Cognition has been defined as 'a generic term embracing the quality of knowing, which includes perceiving, recognizing, conceiving, judging, sensing, reasoning and imaging' (Stedman's Medical Dictionary 1976). Individuals actively process incoming stimuli using pre-existing mental structures (schemas) constructed through experience. These schemas play an important role in organizing and integrating information, including memory processes. Distorted underlying assumptions and errors in information processing can serve to maintain emotional disturbance (Beck 1976). Many different terms are used when referring to cognitive structures. A 'meta-construct' framework (Ingram et al. 1998) suggests three categories for particular groups of constructs: cognitive structures (e.g. memory), and propositions or content (e.g. knowledge) which includes schema-based models; cognitive products (e.g. attributions, thoughts, beliefs), some of which are thought to be accessible to conscious awareness; and cognitive processes (e.g. conditioning, retrieval) which occur at a subconscious level. In short, automatic processes are conceived as largely unconscious and involuntary, requiring a minimum of processing capacity, and being relatively difficult to regulate, whilst controlled processes are conceived as conscious and voluntary, requiring considerable processing capacity, and being easier to adjust (Beck and Clark 1997; McNally 1995; Shiffrin and Schneider 1977). Taken together, the consideration of both implicit and explicit processes in the prediction of any behaviour can contribute to a more thorough and complete understanding of the various components that constitute this particular behaviour.

The application of paradigms from cognitive science to clinical studies has been very productive in contributing to the understanding of the information processing and cognitive content involved in anxiety and depression (e.g. Alloy et al. 1997). One of the aims of cognitive research is to understand individual differences in emotionality, and particularly differences in vulnerability to pathological emotional states. Two general types of studies are therefore of interest: (1) Studies comparing groups differing in trait measures of negative emotionality, and (2) studies contrasting individuals with or without emotional disorders such as anxiety or depression. Information processing approaches to psychopathology propose that cognitive biases contribute to the onset and maintenance of psychopathology. More specifically, individuals' negative affective state or specific concerns are thought to be associated with favouring the processing of information that is congruent to these affective states and concerns, and this selective processing of information is then assumed to guide subsequent behaviour (Beck and Clark 1997; Mathews and MacLeod 1994; Williams et al. 1997).

### 16.2.1 Cognitive biases in chronic pain

Empirical studies of information processing biases in chronic pain have explored selective attention, interpretation of meaning and memory/recall. It has been argued that information-processing biases could maintain or exacerbate pain in different ways: Attentional biases may increase monitoring of physical sensations, hypervigilance, and therefore pain behaviours; interpretation bias may increase interpretation of sensations as painful; recall bias may increase distress and may impact on self-image, which can reduce healthy behaviour and increase actual damage (Pincus 1998; Waddell 1996). Biased information processing has been viewed as a risk factor for the development of chronic disability and has been shown to predict higher health care costs (Pincus and Morley 2002; Pincus and Newman 2001).

### Attention bias

Attention is probably the most extensively investigated cognitive process in relation to pain. Most studies on the detection of attention biases towards pain stimuli have relied on experimental paradigms such as the emotional Stroop task and the visual dot-probe task. Although some studies found support for attention biases in pain patients using these paradigms, these results seemed to be difficult to replicate in other studies and seemed to depend on the specific task and the exact type of stimulus material that were used to assess the bias such as sensory pain words, affective pain words or pictoral stimuli (Asmundson et al. 1997, 2005; Asmundson and Hadjivropoulos 2007; Roelofs et al. 2002, 2005). However, the most recent studies found attentional biases towards sensory-related but not affective words using large sample sizes (Dehghani et al. 2003; Sharpe et al. 2009). In healthy people with elevated levels of pain-related anxiety, results on the occurrence of attention bias towards pain-related stimuli showed more consistency (Asmundson et al. 1997, 2005; Keogh and Cochrane 2002; Keogh et al. 2001a, 2001b), although failures in replicating these findings have been reported as well (e.g. Roelofs et al. 2003a, 2003b). The observation of more consistent findings in healthy people and inconsistent findings in pain patients might suggest that the paradigms tested were not sufficiently difficult for chronic pain patients who might have learned to allocate their attentional resources in the continuous presence of actual pain (Pincus and Morley 2001). In a similar view, Asmundson et al. (2005) proposed that the use of sensory and affective pain words as threatening stimuli might fail in assessing attention biases in patients because these stimuli are not threatening enough for pain patients, in contrast to healthy persons who are not suffering from persistent pain. In conclusion, emotional Stroop and dot-probe paradigms might suffer from low ecological validity due to the use of verbal and pictorial stimulus material. Several studies in which an ecologically more appropriate paradigm has been used (i.e. the primary task paradigm), have demonstrated the attention demanding properties of pain, and the interruptive effect that pain can have on the allocation of attention to other tasks (e.g. Crombez et al. 1998a, 1998b; Eccleston and Crombez 1999; Peters et al. 2002). In the primary task paradigm, the effect of the administration of electrical pain stimuli on the performance of a simple cognitive task (e.g. distinguishing high and low pitch tones) is examined. The resulting interruptive effect of pain on attention has proven to be amplified by the intensity, novelty, unpredictability, and threat value of the pain stimulus (Eccleston and Crombez 1999), and attentional interference has been found to be pronounced in persons high in pain catastrophizing and fear of pain (Carleton et al. 2005; Crombez et al. 1998a, 1998b). Other studies have demonstrated that attention shifts to pain and pain-related cues and, once detected, pain is difficult to disengage from (e.g. Koster et al. 2006; Van Damme et al. 2004a). Based on this line of research, it can be concluded that there is initial evidence that pain demands attention, both in pain patients, but also in healthy individuals with high levels of specific pain-related fears, which has led to the development of a neurocognitive model of attention to pain, including behavioural and neuroimaging evidence (reviewed in Legrain et al. 2009; Van Damme et al. 2010).

In sum, it can be concluded that there is accumulating evidence for a sensory-related attentional bias in chronic pain (Boissevan 1994; Crombez et al. 2000; Pearce and Morley 1989; Snider et al. 2000; Sharpe et al. 2009), and specifically there is some evidence to suggest that anxiety in the presence of pain may be associated with interference (Asmundson et al. 1997; Boissevan 1994; Pincus et al. 1998; Snider et al. 2000).

## Interpretation bias

Data from studies of interpretative biases show consistently a bias for illness- and health-related material; both pain patients and persons with high levels of pain-related fear are inclined to interpret ambiguous and innocuous pain-related stimuli in a threatening or negative fashion (Edwards and Pearce 1994; Pincus et al. 1994; Pincus, et al. 1996a; Vancleef 2007; Vancleef et al. 2009). Recently, Keogh and colleagues (Keogh, Ellery et al. 2001; Keogh, Hamid, Hamid and Ellery 2004) have demonstrated that negative interpretative bias for ambiguous situations mediated the relation between individual levels of anxiety sensitivity and pain tolerance in a cold-pressor test. Nevertheless, it should be noted that studies on interpretive bias in the context of pain have relied on explicit measures predominantly, using homophones (words with the same pronunciation, but a different spelling: e.g. dye/die (McKellar et al. 2003; Pincus et al. 1994), homographs (words with the same spelling, but different meanings: e.g. needle (Pincus et al. 1996), word-stem completion tasks (word stem can be completed in different ways: e.g. ten—: tender/tennis (Edwards and Pearce 1994) or interpretation questionnaires (e.g. Keogh et al. 2001b; Keogh et al. 2004). Consequently, it remains unclear whether the negative bias results from elaborative, constructive, integrative processes at the moment of responding to ambiguity, or if negative interpretations occur actually at an automatic spontaneous level.

## Memory bias

The experimental paradigms used to assess memory biases differ from questionnaire methodology, in that they are likely to tap preconscious, rather than conscious cognitive processes, and are therefore less susceptible to response biases. When these types of experiments are computerized, experimenter effects are additionally minimized (Pincus 1998). These paradigms have been useful in the investigation of diatheses in other populations (see Pincus and Williams 1999).

Experiments into recall bias and chronic pain typically include an 'encoding stage' where partici- pants are presented with a list of words, and a 'recall phase' when they are asked to recall as many of the words as possible within a given timeframe. The words are selected according to their asso- ciation with a particular content category, for instance, pain-related content, or neutral content not associated with pain. The underlying assumption is that people will remember words that are congruent with their emotional state (see Pincus and Morley 2001).

While evidence for recognition bias in pain patients is currently scarce (Pincus and Morley 2001), there seems to be robust evidence for recall bias towards pain-related words. It has also been suggested that memory is an important means of developing representations of the self, and therefore, recall bias can highlight significant information about an individual's cognitive struc- tures (Pincus and Morley 2001). Previous investigations have demonstrated that pain patients recall more pain-related autobiographical memories (Wright and Morley 1995) than people not in pain; however, Eich et al. (1990) found that this effect was entirely mediated by mood. Furthermore, as with similar studies in depression, pain patients' greater autobiographical recall might simply reflect the greater number of pain experiences available to this group.

Experimental methodology (incidental world-list recall) avoids the issue of differences in actual experiences. Chronic pain patients with varying diagnoses recalled more words describing sen- sory aspects of pain than neutral words (Edwards et al. 1992; Johnson and Spence 1997; Pearce et al. 1990). It is further well established that chronic pain patients show greater recall for sensory- pain words encoded in reference to the self than to others (Edwards et al. 1992; Koutanji et al. 1999; Pincus et al. 1993, 1995). Koutanji et al. (1999) applied similar methodology and found similar results in a population of children with chronic pain experience due to arthritis. These results suggest that preferential recall in pain patients is associated with pain words that had been encoded in reference to the self and suggest that an individual's self-schema plays a pivotal role in processing biases.

Differences have also been found in the types of words recalled by chronic pain patients with and without depression. Depressed pain patients have been found to show biased recall towards both sensory and affective (e.g. 'dependent') aspects of pain, whilst non-depressed pain patients show a bias only towards sensory material (Calfas et al. 1997; Clemmey and Nicassio 1997; Edwards et al. 1992; Koutanji et al. 1999). In order to find out which cognitive biases are attribut- able to pain and which to mood, Pincus et al. (1995) further refined this methodology by present- ing depression descriptors and illness-and health-related stimuli that were either positive or negative in meaning (e.g. 'suffering' as a negative health-related word and 'withdrawn' as a nega- tive depression-related word), and found that patients with pain who are depressed or distressed show a bias for illness- and health-related stimuli, but not for depression-related words. However, in the absence of a control group with clinically depressed participants without pain, the conclu- sion that depressed pain patients show a bias towards pain and illness words rather than words associated with depression cannot be conclusively established. Specifically, people with chronic pain show preferential recall for pain-sensory words compared to neutral words when rating the degree to which these words refer to themselves, whereas normal controls show no differential recall (Koutantji et al. 1999; Pincus et al. 1993).

Wells et al. (2003) investigated the impact of diagnostic status on information processing biases among chronic pain and ankylosing spondylitis patients. Results showed that diagnosed chronic pain patients demonstrated a recall bias away from depression-related words, whilst the non- diagnosed chronic pain patients did not. It was suggested that a diagnosis in chronic pain patients might serve as a 'buffering' device against classic depression-related feelings of guilt, shame, and self-blame, which were encapsulated in the depression-related words of the above mentioned study.

Altogether, these findings provide support for the notion that depressed chronic pain patients experience depression that is qualitatively different from that of depression in the conventional psychiatric sense, in which the focus is on guilt, shame, and self-denigration. Pincus et al. (1995) hypothesized that ongoing exposure to pain might result in processing biases towards sensory-pain information, but in some pain patients, there is also an additional bias for pain-distress stimuli, which may be associated with poor self-image and increased levels of depression. Finally, although anxiety has been measured in a number of studies, the relationship between anxiety and memory bias appears to be insubstantial (Pincus and Morley 2001). One suggestion which might account for the inconsistent findings in this area is that the differences may be due to the nature of the words used, which lends further support to the importance of cognitive specificity, sampling biases due to convenience sampling or different recruitment settings (Pincus and Morley 2001). In sum, it can be concluded that memory biases are an important consideration in the onset and exacerbation of maladaptive responses to pain, although further clarification is necessary on the precise structure and impact of these processes in relation to maladaptive responses to physical threat.

## 16.3 Cognitive models of chronic pain

As described in the previous sections of this book, psychological theories work from the perspective that pain, and the disability related to it, are not only influenced by physiological pathology but also by psychological and social factors. Chronic pain is not only a somatic problem. It is influenced by the individual's attitudes and beliefs about their symptoms and the distress and behavioural responses initiated by their experience of pain. There are a number of psychological theories related to chronic pain, however, behavioural and cognitive-behavioural theories are the most relevant ones which have been discussed in previous chapters. The purpose of the following section is to describe predominately cognitive models to pain processing and to review the evidence concerning the cognitive mechanisms by which psychological factors modulate pain in both clinical and experimental contexts. The experience of pain is never an isolated sensory event and it never occurs without the influence of context and meaning. Pain is influenced by beliefs, attention, expectations and emotions, regardless of whether it occurs during the most controlled laboratory circumstances or during circumstances of physical trauma or emotional distress (Price and Bushnell 2004).

### 16.3.1 General model of pain processing

Price (1999) has proposed a conceptual model of pain processing to allow the study of temporal characteristics of sensory-discriminative components, affective, cognitive and behavioural responses. The first stage of this model consists of an initial sensory-discriminative process, which leads to the perceived intensity of the pain sensation. Immediate appraisals are associated with the sensory features of pain, autonomic and somatomotor activation, and perception of the immediate context surrounding the pain. The second stage, the *immediate pain* unpleasantness, reflects immediate affective responses and involves limited cognitive processing. This stage is influenced by the first stage; therefore the immediate unpleasantness can comprise a moment-by-moment unpleasantness, distress, annoyance often closely linked to the intensity of the painful sensation and the accompanying arousal. The third stage of pain processing involves longer-term cognitive processes that relate to the meanings or implications that pain holds for one's life and has been termed *extended pain* affect and conceptualized as suffering, which might include depression, frustration, anxiety and anger. It reflects the personal experience, as opposed to overt behaviour and it is largely autobiographical and directed toward the long-term past and long-term future.

It is influenced by expectations, beliefs, and meanings such as hope for alleviation, belief in one's ability to endure the pain, and perceived control over reducing the pain intensity. Thus, an individual's attitudes, beliefs, and memories about the real or imagined long-term consequences of having pain influence his or her adaptation to this stage. Consequently, these are the mediators that are the focus of cognitive-behavioural interventions and may explain differing levels of adaptation. The final component of the model is the overt behavioural expression of pain, such as moaning, lying down during the day, or declining to participate in daily responsibilities.

Immediate pain unpleasantness, in turn, causes extended emotions related to pain because it can provide an immediate cue for the meanings related to pain-related negative emotions once these meanings have been established over time (Price 1999). For example, the sudden exacerbation of pain in a cancer patient serves as an instant reminder of the progress of the disease, with its implications for deterioration and death. In addition, the difficulty of having to endure immediate pain unpleasantness over long periods of time (days, weeks, months) can lead to pain-related negative emotions. Parallel influences on extended pain-related emotions can also occur as they can be enhanced or diminished by arousal, contextual meanings, and other psychological factors that are present. Pain itself can be conceptualized as both an exteroceptive and interoceptive phenomenon depending on the type of tissue that is stimulated and the types of sensory qualities that are present during pain. Consistent with Damasio's (1994) view of the mechanisms of emotion, pain unpleasantness represents several sources, including pain sensory qualities, arousal, visceral, and somatomotoric responses, which in combination with appraisal of the context in which they occur, give rise to a felt meaning of what is happening to the body and the self, often not necessarily accompanied by specific thoughts. This felt meaning derives largely form the experience of the body and constitutes the immediate unpleasantness of pain (Price and Bushnell 2004).

Rainville et al. (1999) demonstrated this serial interaction by specifically targeting hypnotic suggestions toward unpleasantness, and thereby decreasing or enhancing ratings of the immediate unpleasantness of a hot stimulus, without changing pain sensation intensity. In contrast, when suggestions were directed only toward changing pain sensation intensity, both pain sensation intensity and pain unpleasantness ratings changed in parallel. The combination of these two sets of results helps to establish that pain sensation intensity is a cause of pain unpleasantness and not vice versa. The four-stage model of pain processing is consistent with the neural mechanisms of the sensory and affective dimensions of pain. For example, serial interactions between pain sensation, immediate pain unpleasantness, and extended pain-related affect are respectively associated with serial interactions between somatosensory cortices, insular, and cingulate cortices, and prefrontal and temporal cortical areas (reviewed in Price 1999; Price and Bushnell 2004).

## 16.3.2 Enmeshment and chronic pain

Chronic pain is by its nature prolonged and aversive, generally causing considerable disruption to the sufferer's life. Pain can present overwhelming obstacles to normal activities: work, leisure, and relationships with family and friends. The subjectivity of the experience can impose real isolation, and the personal meaning of pain and its impacts may threaten the individual's sense of who he or she is (Clyde and Williams 2002; Morley and Eccleston 2004). Researchers and clinicians have only recently begun to study the impact of pain on future possible health and self-identity. Reviews consistently show that depression in pain is significantly higher than in the general population, and often higher than in other medically ill populations (Banks and Kerns 1996; Fishbain et al. 1997; Sullivan et al. 1992), which leads to the important issue of what it is about chronic pain that causes such distress.

## Pain and the self

Persistent pain can generate interruptions to attention, memory processes and current thinking, interference with a range of everyday activities, and can pose a threat to identity. Morley and Eccleston (2004) have therefore proposed the framework of the three levels of *interruption, interference,* and *identity*. They referred to the tremendous value of pain as a threat and the capacity to threaten a person at different levels and argue that problem-solving similarly needs to occur at each level. It has been argued that chronic pain establishes itself in the context of an ongoing and unfolding personal dynamic related to the current stage of a life cycle. Pain will impact on ongoing developmental tasks and particular goals determined by motivational states and earlier experiences (Morley and Eccleston 2004). While a wealth of experimental studies have shown that the extent of the interruption is a function of stimulus characteristics and individual differences in threat perception (Eccleston and Crombez 1999), the effect of interference with activities of daily life can be seen in the frequent reports of frustration made by chronic pain patients (Harris et al. 2003; Morley et al. 2005; Price 1999; Wade et al. 1990). More specifically, Morley and Eccleston (2004) suggest the interference with mundane 'low-level' everyday tasks is psychologically significant because they put a burden on others and exert pressure on the sufferer to redefine the self. In addition, there is evidence linking self-reported depression in chronic pain to interference with social roles (Harris et al. 2003; Morley and Eccleston 2004). A key issue in any threat to identity is whether repeated interference with major goals will impact on the self-schemas and therefore on the person's identity (Leventhal et al. 1999). In pain, it has been suggested that current pain interferes with an individual's current tasks, plans, and goals and causes a 'biographical disruption' (Bury 1988) that changes the person's perspective of himself or herself with regard to the past and future (Hellström et al. 2000, 2001). Biographical disruptions appear to enhance emotional distress, and might lead to anxious and depressed mood, which in turn might inhibit active problem-solving (Morley and Eccleston 2004; Morley et al. 2005).

How pain might impact on identity can be further understood by the psychology of motivation and goal-related behaviour, as encompassed in self-regulation and self-discrepancy theories. However it would be beyond the scope of the present chapter to review the various conceptualizations in contemporary psychology (Carver and Scheier 1999; Carver et al. 1999; Karoly 1999; Oatley 1992; Higgins 1997). Goals are often classified into 'approach' goals, a tendency to *reduce* the discrepancy between the current position and the goal, and 'avoidance' goals, which require the person to *increase* the discrepancy between the current state and the goal (Carver and Scheier 1998, 1999). A crucial implication that follows from the frameworks of both Higgins' and Carver and Scheier is that individuals who are dominated by avoidance goals are more likely to experience anxiety and fear when these goals are threatened. In contrast, individuals whose primary goal state is approach-oriented will experience a sense of loss and sadness when these goals are threatened. Self-discrepancy theory (Higgins 1987, 1997) proposes that the self is represented in three domains, *actual, ideal,* and *ought self*. The common method used in self-discrepancy research asks participants to generate a list of descriptors that characterize the various aspects of the self. Studies have confirmed the relationship between self-discrepancies and experienced affect (Higgins 1987, 1997; Higgins and Tykocinski 1992; Higgins et al. 1994). However, self-discrepancy methodology has been criticized on grounds that it does not directly assess particular explicit goals, and attributes represent rather meta-cognition and the representation of a person's motivation and goals (Morley and Eccleston 2004). It has been argued that self-regulation and self-discrepancy theory might provide a useful framework for understanding the variety of emotional experience in chronic pain patients by providing a starting point for more compelling systematic research in this area (Morley and Eccleston 2004). In a first attempt, Morley et al. (2005)

developed a new method of assessing future possible selves (Ross and Buehler 2004) and self-pain enmeshment (Pincus and Morley 2001), which was based on self-discrepancy theory (Higgins 1987, 1997) and the concept of *possible selves*, which was introduced by Markus and Nurius (1986). Chronic pain patients generated characteristics describing their current actual self, hoped-for self, and feared-for self, and made judgements about the degree to which their future possible selves (hoped-for and feared-for) were dependent on the absence or presence of pain, as an indicator for pain enmeshment. Analyses showed that the degree of role interference attributable to pain, and the proportion of hoped-for self characteristics that could be achieved even in the presence of pain predicted the magnitude of depression and acceptance scores. Finally, it should be noted that self-regulation and self-discrepancy theories, which have not been developed in the context of chronic pain, do not appear to make predictions concerning the enmeshment of pain and self as encapsulated in the Schema Enmeshment Model of Pain (SEMP; Pincus and Morley 2001), which is described below, and future research will have to examine its appropriateness for the field of chronic pain.

## The Schema Enmeshment Model of Pain

How can the dynamic interplay between pain, mood and circumstances be represented to understand the observed differences observed in cognitive biases? Clyde and Williams (2002) argued that there is a need for a new model to aid understanding and treatment of pain and depression. Such a model needs to incorporate several factors: (1) the relationship between pain and depression; (2) that the development of depression is not inevitable in the context of chronic pain; (3) there is a need to take into account both vulnerability to depression and the nature of the individual experience of pain (stressor); and (4) there may be several pathways by which pain and depression co-occur, resulting in qualitatively different subtypes of depression.

The SEMP model has been proposed as an extension and refinement of self-discrepancy theory. In reviewing the existing literature on cognitive biases in chronic pain Pincus and Morley (2001) proposed that the degree to which aspects of the self were enmeshed with pain contributed to the observed cognitive bias. In particular the authors proposed that pain patients with concurrent distress/depression exhibited greater enmeshment of self and pain schema, hence causing suffering and disability. It is postulated that three self-schemas interact (see Figure 16.1): those pertaining to pain (sensory features), illness consequences (behavioural and emotional), and self (a dynamic, multifaceted structure including evaluation of self-worth). The SEMP model attempts to account for the variation in psychological adaptation to chronic pain, and aims to explain the different information-processing biases found in people with chronic pain. The pain schema contains the more immediate properties of the experience of pain, and is associated with the interruption of existing behaviour and the initiation of self-protective behaviours. The illness schema incorporates affective and behavioural consequences of illness, and is likely to have an effect on goal attainment, independence, and quality of life. Finally, the self-schema might contain trait-like descriptions of the self or specific behavioural episodes that have been experienced, and is associated with feelings of self-worth (Bradley and Mathews 1983). Importantly, the schema enmeshment model takes account of previous vulnerabilities which might affect an individual's adaptation. For example, a pre-existing vulnerability to depression might mean that an individual's self-worth is more likely to be affected by the experience of pain. This diathesis–stress approach to understanding depression in chronic pain has been described in detail by Banks and Kerns (1996). The schema enmeshment model, however, focuses more specifically on the role of schemas in predisposing an individual to developing depression in the presence of chronic pain.

When the content of two or more schemas is activated simultaneously and repetitively, it is hypothesized that the content of one schema might become incorporated into another schema,

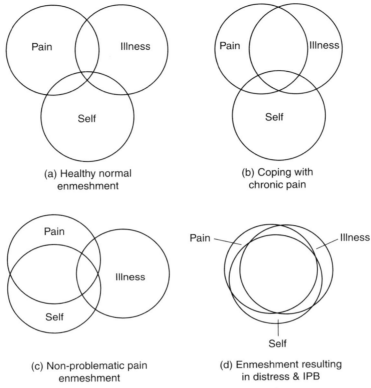

**Fig. 16.1** The Schema Enmeshment Model (Pincus and Morley 2001).

hence causing an 'enmeshment' of the two schemas. Pincus and Morley (2001) suggest that the three schemas always overlap to some extent, but it is the amount of enmeshment, the content of the schemas, and the timing and context of the enmeshment that is important. In adaptive coping, pain and illness are not considered to impact on the person's sense of self-worth, which could be explained by a lack of enmeshment between his/her self-schema and the illness/pain schemas. It is hypothesized that the self-schema is most likely to become enmeshed with the pain and illness schemas if it already contains information about dependence and distress.

In light of the SEMP model, three possibilities of how the self-schema might become vulnerable have been proposed (Pincus and Morley 2001). First, there will be a small percentage of patients who have experienced an episode of depression before the onset of pain. Because of this previously established vulnerability it is likely that they are at risk for the development of chronic distress. Second, other patients might have not experienced a previous episode of depression, but have experienced life events which have compromised their sense of self-worth; previous experiences have made them vulnerable. Even without the onset of pain, people in this group are more likely to experience a depressive episode, and pain could act as a 'trigger' event. This notion is in line with the work of Banks and Kerns (1996), stating that chronic pain is a highly influential stressor, which might cause the reactivation of negative beliefs and cognitions among already vulnerable populations, such as pain patients, resulting in negative cognitive biases. Pincus and Morley (2001) surmise that both these groups of patients should exhibit their vulnerability to depression by showing biases towards stimuli incorporating self-denigration when their self-schema is activated. Finally, the last group consists of those for whom vulnerabilities have not been established earlier, therefore they are less likely to become depressed as a result of chronic pain, but they may become distressed. As a consequence, these patients will not show biases towards material reflecting negative self-worth, but they will show biases towards negative aspects of pain and illness. A more detailed critique of the SEMP model will be provided in the following sections.

## Empirical support for the main components of the SEMP

It has been shown that the application of information processing approaches to the study of chronic pain has proven influential by avoiding the limitations associated with classical self-report measures. Further, it has been shown that conditions such as chronic pain or depression may be distinguished from one another, on the basis of these associated cognitive biases. Most importantly, observations of dysfunctional processing associated with chronic pain hold important implications for the development of new treatment modalities. The SEMP model has been developed through close scrutiny of the existing literature and it provides many testable hypotheses (Pincus and Morley, 2001): (1) processing priorities depend on the salience of information to the content of schemas; (2) all pain patients are proposed to preferentially process pain information; (3) self-referential material is also preferentially processed, especially when congruent with the self-schema; (4) therefore self-referential health-related information would be preferentially recalled, particularly by depressed chronic pain patients, as illness information is enmeshed, and therefore congruent with the self schema; (5) however, enmeshment does not necessarily indicate self-denigratory beliefs, so depressed pain patients would not preferentially recall typical depression-related information, in contrast to clinically depressed patients without chronic pain. Although the SEMP model has been proposed recently, there are already several existing studies, which have directly tested predictions from the SEMP (Davies 2003; Gray 2006; Harris et al. 2003; Morley et al. 2005; Pincus et al. 2007; Read and Pincus 2004; Sutherland and Morley 2008).

As can be seen from the abovementioned research, self-pain enmeshment can be operationalized and measured in different ways. A novel approach for studying self-pain enmeshment and depressive thinking in chronic pain patients has been proposed by Pincus et al. (2007). Beside questionnaires and information-processing methodologies, a sentence completion method has been developed to overcome the limitations of endorsement methodology and elicit idiographic information by describing patients' individual perspectives (Barton and Morley 1999; Barton et al. 2005; Rusu et al. 2009). Briefly, the Sentence Completion Test for Chronic Pain (SCP; Rusu 2008) has been illustrated as a promising approach, which might help to clarify the relationship between pain and depression/distress, contribute to the identification of underlying schemas in depressed pain patients, and might also be of use for case formulation. A first study using a preliminary version of the SCP showed that depressed pain patients generated more negative health-related completions (particularly directed towards the future), than non-depressed pain patients and control participants (Pincus et al. 2007). Non-depressed pain patients focused on health as well, but not necessarily in a negative way. Moreover, the predominance of danger-related thoughts in anxiety patients (Beck et al. 1974; Rachman et al. 1988), contrasts with the themes of loss and self-devaluation in depressive negative automatic thoughts (e.g. Beck et al. 1979), and is the basis of the content-specificity hypothesis (Beck 1987; Beck et al. 1987). In pain, studies have demonstrated that the type of depression experienced by chronic pain patients differs qualitatively from patients with clinical depression by a tendency for health-related negative processing, without the component of self-denigration, shame, and guilt often found in clinical depression (Pincus and Morley 2001; Pincus et al. 1995, 2007). While traditional measures of depressive thinking are based on Beck's (1970) cognitive triad of self, world and future and contain lists of negative thoughts that occur automatically during depressed mood (Beck et al. 1961, 1987; Hamilton 1967; Hollon and Kendall 1980), it has been argued that this kind of measure will approximate a patient's thoughts rather than capture them exactly (Barton and Morley 1999).

Consistent with the SEMP model, Rusu and colleagues (Rusu 2008; Rusu et al. 2008, 2009, in prep.) manipulated self-reference and future reference as a condition during encoding in a recall task and generation of idiographic content in a sentence completion task in a series of experiments, and found that recall biases and cognitive content in pain patients was specific to pain- and illness-related descriptors and themes. More specifically, in depressed pain patients the negative health-related cognitive biases were firmly connected with patients' view of themselves in the future. This might indicate that the experience of chronic pain combined with depressed or distressed mood might lead to a generalization and amplification of cognitive biases, which also extends to the future (see Figure 16.2 for the hypothesized enmeshment for different groups). As both pain groups (whether depressed or not) were involved with pain experiences, one possible explanation for the findings of the depressed pain group would be that the implications of pain go beyond the pain itself, into the domain of health and illness, as presumed by the SEMP model. This explanation would be in line with the results of Pincus et al. (1995), who reported that depressed pain patients showed a marked bias towards illness-related words, which was stronger than for pain-related words. At present it is not known which factors are causing cognitive vulnerabilities, or which processes might lead to the generalization and amplification of cognitive biases, but it is conceivable that factors such as pain catastrophizing, hypervigilance and anxiety sensitivity (Van Damme et al. 2004b), in addition to predisposing factors, might play a crucial role in the development of distress and potentially also the maintenance of chronic pain. There is

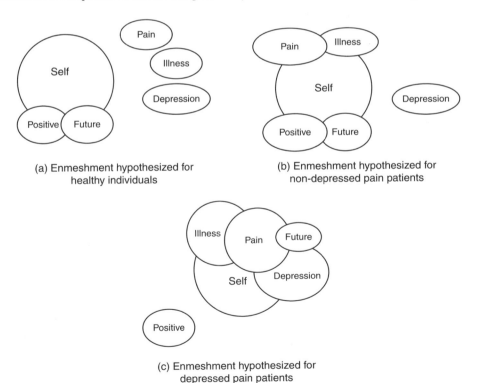

(a) Enmeshment hypothesized for
healthy individuals

(b) Enmeshment hypothesized for
non-depressed pain patients

(c) Enmeshment hypothesized for
depressed pain patients

**Fig. 16.2** Hypothesized enmeshment for different groups (Rusu 2008).

evidence that hypervigilance for pain is associated with a narrowing of the attentional field and a difficulty in disengaging attention from pain and shifting toward other demands in the environment (Van Damme et al. 2002). This effect was more pronounced in persons with high catastrophic thinking. Further research is needed to clarify issues of risk and vulnerability by prospective designs.

The above mentioned findings suggest that the concept of enmeshment as captured in the current measures may provide an alternative approach to explaining distress/depression in chronic pain. Pincus and Morley (2001) note that enmeshment is not a bias in its own right but a structural feature relating the self to pain experience and offered no independent way of assessing the degree of enmeshment, which was essentially a *post-hoc* explanation for the observed data. Whether high levels of enmeshment represent a risk factor for depression or conversely whether low levels of enmeshment act to buffer the individual from depression cannot be distinguished by the present data. However, it should be recognized that a definitive opinion on this must await fuller explication of the concept of enmeshment and prospectively designed tests of the competing theories. Further developments using other methods, e.g. the Implicit Attitude Test (Greenwald et al. 1998) might also be considered. Additionally, the extent to which enmeshment is specific to chronic pain rather than a general characteristic of other chronic health conditions is unknown. It is conceivable that chronic pain is a particularly good model for testing the concept of enmeshment because of the extraordinary capacity of chronic pain to interrupt and interfere with ongoing cognitive and behavioural activity (Banks and Kerns 1996; Eccleston and Crombez 1999; Morley and Eccleston 2004).

## 16.4 **Clinical implications**

The following section discusses the possible implications of this line of research for clinical interventions. Several implications for the assessment and treatment of distress and depression in the context of pain could be outlined, including the following: (1) chronic pain patients should be routinely screened for depressed symptomatology; (2) it may prove useful to distinguish between distress versus depression in chronic pain; and (3) the potential role of cognitive biases as a marker for chronicity.

First, it seems reasonable to assume that the introduction of abovementioned research findings as an educational tool would assist existing strategies of pain management. For example, if pain patients are presented with results indicating the selective focus on negative health or negative future experiences, they could employ this knowledge while attempting to focus on their positive and valued future goals and plans. Presented with the fact that they automatically respond to self-referent cues with pain- and health-related thoughts, such as illustrated in Figure 16.2c, they may become more open to the idea that the process can be employed in reverse by focusing on self-future-positive experiences despite experiencing pain (see Figure 16.2b). In a similar manner, the SCP might be a useful assessment tool to capture the actual thought content and to initialize therapeutic strategies for change. Although the results of the studies presented cannot be interpreted as evidence for the existence of a self-schema, they do show that pain patients selectively process and generate information in reference to themselves; their view of themselves, or self-image is directly connected to their processing and generation of pain- and health-related information. The implications for clinical interventions are that it might prove beneficial to concentrate on patients' self-image instead of concentrating on the pain itself. This would involve attempts to create new associative paths between the self-concept, such as more positive concepts of 'myself as a coping person'. Although many of the standard interventions may contribute to such a process in the long term, there may be more direct routes to contribute to these changes.

Pincus (1998) further proposes that screening for information-processing biases might be a quick and reliable way to assess whether a chronic pain patient needs to be referred on for further psychological treatment. Referral might be warranted where an individual has demonstrated a recall bias for negative health related stimuli, which have been encoded in relation to the self (Pincus, 1998). Thus, information-processing methodologies might provide an effective way to identify distressed chronic pain patients, and so improve outcomes, although this proposition is in need of further research.

From a clinical point of view, it seems important to separate patients with chronic pain who are distressed about the consequences of chronic pain from those who have the additional burden of believing that the negative consequences of pain mean that they are fundamentally flawed and worthless. It is well established that patients with chronic pain rarely endorse self-denigratory statements (Williams and Richardson 1993; Morley and Wilkinson 1995). They are likely to respond more rapidly to focused problem solving as their self-efficacy should be relatively intact, and the more generalized cognitive distortions shown by depressed patients are limited to specific pain-relevant situations in such patients (Smith et al. 1994). Such patients with pain may be construed as being depressed about their pain rather than depressed about depression (Pincus and Morley 2001). The body of literature reviewed in this chapter suggests that traditional cognitive-behavioural interventions may not be optimal for depressed pain patients and that their depression is qualitatively different from that of other groups, involving different concerns and salient concepts. Psychological interventions that focus on these concepts, as many interventions based on Beck's cognitive therapy do, would prove less beneficial for depressed pain patients than interventions that focus on retaining a positive sense of self, for instance. However, cognitive-behavioural interventions have focused so far more on distressed pain patients (Turk and Rudy 1992; Gatchel and Turk 1996), while interventions to specifically target depressed pain patients seem to be underdeveloped. This leads to the question of whether there is a need for psychological therapies such as cognitive-behavioural therapy (CBT) to be specially adapted for depressed pain patients. At present, the demonstrated efficacy of interventions is, at best, modest (Van Tulder et al. 2000). Additionally, Morley et al. (1999) have recently reviewed intervention studies on the effectiveness of CBT in chronic pain and have concluded only modest effect sizes for CBT in chronic pain compared to other conditions like mood and anxiety disorders, with room for improvement. Similarly, researchers in the field have noted the importance of identifying distinct subgroups of patients and to tailor interventions to the specific needs of patients in order to improve treatment outcomes and satisfaction with treatment (Jellema et al. 2005; Turk 2005; Van der Windt et al. 2008; Vlaeyen and Morley 2005).

Despite the recent findings presented in this chapter, it is clear that, as yet, a comprehensive picture of the function and content of depression in chronic pain is lacking, thus limiting the potential for optimally targeted interventions. Overall the existing evidence so far, suggests that there are qualitative differences between clinically depressed patients without pain and depressed pain patients. As long as depressed pain patients are treated in the same way as clinically depressed patients without the physical condition of pain, the treatment outcomes will reflect the non-specificity of the treatment setting for this group of patients. To date, there is little research into specific cognitions and beliefs, which should be targeted and changed through pain management for this substantial group of pain patients. Pincus et al. (2002) reviewed evidence from prospective studies and concluded that current findings constitute a strong indication for the development and testing of clinical interventions specifically targeting psychological distress, depressive mood and somatization. More specifically, Leventhal et al. (1999) argue, in accordance with Pincus and Morley (2001), that living with a chronic illness, such as severely disabling persistent pain, has a powerful impact on self-identity: helplessness, despair, and frustration are associated with a fusion of the self with the disease ('I am pain'), whereas the ability to compartmentalize pain and retain other aspects of the self are important for psychological well-being. However, the main challenge of future research will be to address the question of how to compartmentalize pain or, to express it in schema theory, how to disentangle the enmeshment of self, pain and illness schemas in depressed pain patients (see Figure 16.2c). It has been suggested in the previous chapters that there are a number of plausible mechanisms for how self-pain enmeshment could be reduced and further research is needed to test their clinical utility. In short, reducing self-discrepancies between the actual self and ideal or possible self (e.g. Self-System Therapy; SST) might lead to an improvement in depressed pain patients as well as therapeutic techniques which emphasize the acceptance of pain. SST has recently been introduced as a new approach for patients with unipolar depression (Lau 2008) and is based on regulatory focus theory, which postulates that some depressed individuals are unable to pursue promotion goals effectively (Higgins 1997). A randomized trial compared SST with cognitive therapy (CT), showing that there was no overall difference in efficacy between treatments, but patients whose socialization history lacked an emphasis on promotion goals showed significantly greater improvement with SST (Strauman et al. 2006). There is currently one study underway, which is examining the efficacy of self-system therapy in chronic pain patients (Kindermans et al. in preparation). Similarly, accepting the pain as part of one's present and future life seems to be beneficial for the adjustment to pain and the reduction of depression (e.g. Acceptance and Commitment Therapy). For instance, McCracken (1998) found that acceptance of pain was a significant predictor of several physical and psychosocial variables including depression. The process of acceptance may require abandonment of previous expectations, roles or goals, or their reassessment. Schmitz et al. (1996) found less distress among those pain patients who modified existing goals or substituted new ones (accommodation) than among those who pursed unmodified goals, relying on the eventual relief of pain to enable them to realize them. Along similar lines, MacLeod and Moore (2000) recommended a two-dimensional approach to mental health, which might be also appropriate for chronic pain, by incorporating strategies to work on increasing positive as well as decreasing negative states. Goal setting and planning ability are importantly linked to well-being by having and progressing towards valued goals (Carver and Scheier 1990; Schmuck and Sheldon 2001; Sheldon et al. 2002). Loewenstein et al. (2001) suggested that goal progress and goal attainment is likely to affect well-being though anticipatory effects; people feel good at the moment when they think about experiencing desirable future outcomes. It has been suggested that having meaningful goals and plans to pursue those goals is also likely to result in higher levels of engagement in life tasks and roles (Cantor and Sanderson 1999). MacLeod and colleagues (2008) demonstrated in a recent study that a brief goal-setting and planning skills intervention in a non-clinical sample significantly increased subjective well-being. Similarly, an alternative way of incorporating a positive approach to depressed pain patients would be to work with them to develop identities and interests that are not directly related to their pain problem. However, these kinds of interventions will have to be tested for their pragmatic utility and effectiveness in samples of depressed pain patients, characterized by low levels of well-being. Future work in this area will have to prove *which* of the approaches outlined above will be beneficial under *what circumstances* for depressed pain patients.

To conclude, depression has been identified as a determinant of poor rehabilitation outcomes in individuals with musculoskeletal conditions. However, what remains unclear is why depression in chronic pain is associated with poor rehabilitation outcomes. One possibility is that depressive symptoms might become more treatment resistant as the duration of pain-related disability extends over time. The paucity of research addressing this question has limited conceptual advance in this field, and has probably impacted negatively on the development of effective

## Box 16.1 Implications of cognitive processing for clinical practice

In summary, the value of insights to cognitive biases for clinical practice could be described along the following lines:

◆ Insights into the cognitive content and processing of depressed pain patients can promote the development of tailored pain management techniques that are directed at counteracting dysfunctional response patterns to pain, and promoting functional and adaptive processes.

◆ In providing evidence for the need to focus on self-concept, if long-term cognitive changes are to be achieved.

◆ The identification of assessable psychological vulnerability factors can be helpful for the early screening of individuals who are at risk for developing chronic pain complaints.

◆ The early identification of the presence of vulnerability for developing chronic pain can promote the early application of pain management techniques that are specifically tailored to the needs of the individual at risk.

◆ The assessment of automatic cognitive processing biases might provide a measure to assess change in the salience of emotional concepts after intervention.

intervention programs for individuals with chronic pain and depressive symptomatology. Accumulating evidence highlights the importance of early detection and treatment of depressive symptoms in individuals with painful musculoskeletal conditions. Depression continues to be under-detected and under-treated in individuals with musculoskeletal pain. Delays in referring clients for assessment and treatment of depressive symptoms might mean missing a window of opportunity for effective intervention on depressive symptoms. Surprisingly, there have been few clinical trials examining the efficacy of pain interventions in depressed patients with musculoskeletal pain. Clinicians and researchers alike are encouraged to investigate more systematically the efficacy of different treatment approaches for the management of depressive conditions associated with pain, particularly in more chronic cases where options for effective pain reduction are more limited. In summary, the value of insights into cognitive processing to clinical practice are described in Box 16.1.

## 16.5 Recommendations and future directions

Based on the examination of negative cognitive factors involved in the development and maintenance of chronic pain, the following directions for future research may be proposed.

First, in examining pain-related distress and depression in relation to negative future thinking, it might be valuable to consider the precise object of future-related anxieties and distress, and its impact on self-identity more thoroughly. It is well acknowledged that distress and anxieties in the context of pain can be directed at the presence of physical pain and/or the direct functional consequences of activity or (re)injury, on the exacerbation and continuation of pain. In addition, one might fear the possibility of putative future pain, disability, or physical health problems, the impact of pain on one's social status and relationships, or fears related to the impact of pain on financial resources (McCracken 2004; McNeil and Vowles 2004; Morley and Eccleston 2004). The content and meaning of pain-related depression and anxiety may be proposed to depend upon prior personal learning history, prior knowledge, environmental contexts, and social influences.

For instance, Hadjistavropoulos et al. (2004) suggested that present-oriented fears and anxieties focused on physical pain might be especially predictive of short-term disability and maladaptive responses to pain, whereas future-oriented fears or anxieties, directed at putative physical harm, future long-term disability and the functional and social consequences of injury and illness might be more predictive of long-term disability.

A second direction for further research concerns the further examination of the role of cognitive processing biases in the aetiology and persistence of chronic pain. One of the main limitations of the research reviewed earlier concerns the cross-sectional design of the studies in examining vulnerability factors for developing and maintaining chronic pain problems. Currently, it is unclear whether processing biases result from long-term exposure to pain, or are vulnerability indicators that result in maintenance of pain states. An alternative approach for examining cognitive biases which may provide a more complete picture would be within a prospective study design, which would collect longitudinal data on the development and exacerbation of chronic pain problems. However, such a research design would be difficult to implement, as it requires the selection of participants prior to the experience of pain. One alternative to this option would be to follow up patients from casualty wards, in situations involving acute pain, to see which patients develop chronic pain syndromes, and at what stage do processing biases become evident. Furthermore, it might be suggested that studying the combined effects of multiple cognitive processing biases can add significantly to our understanding of the unique and relative importance of these separate biases as well. Since individuals with chronic pain and associated high levels of depression or anxiety are assumed to be characterized by the propensity to process pain-related information negatively, it seems appropriate to assume that one particular bias will be influenced by other biases or that several biases exert conjunct influences on the maintenance of pain. It is also possible that the pain experience and the information processing biases operate in a cyclical fashion, acting to maintain and strengthen each other (Hirsch et al. 2006). The relationship between processing biases and the prognosis of pain conditions should therefore form the focus of future work. An additional limitation of the studies reviewed concern power problems due to the inclusion of relatively small participant samples. Meta-analyses have shown only small to medium effect sizes for cognitive biases in chronic pain (Pincus and Morley 2001). It is therefore advisable that large enough participant groups are concordantly recruited to test for the influence of these factors.

Another issue that remains to be investigated is the causal linkage between distress/depression, cognitive biases, and the exacerbation of pain complaints. One way of studying causality would be to induce cognitive biases for selective processing of pain- or health-related information in healthy individuals and to study the subsequent effect on pain-related behavioural measures as well as on mood. Evidence for the practicality of inducing cognitive biases successfully has recently been provided with respect to automatic interpretation bias and attentional bias in anxiety disorders (Mathews and MacLeod 2002; Salemink et al. 2007; Yiend and Mackintosh 2004). A first study in student participants has shown that attentional biases towards acute experimentally induced pain could be altered (McGowan et al. 2009). The findings that anxiety-related cognitive biases and attentional biases towards pain can be induced leads to the challenge to examine the extent to which these biases can be conversely reduced, and such techniques may serve as potential valuable additions to the treatment of persons characterized by increased negative cognitive biases towards pain and health information. Future work should also concentrate on recovered groups, as part of outcome studies.

Finally, in addition to studying factors that contribute in a negative fashion to pain and disability, it is proposed that further research devotes attention to the role of psychological factors that might have positive influences on the development and persistence of pain. For instance,

Vancleef (2007) demonstrated, in healthy individuals, the importance of perceived control and self-efficacy beliefs as cognitive factors that have a beneficial influence on the experience of pain by reducing pain intensity and fearfulness of pain. Other cognitive factors presumed to exert positive influences on pain are acceptance (McCracken 2005) as well as several stable personality traits, which have been suggested to have promising value in protecting against the development of chronic pain conditions, for example dispositional optimism, general self-efficacy, and dispositional hope (Arntz and Schmidt 1989; Carver and Scheier 2005; Peters et al. 2007; Peters and Vancleef 2008; Schwarzer et al. 2005). Accumulating knowledge on processes and factors that might contribute to adjustment and adequate coping with pain provides useful information for theoretical and management perspectives on chronic pain.

In conclusion, taking a broader perspective on the role and meaning of depression in pain and studying the interplay between various constructs on an idiographic and nomothetic level, allows for the identification of the unique and relative importance of each of these constructs for specific components of the pain problem. It is suggested that the SEMP model might serve as a useful framework within which findings of divergent influences can be understood and interpreted, and further formal testing of this model is warranted.

## Acknowledgements

The contribution of Adina C. Rusu and Tamar Pincus was supported by Back Care, United Kingdom. Work on this chapter was also partially supported by a grant from the Research Committee, University of Bochum, Germany, awarded to the first author.

## References

Alloy, L. B., Abramson, L. Y., Murray, L. A., Whitehouse, W. G. & Hogan, M. E. (1997). Self-referent information processing in individuals at high and low cognitive risk for depression. *Cognition and Emotion,* **11**, 539–68.

Arntz, A. & Schmidt, J. M. (1989). Perceived control and the experience of pain. In A. Steptoe & A. Appels (Eds.), *Stress, personal control, and health* (pp. 131–62). Chichester: Wiley.

Asmundson, G. J. G., & Hadjivropoulos, H. D. (2007). Is high fear of pain associated with attentional biases for pain-related or general threat? A categorical reanalysis. *Journal of Pain,* **8**, 11–18.

Asmundson, G. J. G., Kuperos, J. L. & Norton, G. R. (1997). Do patients with chronic pain selectively attend to pain-related information? Preliminary evidence for the mediating role of fear. *Pain,* **72**, 27–32.

Asmundson, G. J. G., Carleton, N. R. & Ekong, J. (2005). Dot-probe evaluation of selective attentional processing of pain cues in patients with chronic headaches. *Pain,* **114**, 250–6.

Banks, S. M., & Kerns, R. D. (1996). Explaining high rates of depression in chronic pain: A diathesis stress framework. *Psychological Bulletin,* **199**, 95–110.

Barton, S. B. & Morley, S. (1999). Specificity of reference patterns in depressive thinking: agency and object roles in self-representation. *Journal of Abnormal Psychology,* **108**(4), 655–61.

Barton, S. B., Morley, S., Bloxham, G., Kitson, C. & Platts, S. (2005). Sentence completion test for depression (SCD): An idiographic measure of depressive thinking. *British Journal of Clinical Psychology,* **44**(1), 29–46.

Beck, A. T. (1970). The core problem in depression: The cognitive triad. In J. H. Masserman (Ed.), *Depression: Theories and therapies* (pp. 47–55). New York: Grune and Statton.

Beck, A. T. (1976). *Cognitive Therapy and the Emotional Disorders.* New York: International Universities Press.

Beck, A. T. (1987). Cognitive models of depression. *Journal of Cognitive Psychotherapy,* **1**, 5–37.

Beck, A. T. & Clark, D. A. (1997). An information processing model of anxiety: Automatic and strategic processes. *Behaviour Research and Therapy,* **35**, 49–58.

Beck, A. T., Ward, C. H., Mendelson, M., Mock, J. E. & Erbaugh, J. K. (1961). An inventory for measuring depression. *Archives of General Psychiatry,* **4,** 561–71.

Beck, A. T., Laude, R. & Bohnert, M. (1974). Ideational components of anxiety neurosis. *Archives of General Psychiatry,* **31,** 319–25.

Beck, A. T., Rush, A. J., Shaw, B. F. & Emery, G. (1979). *Cognitive Therapy for Depression.* New York: Guilford.

Beck, A. T., Brown, G., Steer, R. A., Eidelson, J. I. & Riskind, J. H. (1987). Differentiating anxiety and depression: A test of the cognitive content-specificity hypothesis. *Journal of Abnormal Psychology,* **96,** 179–83.

Boissevan, M. (1994). Information processing in chronic pain. Unpublished doctoral dissertation. London, Ontario, Canada: University of Western Ontario.

Bradley, B., & Mathews, A. (1983). Negative self-schemata in clinical depression. *British Journal of Clinical Psychology,* **22,** 173–81.

Bury, M. (1988). Meaning at risk: The experience of arthritis. In R. Anderson & M. Bury (eds.), *Living with Chronic Illness: The Experience of Patients and their Families* (pp. 89–116). London: Unwin Hyman.

Calfas, K. J., Ingram, R. E. & Kaplan, R. M. (1997). Information processing and affective distress in osteoarthritis patients. *Journal of Consulting and Clinical Psychology,* **65,** 576–81.

Cantor, N. & Sanderson, C. A. (1999). Life task participation and well-being: The importance of taking part in daily life. In D. Kahneman, E. Diener, & N. Schwartz (Eds.), *Well-being: The foundations of hedonic psychology* (pp. 230–43). New York: Russell Sage Foundation.

Carleton, N. R., Asmundson, G. J. G. & Taylor, S. (2005). Fear of physical harm: factor structure and psychometric properties of the injury/illness sensitivity index. *Journal of Psychopathology and Behavioural Assessment,* **27,** 235–41.

Carver, C. S. & Scheier, M. F. (1990). Origins and functions of positive and negative affect: A control process view. *Psychological Review,* **97,** 19–35.

Carver, C. S. & Scheier, M. F. (1998). *On the self-regulation of behavior.* Cambridge, MA: Cambridge University Press.

Carver, C. S. & Scheier, M. F. (1999). Themes and issues in self regulation. In R. S. Wyer, Jr. (ed.), *Perspectives on Behavioural Self-regulation,* Vol. XII, pp. 1–105. Mahwah, NJ: Lawrence Erlbaum Associates.

Carver, C. S. & Scheier, M. F. (2005). Optimism. In C. R. Synder & S. J. Lopez (Eds.), *Handbook of positive psychology* (pp. 231–43). Oxford: University Press.

Carver, C. S., Lawrence, J. W. & Scheier, M. F. (1999). Self-discrepancies and affect: Incorporating the role of feared selves. *Personality and Social Psychology Bulletin,* **25,** 783–92.

Clemmey, P. A. & Nicassio, P. M. (1997). Illness self-schemas in depressed and nondepressed rheumatoid arthritis patients. *Journal of Behavioural Medicine,* **20,** 273–90.

Clyde, Z. K. & Williams, A. C. (2002). Depression and mood. In: S. J. Linton (Ed.), *New avenues for the prevention of chronic musculoskeletal pain and disability. Pain Research and Clinical Management,* Vol. 12 (pp. 105–21). Amsterdam: Elsevier.

Crombez, G., Eccleston, C., Baeyens, F. & Eelen, P. (1998a). Attentional disruption is enhanced by the threat of pain. *Behaviour Research and Therapy,* **36,** 195–204.

Crombez, G., Eccleston, C., Baeyens, F. & Eelen, P. (1998b). When somatic information threatens, catastrophic thinking enhances attentional interference. *Pain,* **75,** 187–98.

Crombez, G., Hermans, D. & Andriaensen, H. (2000). The emotional Stroop task and chronic pain: What is threatening for chronic pain sufferers? *European Journal of Pain,* **4,** 37–44.

Damasio, A. (1994). *Descartes Error.* New York: Avon Books.

Davies, C. (2003). Self-discrepancy Theory and Chronic Pain. Unpublished Dissertation in Clinical Psychology, University of Leeds, Leeds.

Dehghani, M., Sharpe, L. & Nicholas, M. K. (2003). Selective attention to pain-related information in chronic musculoskeletal pain patients. *Pain,* **105,** 37–46.

Eccleston, C. & Crombez, G. (1999). Pain demands attention: a cognitive-affective model of the interruptive function of pain. *Psychological Bulletin,* **125**, 356–66.

Edwards, L. & Pearce, S. A. (1994). Word completion in chronic pain: Evidence for schematic representation of pain? *Journal of Abnormal Psychology,* **103**, 379–82.

Edwards, L., Pearce, S. A., Collett, B. J. & Pugh, R. (1992). Selective memory for sensory and affective information in chronic pain and depression. *British Journal of Clinical Psychology,* **31**, 239–48.

Eich, E., Rachman, S. & Lopatka, C. (1990). Affect, pain, and autobiographical memory. *Journal of Abnormal Psychology,* **99** (2), 174–78.

Fishbain, D. A., Cutler, R., Rosomoff, H. L. & Rosomoff, R. S. (1997). Chronic pain-associated depression: antecedent or consequence of chronic pain? A review. *Clinical Journal of Pain,* **13**, 116–37.

Gatchel, R. J. & Turk, D. C. (1996). *Psychological approaches to pain management: A practitioner's handbook.* New York: Guilford Press.

Gray, E. (2006). Cognitive bias and positive affect in chronic pain. Unpublished Dissertation in Clinical Psychology, Royal Holloway, University of London, London.

Greenwald, A. G., McGhee, D. E. & Schwartz, J. L. K. (1998). Measuring individual differences in implicit cognition: the implicit association test. *Journal of Personality and Social Psychology,* **74**, 1464–80.

Hadjistavropoulos, T. & Craig, K. D. (2004). An Introduction to Pain: Psychological Perspectives. In T. Hadjistavropoulos & K. D. Craig (Eds.), *Pain: psychological perspectives* (pp. 1–12). New Jersey: Lawrence Erlbaum Associates.

Hamilton, M. (1967). Development of a rating scale for primary depressive illness. British *Journal of Social and Clinical Psychology,* **6**, 278–96.

Harris, S., Morley, S. & Barton, S. B. (2003). Role loss and emotional adjustment in chronic pain. *Pain,* **105**, 363–70.

Hellström, C., Jansson, B. & Carlsson, S. G. (2000). Perceived future in chronic pain: the relationship between outlook on future and empirically derived psychological patient profiles. *European Journal of Pain,* **4**, 283–90.

Hellström, C. (2001). Temporal dimensions of the self-concept: entrapped and possible selves in chronic pain. *Psychology and Health,* **16**, 111–24.

Higgins, E. T. (1987). Self-discrepancy: A theory relating self and affect. *Psychological Review,* **94**, 319–40.

Higgins, E. T. (1997). Beyond pleasure and pain. *American Psychologist,* **52**, 1280–1300.

Higgins, E. T. & Tykocinski, O. (1992). Self-discrepancies and biographical memory: Personality and cognition at the level of psychological situation. *Personality and Social Psychology Bulletin,* **18**, 527–35.

Higgins, E. T., Roney, C. J. R., Crowe, E. & Hymes, C. (1994). Ideal versus ought predilections for approach and avoidance distinct self-regulatory systems. *Journal of Personality and Social Psychology,* **66**, 276–86.

Hirsch, C., Clark, D. M. & Mathews, A. (2006). Imagery and interpretation in social phobia: support for the combined cognitive bias hypothesis. *Behavior Therapy,* **37**, 223–36.

Hollon, S. D. & Kendall, P. C. (1980). Cognitive self-statements in depression: Development on an automatic thoughts questionnaire. *Cognitive Therapy and Research,* **4**, 383–95.

Ingram, R. E., Miranda, J. & Segal, Z. V. (1998). *Cognitive Vulnerability to Depression.* New York: Guilford Press.

Jellema, P., van der Windt, D. A. W. M., van der Horst, H. E., Blankenstein, A., Bouter, L. M. & Stalman, W. A. B. (2005). Why is a treatment aimed at psychosocial factors not effective in patients with (sub)acute low back pain? *Pain,* **118**, 350–59.

Johnson, R. & Spence, S. (1997). Pain, affect and cognition in children: recall bias associated with pain. In G. F. Gebhart, D. L. Hammond & T. S. Jensen (Eds.), *Progress in Pain Research and Management 2: Proceedings of the 7th World Congress on Pain* (pp. 877–84). Seattle: IASP Press.

Karoly, P. (1999). A goal systems-self-regulatory perspective on personality, psychopathology, and change. *Review of General Psychology,* **3**, 264–91.

Keogh, E. & Cochrane, M. (2002). Anxiety sensitivity, cognitive biases, and the experience of pain. *Journal of Pain*, **3**, 320–29.

Keogh, E., Dillon, C., Georgiou, G. & Hunt, C. (2001a). Selective attentional biases for physical threat in physical anxiety sensitivity. *Journal of Anxiety Disorders*, **15**, 299–315.

Keogh, E., Ellery, D., Hunt, C. & Hannent, I. (2001b). Selective attentional bias for pain-related stimuli amongst pain fearful individuals. *Pain*, **91**, 91–100.

Keogh, E., Hamid, R., Hamid, S. & Ellery, D. (2004). Investigating the effect of anxiety sensitivity, gender and negative interpretative bias on the perception of chest pain. *Pain*, **111**, 209–217.

Koster, E. H. W., Crombez, G., Verschuere, B., Van Damme, S. & Wiersema, J. R. (2006). Components of attentional bias to threat in high trait anxiety: Facilitated engagement, impaired disengagement, and attentional avoidance. *Behaviour Research and Therapy*, **44**, 1757–71.

Koutanji, M., Pearce, S., Oakley, D. A. & Feinmann, C. (1999). Children in pain: an investigation of selective memory for pain and psychological adjustment. *Pain*, **81**, 237–44.

Lau, M. A. (2008). New developments in psychosocial interventions for adults with unipolar depression. *Current Opinion in Psychiatry*, **21**(1), 30–6.

Legrain, V., Van Damme, S., Eccleston, C., Davis, K. D., Seminowicz, D. A. & Crombez, G. (2009). A neurocognitive model of attention to pain: Behavioral and neuroimaging evidence. *Pain*, **144**, 230–2.

Leventhal, H., Idler, E. L. & Leventhal, E. A. (1999). The impact of chronic illness on the self system. In R. J. Contrada & R. D. Ashmore (Eds.), *Self, social identity, and physical health. Interdisciplinary explorations* (pp. 185–208). Oxford: Oxford University Press.

Loewenstein, G. F., Weber, E. U., Hsee, C. K. & Welch, N. (2001). Risk as feelings. *Psychological Bulletin*, **127**, 267–86.

MacLeod, A. K. & Moore, R. (2000). Positive Thinking Revisited: Positive Cognitions, Well-being and Mental Health. *Clinical Psychology and Psychotherapy*, **7**, 1–10.

MacLeod, A. K., Coates, E. & Hetherton, J. (2008). Increasing well-being through teaching goal-setting and planning skills: results of a brief intervention. *Journal of Happiness Studies*, **9**, 185–96.

Markus, H. & Nurius, P. (1986). Possible selves. *American Psychologist*, **41**, 954–69.

Mathews, A. & MacLeod, C. (1994). Cognitive approaches to emotion and emotional disorders. *Annual Review of Psychology*, **45**, 25–50.

Mathews, A. & MacLeod, C. (2002). Induced processing biases have causal effects on anxiety. *Cognition and Emotion*, **16**, 331–54.

McCracken, L. M. (1998). Learning to live with the pain: acceptance of pain predicts adjustment in persons with chronic pain. *Pain*, **74**, 21–27.

McCracken, L. M. (2004). A behavioural analysis of pain-related fear responses. In G. J. G. Asmundson, J. W. S. Vlaeyen & G. Crombez (Eds.), *Understanding and treating fear of pain* (pp. 51–69). New York: Oxford University Press.

McCracken, L. M. (2005). *Contextual Cognitive-Behavioral Therapy for Chronic Pain*. Seattle: IASP Press.

McCracken, L. M. & Turk, D. C. (2002). Behavioral and cognitive behavioral treatment for chronic pain: outcome, predictors of outcome, and treatment process. *Spine*, **27**, 2564–73.

McGowan, N., Sharpe, L., Refshauge, K. & Nicholas, M. K. (2009). The effect of attentional re-training and threat expectancy in response to acute pain. *Pain*, **142**, 101–107.

McKellar, J. D., Clark, M .E. & Shriner, J. (2003). The cognitive specifity of associative responses in patients with chronic pain. *British Journal of Clinical Psychology*, **42**, 27–39.

McNally, R. J. (1995). Automaticity and the anxiety disorders. *Behaviour Research and Therapy*, **33**, 747–54.

McNeil, D. W. & Vowles, K. E. (2004). Assessment of fear and anxiety associated with pain: Conceptualization, methods, and measures. In G. J. G. Asmundson, J. W. S. Vlaeyen & G. Crombez (Eds.), *Understanding and treating fear of pain* (pp. 189–211). New York: Oxford University Press.

Morley, S. & Eccleston, C. (2004). The object of fear in pain. In G. J. Asmundson, J. Vlaeyen, & G, Crombez (Eds.), *Understanding and treating fear of pain* (pp. 163–88). Oxford: Oxford University Press.

Morley, S. & Wilkinson, L. (1995). The pain beliefs and perceptions inventory: A British replication. *Pain*, **61**, 427–33.

Morley, S., Eccleston, C. & Williams, A. (1999). Systematic review and meta-analysis of randomized controlled trails of cognitive behaviour therapy and behaviour therapy for chronic pain in adults, excluding headache. *Pain*, **80**, 1–13.

Morley, S., Davies, C. & Barton, S. (2005). Possible selves in chronic pain: self-pain enmeshment, adjustment and acceptance. *Pain*, **115**, 84–94.

Oatley, K. (1992). *Best Laid Schemes: The Psychology of Emotions*. Cambridge: Cambridge University Press.

Pearce, J. & Morley, S. (1989). An experimental investigation of the construct validity of the McGill Pain Questionnaire. *Pain*, **39**, 115–21.

Pearce, S., Isherwood, S., Hrouda, D., Richardson, P. H., Erskine, A. & Skinner, J. (1990). Memory and pain: test of mood congruity and state-dependent learning in experimentally induced and clinical pain. *Pain*, **43**, 187–93.

Peters, M. L. & Vancleef, L. M. G. (2008). The role of personality traits in pain perception and disability. *Reviews in Analgesia*, 10, 11–22.

Peters, M. L., Vlaeyen, J. W. S. & Kunnen, A. M. W. (2002). Is pain-related fear a predictor of somatosensory hypervilance in chronic low back pain patients? *Behaviour Research and Therapy*, **40**, 85–103.

Peters, M. L., Sommer, M., de Rijke, J. M., *et al.* (2007). Somatic and psychological predictors of long-term unfavourable outcome after surgical intervention. *Annals of Surgery*, **245**, 487–94.

Pincus, T. (1998). Assessing psychological factors in chronic pain–a new approach. *Physical Therapy Review*, **3**, 1–5.

Pincus, T. & Morley, S. (2001). Cognitive-processing bias in chronic pain: a review and integration. *Psychological Bulletin*, **127**, 599–627.

Pincus, T. & Morley, S. (2002). Cognitive appraisal. In S.J. Linton (Ed.), *New Avenues for the Prevention of Chronic Musculoskeletal Pain and Disability, Pain Research and Clinical Management, Vol. 12* (pp. 123–41). Amsterdam: Elsevier.

Pincus, T. & Newman, S. (2001). Recall bias, pain, depression and cost in back pain patients. *British Journal of Clinical Psychology*, **40**, 143–56.

Pincus, T. & Williams, A. C. deC. (1999). Models and measurements of depression in chronic pain. *Journal of Psychosomatic Research*, **47**, 211–19.

Pincus, T., Pearce, S., McClelland, A. & Turner-Stokes, L. (1993). Self-referential selective memory in pain patients. *British Journal of Clinical Psychology*, **32**, 365–75.

Pincus, T., Pearce, S., McClelland, A., Farley, S. & et al. (1994). Interpretation bias in responses to ambiguous cues in pain patients. *Journal of Psychosomatic Research*, **38**, 347–53.

Pincus, T., Pearce, S., McClelland, A. & Isenberg, D. (1995). Endorsement and memory bias of self-referential pain stimuli in depressed pain patients. *British Journal of Clinical Psychology*, **34**, 267–77.

Pincus, T., Pearce, S. & Perrott, A. (1996a). Pain patients' bias in the interpretation of ambiguous homophones. *British Journal of Medical Psychology*, **69**, 259–66.

Pincus, T., Griffith, J., Pearce, S. et al. (1996b). Prevalence of self-reported depression in patients with rheumatoid arthritis. *British Journal of Rheumatology*, **35**, 879–83.

Pincus, T., Fraser, L. & Pearce, S. (1998). Do chronic pain patients 'Stroop' on pain stimuli? *British Journal of Clinical Psychology*, **37**, 49–58.

Pincus, T., Burton, A.K., Vogel, S. & Field, A.P. (2002). A systematic review of psychological factors as predictors of chronicity/disability in prospective cohorts of low back pain. *Spine*, **27** *(5)*, 109–20.

Pincus, T., Santos, R. & Morley, S. (2007). Depressed cognitions in chronic pain patients are focused on health: Evidence from a sentence completion task. *Pain*, **130**, 84–92.

Price, D. D. (1999). *Psychological mechanisms of Pain and Analgesia, Progress in Pain Research and Management, Vol. 15*. Seattle: IASP Press.

Price, D. D. & Bushnell, M. C. (2004). *Psychological methods of pain control: basic science and clinical perspectives, Progress in Pain Research and Management, Vol. 29*. Seattle: IASP Press.

Rachman, S., Lopatka, K. & Levitt, L. (1988). Experimental analysis of panic 2: Panic patients. *Behaviour Research and Therapy*, **26**, 33–40.

Rainville, P., Carrier, B., Hofbauer, R. et al. (1999). Dissociation of sensory and affective dimensions of pain using hypnotic modulation. *Pain*, **82** (2), 159–71.

Read, J. & Pincus, T. (2004). Cognitive bias in back pain patients attending osteopathy: testing the enmeshment model in reference to future thinking. *European Journal of Pain*, **8**, 525–31.

Roelofs, J., Peters, M. L., Zeegers, M. P.A. & Vlaeyen, J. W. S. (2002). The modified stroop paradigm as a measure of selective attention towards pain-related stimuli among chronic pain patients: a meta-analysis. *European Journal of Pain*, **6**, 273–81.

Roelofs, J., Peters, M. L. & Vlaeyen, J. W. S. (2003a). The modified Stroop paradigm as a measure of selective attention towards pain-related information in patients with chronic low back pain. *Psychological Reports*, **92**, 707–715.

Roelofs, J., Peters, M. L., van der Zijden, M., Thielen, F. G. J. M. & Vlaeyen, J. W. S. (2003b). Selective Attention and Avoidance of Pain-Related Stimuli: A Dot-Probe Evaluation in a Pain-Free Population. *Journal of Pain*, **4**, 322–28.

Roelofs, J., Peters, M. L., Fassaert, T. & Vlaeyen, J. W. (2005). The role of fear of movement and injury in selective attentional processing in patients with chronic low back pain: a dot-probe evaluation. Journal of Pain, 6, 294–300.

Ross, M. & Buehler, R. (2004). Identity through time: constructing personal pasts and futures. In M. B. Brewer, & M. Hewstone (eds.), *Self and social identity* (pp. 25–51). Oxford: Blackwell,

Rusu, A. C. (2008). Cognitive biases and future thinking in chronic pain. Unpublished doctoral thesis, London, UK: University of London.

Rusu, A. C. Pincus, T. & Morley, S. J. (2008). Measuring depressive thinking in chronic pain: Development and preliminary validation of the Sentence Completion Test for Chronic Pain (SCP). Abstracts of the 12th World Congress on Pain, International Association for the Study of Pain, *Glasgow, U.K.*: PH 317.

Rusu, A.C., Vogel, S., Van der Merwe, J., Pither, C. & Pincus, T. (2009). Testing the Schema Enmeshment Model of Pain (SEMP): cognitive biases, depressed mood and future thinking in chronic pain. *European Journal of Pain*, **13**, Suppl.1, S 139.

Rusu, A. C., Barton, S., Morley, S. & Pincus, T. Sentence Completion Test for Chronic Pain (SCP): Development of an idiographic measure of depressive thinking. Manuscript in preparation.

Salemink, E., van den Hout, M. A. & Kindt, M. (2007). Trained interpretative bias: Validity and effects on anxiety. *Journal of Behavior Therapy and Experimental Psychiatry*, **38**, 212–24.

Schmitz, U., Saile, H. & Nilges, P. (1996). Coping with chronic pain: flexible goal adjustment as an interactive buffer against pain-related distress. *Pain*, **67**, 41–51.

Schmuck, P. & Sheldon, K. M. (Eds.). (2001). *Life goals and well-being. Towards a positive psychology of human striving*. Seattle: Hogrefe & Huber.

Schwarzer, R., Boehmer, S., Luszczynska, A., Mohamed, N. E. & Knoll, N. (2005). Dispositional self-efficacy as a personal resource factor in coping after surgery. *Personality and Individual Differences*, **39**, 807–18.

Sharpe, L., Dear, B. F. & Schrieber, L. (2009). Attentional biases on chronic pain associated with rheumatoid arthritis: hypervigilance or difficulties disengaging? *Journal of Pain*, **10**, 329–35.

Sheldon, K. M., Kasser, T., Smith, K. & Share, T. (2002). Personal goals and psychological growth: Testing an intervention to enhance goal-attainment and personality integration. *Journal of Personality*, **70**, 5–31.

Shiffrin, R. M. & Schneider, W. (1977). Controlled and automatic human information processing–II. Perceptual learning, automatic attending, and a general theory. *Psychological Review*, **84**, 127–90.

Smith, T. W., O'Keeffe, J. L. & Christensen, A. J. (1994). Cognitive distortion and depression in chronic pain: Association with diagnosed disorders. *Journal of Consulting and Clinical Psychology*, **62**, 195–98.

Snider, B. S., Asmundson, G. J. G. & Wiese, K. C. (2000). Automatic and strategic processing of threat cues in patients with chronic pain: A modified-Stroop evaluation. *Clinical Journal of Pain*, **16**, 144–54.

**Stedman's Medical Dictionary.** (1976). 23rd edition. Baltimore: Williams & Wilkins.

Strauman, T. J., Vieth, A. Z., Merrill, K. A., *et al.* (2006). Self-system therapy as an intervention for self-regulatory dysfunction in depression: a randomized comparison with cognitive therapy. *Journal of Consulting and Clinical Psychology,* **74**(2), 367–76.

Sullivan, M. J. L., Reesor, K., Mikail, S. & Fisher, R. (1992). The treatment of depression in chronic low back pain: review and recommendations. *Pain,* **50,** 5–13.

Sutherland, R. & Morley, S. (2008). Self-pain enmeshment: Future possible selves, sociotropy, autonomy and adjustment to chronic pain. *Pain,* 137, 366–77.

Turk, D.C. (2005). The potential of treatment matching for subgroups of chronic pain patients: lumping vs. splitting. *Clinical Journal of Pain,* **21,** 44–55.

Turk, D. C. & Okifuji, A. (2002). Psychological factors in chronic pain: evolution and revolution. *Journal of Consulting and Clinical Psychology,* **70,** 678–90.

Turk, D. C. & Rudy, T. E. (1992). Cognitive factors and persistent pain: A glimpse into Pandora's box. Cognitive *Therapy and Research,* **16,** 99–122.

Van Damme, S., Crombez, G. & Eccleston, C. (2002). Retarded disengagement from pain cues: The effects of pain catastrophizing and pain expectancy. *Pain,* **100,** 111–18.

Van Damme, S., Crombez, G. & Eccleston, C. (2004a). Disengagement from pain: the role of catastrophic thinking about pain. *Pain,* **107,** 70–6.

Van Damme, S., Crombez, G., Eccleston, C. & Roelofs, J. (2004b). The role of hypervigilance in the experience of pain. In G.J.G. Asmundson, J.W.S. Vlaeyen & G. Crombez (Eds.), *Understanding and treating fear of pain.* Oxford: Oxford University Press, p. 71–90.

Van Damme, S., Legrain,V., Vogt, J. & Crombez, G. (2010). Keeping pain in mind: A motivational account of attention to pain. *Neuroscience and Biobehavioral Reviews,* **34** (2), 204–213.

Van der Windt, D., Hay, E., Jellema, P. & Main, C. (2008). Psychosocial Interventions for low back pain in primary care: Lessons learned from recent trials. *Spine,* **33,** 81–89.

Van Tulder, M. W., Ostelo, R., Vlaeyen, J. W., Linton, S. J., Morley, S. J. & Assendelft, W. J. (2000). Behavioral treatment for chronic low back pain: a systematic review within the framework of the Cochrane Back Review Group. *Spine,* **25,** 2688–99.

Vancleef, L. (2007). *At Risk for Pain: Pain-related Anxiety, Cognition, and Processing Biases.* Maastricht: Universitaire Pers Maastricht.

Vancleef, L., Peters, M. L. & De Jong, P. J. (2009). Interpreting ambiguous health and bodily threat: are individual differences in pain-related vulnerability constructs associated with an on-line negative interpretation bias? *Journal of Behavioural Therapy and Experimental Psychiatry,* **40,** 59–69.

Vlaeyen, J. W. S. & Morley, S. (2005). Cognitive-behavioral treatments for chronic pain: what works for whom? *Clinical Journal of Pain,* **21,** 1–8.

Waddell, G. (1996). Low back pain: a 20th century health care enigma. *Spine,* **21,** 2820–25.

Wade, J. B., Price, D. D., Hamer, R. M., Schwartz, S. M. & Hart, R. P. (1990). An emotional component analysis of chronic pain. *Pain,* **40,** 303–10.

Wells, H. J., Pincus, T. & McWilliams, E. (2003). Information processing biases among chronic pain patients and ankylosing spondylitis patients: the impact of diagnosis. *European Journal of Pain,* **7,** 105–11.

Williams, A. C. deC. & Richardson, J. M. (1993). What does the BDI measure in chronic pain? *Pain,* **55,** 259–66.

Williams, J. M. G., Watts, F. N., MacLeod, C. & Mathews, A. (1997). *Cognitive Psychology and Emotional Disorders* (2nd edn.). Chichester: Wiley.

Wright, J. & Morley, S. (1995). Autobiographical memory and chronic pain. *British Journal of Clinical Psychology,* **34** (2), 255–65.

Yiend, J. & Mackintosh, B. (2004). The experimental modification of processing biases. In J. Yiend (Ed.), *Cognition, emotion and psychopathology: Theoretical, empirical and clinical directions* (pp. 190–210). New York: Cambridge University Press.

Chapter 17

# Significant Others in the Chronicity of Pain and Disability

Annmarie Cano and Laura Leong

Pain occurs within an interpersonal context. Indeed, interpersonal processes including marital functioning are associated with physiological and immune processes that affect health and pain (Kiecolt-Glaser & Newton 2001). Marital distress, as well as maladaptive interaction, is associated with pain, interference, and depression in persons with chronic pain (Leonard et al. 2006). Family members can also be affected by pain, in turn contributing to patients' adjustment (Coyne & Fiske 1992; Leonard et al. 2006). The purpose of this chapter is to examine the manner in which the social context might contribute to the chronicity of pain. Unfortunately, this is a topic that has received little attention in the literature. To address this topic, we provide an overview of the theoretical and empirical literature that suggests pathways through which relationships with significant others may foster the development of chronic pain from acute states. We also review theoretical work that suggests other mechanisms through which relationships may play a role in the development of chronic pain. We conclude by offering an integrative model and recommendations for further research that might contribute to the knowledge on the extent to which close relationships impact pain over time.

## 17.1 Support for theoretical conceptualizations of the role of close relationships in pain

### 17.1.1 Operant model

The operant model of pain (Fordyce 1976) is best known as advancing the notion that significant others including spouses have active roles in the experience of pain. Fordyce (1976) argued that the reinforcement of pain behaviours and the extinction of well behaviours may explain why acute pain behaviours from surgeries or injuries can persist over time. Reinforcement may also explain the persistence of pain behaviours once such behaviours become chronic. Specifically, spouses may reinforce pain behaviours by providing attention or help. Reinforcing or solicitous pain behaviours such as these may lead to increases or at least the maintenance of chronic pain behaviours including verbal expressions of pain, excessive rest, or ambulation problems. As a result, solicitous behaviours may actually encourage pain behaviours, which can lead to greater disability. Spouses may also punish pain behaviours by expressing anger or other forms of negative affect. Finally, spouses may ignore pain behaviours and reinforce well behaviours, both of which would theoretically lead to an extinction of pain behaviours and an increase in activity.

Very little research has tested the operant model in couples facing acute pain. One study examined pain, depression, and spouse social support after a laparoscopic radical prostatectomy as a treatment for prostate cancer (Knoll et al. 2007). Higher levels of pain as reported by patients at two days post-surgery were associated with a drop in their spouses' provision of instrumental support from 2 days to 2 weeks following the surgery. This was only for pain in other body sites, not at the site of the surgery. The authors suggest that spouses may have interpreted these pains (e.g. headache, sore throat) as attention-seeking behaviours rather than genuine ailments, and so they deliberately reduced their instrumental support as a way to prevent the patients from adopting the sick role.

To date, the strongest evidence for the operant model is found in studies of chronic pain couples, which have been conducted by Romano and colleagues (1991, 1992, 1995, 2000). These studies are of particular value because they are observational studies, and thus, they are a more rigorous test of the model. Couples in which one member had a chronic pain condition were compared to healthy control couples (Romano et al. 1991, 1992, 1995). Participants were videotaped in the laboratory doing a series of routine household activities: sweeping the floor, changing bed sheets, bundling newspapers, and carrying fire logs across the room. They were instructed to perform the tasks together, stressing that the pain patient must be involved at all times. Trained raters coded the videos for six categories of behaviours: Non-verbal pain, verbal pain, solicitous, facilitative, aggressive, and distressed. Non-verbal pain behaviours included facial expressions, such as grimacing, and bodily actions such as limping or groaning; verbal pain behaviours included statements that indicated pain or functional limitations; solicitous behaviours included offering or giving assistance, and statements that expressed concern for the other; facilitative behaviours included compliments, encouragement, and humour; aggressive behaviours involved negative affect directed towards the other (e.g. disapproval, threats, arguments, disagreement); and distressed behaviours included complaints not directed towards the spouse, sadness, and whining. Preliminary analyses revealed that pain patients showed higher rates of overt verbal and non-verbal pain behaviours, and their spouses showed higher rates of solicitous behaviour, compared to control couples (Romano et al. 1991). In addition, pain patients and their spouses both showed significantly lower rates of facilitative behaviours than the control couples, though groups did not differ on the rate of aggression or distressed behaviours (i.e. negative affect). In subsequent analyses, the authors found that solicitous spouse behaviours preceded and followed both verbal and non-verbal pain behaviours more often in the pain couples than in the control couples (Romano et al. 1992). When they examined additional pain adjustment variables, they found that the sequence of spouse solicitousness in response to the patient's non-verbal pain behaviour was a significant predictor of physical dysfunction, but only in more depressed patients (Romano et al. 1995).

Another study with similar methodology but using additional household chore tasks (folding laundry, cleaning up toys, building a bookcase from bricks and boards, then loading books out of boxes onto the bookcase) confirmed earlier findings: partner solicitous responses to the patient's pain behaviours were significantly positively associated with the rate of patient non-verbal pain behaviours, while negative partner responses were significantly inversely associated with patient pain non-verbal behaviour rates (Romano et al. 2000). Regression analyses revealed that the rate of partner solicitous behaviours significantly contributed to the prediction of rates of both patient verbal and non-verbal pain behaviours, but partner negative behaviours did not. Taken together, the results of these studies suggest that spouse solicitous behaviours influence patients' non-verbal pain behaviours. It was noted that the rate of verbal pain behaviours in these studies were low, so the results may have been dampened by restriction of range. Different kinds of interaction tasks may be more appropriate for analysing verbal behaviours, such as a discussion. Another limitation to these studies is that the sequential data were analysed using z scores, which are affected by the number of behaviours that are observed. In other words, couples should not be compared on z scores unless they exhibit exactly the same number of behaviours (Bakeman & Gottman 1997).

Nevertheless, these observational studies are invaluable because they provide convincing evidence that solicitous spouses can maintain pain and disability in chronic pain patients. The results were also confirmed by Paulsen and Altmaier (1995) who found, using similar tasks which only the patient completed, that patient- and spouse-reported spouse solicitousness were consistently associated with higher levels of observed patient pain behaviours. Patients with solicitous spouses engaged in more pain behaviours than patients with non-solicitous spouses, regardless of whether the spouse was present or not. A study by Lousberg and colleagues (1992) also sought to examine this relationship using a different behavioural task. Chronic low back pain patients engaged in a walking-to-tolerance treadmill test during which they walked on a treadmill that became gradually steeper. They were instructed to continue until they had to stop due to pain or fatigue. Each participant performed the test twice: once in the presence of his/her spouse, and once without the spouse. Pain behaviours were measured as pain intensity on a visual analogue scale and the total time spent on the treadmill, while spouse solicitousness was reported by both patients and spouses on a self-report measure. Patients who had solicitous spouses (as rated by the spouse, after a median split) reported increased pain intensity, and they spent less time on the treadmill when their spouse was present, compared to when they were alone. Patients with non-solicitous spouses showed the opposite effect; they spent more time on the treadmill and reported less pain. The authors interpret this as an increase in pain behaviours in the presence of a solicitous spouse. These results, however, were not found when they used the patients' ratings of spouse solicitousness: regardless of the patient's rating of spouse solicitousness, the presence of the spouse during the walking test resulted in more pain and shorter walking time. It is possible that patients and spouses had widely different perceptions of the spouse's solicitousness with varying degrees of accuracy, which caused these discrepant results.

There are some limitations to how these observational studies can be interpreted. Most importantly, the data are cross-sectional and cannot be interpreted causally. Also, the patients who participated already had chronic pain conditions, so it is not certain that the observed behaviours were related to the progression of an acute condition to a chronic one. Finally, observational studies do not account for how patients interpret spousal behaviours. Nevertheless, the evidence generally supports the operant model's hypothesis that solicitous spouse behaviours should be detrimental to patients' pain adjustment.

## 17.1.2 Cognitive-behavioural models

The next generation of models that includes a role for spouses are the cognitive-behavioural models of pain (Sharp 2001; Turk & Kerns 1985; Turk et al. 1983). These models have in common the idea that perceptions and thoughts, including those focused on spouse behaviour, play an important role in pain adjustment. For instance, a spouse may respond solicitously to a patient's pain behaviour. However, the spouse's response may not reinforce the pain behaviour if the patient interprets that behaviour as fake or hostile. Similarly, negative spouse responses might not punish pain behaviour if patients interpret the behaviour as a sign of the spouse's concern for the patient's health.

One cognitive-behavioural model, the Transactional Model of Health (Turk & Kerns 1985), was developed for health and illness in families more broadly and is easily applied to chronic pain conditions and spouses. It builds on the work of Turk et al. (1983) by expanding its treatment of coping with illness and by focusing on the active interactions between spouses and between the partners and their environment. Couples are said to develop schemata about the world and about themselves. These, along with their resources, influence how they respond to health threats: situations are deemed stressful based on the couples' appraisals and available resources. Coping is seen as the complement to stress; it is an active process that involves appraising events and determining what will happen in the future. Spouses' coping efforts can benefit each partner, or they can further deteriorate the situation. For example, in pain patients, a solicitous spouse may ameliorate the situation by providing emotional support, or they may reinforce pain behaviours and prolong recovery.

Though the cognitive-behavioural models purport to account for unique aspects of the pain experience, Sharp (2001) has raised some criticisms. He argues that the so-called cognitive-behavioural theories have failed to successfully incorporate cognitions, and that they are still heavily based on operant theory. As a result, he proposed a reformulated cognitive-behavioural model of pain. Sharp asserts that patients who are distressed react to their pain differently than those who are not distressed. In his model, these reactions include all cognitions as well as observable behaviours. The main tenet of this model, as it is for the other cognitive-behavioural models of pain, is that patients' appraisals and interpretations of their pain are fundamental to their distress. Many factors contribute to their appraisals, including sensations, learning history, culture, physiological responses, mood, motor behaviours, iatrogenic causes, and environmental contingencies. Environmental contingencies include responses of family members and significant others. Sharp explains that these responses can provide evidence for or against patients' beliefs. For example, a solicitous spouse may confirm a patient's belief that he/she is disabled.

Other cognitive models, though not explicitly including significant others, suggest that environmental factors more generally play an important role in pain adjustment. For example, fear-avoidance models feature the notion that people with pain have a fear that physical activity will cause (re)injury (Severeijns et al. 2004; Vlaeyen & Crombez 1999). There are two potential responses to this fear: confrontation (continuing with motor activities despite the pain, an adaptive response), or avoidance (maintaining fear, leading to exacerbated physical and psychological symptoms). The model starts with a patient experiencing pain (possibly as the result of an injury). Some patients do not experience a fear of (re)injury, so they confront the pain and recover. Others, however, enter a detrimental cycle: they catastrophize about the pain, become fearful, and avoid activities. This avoidance results in increased disability and depression over time (e.g. via loss of muscle strength and self-esteem). These have been shown to decrease pain tolerance, resulting in increased pain experiences, and the cycle restarts. One could imagine that fears expressed by spouses might contribute to patients' fears and contribute to their avoidance behaviours.

As with the operant model, very little research has tested the cognitive-behavioural perspective in couples with acute pain. However, one study on postoperative pain and speed of recovery after coronary bypass surgery may provide some clues (Kulik & Mahler 1989). Men who had bypass surgery were divided into two groups based on their perceptions of marital quality: those who rated their marital quality as excellent and those who rated quality as less than excellent. Hospital staff also counted the number of times they were visited by their wives, and divided this by the total number of days hospitalized to obtain a measure of support. Men with high levels of support took significantly fewer pain medications as recorded in their charts and spent less time both in the surgical intensive care unit and in the hospital overall whereas perceived marital quality was an insignificant factor. It is possible that much of the support was emotional and that it was perceived by husbands as caring and encouraging behaviour. This interpretation would be consistent with cognitive-behavioural models of pain, in which spouse encouragement helps to foster the patient's own coping skills and autonomy. Follow-up data would be extremely useful for determining whether these relationship between perceived support and pain hold over time.

Much of the work on perceptions of spousal behaviour has focused on solicitous and punishing responses in chronic pain couples. Patient perceptions of spousal solicitousness (i.e. getting the patient medication or something to eat or drink when in pain) are related to poorer pain adjustment including increased pain severity, physical disability, and depression (for a review, see Leonard et al. 2006). However, patients' reports of spouses' punishing responses (e.g. anger, irritability) to patient pain behaviours are related to increased pain severity and depressive symptoms (Cano et al. 2000, 2004a; Kerns et al. 1990; Stroud et al. 2006; Turk et al. 1992; Williamson et al. 1997). This latter finding is not entirely consistent with the operant model, which suggests that punishing responses would contribute to a decline in pain behaviours. However, these responses may represent a loss of reinforcement of positive interaction, thereby contributing to depression.

More recent research has focused on patients' perceptions of spousal reinforcement of well behaviours. Facilitative responses to well behaviours (e.g. encouraging activity and exercise) are negatively related to physical disability whereas negative responses to well behaviour (e.g. discouraging activity) are positively related to pain behaviours and physical disability in chronic musculoskeletal pain and headache patient samples (Pence et al. 2008; Schwartz et al. 2005). The interrelationships between different behaviours were also quite interesting. Facilitative responses to well behaviour were positively associated with solicitous responses to pain behaviour in both studies. Facilitative responses to well behaviour and solicitous responses were also negatively related to punishing spouse responses to pain. Thus, spouses who respond in a supportive manner to both types of behaviours may not respond in a negative manner to pain behaviours. However, punishing spouse responses to pain behaviours and negative responses to well behaviours were not significantly correlated. It is possible that the greater differentiation is between spouses who respond negatively to pain behaviours versus spouses who respond negatively to well behaviours. The former may either feel helpless about being able to aid their partners or may be irritated about how the relationship has changed due to pain. In contrast, spouses who respond negatively to well behaviours may be fearful that their partners will reinjure themselves. These studies provide the first evidence that spousal responses to pain and well behaviours must be taken into account when determining the manner in which spouses may influence patient outcomes.

In sum, research has demonstrated that perceptions of spouse responses appear to be related to patients' pain adjustment. However, the extent to which this research can be applied to the transition from acute to chronic pain is limited. Like the observational work, much of this research is cross-sectional in nature and has been conducted with persons experiencing chronic pain. Thus the findings are correlational, not causal, and for now, only apply to persons experiencing chronic pain. Furthermore, while patients' interpretations and attributions of spouse responses are argued to be crucial to the reinforcement process, very little research has examined these attributions.

## 17.1.3 Communal coping model

Other models of pain have begun to integrate interpersonal and cognitive-behavioural perspectives. The communal coping model of pain catastrophizing (Sullivan et al. 2001; Thorn et al. 2003) is one such model. Pain catastrophizing is a negative cognitive process that consists of rumination, magnification, and helplessness about pain (Sullivan et al. 1995). Patients may engage in catastrophizing to communicate their distress about pain to close others who may be able to help. Catastrophizing is thought to result in behaviours aimed at communicating distress and eliciting support. This model has been tested in experimental paradigms of acute pain. Sullivan and colleagues found that observers' ratings of participants' pain severity during a cold pressor task was explained by the pain behaviour exhibited by participants (Sullivan et al. 2006). In another cold pressor task study, greater catastrophizing was associated with longer displays of communicative pain behaviours such as facial expressions of pain when someone was present during the task than when the participant was alone in the room (Sullivan et al. 2004). A study of chronic pain patients and their spouses yielded somewhat different results regarding the communication of pain. In this study, pain behaviours did not enhance the spouse's ability to estimate the pain experienced by the patient partner (Gauthier et al. 2008). Rather, pain adjustment variables were correlated with the spouses' ability to infer patients' pain. It appears that spouses attend to patient characteristics to estimate pain but not to behaviours expressed during the task. This collection of studies shows that observers may use pain behaviours to interpret pain during the acute phase but not during the chronic phase. However, the acute pain studies investigated strangers whereas the chronic pain study investigated close others. Therefore, it is not clear if the differences among studies are due to the relationship of the participants and observers, differences between acute and chronic pain, or both.

Indirect support for the communal coping model also comes from work conducted on catastrophizing and social support. Pain catastrophizing is positively associated with solicitous responses from significant others in samples of patients with spinal cord injuries and chronic musculoskeletal pain (Cano 2004; Giardino et al. 2003). Pain duration also matters in the association between catastrophizing and support. In a study of persons with chronic pain, catastrophizing was associated with greater solicitous spouse responses at shorter pain durations (Cano 2004). In contrast, catastrophizing was associated with less social support from the spouse at longer pain durations. Taken together, these findings suggest that spouses provide pain-specific support in response to patient catastrophizing; however, catastrophizing over the long-term may cause partners to withdraw from patients, resulting in a loss of intimacy in couples. Buenaver et al. (2007) found similar results. Although shorter pain durations in these studies are still considered chronic, it is possible that the effect of catastrophizing on pain-specific support occurs in acute pain episodes and contributes to changes in the relationship as pain persists over time.

### 17.1.4 Empathy models

Empathy is an interpersonal concept that has received increasing amounts of attention in the pain literature. Goubert et al. (2005) argued that the pain empathy process involves characteristics of patients and observers. The observer's characteristics, including personal experience with pain or catastrophizing about the observed person's pain, may contribute to the observer's understanding or 'sense of knowing' about the pain. Patient characteristics including facial expressions or verbalizations of pain may also contribute to the observer's knowledge. In turn, the observer may engage in a variety of behavioural and emotional responses. For example, observers may validate the patient's experience of pain, withdraw from the patient, feel personal distress about witnessing pain, or feel distress or sympathy for the patient. This model was developed to account for empathy in acute as well as chronic pain.

Support for this model of pain empathy comes from a study of chronic pain couples. Leonard and Cano (2006) found that one observer characteristic, spousal catastrophizing about the partner's pain, was related to greater spousal distress for those spouses who also had personal experience with pain (i.e. reported chronic pain). This association was not found for spouses without chronic pain. Patient depression also appears to vary depending on spousal catastrophizing. Depressive symptoms in patients are most elevated when both partners have high levels of catastrophizing about the patient's pain (Cano et al. 2005). Thus, spousal characteristics such as catastrophizing may promote emotional distress in both partners, perhaps because such cognitions heighten one's understanding of the other's pain. In turn, awareness could affect a couple's interactions and distress. It is possible that spousal catastrophizing promotes distress in acute pain, which could lead to decreases in activity that contribute to functional impairment and disability over time.

Some work has also investigated empathic responses toward patients with pain. Newton-John and Williams (2006) demonstrated that some solicitous spouse responses are interpreted as hostile responses. Furthermore, these researchers have argued that talking about the pain experience may be helpful for some patients. These ideas are consistent with the pain empathy model (Goubert et al. 2005). Perhaps talking about pain-related distress is a form of emotional disclosure that provides spouses with the information they need to understand the pain. In turn, the spouse may be able to engage in empathic and validating responses to the patient. These ideas are also consistent with emotion regulation models of interaction (Fruzzetti & Iverson 2004, 2006) and intimacy research (Laurenceau et al. 1998); however, these conceptualizations of emotional disclosure and empathic response are not entirely consistent with the operant model's conceptualization of verbal pain behaviour and solicitous responses.

Preliminary research on empathic responses suggests that such responses are indeed conceptually distinct from solicitous responses. Cano et al. (2008) conducted a study in which couples attended a lab session and were videotaped while discussing the impact of pain on their lives. Validating responses were responses that conveyed one spouse's attempts to understand the thoughts and feelings of the other. Invalidating responses were responses that communicated a general disregard for the feelings of the other and included behaviours such as eye rolls and changing the subject. Marital quality was negatively correlated with invalidation and positively correlated with validation behaviours. An exploratory factor analysis was also conducted to understand the intercorrlations among spousal validating and invalidating responses, and reports of spousal solicitous, distracting, and punishing responses. A two-factor solution that accounted for 57% of the variance in the data was found in which both partners' reports of solicitous and distracting spouse responses loaded on a 'Solicitous Responding' factor. Couples' reports of punishing spouse responses as well as observed spousal invalidation and validation loaded on an 'Empathic Responding' factor. The factors were weakly related to one another (r=−0.17). Both factors correlated with marital satisfaction and spousal support in both partners but the Empathic Responding factor was more strongly correlated with these measures of marital quality. These findings suggest that validation and solicitousness are related but distinct concepts. Validation may work to enhance intimacy and emotion regulation in couples whereas solicitous responses may have a rather pain-specific function. This study points to the importance of using more than one theoretical approach to understand the function of interaction in couples facing pain. It is likely that similar processes are present in couples with acute pain but future research will need to address this issue.

While not specifically examining empathic responses, Johansen and Cano (2007) investigated the role of hostility, one form of invalidation, and sadness in couples' interactions. Interactions characterized by hostility or disregard for partners' emotional responses are thought to disrupt emotion regulation attempts (Fruzzetti & Iverson 2004, 2006). Couples engaged in a 15-minute marital problem-solving task. Approximately half of the couples displayed anger/contempt, a form of emotional invalidation, and sadness whereas humour was normally distributed. The association between negative interaction codes and depressive symptoms depended on whether one or both spouses reported chronic pain. Specifically, patient sadness was associated with greater pain and depression when only he or she reported pain. In contrast, patient sadness was associated with less pain and depression when patients' spouses also reported pain. Perhaps, expressing sadness in the context of an empathic spouse may help patients in their attempts to regulate their emotions. Spouses' expressions of anger/contempt were associated with their own depressive symptoms only when they did not report pain and their partners (i.e. the patients) also expressed anger/contempt. In these couples, it is possible that the absence of pain in the spouse interferes with the couple's ability to talk about pain in an accepting environment. In any event, these results suggest that empathic processes depend on the partner's personal experience with pain, which supports the importance of spouses' personal characteristics in the empathy process (Goubert et al. 2005).

In sum, research has borne out that spouses play an important role in pain. Spouses' behavioural responses to patients as well as patients' perceptions of these responses may contribute to pain adjustment and psychological well-being. Furthermore, patients' and spouses' thoughts about the pain, including pain catastrophizing, may influence social support over time. Much of the research has been conducted on chronic pain and none of the research to date has examined acute clinical pain in a couples context. These gaps in the research offer exciting new opportunities for researchers interested in the social factors involved in the progression of acute to chronic pain over time.

## 17.2 **Treatment research on couples and spouses**

We now turn our discussion to pain interventions that involve spouses and couples. Although there are no chronic pain prevention programmes of which we are aware that involve acute pain patients and spouses, the effectiveness of couple-based treatments for chronic pain implies that spouses can help alter the course of pain.

### 17.2.1 **Spouse involvement in education and coping skills training**

Keefe and colleagues have developed a programme called spouse-assisted coping skills training (S-CST), which is a cognitive-behavioural treatment for chronic pain that actively involves spouses (Keefe et al. 1996, 1999, 2004). S-CST is typically led by a clinician in a group setting with 10–12 2-hour weekly sessions. Clinicians provide education about pain and teach couples various techniques and use behavioural rehearsal (i.e. practise) so that couples can master skills. Skills include communication training and coping skills such as relaxation, imagery, and distraction techniques. In addition, spouses are encouraged to provide feedback to each other and to practise skills between sessions during activities that might elicit pain.

A series of studies have examined the effectiveness of S-CST in pain management. S-CST has been compared to coping skills training without spouse involvement (CST) and a control group that involved education about arthritis and spousal support in a sample of chronic osteoarthritic knee patients and their spouses (Keefe et al. 1996, 1999). Results showed few differences between the two CST groups. Results suggested that the S-CST group performed better than the CST group on self-reported outcome measures at post-treatment and follow-up (i.e. pain severity, psychological disability, pain behaviour, marital adjustment, coping). However, the CST groups did not differ significantly on these measures. Both CST groups experienced better outcomes than the control group.

Additional analyses suggested that differences are more apparent when examining how change occurs during treatment. Specifically, initial improvements in marital satisfaction were associated with to better adjustment at 12-month follow-up in the S-CST group (Keefe et al. 1999). This was not the case in the other two groups, where initial improvement in marital satisfaction was actually related to poor pain adjustment. Participants in S-CST with or without an exercise component reported greater self-efficacy and coping skills compared to participants undergoing exercise training alone or standard care (Keefe et al. 2004). In this study, however, no significant group differences were found on marital satisfaction, pain, or psychological disability. It appears that the S-CST approach may lead to some improvements in marital quality and coping that are beneficial for patient functioning in chronic pain.

Martire et al. (2007) compared an education plus support intervention that involved couples with patient-oriented education plus support involving patients only, and usual care in an older adult sample with osteoarthritis. Participants in the education and support interventions attended six weekly group sessions that last 2 hours each. The education and support conditions were similar to S-CST in that the sessions included arthritis education and the teaching of effective coping skills. Participants were encouraged to rely on each other for support. The couple intervention also presented this information from a couple's perspective rather than an individual perspective. Like the S-CST research, there were few differences among the three groups from baseline to 6-month follow-up. However, participants in the patient-oriented group experienced greater improvements in pain adjustment than participants in the couple intervention whereas the couple-oriented group experienced greater improvements in psychological outcomes including perceived stress and critical attitudes. Patients' spouses also experienced some improvements depending on their gender and relationship satisfaction. Specifically, in the couple-oriented group, maritally satisfied spouses experienced decreases in depressive symptoms whereas maritally dissatisfied spouses reported increases in depression. In addition, patients' wives reported lower stress over time if they participated in the couple-oriented group. These results suggest that the couples approach is more appropriate for psychologically distressed patients who are married to relatively satisfied spouses. An individual approach may be more appropriate for patients experiencing poor pain adjustment.

S-CST has also been adapted as a brief intervention for pain in individuals with advanced cancer diagnoses (Keefe et al. 2005). In this study, couples participated in three home-based sessions over the course of approximately 2 weeks. The sessions included education about cancer pain management and pain coping skills (e.g. relaxation training, imagery). Instructors taught couples to pace activity. Behavioural rehearsal techniques were used to train couples on how to maintain skills over time. This intervention was compared against a usual care condition. Similar to traditional S-CST for knee pain, there were no group differences in patients' pain severity. However, partners in the partner-guided condition reported greater self-efficacy in assisting their partners with pain and other symptoms. In addition, partners reported slightly less caregiver burden in the partner-guided group than in the usual care group.

In sum, these studies demonstrate that the involvement of significant others may have beneficial psychological and relational effects on persons with pain and their partners although effects on pain appear to be limited. Most of these studies have been conducted in chronic pain samples; however, these findings suggest that education and couples-based coping skills training during the acute phase of pain may help prevent distress that could contribute to the persistence of pain over time.

## 17.2.2 Couple therapy

Insight-oriented therapy has also been tested as a treatment for chronic pain. Insight-oriented therapy explores historical and current relationship processes rather than focusing on pain coping skills. Saarijarvi (1991) compared couples who attended five monthly sessions of insight-oriented couple therapy with couples in a no-treatment control group. Marital satisfaction in both groups declined over a 12-month follow-up but the decline was significantly smaller in the insight couple therapy group. The couple therapy group reported that their communication improved whereas the control group reported communication declines. However, there were no significant group differences on pain or disability at the 12-month follow-up (Saarijarvi et al. 1991). At 5-year follow-up, the therapy group reported significantly better psychological health than the control group but the groups did not differ significantly on marital satisfaction, pain, or disability (Saarijarvi et al. 1992). These results suggest that insight-oriented therapy may be appropriate to treat psychological distress and relationship satisfaction but it does not appear to relate to improvement in pain adjustment. Applied to the problem of acute pain, such treatment may promote relationship and psychological health, which might indirectly relate to pain adjustment over time.

Integrative behavioural couple therapy (IBCT) may also have beneficial effects for couples with chronic pain (Cano & Leonard 2006). IBCT therapists use behavioural strategies often used in traditional behavioural couple therapy (e.g. behaviour exchange, communication training). In addition, therapists promote emotional acceptance, which involves changes in how partners perceive undesirable partner behaviours (Christensen et al. 1995; Jacobson & Christensen 1998). For example, personality or behaviour patterns (e.g. need for spontaneity, need for order) that have become irritating to the partner may be reinterpreted in a positive light.

IBCT results in improvements in psychological and marital distress (Christensen et al. 2004, 2006; Jacobson et al. 2000). It has been argued that IBCT is appropriate for chronic pain (Cano & Leonard 2006). First, IBCT addresses the psychological distress that is reported by couples with pain (Leonard et al. 2006). Second, such therapy might address spouses' difficulties in understanding the pain of their partners. Spouses under- and overestimate the pain and disability experienced by their partners (Cano et al. 2005, 2004b) and patients often think their partners do not understand their pain and emotional suffering (Herbette & Rime 2004). IBCT could be used to promote empathic understanding of each partner's experience of the pain and its impact on the relationship. Greater empathic understanding and improved communication skills might also alleviate patients' fear of rejection or lack of self-efficacy in discussing the pain (Morley et al. 2000; Porter et al. 2008). IBCT has not been empirically tested in acute or chronic pain couples. However, this treatment offers promising avenues through which to improve relationship functioning in pain patients and their partners.

In sum, cognitive-behavioural approaches have dominated the research on couples-based treatments for pain. The most effective interventions focus on building communication and pain coping skills and result in improvements in marital and psychological well-being. However, much is unknown about what is actually being changed in these interventions. For instance, it is assumed that spousal beliefs about pain are targeted during treatment but these beliefs are often not assessed. It will be important for researchers to continue this work by measuring spousal pain beliefs and investigating change in such beliefs (Cano et al. 2009). Furthermore, existing couple-based treatments, whether they focus on coping skills or insight, have little direct effect on pain severity and disability and do not consistently outperform similar treatments that focus solely on patients. It is possible that couples-based treatments should be considered an adjunct to other forms of pain management that more directly impact pain and disability. Alternatively, the mechanisms through which these treatments work may need to be further investigated. Perhaps, couple-based treatment is more important during the acute phase of pain in order to promote healthy communication and pain coping skills in both partners, set realistic expectations regarding pain, and promote healthy emotion regulation, all of which might prevent pain from adversely impacting the relationship and resulting in depression and pain behaviour.

## 17.3 **Recommendations and future directions**

Operant and cognitive-behavioural theories have received quite a bit of attention in the research on the social context of pain. Indeed, the empirical literature has demonstrated that spouse responses to pain behaviours as well as patients' perceptions of those behaviours are related to pain adjustment. Other cognitions such as patient and spouse pain catastrophizing also appear to have a role in patients' pain adjustment. Existing treatments focusing on cognition and behaviour appear to be somewhat beneficial in treating the psychological and emotional consequences of pain. Furthermore, recent research drawing from interpersonal and empathy models suggests

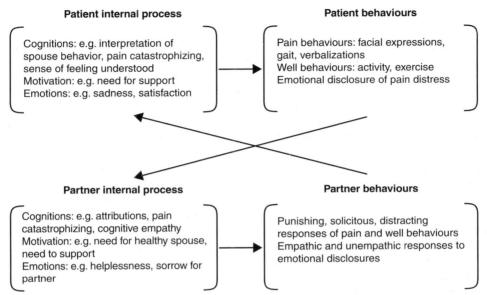

**Fig. 17.1** Pain-related interaction process that might explain the progression of acute to chronic pain in couples.

that it is necessary to go beyond a conceptualization of spouse responses that focuses solely on an operant formulation. Specifically, empathic spouse responses that build intimacy and understanding may also enhance adjustment to pain.

Following existing research and theory, we developed a model of the couple interaction process that may account for the progression of acute to chronic pain (see Figure 17.1). A key feature of the interaction process is that each partner's behaviours trigger intrapersonal processes aimed at understanding partner behaviour. In turn, these intrapersonal processes translate into behaviours. For instance, a patient may feel helpless about their pain and is motivated to seek support from his spouse. These cognitions and motivations may lead the patient to engage in more facial expressions of pain and reduced activity. The wife observes these behaviours and tries to make sense of them. She may attribute his behaviours to heightened pain and she may be frustrated that his pain is not diminishing over time. In turn, she may react with behaviours that show her frustration at the patient for not getting better. This type of interaction fits with the traditional operant approach of viewing interaction in pain. The model presented in Figure 17.1 can also be used to explain the role of empathic spouse responses. A patient may engage in facial expressions of pain as well as self-disclosures about pain-related distress because she is motivated to obtain support from her husband. The husband may understand these behaviours to indicate heightened pain and he may take her perspective and feel moved to empathize with her. He then may react with empathic responses such as validation. In this case, intimacy would be enhanced. Of course, some behaviours may reinforce pain or well behaviours while affecting intimacy levels. For example, some behaviours may reinforce pain and also enhance intimacy (e.g. solicitousness expressed with sympathy). Other responses may reinforce pain but lead to deteriorations in intimacy (e.g. hostile solicitousness). Still other reactions may reinforce well behaviours and enhance intimacy (e.g. praise for activity and validation for difficulty in initiating activity). Research has yet to demonstrate how the various unique combinations of responses may influence chronic pain behaviour over time, let alone the progression of acute pain to chronic pain. This is likely to be an especially fruitful area of research.

As noted several times in this review, the bulk of the research on spousal influences on pain has been conducted with patients with *chronic* pain. It is possible that spousal and family influences would be quite similar in acute pain. Clearly, research is needed in this area to identify how interactions between patients and spouses may actually prevent the progression of acute to chronic pain. One avenue for this research is to recruit acute pain patients and their families and track them over time. To minimize cost, patients could be chosen who are at risk for developing persistent pain. For instance, persons who have undergone cardiac or breast surgery (Bruce et al. 2003; Lahtinen et al. 2006; Vilholm et al. 2008) or who have had traumatic brain injury injuries (Nampiaparampil 2008) are more likely to develop chronic pain compared to persons with low back pain (Pengel et al. 2003). However, patients recovering from surgery or brain injuries may have other difficulties (e.g. difficulty communicating, hospital stay or rehabilitation) that would preclude their participation in research. Thus, it may be difficult to recruit these participants within 1–2 months of pain onset. Another possibility is to recruit primary care patients with acute pain and follow them over time. Because most of these patients are likely to be ambulatory, their participation might be more feasible. However, a very large initial sample size will be needed to identify those who transition to chronic pain. Successful research study recruitment may also be more likely if participation compensation includes some sort of intervention or prevention programme.

In terms of intervention research, acute pain patients may not be motivated to seek treatment with their spouses because they might envision that any behavioural changes will be short-lived until the pain is cured. It is only when the pain becomes chronic and couples come to understand that long-lasting changes are likely that couples may begin to seek ways to cope with the illness and its related effects on the relationship. Physicians and nurses may be able to educate acute pain patients about the importance of maintaining healthy relationships during all phases of treatment, not just when the pain becomes chronic. Most family-based interventions for chronic illness focus on relationship issues, with many of these being treatments involving spouses (Martire et al. 2004). Acute pain interventions can build on existing treatments available for couples facing chronic pain. For instance, couples can be taught about the issues associated with a particular acute pain problem. The effective use of pain coping skills including the spouse's role in encouraging the use of such skills is also likely to be helpful in an acute pain situation. Communication training and careful use of empathic responses may be beneficial as well. As discussed earlier, couple-based treatments have direct effects on marital and individual well-being but more limited effects on pain and disability. Research will be needed to determine if early couple-based intervention can be used to prevent the acute pain problem from becoming chronic. Perhaps such interventions do not have direct effects on pain but have an indirect effect on the pain problem by promoting activity, couples' coping, and empathic understanding while preventing depression and marital distress.

## Acknowledgements

Work on this chapter was partially supported by grant K01 MH61569 awarded to the first author.

## References

Bakeman, R. & Gottman, J. M. (1997). *Observing interaction: An introduction to sequential analysis* (2nd edn.). New York: Cambridge University Press.

Bruce, J., Drury, N., Poobalan, A. S., Jeffrey, R. R., Smith, W. C. S., & Chambers, W. A. (2003). The prevalence of chronic chest and leg pain following cardiac surgery: A historical cohort study. *Pain,* **104**, 265–73.

Buenaver, L. F., Edwards, R. R., & Haythornthwaite, J. A. (2007). Pain-related catastrophizing and perceived social responses: Inter-relationships in the context of chronic pain. *Pain*, 127, 234–42.

Cano, A. (2004). Pain catastrophizing and social support in married individuals with chronic pain: The moderating role of pain duration. *Pain*, 110, 656–64.

Cano, A. & Leonard, M. T. (2006). Integrative behavioral couple therapy for chronic pain: Promoting behavior change and emotional acceptance. *Journal of Clinical Psychology: In Session*, 62, 1409–18.

Cano, A., Weisberg, J., & Gallagher, M. (2000). Marital satisfaction and pain severity mediate the association between negative spouse responses to pain and depressive symptoms in a chronic pain patient sample. *Pain Medicine*, 1, 35–43.

Cano, A., Gillis, M., Heinz, W., Geisser, M., & Foran, H. (2004a). Marital functioning, chronic pain, and psychological distress. *Pain*, 107, 99–106.

Cano, A., Johansen, A., & Geisser, M. (2004b). Spousal congruence on disability, pain, and spouse responses to pain. *Pain*, 109, 258–65.

Cano, A., Johansen, A., & Franz, A. (2005). Multilevel analysis of spousal congruence on pain, interference, and disability. *Pain*, 118, 369–79.

Cano, A., Barterian, J., & Heller, J. (2008). Empathic and nonempathic interaction in chronic pain couples. *Clinical Journal of Pain*, 24, 678–84.

Cano, A., Miller, L.R., & Loree, A. (2009). Spouse beliefs about partner chronic pain. *Journal of Pain*, 10, 486–92.

Christensen, A., Jacobson, N., & Babcock, J. (1995). Integrative behavioral couple therapy. In N. Jacobson & A. S. Gurman (Eds.), *Clinical handbook of marital therapy* (2nd edn), pp. 31–64. New York: Guilford Press.

Christensen, A., Atkins, D., Berns, S., Wheeler, J., Baucom, D., & Simpson, L. (2004). Traditional versus integrative behavioral couple therapy for significantly and chronically distressed married couples. *Journal of Consulting and Clinical Psychology*, 72, 176–91.

Christensen, A., Atkins, D. C., Yi, J., Baucom, D. H., & George, W. H. (2006). Couple and individual adjustment for 2 years following a randomized clinical trial comparing traditional versus integrative behavioral couple therapy. *Journal of Counseling and Clinical Psychology*, 74, 1180–91.

Coyne, J. C. & Fiske, V. (1992). Couples coping with chronic and catastrophic illness. In T. J. Takamatsu, M. A. P. Stephens, S. E. Hobfall, & J. H. Crowther (Eds.) *Family health psychology. Series in applied psychology: Social issues and questions*, pp. 129–49. Washington, DC: Hemisphere Publishing Corp.

Fordyce, W. E. (1976). *Behavioral methods for chronic pain and illness*. St. Louis, MO: C.V. Mosby.

Fruzzetti A. E. & Iverson, K. M. (2004). Mindfulness, acceptance, validation, and 'individual' psychopathology in couples. In S. C. Hayes, V. M. Follette, & M. M. Linehan (Eds.) *Mindfulness and acceptance: expanding the cognitive-behavioral tradition*, pp. 168–91. New York: Guilford Press.

Fruzzetti A. E. & Iverson, K. M. (2006). Intervening with couples and families to treat emotion dysregulation and psychopathology. In D.K. Snyder, J. A. Simpson, & J.N. Hughes (Eds.) *Emotion regulation in couples and families: Pathways to dysfunction and health*, pp. 249–67. Washington, DC: American Psychological Association.

Gauthier, N., Thibault, P., & Sullivan, M. J. L. (2008). Individual and relational correlates of pain-related empathic accuracy in spouses of chronic pain patients. *Clinical Journal of Pain*, 24, 669–77.

Giardino, N. D., Jensen, M. P., Turner, J. A., Ehde, D. M., & Cardenas, D. D. (2003). Social environment moderates the association between catastrophizing and pain among persons with a spinal cord injury. *Pain*, 106, 19–25.

Goubert, L., Craig, K. D., Vervoort, T., *et al.* (2005). Facing others in pain: The effects of empathy. *Pain*, 118, 285–8.

Herbette, G. & Rime, B. (2004). Verbalization of emotion in chronic pain patients and their psychological adjustment. *Journal of Health Psychology*, 9, 661–76.

Jacobson, N. & Christensen, A. (1998). *Acceptance and change in couple therapy: A therapist's guide to transforming relationships*. New York: Norton.

Jacobson, N., Christensen, A., Prince, S., Cordova, J., & Eldridge, K. (2000). Integrative behavioral couple therapy: An acceptance-based, promising new treatment for couple discord. *Journal of Consulting and Clinical Psychology,* **68,** 351–5.

Johansen, A. & Cano, A. (2007). A preliminary investigation of affective interaction in chronic pain couples. *Pain,* **132,** S86–95.

Keefe, F., Blumenthal, J., Baucom, D., *et al.* (2004). Effects of spouse-assisted coping skills training and exercise training in patients with osteoarthritic knee pain: A randomized controlled study. *Pain,* **110,** 539–49.

Keefe, F., Caldwell, D., Baucom, D., & Salley, A. (1996). Spouse-assisted coping skills training in the management of osteoarthritic knee pain. *Arthritis Care & Research,* **9,** 279–91.

Keefe, F., Caldwell, D., Baucom, D., *et al.* (1999). Spouse-assisted coping skills training in the management of knee pain in osteoarthritis: Long-term followup results. *Arthritis Care & Research,* **12,** 101–11.

Keefe, F. J., Ahles, T. A., Sutton, L., *et al.* (2005). Partner-guided cancer pain management at the end of life. *Journal of Pain and Symptom Management,* **29,** 263–72.

Kerns R. D., Haythornthwaite J., Southwick S., Giller, E. L. (1990). The role of marital interaction in chronic pain and depressive symptom severity. *Journal of Psychosomatic Research,* **34,** 401–8.

Kiecolt-Glaser J. & Newton, T. (2001). Marriage and health: His and hers. *Psychological Bulletin,* **127,** 472–503.

Knoll, N., Burkert, S., Rosemeier, H. P., Roigas, J., & Gralla, O. (2007). Predictors of spouses' provided support for patients receiving laparoscopic radical prostatectomy peri-surgery. *Psycho-Oncology,* **16,** 312–19.

Kulik, J. A. & Mahler, H. I. M. (1989). Social support and recovery from surgery. *Health Psychology,* **8,** 221–38.

Lahtinen, P., Kokki, H., Hynynen, M. (2006). Pain after cardiac surgery – a prospective cohort study of 1-year incidence and intensity. *Anesthesiology,* **105,** 794–800.

Laurenceau, J., Feldman Barrett, L., & Pietromonaco, P. R. (1998). Intimacy as an interpersonal process: The importance of self-disclosure, partner disclosure, and perceived partner responsiveness in interpersonal exchanges. *Journal of Personality and Social Psychology,* **74,** 1238–51.

Leonard, M. T. & Cano. A. (2006). Pain affects spouses too: Personal experience with pain and catastrophizing as correlates of spouse distress. *Pain,* **126,** 139–46.

Leonard, M., Cano, A., & Johansen, A. (2006). Chronic pain in a couples context: A review And integration of theoretical models and empirical evidence. *Journal of Pain,* **7,** 377–90.

Lousberg, R., Schmidt, A. J. M., & Groenman, N. H. (1992). The relationship between spouse solicitousness and pain behavior: Searching for more experimental evidence. *Pain,* **51,** 75–9.

Martire, L. M., Lustig, A. P., Schulz, R., Miller, G. E., & Helgeson, V. S. (2004). Is it beneficial to involve a family member? A meta-analysis of psychosocial interventions for chronic illness. *Health Psychology,* **23,** 599–611.

Martire, L. M., Schulz, R., Keefe, F. J., Rudy, T. E., Starz, T. W. (2007). Couple-oriented education and support intervention: Effects on individuals with osteoarthritis and their spouses. *Rehabilitation Psychology.* **52,** 121–32.

Morley, S., Doyle, K., & Beese, A. (2000). Talking to others about pain: Suffering in silence. In M. Devor, M. Rowbothan, & Z. Wiesenfeld-Hallin (Eds.) *Proceedings of the ninth world congress on pain: Progress in pain research and management,* pp. 1123–29. Seattle, WA: IASP Press.

Nampiaparampil, D. D. (2008). Prevalence of chronic pain after traumatic brain injury: A systematic review. *Journal of the American Medical Association,* **300,** 711–19.

Newton-John, T. R. & Willams, A. C. de C. (2006). Chronic pain couples: Perceived marital interactions and pain behaviours. *Pain,* **123,** 53–63.

Paulsen, J. S., & Altmaier, E. M. (1995). The effects of perceived versus enacted social support on the discriminative cue function of spouses for pain behaviors. *Pain,* **60,** 103–10.

Pence L. B., Thorn, B. E., Jensen, M. P., Romano, J. M. (2008). Examination of perceived spouse responses to patient well and pain behavior in patients with headache. *Clinical Journal of Pain*, **24**, 654–61.

Pengel, L. H. M., Herbert, R. D., Maher, C. G., & Refshauge, K. M. (2003). Acute low back pain: Systematic review of ifs prognosis. *British Medical Journal*, **327**, 323–7.

Porter, L. S, Keefe, F. J., Wellington, C., & Williams, A. C. de C. (2008). Pain communication in the context of osteoarthritis: Patient and partner self-efficacy for pain communication and holding back from discussion of pain and arthritis-related concerns. *Clinical Journal of Pain*, **24**, 662–8.

Romano, J. M., Turner, J. A., Friedman, R. A., Jensen, M. P., & Hops, H. (1991). Observational assessment of chronic pain patient-spouse behavioral interactions. *Behavioral Therapy*, **22**, 549–67.

Romano, J. M., Turner, J. A., Friedman, L. S., *et al.* (1992). Sequential analysis of chronic pain behaviors and spouse responses. *Journal of Consulting and Clinical Psychology*, **60**, 777–82.

Romano, J. M., Turner, J. A., Jensen, M. P., *et al.* (1995). Chronic pain patient-spouse behavioral interactions predict patient disability. *Pain*, **63**, 353–60.

Romano, J. M., Jensen, M. P., Turner, J. A., Good, A. B., & Hops, H. (2000). Chronic pain patient-partner interactions: Further support for a behavioral model of chronic pain. *Behavior Therapy*, **31**, 415–40.

Saarijarvi, S. (1991). A controlled study of couple therapy in chronic low back pain patients: Effects on marital satisfaction, psychological distress and health attitudes. *Journal of Psychosomatic Research*, **35**, 265–72.

Saarijarvi, S., Rytokoski, U., Alanen, E. (1991). A controlled study of couple therapy in chronic low back pain patients: No improvement of disability. *Journal of Psychosomatic Research*, **35**, 671–7.

Saarijarvi, S., Alanen, E., Rytokoski, U., & Hyyppa, M. (1992). Couple therapy improves Mental well-being in chronic low back pain patients: A controlled, five year follow up study. *Journal of Psychosomatic Research*, **36**, 651–6.

Schwartz, L., Slater, M. A., & Birchler, G. R. (1996). The role of pain behaviors in the modulation of marital conflict in chronic pain couples. *Pain*, **65**, 227–33.

Schwartz, L., Jensen, M. P., & Romano, J. M. (2005). The development and psychometric evaluation of an instrument to assess spouse responses to pain and well behavior in patients with chronic pain: The Spouse Response Inventory. *The Journal of Pain*, **6**(4), 243–52.

Severeijns, R., Vlaeyen, J. W. S., & van den Hout, M. A. (2004). Do we need a communal coping model of pain catastrophizing? An alternative explanation. *Pain*, **111**, 226–9.

Sharp, T. J. (2001). Chronic pain: A reformulation of the cognitive-behavioural model. *Behaviour Research and Therapy*, **39**, 787–800.

Stroud, M. W., Turner, J. A., Jensen, M. P., & Cardenas, D. D. (2006). Partner responses to pain behaviors are associated with depression and activity interference among persons with chronic pain and spinal cord injury. *The Journal of Pain*, **7**, 91–9.

Sullivan, M. J. L., Bishop, S., & Pivik, J. (1995). The Pain Catastrophizing Scale: Development and Validation. *Psychological Assessment*, **7**, 524–32.

Sullivan, M. J. L., Thorn, B. E., Haythornthwaite, J. A., Keefe, F. J., Martin, M., & Bradley, L. A. (2001). Theoretical perspectives on the relation between catastrophizing and pain. *Clinical Journal of Pain*, **17**, 52–64.

Sullivan, M. J. L., Adams, H., & Sullivan, M. E. (2004). Communicative dimensions of pain catastrophizing: Social cueing effects on pain behaviour and coping. *Pain*, **107**, 220–6.

Sullivan, M. J. L., Martel, M. O., Tripp, D., Savard, A., & Crombez, G. (2006). The relation between catastrophizing and the communication of pain experience. *Pain*, **122**, 282–8.

Thorn B. E., Ward L. C., Sullivan M. J. L., & Boothby J. L. (2003). Communal coping model of catastrophizing: Conceptual model building. *Pain*, **106**, 1–2.

Turk, D. C. & Kerns, R. D. (1985). The family in health and illness. In D. C. Turk & R. D. Kerns (Eds.), *Health, illness, and families: A life-span perspective*, pp. 1–22. New York: Wiley.

Turk D. C., Meichenbaum D., Genest, M. (1983). *Pain and behavioral medicine: A cognitive-behavioral perspective*. New York: Guilford Press.

Turk, D. C., Kerns, R. D., Rosenberg, R. (1992). Effects of marital interaction on chronic pain and disability: Examining the down side of social support. *Rehabilitation Psychology, 37*, 259–74.

Vilholm, O. J., Cold, S., Rasmussen, L., & Sindrup, S. H. (2008). The postmastectomy pain syndrome: an epidemiological study on the prevalence of chronic pain after surgery for breast cancer. *British Journal of Cancer, 99*, 604–10.

Vlaeyen, J. W. S. & Crombez, G. (1999). Fear of movement/(re)injury, avoidance and pain disability in chronic low back pain patients. *Manual Therapy, 4*, 187–95.

Williamson, D., Robinson, M. E., & Melamed, B. (1997). Pain behavior, spouse responsiveness, and marital satisfaction in patients with rheumatoid arthritis. *Behavior Modification, 21*, 97–118.

Chapter 18

# Effects of Workers' Compensation Systems on Recovery from Disabling Injuries

James P. Robinson and John D. Loeser

## 18.1 Introduction

Many observers have argued that disability systems have adverse effects on the people whom they serve (Harris et al. 2005; Atlas 2007; Gabbe 2007). The purpose of this chapter is to evaluate these claims, and consider ways in which disability systems might affect the behaviour of their beneficiaries.

Any discussion of the effects of disability systems is complicated by the fact that there are many types of disability, and many organizations that provide disability benefits. For example, some people (e.g. ones with C4 quadriplegia or severe mental retardation) require personal attendants or long term institutionalization because they cannot perform basic activities of daily living (ADLs). Others are able to perform basic ADLs, but are disabled in the sense that they are unable to work. Among work-disabled individuals, some have life-long disabilities, whereas others function in the work place for an extended period of time, and then develop medical conditions that disable them. These conditions might be results of their work activities (e.g. a logger who sustains a spinal fracture when a tree falls on him), or might be unrelated (e.g. a worker who has a myocardial infarction). Corresponding to the multiplicity of types of disability and circumstances under which people become disabled, there are several organizations that provide assistance to them. In the USA these include workers' compensation (WC), programmes run by the Social Security Administration, disability programmes run through the Veterans Administration system, private disability programmes, and welfare programmes. It is not uncommon for a disabled person to interact with several of these—e.g. he might start with a workers' compensation claim, but later receive Social Security Disability Insurance benefits.

For simplicity, this chapter focuses on individuals who sustain injuries at work and receive benefits through a WC system in the USA. Several other caveats are in order. First, it should be noted that the majority of work injuries (approximately 70%) (Bureau of Labor Statistics 2008) resolve uneventfully, and do not lead to work disability. A WC system is more likely to affect the recovery of an injured worker (IW) if the worker has a significant amount of contact with it. Thus, this chapter focuses on work injuries that lead to work disability, and especially ones associated with protracted work disability. Second, there are workers' compensation systems for each of the 50 states, as well as federal systems (Williams 1991). These systems vary substantially. It is beyond the scope of this chapter to explore this variation (Analysis of workers' compensation laws 1996). But it is important to note that an IW's behaviour is likely to be influenced by specific rules and regulations pertaining to the WC system with which he/she interacts.

Two basic questions need to be asked regarding the influence of the WC system on IWs: (1) are IWs affected by their interactions with the WC system, and if so, (2) what are the mechanisms by which the effects take place?

## 18.2 **Is there an effect?**

Three kinds of evidence suggest that the behaviour of IWs is affected by their interactions with WC systems. As noted below, though, each kind of evidence is subject to more than one interpretation.

### 18.2.1 **Shape of the recovery curve**

Informal observation suggests that as time goes on following a disabling work injury, IWs become progressively more resistant to treatment, and more 'stuck' in their disability. Some observers have used the term 'disability syndrome' to describe the constellation of behavioural issues that chronically disabled IWs often demonstrate (Robinson et al. 1997). The hypothesis that chronically disabled IWs develop disability syndromes is at least compatible with large-scale data regarding recovery from work injuries. As demonstrated by Cheadle et al. (Cheadle et al 1994) and several other investigators, the recovery curve following disabling injuries follows a negative exponential curve (see Figure 18.1). Thus, for example, among workers who go on disability

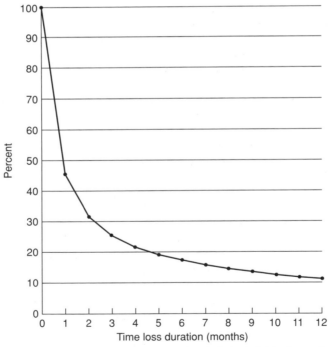

**Fig. 18.1** Probability of continued disability payments as a function of time in a cohort of injured workers who were initially disabled by a work injury. Reproduced from Cheadle A, Franklin G, Wolfhagen C, et al. Factors influencing the duration of work-related disability: a population-based study of Washington State workers' compensation, *Am J Public Health*, **84**(2), 190–6, 1994 with permission from The Sheridan Press.

following an injury, approximately 70% go off disability within 2 months. However, at about 4 months, the recovery curve flattens out. A worker who is on disability at 4 months has about of 50% chance of still being on disability at 1 year following injury. Based on this curve, one might conclude that workers who are disabled at 4 months become more resistant to rehabilitation, perhaps because of interactions that they have with the WC system. However, at least two other explanations of the curve are also possible. One is that IWs who end up in the tail of the curve had risk factors at the time of injury that made them less likely to recover. Thus, their paths might be determined by pre-injury or injury factors, rather than by subsequent interactions with a WC system (Mustard and Hertzman 2001). Second, as time elapses following a disabling injury, IWs face the kinds of stresses that impact all people who are dislodged from the work place. The importance of such dislodgement is demonstrated by research on the psychological effects of prolonged absence from work that has nothing to do with injuries or disability (Bartley 1994; Dooley et al 1996; Murphy and Athanasou 1999; Fryer and Fagen 2003; Leino-Loison et al. 2004). It is reasonable to presume that IWs who have lost their confidence and have become depressed as a result of prolonged separation from the work force will view their prospects for success in the workplace negatively. Their emotional dysfunction and loss of confidence might delay recovery from their work injury, regardless of their interactions with WC.

## 18.2.2 **Moral hazards**

Studies on the effects of insurance indicate that when people have insurance that indemnifies them against certain events, they tend to behave in ways that make these events more likely to occur. The term 'moral hazard' has been used to describe this effect. For example, if individuals are indemnified against the loss of their home in a fire, they may become careless in the safety procedures they employ at home to prevent fires, or may even set fires deliberately in order to receive insurance benefits. In the context of WC, there is evidence that as benefits to IWs increase, the probability of filing WC claims increases, as does the duration of claims (Loeser et al. 1995; Dembe and Boden 2000). As noted by Dembe and Boden (2000), when the term moral hazard was introduced in the 19th century, it was widely believed that the changes in behaviour elicited by insurance benefits were attributable to carelessness, deceit or fraud on the part of insurance beneficiaries. These authors document that the term continues to be used in ways that disparage IWs by suggesting that many of them file claims that are unnecessary or fraudulent. Thus, the statistical finding of an association between insurance benefits and aggregate behaviours of beneficiaries is congruent with explanations for protracted disability that focus on worker malingering and/or 'secondary gain'. These explanations will be described below.

It is beyond the scope of this chapter to discuss the concept of moral hazard in any depth. However, a few comments are appropriate. First, as Dembe and Boden (2000) point out, much of the research on moral hazards has been carried out by economists. An implicit assumption in economic analyses of work behaviour is that workers voluntarily choose employment in order to make money, and voluntarily choose when to leave their jobs. Thus, when a worker files a WC claim, this is viewed as a voluntary, calculated act rather than as a response to an injury that actually incapacitates the worker. If workers' decisions to file claims are construed as calculated, it is a short conceptual leap to construe them as fraudulent. Moreoever, as Dembe and Boden forcefully argue, moral hazard research has tended to focus on the suspicious behaviour of IWs rather than on the behaviour of employers, insurance adjusters, and others who participate in WC claims. They state:

> In the economist's model of the labor market, workers freely sell their labor to employers, control their working conditions, decide when they are injured and how long they need to recuperate, choose their

medical care provider, and decide on the type and amount of care that they receive ... They become injured (or claim that they are injured when they are not), and the defenseless employer or insurer must pay them until the injured workers decide it's time to return to work, perhaps after taking a vacation in sunny Florida, running in a marathon in Hawaii, and painting their houses. Consider another possibility. Workers who are injured frequently do not file workers' compensation claims, worrying that they will be fired, that their fellow workers will think of them as malingerers and cheats, and that they will carry with them the social stigma formerly only associated with people on welfare. If they file and take time from work to recover, they may not have a job when they are ready to return. Potential future employers will know that they have filed workers' compensation claims and may decide that it is too risky to hire them. If the employer or insurer contests the claim, they then have to decide to give up their benefits or deal with their anxiety and discomfort around lawyers and the legal system (Dembe and Boden 2000, p. 269).

Also, it should be noted that even if generous benefits influence workers to exaggerate their incapacitation or file fraudulent claims ('Retirees' disability epidemic' 2008), the relevance of this phenomenon to IWs is questionable. The reason for this is that WC benefits are generally modest, and do not cover the costs that IWs incur as a result of their injuries (Hunt 2003; Reville et al. 2005). Thus, it is hard to understand the economic benefits that IWs receive when they file claims. It is also noteworthy that a very substantial proportion of workers do not file claims for work injuries or occupational illnesses (Morse et al. 2000; Shannon and Lowe 2002; Scherzer et al. 2005). Investigators have attributed this under-reporting of injuries to a variety of factors, such as fear of retaliation from employers or pressure from co-workers. But it is also likely that workers realize that they are likely to suffer adverse financial consequences if they file a WC claim and go off work. These data put the issue of moral hazards in WC in a different light. A reasonable interpretation is that WC benefits are generally so low that they contribute to under-reporting of injuries by workers, but that the under-reporting is less pronounced in WC systems that provide relatively generous benefits.

### 18.2.3 Comparisons between IWs and other patient groups

The most convincing evidence for adverse effects associated with participation in WC systems comes from studies comparing patients with WC to patients without WC regarding response to treatment. A recent meta-analysis performed by Harris et al. (2005) included 211 studies. In 175 of them, it was found that compensation/litigation was associated with poorer surgical outcome. Thirty five studies showed no association between compensation/litigation status and outcome, while only 1 study found that patients with compensation/litigation had better outcomes than others. A formal meta-analysis performed on 129 studies with appropriate data revealed on odds ratio of 3.79 for an unsatisfactory surgical outcome among patients with compensation/litigation.

It is worth noting that the non-compensation patients were often not clearly described in the studies reviewed, although it is likely that for the most part they were patients who received treatments under private insurance coverage and were not involved in litigation. Here they are designated as 'private pay' patients. Also, within the compensation cohort, the authors of individual studies and Harris et al. did not clearly distinguish between compensation status and litigation status, or between different types of compensation. However, since the 'compensation' cohort in most of the studies consisted of injured workers, the results of the review are relevant to the present discussion.

At first glance, the above data seem to provide convincing evidence for an adverse effect of WC on the recovery of IWs. However obvious this conclusion appears to be, it is important to consider alternative ways of interpreting the findings reviewed by Harris et al. First, studies that compare recovery trajectories of injured workers vs. 'private pay' patients essentially never control adequately for baseline, pre-injury variables on which these two types of patients may differ. There is evidence that important differences exist between the two types of patients. For example, Atlas et al. (2000) found that in comparison to private pay patients, WC patients at baseline were more likely to be young, male, and employed as labourers. Moreover, there is evidence that compared to IWs in general, ones with protracted WC claims are relatively likely to have pre-injury histories characterized by high health care utilization and a high risk of receiving welfare benefits (Mustard and Hertzman 2001) Also, longitudinal studies show that among workers who are initially asymptomatic, ones who report new onset of symptoms and/or file a claim for a new injury are more likely than other workers to report job-related psychosocial stressors such as monotony of the job (Harkness et al. 2003) or job dissatisfaction (Bigos et al. 1992). These data strongly suggest that individuals with risk factors for protracted disability and health problems are over-represented among workers who file WC claims.

It is also likely that WC and private pay patients differ on a wide range of variables related to employment. As noted above, Atlas et al. (2000) found that WC patients treated for disc herniations were more likely than private pay patients to be labourers. Also, they found that 80% of their private pay patients reported working during the 4 weeks prior to their baseline assessments vs. only 35% of WC patients. It might seem that these work-related variables have nothing to do with patients' clinical status following surgery. However, this assumption ignores the fact that for many IWs, employment issues, clinical status of the work injury, and access to medical care can be intertwined in complex ways. The reason for this is that WC claims are typically closed when an IW's clinical status has reached medical stability, and disability benefits are terminated if the worker is judged to be capable of working. Given these rules, IWs who believe that they are unable to return to the workforce have an incentive to extend their benefits by reporting ongoing symptoms following treatments.

## 18.3 **How does the workers' compensation affect the behaviour of IWs?**

Despite the caveats given above, the most parsimonious way to explain the findings of studies on recovery curves, moral hazards, and surgical outcomes for WC vs. private pay patients is that WC systems adversely affect the recovery of IWs. Assuming this is true, what are the processes that mediate this adverse effect?

In addressing this question, it should be noted that the factors influencing IWs' recovery and return to work are multiple and complex. They may well include the workers' interactions with representatives of their WC carrier, but they also include the severity and functional consequences of the work injuries, the demands of the workers' jobs at the time of injury, their opportunities for alternative employment based on prior education and training, their motivation to return to work, their resourcefulness in overcoming barriers to return to the job they had at the time of injury or find alternative employment, their relationships with co-workers and managers at the job, information they receive from medical professionals about the risks they take by engaging in various kinds of activity, and advice they receive from their attorneys. Thus, we should not expect simple explanations when we try to abstract the role of the WC system from the myriad of influences on an IW's recovery, and determine exactly how the worker's interactions with the system affect him/her.

## 18.4 **Possible explanations for the negative effect of WC**

Several hypotheses have been advanced to explain the negative effect of WC on the recovery of IWs. Many of the studies bearing on these hypotheses combine individuals with different types of compensation (e.g. WC and Social Security Disability Insurance), and combine compensation claimants with litigants in tort cases. However, since IWs with WC claims are well represented in these studies, they will be considered below without any effort to isolate the effect of WC.

### 18.4.1 **Malingering and secondary gain**

### Malingering

Many publications, often appearing in industry journals, have titles that suggest an epidemic of fraud/malingering perpetrated by IWs—e.g. 'Employers must be alert to comp fraud' (Auth 2005), 'Reducing workers' compensation fraud: a deterrent approach' (Mah 1998), and 'Screen patients quickly for workers' comp fraud' (Easton 1997). The concern implied by these titles is consistent with results of a recent review by Aronoff et al. (2007). These authors reported an astonishingly high prevalence of malingering in settings where compensation or litigation are involved—for example, some of the studies they reviewed reported a 36–50% rate of malingering among compensation/litigation patients with chronic pain.

The literature on malingering among compensation recipients dovetails with the previously described literature on the moral hazard associated with compensation for work injuries. Both areas of research suggest that the negative effect of compensation on recovery can be explained in terms of wilful deceit on the part of IWs. If this explanation is valid, it provides a conceptually simple, though somewhat distasteful, explanation of the compensation effect.

However, serious questions can be raised about the validity of the research on malingering summarized by Aronoff et al. Malingering is best defined as fraud in a medical context. As such, it is a criminal activity, and involves planned feigning of incapacitation from a medical condition in order to receive some kind of reward (typically a monetary reward). Thus, in order to demonstrate malingering, an investigator must: (1) show evidence that a suspect is deliberately feigning his/her medical condition, and (2) provide evidence that the feigning is designed to help the suspect secure a monetary award. The malingering research mentioned above runs into problems with respect to both criteria.

One key issue is that most of the studies cited by Aronoff et al. as proof of malingering involve the behaviour of claimants on paper and pencil tests of various kinds. In general, malingering is identified when patients perform very poorly on the tests, or when their test performance is dramatically altered by instructions given by an experimenter. It is beyond the scope of this chapter to discuss the validity of these tests among individuals who claim to have brain injuries or other work-related conditions that would directly affect their test taking abilities. But regardless of the validity of the tests among people with purported neurocognitive impairment, their relevance to work injuries in general is highly suspect. The reason for this is that epidemiologic data clearly indicate that musculoskeletal injuries dominate all other categories of work related disorders. For example, the Bureau of Labor Statistics compiles data on various categories of injuries/illnesses and indicates the percentage of total injuries/illnesses represented by each category. Data for 2005 indicate that 40.8% of all injuries/illnesses were coded as sprains/strains, 7.8% as fractures, 2.9% as back pain, 1.3% as carpal tunnel syndrome, and 0.5% as tendonitis (Bureau of Labor Statistics 2005). Thus, at least 53.5% of all work injuries/illnesses in 2005 were musculoskeletal in nature. In these conditions, workers remain disabled because of limitations in physical capacities, rather than limitations in their ability to perform cognitive tasks. Thus, the detection of malingering must rest on observations of claimants' physical activities, as demonstrated, for example, in surveillance videotapes. Although surveillance videotaping is used in WC, there are very few publications on the procedure in the medical literature (Kay and Morris-Jones 1998; 'Phoney worker's comp. claim?' 2007), and the pick up rate of malingering by video surveillance is uncertain. Dembe and Boden (2000) mention a series of newspapers articles on surveillance videotaping in California during the late 1990s—the activity was reportedly disbanded because evidence of malingering was found so rarely (Fricker 1997).

As far as incentives for malingering are concerned, literature mentioned above in the discussion of moral hazards is relevant. This literature clearly demonstrates that the monetary benefits that IWs receive—either during the course of their claims or when their claims are closed—do not compensate for the financial losses they incur as a result of being out of the work force, or being re-employed in low paying jobs after their claims have been closed. Thus, assertions that malingering is rampant among IWs fail to give a satisfactory answer to a very basic question: why would an IW engage in criminal activity in order to gain such a paltry sum of money?

## Secondary gain and related terms

There is a substantial literature related to the hypothesis that individuals involved in compensation or litigation are influenced by 'secondary gain' (Fishbain et al. 1995). This term has its origin in the writings of Freud, who distinguished between the primary gain in a neurosis (management of unconscious impulses) and various secondary gains (such as enjoying the nurturance that one can get for being sick). In the context of compensation/litigation, multiple potential rewards for failure to recover and protracted disability have been proposed (Box 18.1) (Dersh et al. 2004). Most writers, however, discuss secondary gain in relation to financial rewards that a claimant can get.

Some observers emphasize that secondary gain describes the behaviour of claimants who are influenced unconsciously by potential rewards in their environment (Fishbain 1994). The idea that secondary gain involves unconscious behaviour makes it morally less objectionable than malingering, which refers to conscious fabrication in order to achieve some reward. However, this seemingly clear distinction between secondary gain and malingering has been challenged by other writers. For example, Dersh et al. (2004) address several conceptual conundrums regarding the secondary gain construct, and indicate that IWs sometimes consciously engage in behaviours designed to achieve secondary gains. They do not provide a specific definition of secondary gain, but, rather describe its features (see Box 18.2).

The disagreements among different observers in the conceptualization of secondary gain highlight the elusiveness of the concept. It is best to think of the terms 'malingering' and 'secondary gain' as alternative ways to describe the effect of environmental rewards on the behaviour of claimants, with the difference being one of the moral opprobrium assigned to a claimant's behaviour. While neither term is flattering, a clinician or adjudicator who accuses a claimant of malingering is rendering a much harsher judgment than one who says the claimant's behaviour is motivated by secondary gain.

A myriad of other terms have been used to describe the behaviours of claimants as they interact with the compensation systems or legal systems. Mendelson (1988) listed several of these (See Box 18.3). All of them are unflattering, and in some way embody the perception by some observers that compensation/litigation patients tend to behave in ways that are self-serving.

It is worth noting that some observers have talked about the secondary losses that compensation/litigation claimants sustain, rather than just the gains they seek (Fishbain 1994; Gatchel et al. 2002). Box 18.4 lists possible losses suggested by Dersh et al. The concept of secondary losses

## Box 18.1 Types of secondary gains

### Internal

1. Gratification of pre-existing unresolved dependency strivings or affiliation needs.

2. Gratification of pre-existing unresolved revengeful strivings (e.g. revenge directed toward insurance carriers or adjustors who gave patient a hard time; revenge directed toward spouse/partner who was perceived as not living up to his or her responsibilities in the relationship).

3. An attempt to elicit care-giving, sympathy, and concern from family and friends.

4. Family anger because of patient's disability may increase patient resentment and determination to get his or her due to prove entitlement.

5. Obtaining one's entitlement for years of struggling, dutiful attention to responsibilities, and a 'much-earned' recompense.

6. Ability to withdraw from unpleasant or unsatisfactory life roles, activities, and responsibilities, including those of 'breadwinner', spouse, and parent.

7. Adoption of 'sick role' allows the patient to communicate and relate to others in a new, socially sanctioned manner.

8. Converting a socially unacceptable disability (psychological disorder) to a socially acceptable disability (injury or disease)

9. Displacing the blame for one's failures from oneself to an apparently disabling illness beyond one's control.

10. Maintenance of status in family.

11. Holding a spouse/partner in a marriage/relationship.

12. Avoiding sex.

13. Contraception.

14. Obtaining drugs.

15. Denial of the randomness of events.

### External

1. Obtaining financial awards associated with disability.
   a. Wage replacement (short- and long-term disability, social security disability insurance, workers' compensation benefits).
   b. Settlement (disability- or impairment-based).
   c. Disability-based debt protection (e.g. credit cards, mortgage, auto loan).
   d. Subsidized child and family care, housing, and food.

2. Protection from legal and other obligations (e.g. child support payments, court appearances, parole or probation demands).

3. Job manipulation (e.g. promotion or transfer, handling personnel or work adjustment difficulties, prevention of lay-off or termination).

4. Vocational retraining and skills upgrade.

With kind permission from Springer Science+Business Media: *Journal of Occupational Rehabilitation*, The Management of Secondary Gain and Loss in Medicolegal Settings: Strengths and Weaknesses, **14**(4), 2004, Jeffrey Dersh.

## Box 18.2 Features of secondary gain

- Secondary gain issues are prominent factors in illness, particularly chronic illness and illness being evaluated and treated in a medicolegal context.

- Secondary gain issues are rarely suggestive of 'pure' malingering or factitious disorder.

- Disability/illness exaggeration is frequently associated with secondary gain, and can often be inferred from abnormal illness behavior.

- Conscious, unconscious, and preconscious processes are involved in secondary and tertiary gain.

- Unconscious and conscious processes are better conceptualized from a dimensional perspective, rather than a dichotomous one.

- When conscious processes are primary, the patient may conceal secondary gains from others (resulting in hidden agendas). On the other hand, the patient may be quite open and transparent about his or her agendas.

- All chronic illnesses (physical and psychiatric) involve secondary gains and losses, as well as tertiary gains and losses.

- In almost all cases, there are multiple gains and losses, resulting in multiple agendas.

- Understanding the gain and loss issues (the secondary and tertiary economies) will lead to the most effective management of these patients.

- Operant conditioning (reinforcement) principles will often be effective in altering this economy in a positive direction.

- However, these economies cannot be understood in a purely mechanistic, operant conditioning, or rational manner.

- Psychodynamic and sociocultural factors are also important factors to be considered in understanding gain and loss issues.

With kind permission from Springer Science+Business Media: *Journal of Occupational Rehabilitation*, The Management of Secondary Gain and Loss in Medicolegal Settings: Strengths and Weaknesses, **14**(4), 2004, Jeffrey Dersh.

associated with injury and participation in compensation systems dovetails with the findings in studies cited above—i.e. ones demonstrating that the financial remuneration IWs receive from WC systems almost never matches the financial losses they incur as a result of their injuries.

## Cured by a verdict?

Kennedy famously described compensation neurosis as 'A state of mind, born out of fear, kept alive by avarice, stimulated by lawyers, and cured by a verdict' (Kennedy 1946). The idea that the apparent disability of a person with a compensation/litigation claim suddenly resolves after some decision or verdict has been reached regarding his/her claim is congruent with the view that the prior apparent incapacitation reflected malingering or seeking secondary gain. As Mendelson documented in his 1988 book *Psychiatric aspects of injury claims*, the empirical evidence to that point in time did not support Kennedy's assertion. A later review by Fishbain et al. (1995) reached the same conclusion. A recent study by Overman et al. (2008) also questions the validity of the 'cured by a verdict' hypothesis. These investigators examined health complaints among a large cohort of Norwegians several years before, around the time of, and several years after they were

## Box 18.3 Terms related to secondary gain

- Accident aboulia
- Accident neurosis
- Accident victim syndrome
- Aftermath neurosis
- American disease
- Attitudinal pathosis
- Compensation hysteria
- Compensationitis
- Compensation neurosis
- Entitlement neurosis
- Erichsen's disease
- Functional overlay
- Fright neurosis
- Greek disease
- Greenback neurosis
- Justice neurosis
- Litigation neurosis
- Mediterranean back
- Mediterranean disease
- Neurotic neurosis
- Postaccident anxiety syndrome
- Postaccident syndrome
- Post-traumatic syndrome
- Profit neurosis
- Railway brain
- Railway spine
- Secondary gain neurosis
- Syndrome of disproportionate disability
- Traumatic hysteria
- Traumatic neurasthenia
- Traumatic neurosis
- Triggered neurosis
- Unconscious malingering
- Vertebral neurosis
- Wharfie's back
- Whiplash neurosis

From Mendelson, G., *Psychiatric Aspects of Personal Injury Claims*, Table 1, pp. 13, Copyright 1988. Courtesy of Charles C Thomas Publisher, Ltd., Springfield, IL.

## Box 18.4 Types of secondary loss

1. Economic loss.

2. Loss of meaningfully relating to society through work.

3. Loss of work social relationships.

4. Loss of social support network.

5. Loss of meaningful and enjoyable family roles and activities.

6. Loss of recreational activities.

7. Loss of respect from family and friends.

8. Negative sanctions from family.

9. Loss of community approval.

10. Loss of respect from those in helping professions (e.g. physicians).

11. New role not comfortable and not well defined.

12. Social stigma of being chronically disabled.

13. Guilt over disability.

14. Communications of distress become unclear.

With kind permission from Springer Science+Business Media: *Journal of Occupational Rehabilitation*, The Management of Secondary Gain and Loss in Medicolegal Settings: Strengths and Weaknesses, **14**(4), 2004, Jeffrey Dersh.

awarded disability benefits. 'Somatic symptoms' and 'pain distribution' tended to worsen as the time when disability was granted approached, with improvement during the 7 years after awards were granted. However, during the post-award period, the complaints of respondents did not disappear; rather, they generally returned to the baseline levels that had existed years prior to the awards. When differences between pre and post award indices were noted, they were in the direction of being worse following awards than prior to the awards. These data suggest that claimants' increased symptom levels shortly before disability determinations are made reflect stress associated with the disability evaluation process. Other large scale studies document relatively high morbidity and mortality rates among disability beneficiaries (Kivimaki 2003; Vahtera et al 2004; Wallman et al 2006). In sum, the balance of evidence argues against the conclusion that claimants are cured by a verdict.

### 18.4.2 Perceptions of IWs

Whereas research on malingering and secondary gain suggest that workers consciously or unconsciously exaggerate their disability in order to achieve financial gains, a very different picture emerges from qualitative studies in which the perceptions of IWs are assessed by interview (Cole et al. 2002; Cromie et al. 2003; Strunin and Boden 2004; Beardwood et al 2005; Cacciacarro and Kirsh 2006; Lippel 2007; MacEachen et al. 2007; Soeker et al. 2008). These document recurring themes and concerns of the workers. Since the qualitative studies do not provide statistical data, quotations from the studies are given below to describe themes that commonly emerged during interviews with IWs. Four themes were prominent in the majority of qualitative studies.

## Sense of being distrusted

Many subjects felt that they were disbelieved by physicians and WC claims managers. They expressed the view that they had to prove their incapacitation to sceptical observers. Some of them expressed concern that they might be put under surveillance, and that any behaviours that were documented in surveillance tapes might be used against them. For example, Cromie et al. (2003, pp. 1086–7) write:

> Medical examiners made comments in their medical reports that had consequences for the financial and physical well-being of their patients. In some cases, they were quite judgmental and damning. Louise reported how a physician attributed her symptoms to a familial condition 'which was a total and outright lie' (p. 6). Denise described a situation where a neurologist decided she was 'swinging the lead . . . malingering . . .' She said: 'It was written on my history that I was a malingerer . . . they virtually withdrew all pain-killing drugs . . . and I actually got treated very badly from that point in time' (p. 10). Medical examiners, and in particular those to whom participants were referred by insurers, seemed to reflect some of the stereotypical prejudices toward claimants described by Quintner. . . The attitude of some medical practitioners led Jane to the point that she wanted to terminate her claim. Jane stated that a rheumatologist had written in a report that she was using her injury as an excuse not to have children and that in choosing not to have children she was avoiding her duty to her husband (Jane, p. 5). The rheumatologist implied that her problem was primarily psychological (Jane, p. 5). The rheumatology report was 'amazingly hostile . . . and . . . out of sync [sic] with any of the other reports I've got myself' (Jane, p. 6). She found the rheumatologist's report 'profoundly offensive' and said that it made her 'so angry,' but at the same time she felt unable to show the report to anybody else (Jane, p 15).

## Conflict with the WC system

Workers repeatedly talked about the difficulties they had in their interactions with WC systems. Problems ranged from personal insults by claims managers to fears about having benefits cut off. For example, Beardwood et al. (2005, pp. 40–2) state:

> Stories of difficulties with the compensation system were abundant. However, the major areas of tension could best be categorized as concern regarding the adversarial nature of the relationship with the compensation system; the lack of information, control, and choice provided by the system; and the fear and paranoia that were evoked through interaction within this system. Many workers found themselves entangled in an adversarial relationship, which was characterized by a lack of trust, misinterpretation of information provided, and a perception of inappropriate responses of workers within the system . . . A worker provided an analysis of the power structures in this way: 'It's fear. They instill fear in you. They're experts at that. They know how to instill fear in the person that's injured. You're already injured so your defenses are down. You're now sort of backed into a corner because they're the ones that are supposed to be paying the money. And yet they're not paying you properly. Or they're threatening to take it away. So you feel like you're alone and you have no recourse. You know. And it's a rotten position to be in.

## Stress; personal loss; family loss

IWs repeatedly talked about the emotional stresses they experienced, and about the impact of their injuries on their finances and their families. Beardwood et al. (2005, p. 43) state:

> The final stage was the impact on workers' lives and the nature of living as an injured worker. Themes included financial and social impacts, mental and emotional impacts, impacts on activities of daily living, and living with pain.
>
> Not surprisingly, workers described the financial hardships they experienced as a result of losing their regular wages. Some incurred medical expenses alongside these losses, which further increased their debt . . . The effects on family life and social inclusion were severe, as exemplified by this worker's

report: 'It has caused the end of my marriage. I do still have the custody of my children, but my injury affects them. If I have some sort of painful episode, my five-year-old starts to cry. My twelve-year-old really helps me out a lot by dealing with some things that I physically can't do. I get a lot of help from my parents. I've been forced to move in with them because of the injury, and I'll probably be stuck there for a while until I'm able to be completely independent.' Many workers revealed that their psychological state had deteriorated through the process of becoming injured and dealing with the system. They discussed the effects of poverty, role disruption, and stress on their mental and emotional health. Depression was a common experience.

## Anger with the WC system

Interviewees often talked about their anger with the WC system. This was articulated best by an IW who became an activist, and wrote an entire article about her experiences (Hammer 2000). She pointed out that although attention was often given to fraud/malingering on the part of IWs, misbehaviour by other participants in WC claims needed more attention:

> *Employer fraud* is rampant in under-reporting and not having any insurance at all. Workers know when their employer waits to report their injury way past the required time. The employer hopes that the injury will improve with care from just the company doctor. Then the employer doesn't report the claim at all. Employers are famous for declaring a worker an independent contractor to avoid Workers'Compensation coverage as well as misclassifying their workers to reduce insurance premiums. Employers have under-reported work as less hazardous than it really is. We've seen examples of employers underestimating employment projections at the beginning of the premium year to receive a better rate from the insurer, which, in effect, gives them more money to use during the year. Legitimately injured workers are discouraged and intimidated into not reporting their injuries . . . *Insurance fraud* is endless. They often misinform the injured workers of their rights, attempt to trick them into signing away their rights without their knowledge, deny/delay approval, deny/delay payment just to work 'the float.' We also see high numbers of unpaid benefits as well as inaccurate benefit notices. In some states, insurance companies have far outspent investigation of worker fraud than any other fraud in the Workers' Compensation system. A Texas study of Worker's Compensation fraud conducted by the state's Research and Oversight Council on Workers' Compensation found that, 'of the 4,077 cases of claimant fraud that were investigated, only 18 were prosecuted criminally.' The report concluded: 'It is clear that more resources should be spent fighting the most expensive and overlooked types of Workers' Compensation fraud: employer premium and health care provider fraud.' However, they do spend plenty of money to pay for video surveillance, private investigators, and a large staff—all of which is used to intimidate the injured worker out of their rights. When will they begin to seriously investigate insurance fraud? (pp. 295–6).

Although findings of different qualitative studies are difficult to aggregate, the thematic similarities among several of them are quite striking. In a very general way, the participants in the studies clearly indicated that they were suffering financially and emotionally, and that they felt victimized.

The studies do not provide any direct information about reasons why IWs do not recover from their injuries as rapidly or completely as private pay patients. (The interviewees in these studies communicated the sense that they were doing the best they could under very adverse circumstances.) However, given workers' descriptions of the severe stress they experienced in relation to their work injures, it is plausible to infer that their slow recoveries were products of stress. This hypothesis is consistent with a vast literature demonstrating adverse effects of emotional stress on health (Finestone et al. 2008; Schmidt et al. 2008).

A key problem in interpreting the many qualitative studies on IWs is that the study participants may not have been representative of IWs. For example, Beardwood et al. (2005) selected IWs who were going through training to become peer researchers; Crombie et al. (2003) informally gathered a cohort of physical therapists with work injuries; Cacciacarro and Kirsh (2006) recruited participants from an IW support group. It is certainly possible that the IWs who agreed to participate in the studies were particularly bitter ones who were not representative of IWs as a whole.

In principle, this possibility could be tested via systematic research on the satisfaction of IWs with WC systems. Such research could provide insights into whether the negative attitudes expressed by participants in the qualitative studies were representative of those of IWs in the aggregate, or reflected the views of a disgruntled minority. Unfortunately, very little research has been done on this issue. In one population based study that addressed attitudes of IWs toward the claim process (Wickizer et al. 2004a, 2004b), investigators found that while approximately 70% of the 804 study participants were very satisfied with the medical care they received, only 42% were very satisfied with the handling of their claim. These results suggest that IWs were modestly satisfied with administrative aspects of their claims. It should be noted that the 42% 'very satisfied' rate may overstate the degree of satisfaction that would be expressed by IWs with protracted claims. A key issue is that only 60% of the 804 study participants went on work disability because of their injuries, and only 13% were work disabled more than 6 months. The participants with prolonged work disability were significantly less satisfied with their care than ones with no or short term work disability. This subgroup of 13% was probably more comparable to participants in the qualitative studies than was the cohort as a whole.

If the results of qualitative studies on IWs are compared to results from more rigorous research done on moral hazards, malingering, and secondary gain, a striking mismatch becomes obvious. Moral hazard/malingering/secondary gain studies suggest that IWs are doing something deceitful in order to get financial gain. The behaviour of IWs might be unconscious, but nonetheless it is somewhat unseemly. The common thread in this research is that IWs (deliberately or unconsciously) drag their feet. In contrast, the qualitative studies document that IWs experience severe emotional distress and a sense of victimhood as they interact with WC systems. Although these studies do not address the issue of delayed recovery, they suggest that chronic, severe emotional distress contributes heavily to the delayed recoveries of IWs.

There is no simple way to integrate these two lines of research into a coherent theory that explains the delayed recovery of IWs. At first glance, it might seem appropriate to accept conclusions from moral hazards/malingering/secondary gain research, since it is more rigorous and more extensive than qualitative research on IWs. However, such a conclusion overlooks a fundamental point. As Hammer (2000) pointed out, it is quite possible that participants in WC other than IWs are engaged in unseemly behaviour. But essentially no systematic research has been on supervisors or owners of businesses, or on WC claims managers. Thus, the unflattering results of studies on IWs reflect in part the fact that the behaviour of IWs has been carefully scrutinized by numerous investigators. Representatives of the business community and WC systems have simply not been scrutinized.

The different pictures of IWs provided by qualitative studies vs. more formal studies on moral hazards/malingering/secondary gain highlight basic problems in untangling the factors that lead to delayed recovery among IWs. One basic problem is that the clinical recovery from an injury is affected not only by objectively measurable medical features of the injury, but also by a variety of host and environmental factors that are more difficult to measure. Similarly, the ability of an IW to return to work (or the probability that he/she will return to work) is influenced by a variety of factors other than strictly objective medical data about the worker's initial injury or response to treatment. Thus, while it is administratively convenient for WC carriers to focus on objective medical data when they make decisions about benefits (Robinson 2005), reliance on these data vastly oversimplifies the processes involved in recovery from an injury. Subjective data from

IWs—such as reports of continuing pain—can give a more realistic picture of the recovery process, but the reports can be manipulated by IWs in order to prolong their claims or receive unwarranted settlements. Physicians, claims managers, and others given the responsibility to make decisions about IWs have the difficult task of determining the veracity of statements by IWs about their clinical status and ability to work. Sceptics are likely to see evidence of foot dragging or outright fraud in these workers; advocates for IWs are likely to perceive the IWs as doing the best they can under very difficult circumstances. Evidence to date suggests that determining the 'true motives' of these IWs is difficult for the simple reason that the interpersonal appraisals needed to make such determinations are fraught with error (Robinson 2010).

## 18.4.3 **Other possible causes of the negative effect of WC**

### Lack of access to care

Some observers have noted that because of the poor reimbursement offered by WC carriers and the high burden of paper work imposed on physicians who treat IWs, experienced physicians with well established practices may refuse to treat these patients (Bellamy 2001; Pourat 2007). Thus, one possible explanation for poorer outcomes of IWs compared to private pay patients is that IWs do not receive comparable care. Although this is certainly a possibility, it would not account for the negative effect of WC documented by Harris et al. (2005), since in most of the studies in this review, the same physicians treated IWs and private pay patients.

### Involvement of unions

There is evidence that workers are more likely to file claims if they are union members (Morse et al. 2003). The authors of this study suggested several hypotheses to explain this effect, including: (1) high filing rates could be spurious byproducts of the fact that industries and occupations with high injury rates are relatively likely to be unionized; (2) unions might create a culture in which filing work injuries is views as legitimate; (3) unions might protect workers who file claims from retaliation.

### Involvement of attorneys

Involvement of an attorney may influence the course of a claim. In various studies, attorney involvement has been shown to be negatively associated with outcomes of a WC claim (Bernacki 2004; Katz et al. 2005; Bernacki et al. 2007; LaCaille et al. 2007; Bernacki and Tao 2008; Welch and Boden 2009). There is a problem of cause and effect, however. In particular, it is quite possible that IWs seek assistance from an attorney because they are not recovering from their injury, or are having adversarial interactions with their WC carrier. From this perspective, attorney involvement should be viewed as a marker of failure to recover rather than as a cause of failure to recover (Welch and Boden 2009). Consistent with this hypothesis, Wickizer et al. (2004b) found that in a cohort of 804 IWs, 46 retained an attorney. The median time between onset of the claim and retention of an attorney was 288 days. Thus, IWs tended to retain attorneys only after their claims had been opened for an extended period of time.

### The need to prove incapacitation

Norton Hadler has written extensively on contradictions within the WC system (Hadler 1995, 2005; Hadler et al. 2007). He has not articulated an easily summarized list of the ways in which WC negatively impact IWs, but one dynamic he has highlighted involves a paradox that individuals face as they interact with disability systems. He points out that it is difficult for individuals with medical problems to recover if, in order to maintain medical or disability benefits, they must repeatedly convince others that they are incapacitated (Hadler 1996). Although this assertion is difficult to prove in relation to WC, it is certainly consistent with research demonstrating that when people play various roles, they take on attitudes and beliefs consistent with these roles (Knapp et al. 1989; Smith et al. 1995). In the case of medical disorders, a patient who is forced by the WC system to play the role of a disabled person is likely to adopt the attitudes, beliefs, and behaviours of such a person.

## 18.5 **Moral hazards: another look**

As noted above, research on moral hazards has focused on the ways in which insurance benefits influence the behaviour of beneficiaries. This narrow focus obscures the fact all participants in WC can be influenced by moral hazards.

Employers may have overt or covert policies that influence claims behaviour. Injuries may not be reported in an attempt to avoid sanctions, increased insurance rates and increased healthcare costs. Workers who are deemed ready to return to partial or limited employment may be denied such opportunities by 'company policy' and thereby have their disabilities prolonged. Various forms of retaliation can follow claim for injury submission. In short, employers are just as suscep- tible to moral hazards influencing their behaviours as are the workers. We live in a capitalist system whose underlying principle is 'money motivates behaviour'.

Workers Compensation plan administrators are not immune to moral hazards. It has been our observation that plan administrators are more likely to identify with and support the employers' viewpoints than the workers'. They may support a range of policies that work to the disadvantage of IWs, including delaying treatment authorizations and imposing paperwork hurdles. Also, they may use a simple but effective method to encourage claims managers to close claims quickly. The claims managers continue to be assigned new claims regardless of rate at which they close claims. Thus, claims managers who do not move aggressively to close claims can be inundated by a mountain of new and old claims.

Physicians are also susceptible to moral hazards when a fee for service system gives them unlim- ited opportunities to provide services to injured workers. On the other hand, prepaid plans have the opposite effect of pushing providers to offer services as limited as possible. The effects of incentives often play out in forensic settings, where each physician expert swears that his testi- mony is the truth and nothing but the truth, but always reinforces the viewpoint of the attorney who has hired him.

Attorneys involved in WC have incentives that almost certainly influence their behaviour. Ones representing IWs typically work on contingency basis. If, for example, an attorney's client is awarded a pension by the WC carrier, the attorney gets a proportion of the award. Thus, attorneys representing IWs have an incentive to emphasize how disabled their clients are. In contrast, attor- neys representing WC carriers have incentives to minimize the exposure of their clients by doing what they can to minimize the benefits that IWs receive.

One might think that researchers are above the fray, and impartially seek to determine 'the truth' about the WC system. Unfortunately, new research has convincingly demonstrated that authors of scientific, economic, and philosophic papers might be influenced by the sources of funding for their research and writings. One obvious influence involves the choice of topics for research projects. As noted above, research funded by insurance companies and WC agencies focuses heavily on the behaviour of IWs. It rarely studies the behaviour of employers, and almost never examines the adverse effects that the companies and agencies might have on the recovery of IWs. At a more subtle level, there is evidence that the research results reported by investigators are statistically linked to the sources of support for their research. This effect has been demonstrated in relation to studies on the effectiveness of drugs (Bekelman et al. 2003; Bhandari et al. 2004;

Tereskerz and Moreno 2005; Fenton et al. 2007) For example, Lexchin et al. (2005) reviewed 30 publications that reported results from drug studies funded by pharmaceutical companies vs. ones with other sources of funding. The studies in the review considered a wide range of drugs, including tacrine, clozapine, third-generation oral contraceptives, erythropoietin, antidepressants, and topical glucocorticosteroids. The authors found that: 'Studies sponsored by pharmaceutical companies were more likely to have outcomes favouring the sponsor than were studies with other sponsors (odds ratio 4.05; 95% confidence interval 2.98 to 5.51; 18 comparisons). None of the 13 studies that analysed methods reported that studies funded by industry were of poorer quality' (p. 1167). Concerns about the potential for bias as a result of industry sponsorship have recently reached the political arena, with calls for a sunshine law in the US Senate (Grassley 2008), and requirements by journal editors that authors of papers provide information about sources of financial support for their work (Fontanarosa 2005).

Although the studies on industry sponsorship cited above deal with medicines and medical devices, they have clear implications for research on WC. Specifically, they suggest that research sponsored by WC carriers is likely to be biased in ways that are favourable toward the carriers and unfavourable toward IWs.

Thus, all of the players in the WC system are influenced by the systems in which they live and work and play. Workers are not uniquely influenced by the opportunities provided by a moral hazard. Studies should encompass the full range of such hazardous behaviours, including the behaviours of employers, WC claims managers, and other participants in the WC system. Moreover, researchers cannot be considered immune to the moral hazard effect. Thus, future research on the effects of incentives in the WC system should not only be more inclusive with respect to the topics investigated, but also should be funded by agencies other than WC carriers.

## 18.6 **Conclusions: implications for social policy**

An extensive body of literature supports the conclusion that WC systems exert an adverse effect on recovery from work injuries. As discussed above, several possible explanations for this negative effect have been proposed. A key question is: Does the research to date provide insights into how WC systems might be changed so as to encourage recovery among IWs?

Unfortunately, attempts to improve WC on the basis of the research discussed in this chapter run into at least 3 problems. First, different participants in and observers of the WC systems have profoundly different perspectives regarding the reasons why IWs demonstrate delayed recoveries. On one side of this divide are industry supporters, who in effect argue that IWs are at best careless and at worst fraudulent. In sharp contrast, advocates for IWs portray these people as victims and emphasize the suffering that they experience as they try to recover from work injuries. They express the view that there are abusers in the WC system, but that the abusers are employers and claims managers rather than employees. The key point here is that questions about causes of the negative effect of the WC system are anything but questions simply of science and research. Rather they are fundamentally intertwined with perceptions of social justice and ongoing conflicts between labour and management.

Second, it is inherently difficult to develop large scale programmes to support IWs that are efficient and sensitive to the emotional needs of individuals whose livelihoods are threatened by work injuries. Large, bureaucratic systems have inherent inefficiencies. In this regard, it is noteworthy that although several observers have criticized the WC systems in the United States and other Western countries, they have generally not offered concrete ideas about how to improve the systems.

Finally, research on moral hazards suggests an inherent contradiction in the social goals of WC systems. The contradiction can be seen when one ponders the question: How can a WC system provide support to IWs that eases their suffering without creating incentives for them to take advantage of this support?

Although the above points suggest that dramatic improvements in WC may be hard to achieve, there are certainly modest steps that could be taken. One important step would be to have research that is funded by agencies other than WC carriers, and that examines the behaviour of all participants in the WC system. Second, it would be interesting to examine the breadth of the negative effects of WC. For example, it would be interesting to see if the negative effect of WC documented by Harris et al. for surgical treatments also applies to rehabilitative treatments and other conservative therapies for various injuries.

Thirdly, it would be helpful to study experiments of nature in which fundamental principles of WC have been altered. For example, during the 1970s New Zealand's national health system eliminated the distinction between work-related and non-work-related medical conditions (McNaughton et al. 2000). It would be interesting to examine the impact of this change in social policy on the recovery from injuries and illnesses among citizens of New Zealand.

Finally, more systematic research is needed on the perceptions of IWs regarding WC systems. As noted above, Wickizer et al. (2004a) studied satisfaction of IWs in Washington State with their medical treatment and their interactions with the WC system. This kind of research should be replicated in other WC systems. At one extreme, it might demonstrate that from the perspective of IWs, WC systems usually function quite well. In that event, administrators of WC systems would be justified in continuing policies that already exist. Alternatively, research might confirm the negative attitudes voiced by IWs in the qualitative studies described above. If these attitudes turn out to be widespread among IWs, rather than limited to a few particularly bitter ones, it would be incumbent upon WC carriers to look carefully at their procedures, and modify them so as to become more 'customer-friendly'.

## References

**Analysis of workers' compensation laws.** (1996). Washington, DC: U.S. Chamber of Commerce, 1996.

**Aronoff GM, Mandel S, Genovese E, *et al.*** (2007). Evaluating malingering in contested injury or illness. *Pain Practice* **7** (2), 178–204.

**Atlas SJ, Chang Y, Kammann E, Keller RB, Deyo RA, Singer DE.** (2000). Long-term disability and return to work among patients who have a herniated lumbar disc: the effect of disability compensation. *J Bone Joint Surg Am* **82**(1), 4–15.

**Atlas SJ, Tosteson TD, Hanscom B, *et al.*** (2007). What is different about worker's compensation patients? *Spine* **32** (18), 2019–26.

**Auth J.** (2005). Employers must be alert to comp fraud. *Occup Health Saf* **74**(5), 12.

**Bartley MU.** (1994). Unemployment and ill health: understanding the relationship. *J Epidemiol Community Health* **48**(4), 333–7.

**Beardwood BA, Kirsh B, Clark NJ.** (2005). Victims twice over: perceptions and experiences of injured workers. *Qual Health Res* **15**(1), 30–48.

**Bekelman JE, Li Y, Gross CP.** (2003). Scope and impact of financial conflicts of interest in biomedical research. *JAMA* **289**, 454–65.

**Bellamy RE.** (2001). Workers' compensation: the patient, the physician, and the system. *J Bone Joint Surg Am* **83-A**(5), 781–3

**Bernacki EJ, Tao XG.** (2008). The relationship between attorney involvement, claim duration, and workers' compensation costs. *J Occup Environ Med* **50**(9), 1013–18.

**Bernacki EJ, Yuspeh L, Tao X.** (2007). Determinants of escalating costs in low risk workers' compensation claims. *J Occup Environ Med* **49**(7), 780–90.

Bernacki EJ. (2004). Factors influencing the costs of workers' compensation. *Clin Occup Environ Med* **4**(2), v–vi, 249–57.

Bhandari M, Busse JW, Jackowski D, *et al.* (2004). Association between industry funding and statistically significant pro-industry findings in medical and surgical randomized trials. *CMAJ* **170**, 477–80.

Bigos SJ, Battie MC, Spengler DM, *et al.* (1992). A longitudinal, prospective study of industrial back injury reporting. *Clin Orthop Relat Res* **279**, 21–34.

Bureau of Labor Statistics. (2008). Workplace injuries and illnesses in 2007. Bureau of Labor Statistics. http://www.bls.gov/iif/oshwc/osh/os/osnr0030.pdf. [Accessed 25 January 2009.]

Bureau of Labor Statistics. (2005). *Distribution of Injuries and Illnesses, by Nature,* 2005. http://www.bls. gov/iif/oshwc/osh/os/osh05_28.pdf [Accessed 30 January 2009.)

Cacciacarro L, Kirsh B. (2006). Exploring the mental health needs of injured workers. *Can J Occup Ther* **73**(3):178–87.

Cheadle A, Franklin G, Wolfhagen C, Savarino J, Liu PY, Salley C, Weaver M. (1994). Factors influencing the duration of work-related disability: a population-based study of Washington State workers' compensation. *Am J Public Health* **84**(2), 190–6.

Cole DC, Mondloch MV, Hogg-Johnson S. (2002). Listening to injured workers: how recovery expectations predict outcomes—a prospective study. *CMAJ* **166**(6), 749–54.

Cromie JE, Robertson VJ, Best MO. (2003). Physical therapists who claimed workers' compensation: a qualitative study. *Phys Ther* **83**(12), 1080–9.

Dembe AE, Boden LI. (2000). Moral hazard: a question of morality? *New Solut* **10**(3), 257–79.

Dersh J, Polatin PB, Leeman G, Gatchel RJ. (2004). The management of secondary gain and loss in medicolegal settings: strengths and weaknesses. *J Occup Rehabil* **14**(4), 267–79.

Dooley D, Fielding J, Levi L. (1996). Health and unemployment. *Annu Rev Public Health* **17**, 449–65.

Easton R. (1997). Screen patients quickly for workers' comp fraud. *Manag Care* **6**(4), 49–50.

Fenton JJ, Mirza SK, Lahad A, Stern BD, Deyo RA. (2007). Variation in reported safety of lumbar interbody fusion: influence of industrial sponsorship and other study characteristics. *Spine* **32**, 471–80.

Finestone HM, Alfeeli A, Fisher WA. (2008). Stress-induced physiologic changes as a basis for the biopsychosocial model of chronic musculoskeletal pain: a new theory? *Clin J Pain* **24**(9):767–75.

Fishbain D. (1994). Secondary gain concept: Definition problems and its abuse in medical practice. *Am Pain Soc J* **3**(4), 264–73.

Fishbain DA, Rosomoff HL, Cutler RB, *et al.* (1995). Secondary gain concept: A review of the scientific evidence. *Clin J Pain* **11**, 6–21.

Fishbain DA, Rosomoff HL, Cutler RB, Rosomoff RS. (1995). Secondary gain concept: A review of the scientific evidence. *Clin J Pain* **11**(1),: 6–21.

Fontanarosa PB, Flanagin A, DeAngelis CD. (2005). Reporting conflicts of interest, financial aspects of research, and role of sponsors in funded studies. *JAMA* **294**, 110–11.

M. Fricker M. (1997). , Widespread Fraud: Bogus Claim, *The Press Democrat,* December 7, 1997. [Cited in; Dembe AE, Boden LI. (2000). Moral hazard: a question of morality? *New Solut* **10**(3), 257–79.]

Fryer D, Fagan R. (2003). Toward a critical community psychological perspective on unemployment and mental health research. *Am J Community Psychol* **32**(1–2), 89–96.

Gabbe BJ, Cameron PA, Williamson OD, *et al.* (2007). The relationship between compensable status and long-term patient ourtcomes following orthopaedic trauma. *MJA* **187**(1), 14–7.

Gatchel RJ, Adams L, Polatin PB, *et al.* (2002). Secondary loss and pain-associated disability: theoretical overview and treatment implications. *J Occup Rehabil* **12**, 99–110.

Grassley C. (2008). Straight talk with . . . Charles Grassley. Interview by Meredith Wadman. *Nat Med* **14**(10):1006–7.

Hadler NM, Tait RC, Chibnall JT. (2007). Back pain in the workplace. *JAMA* **298**(4), 403–4

Hadler NM. (1995). The disabling backache. An international perspective. *Spine* **20**(6), 640–9.

Hadler NM. (1996). If you have to prove you are ill, you can't get well. The object lesson of fibromyalgia. *Spine* **21**(20), 2397–400

Hadler NM. (2005). The health assurance-disease insurance plan: harnessing reason to the benefits of employees. *J Occup Environ Med* **47**(7), 655–7

Hammer A. (2000). Word from the front lines: injured worker organizations speak out. *New Solut* **10**, 293–9.

Harkness EF, Macfarlane GJ, Nahit ES, Silman AJ, McBeth J. (2003). Risk factors for new-onset low back pain amongst cohorts of newly employed workers. *Rheumatology* **42**(8), 959–68.

Harris I, Mulford J, Solomon M *et al.* (2005). Association between compensation status and outcome after surgery: A meta-analysis. *JAMA* **293** (13), 1644–52.

Hunt HA. (2003).Benefit adequacy in state workers' compensation programs. *Soc Secur Bull* **65**(4), 24–30.

Katz JN, Amick BC 3rd, Keller R, Fossel AH, Ossman J, Soucie V, Losina E. (2005). Determinants of work absence following surgery for carpal tunnel syndrome. *Am J Ind Med* **47**(2), 120–30.

Kay N, Morris-Jones H. (1998). Pain clinic management of medico-legal litigants. *Injury* **29**, 305–8.

Kennedy F. (1946). The mind of the injured worker: its effect on disability periods. *Compensation Med* 1946; **1**, 19–24.

Kivimaki M, Head J, Ferrie JE, *et al.* (2003). Sickness absence as a global measure of health: evidence from mortality in the Whitehall II prospective cohort study. *BMJ* **327**(7411), 364–8.

Knapp, Patricia A.; Deluty, Robert H. (1989). Relative effectiveness of two behavioral parent training programs. *J Clin Child Psychol* **18**(4), 314–22.

LaCaille RA, DeBerard MS, LaCaille LJ, Masters KS, Colledge AL. (2007). Obesity and litigation predict workers' compensation costs associated with interbody cage lumbar fusion. *Spine J* **7**(3), 266–72.

Leino-Loison K, Gien LT, Katajisto J, Välimäki M. (2004). Sense of coherence among unemployed nurses. *J Adv Nurs* **48**(4), 413–22.

Lexchin J, Bero LA, Djulbegovic B, Clark O. (2005). Pharmaceutical industry sponsorship and research outcome and quality: systematic review. *BMJ* **326**, 1167–70.

Lippel K. (2007). Workers describe the effect of the workers' compensation process on their health: a Québec study. *Int J Law Psychiatry* **30**(4–5), 427–43.

Loeser JD, Henderlite SE, Conrad DE. (1995). Incentive effects of workers' compensation benefits: A literature synthesis. *Med Care Res Rev* **52**(1):34–59.

MacEachen E, Kosny A, Ferrier S. (2007). Unexpected barriers in return to work: lessons learned from injured worker peer support groups. *Work* **29**(2), 155–64.

Mah DR. (1998). Reducing workers' compensation fraud: a deterrent approach. *Occup Med* **13**(2), 429–38.

McNaughton HK, Sims A, Taylor WJ. (2000). Prognosis for people with back pain under a no-fualt 24-hour-cover compensation scheme. *Spine* 2000; **25**, 1254–8.

Mendelson G. (1988). *Psychiatric aspects of personal injury claims.* Springfield, IL: Charles C. Thomas.

Morse T, Dillon C, Warren N. (2000). Reporting of work-related musculoskeletal disorder (MSD) to workers Compensation. *New Solut* **10**(3), 281–92.

Morse T, Punnett L, Warren N, *et al.* (2003). The relationship of unions to prevalence and claim filing for work-related upper-extremity musculoskeletal disorders. *Am J Ind Med* 2003; **44**, 83–93.

Murphy GC, Athanasou JAT. (1999). The effect of unemployment on mental health. *J Occup Organisational Psychol* **72**, 83–100.

Mustard C, Hertzman C. (2001). Relationship between health services outcomes and social and economic outcomes in workplace injury and disease: data sources and methods. *Am J Ind Med* **40**(3), 335–43.

Overland S, Glozier N, Henderson M, *et al.* (2008). Health status before, during and after disabilkty pension award: the Hordaland Health Study (HUSK). *Occup Environ Med* **65**, 769–73.

Phoney worker's comp. claim?: smile, you may be on video (2007). *Nurs Law Regan Rep* **47**(11), 4.

Pourat N, Kominski G, Roby D, Cameron M. (2007). Physician perceptions of access to quality care in California's workers' compensation system. *J Occup Environ Med* **49**(6), 618–25.

'Retirees' disability epidemic'. (2008). *New York Times* 21 September, A1.

Reville RT, Seabury SA, Neuhauser FW, Burton JF, Greenberg MD. (2005). *An evaluation of California's permanent disability rating system*. Santa Monica, CA: RAND Corporation, MG-258.

Robinson J.P., Rondinelli R.D., & Scheer, S.J. (1997). Industrial rehabilitation medicine 1: Why is industrial rehabilitation medicine unique? *Arch Phys Med Rehabil*, **78**(3S), S3–S9.

Robinson, J.P. (2005). Disability management in primary care. In B. McCarberg & SD Passik (Ed.). *Expert guide to pain management*. Philadelphia, PA: American College of Physicians.

Robinson JP, Tait RC. (2010). Disability evaluation in painful conditions. In JC Ballantyne JP Rathmell, SM Fishman (Eds.) *Bonica's Management of Pain* (4th edn.). Philadelphia, PA: Lippincott Williams & Wilkins.

Scherzer T, Rugulies R, Krause N. (2005). Work-related pain and injury and barriers to workers' compensation among Las Vegas hotel room cleaners. *Am J Public Health* **95**(3), 483–8.

Schmidt MV, Sterlemann V, Müller MB. (2008). Chronic stress and individual vulnerability. *Ann N Y Acad Sci* **1148**, 174–83.

Shannon HS, Lowe GS. (2002). How many injured workers do not file claims for workers' compensation benefits? *Am J Ind Med* **42**, 467–73.

Smith, Mike U.; Katner, Harold P. (1995). Quasi-experimental evaluation of three AIDS prevention activities for maintaining knowledge, improving attitudes, and changing risk behaviors of high school seniors. *AIDS Educ Prev*, **7**(5), 391–402.

Soeker MS, Wegner L, Pretorius B. (2008). I'm going back to work: back injured clients' perceptions and experiences of their worker roles. *Work* **30**(2), 161–70.

Strunin L, Boden LI. (2004). The workers' compensation system: worker friend or foe? *Am J Ind Med* **45**, 338–45.

Tereskerz PM, Moreno J. (2005). Ten steps to developing a national agenda to address financial conflicts of interest in industry sponsored clinical research. *Account Res* **12**, 139–55.

Vahtera J, Pentti J, Kivimaki M. (2004). Sickness absence as a predictor of mortality among male and female employees. *J Epidemiol Community Health* **58**(4), 321–6.

Wallman T, Wedel H, Johansson S, *et al.* (2006). The prognosis for individuals on disability retirement. An 18-year mortality follow-up study of 6887 men and women sampled from the general population. *BMC Public Health* **6**(1), 103.

Welch LS, Boden LI. (2009). Attorney involvement, claim duration, and workers' compensation costs. *J Occup Environ Med* **51**(1), 1–2.

Wickizer TM, Franklin G, Fulton-Kehoe D, Turner JA, Mootz R, Smith-Weller T. (2004a). Patient satisfaction, treatment experience, and disability outcomes in a population-based cohort of injured workers in Washington State: implications for quality improvement. *Health Serv Res* **39**(4 Pt 1), 727–48.

Wickizer TM, Franklin G, Turner J, Fulton-Kehoe D, Mootz R, Smith-Weller T. (2004b). Use of attorneys and appeal filing in the Washington State workers' compensation program: does patient satisfaction matter? *J Occup Environ Med* **46**(4), 331–9.

Williams CA. (1991). *An international comparison of workers' compensation*. Boston, MA: Kluwer Academic Publishers.

# Chapter 19

# Work-Related Risk Factors for Transition to Chronic Back Pain and Disability

William S. Shaw, Glenn S. Pransky, and Chris J. Main

## 19.1 **Introduction**

Low back pain (LBP) is a common cause of suffering and disability in workers. As many as 85% of workers will experience at least one episode of back pain severe enough to limit their ability to work. Yet, most do recover, returning to normal function at work and at home, although bothersome symptoms may persist or intermittently recur. Among those recovered from an acute episode of work-related LBP, the prevalence of recurrent pain over the following year is 50–60%, but recurring sickness absence from work occurs in only 12–15% of cases (Marras et al. 2007; Wasiak et al. 2003). Approximately 10% of those with an acute episode of disabling back pain progress to develop long-term problems that include both significant pain and limitations in their ability to function at work and at home (Nachemson et al. 2000; Waddell et al. 2002). This small group accounts for the majority of LBP-related suffering and associated costs in working-age persons. In the USA, 18% of workers lose an estimated 149 million days of work due to LBP annually (Guo et al. 1995). There are comparable figures in other industrialized countries (van Tulder et al. 1995). This significant burden has attracted the attention of workers, employers, providers, insurers, and governments, who are seeking better ways to prevent pain and disability in those who would otherwise be contributing to economic productivity.

The workplace has a number of features of specific relevance to LBP occurrence, treatment, and consequences. First, it is important to distinguish chronic pain (persistent symptoms) from chronic disability (inability to function at work), because these outcomes are often independent (Volinn et al. 1988). Indeed, in countries with a workers' compensation system, the distinction between injuries caused by work and those of non-occupational origin is of legal necessity, although this distinction is not always supported by scientific evidence. LBP that is persistent or intermittent, but does not result in significant pain, functional limitations, or work disability, may be troublesome but of much less importance to workers as long as they can maintain employment. Thus return-to-work (RTW) in those off work may be the most salient outcome for workers with acute LBP, as these outcomes are directly linked to key social roles and economic status for working-age adults (Cats-Baril and Frymoyer 1991).

It is difficult to quantify the precise relationship between LBP and work since working adults with LBP may encounter issues unique to the nature of their work and workplace. LBP-related functional limitations may lead to inability to do some jobs, but they may have little or no impact on other jobs. Similarly, on-site healthcare services, employer accommodations, and co-worker support can enable rapid recovery and RTW, but there is huge variation in the assistance and support available to injured workers. Finally, on a macro level, the involvement of a workers' compensation or disability insurer may also facilitate RTW, but insurance systems can also lead to legal conflicts that can prolong work disability.

Across disparate insurance and governmental benefit systems, a number of work-related factors have been consistently associated with poor outcomes in LBP, including progression to chronic disability, and these are the focus of this chapter. Even after controlling for a number of health, psychosocial, and demographic variables, characteristics of work and the work environment are significant predictors of continued symptoms, functional incapacity, and prolonged disability (Shaw et al. 2001). These factors can be identified early on, before chronicity has developed. We review the evidence supporting these workplace factors, appraise methods for identifying them and explore the opportunity for subsequent interventions to prevent long-term, chronic disability. Although research on workplace interventions is somewhat limited, enough information is available to provide some well-supported recommendations to healthcare providers, employers, and others. Nonetheless, a caveat is necessary: these work factors have been primarily studied in relationship to workplace-relevant outcomes, commonly RTW, recurrent disability, and function at work. Their association with other outcomes such as pain or overall quality of life tends to be weaker (Franche et al. 2005; Hasenbring et al. 1994).

## 19.2 **Workplace risk factors**

There are now numerous cross-sectional, retrospective, and prospective cohort studies that have examined the effects of various factors on the progression from acute to chronic LBP. The most commonly supported disability risk factors include demographic variables, pain and pain beliefs, perceptions of function and expected recovery, and workplace physical and psychosocial environment (Waddell 2004). For the outcome of back disability, psychosocial variables (including perceptions of the work environment) seem to be better overall prognostic indicators than either demographic or clinical exam findings. Thus, individual and workplace psychosocial factors have been highlighted as crucial in the development of long-term disability (Crook et al. 2002). These factors reflect some of the greatest challenges facing workers with LBP—managing symptoms while at work, overcoming the frustrations of having to ask for help, lacking the job flexibility to modify physical demands, and failing to meet productivity demands (Shaw and Huang 2005).

To identify the most important workplace risk factors for prolonged LBP chronicity and disability, we searched for English language scientific reviews that summarized workplace risk factors for LBP and disability, published since the year 2000. Studies of both work-related and non-work related LBP were included. We identified six reviews that met these criteria. Most of the reviewers focused on those factors supported by prospective cohort studies. Some reviews were limited to workplace risk factors, but most included both individual and workplace factors. As these reviews have applied different methods for synthesizing results, there are some conflicting conclusions. As examples, job satisfaction was supported in four of six reviews, job stress and social support were supported in some reviews and not by others; and only one review took magnitude of effect (relative risk) into account (Hartvigsen et al. 2004).

We compiled a list of the risk factors supported by the scientific evidence in at least one review, resulting in the 24 variables identified in Table 19.1. For convenience we have grouped these under four types of factors: physical work demands, social climate at work, perceptions about health and work, and workplace disability management. Each of the four groupings is described below:

*Physical work demands.* The five job physical demand factors all relate to the likelihood that a worker with diminished capacity due to LBP will be unable to meet significant job demands. The advantage of jobs in the public sector may relate to larger workforces where additional help is more readily available; the opposite is true for jobs where a worker has to drive to a remote location, and thus may often be working alone. The availability of modified duty can address the

**Table 19.1** Variables described and supported as modifiable risk factors for chronic LBP disability in recent literature reviews (2000–2005)

| Factors | Hartvigsen et al. (2004) | Crook et al. (2002) | Hoogendoorn et al. (2000) | Linton (2001) | Shaw et al. (2001) | Steenstra et al. (2005) |
|---|---|---|---|---|---|---|
| Workplace—physical demands | | | | | | |
| Fast work pace | ✓ | ✓ | | ✓ | | |
| Heavier physical demands | | | | | ✓ | ✓ |
| Work demands > capacity | | ✓ | | ✓ | | |
| Private industry (versus public) | | ✓ | | | | |
| Driving (as majority of job) | | | | | | ✓ |
| Workplace—social/managerial | | | | | | |
| Social support or dysfunction | | ✓ | | ✓ | ✓ | ✓ |
| Supervisor support | | | | | | ✓ |
| Lack of control | ✓ | ✓ | ✓ | ✓ | | ✓ |
| Short job tenure | | ✓ | | | ✓ | |
| Conflict at work | | | ✓ | | | |
| Inability to take breaks at will | | ✓ | | | | |
| Workplace—worker perceptions | | | | | | |
| Job dissatisfaction | ✓ | ✓ | ✓ | ✓ | | |
| Monotonous work | | | | ✓ | | ✓ |
| Job stress | | | | ✓ | ✓ | ✓ |
| Belief work is dangerous | | | | ✓ | | |
| Emotional effort of work | | | | ✓ | | |
| Belief should not work with pain | | | | ✓ | | |
| Work-related disability issues | | | | | | |
| WC claim (vs. non-wk related) | | ✓ | | | | ✓ |
| Prior work disability claim | | ✓ | | | | |
| Discouraging claim reporting | | | | | | ✓ |
| Delayed report of injury | | ✓ | | | ✓ | |
| Lower quality immediate medical care | | | | | | ✓ |
| Lack of modified duty | | ✓ | | | ✓ | ✓ |
| Higher wage replacement rate | | ✓ | | | | ✓ |

Notes: ✓=review found at least moderate evidence supporting this risk factor.

RTW barrier of high work demands, and thus potentially counteract its negative effect (Weir and Nielson 2001). While there is evidence of an interaction between job demands and psychosocial work environment in the development of musculoskeletal symptoms (Devereux et al. 1999; Devereux et al. 2002), few prospective studies of RTW outcomes have tested or reported such interactions.

*Social climate at work.* Social or managerial issues may influence disability outcomes in several ways. Workers who experience low levels of social support at work, from co-workers or supervisors, may be concerned that no one will look after their interests after they return to work. Jobs that are structured so that workers have little control, or an inability to take breaks, may reflect adverse or unsupportive labor-management relationships. Conflicts at work might be a result of poor social relationships. Those with short job tenure may not have had adequate time or opportunity in the workplace to develop supportive relationships. Some have theorized that lack of social support leads to more anxiety and arousal in the context of LBP, with higher levels of pain and dysfunction, and subsequent delays in RTW (Brouwer et al. 2009; Marhold et al. 2002) (see also Chapter 17).

*Perceptions about health and work.* Worker perceptions are important, as they can all contribute to a negative attitude towards the workplace, and subsequent reluctance to pursue RTW. Jobs that are perceived as stressful or monotonous, emotionally exhausting, unsatisfying or dangerous, may be undesirable even before onset of low back pain; thus, workers in these positions may actively seek other alternatives rather than return to the same position. A worker's beliefs that he or she should not return to work until completely pain-free may reflect some of these underlying perceptions about the job (Linton 2001).

*Workplace disability management.* The last category comprises policies about low back pain in the workplace- how it is identified, treated, and how the disability consequences are managed. Workplaces that are most successful in minimizing LBP disability usually have several of the following characteristics: (1) encouraging workers with LBP concerns to come forward; (2) a systematic approach that includes supervisor support and access to evidence-based initial care; (3) early attention to disability issues through communication and offer of alternate duty to avoid disability; and (4) appropriate organization of economic incentives (for workers and supervisors) to insure that it's worthwhile for workers to come back to work as soon as possible (Westmorland et al. 2005).

## 19.3 **Screening for workplace factors**

The evidence-based workplace factors listed above, as well as additional items (both work-related and non-occupational factors), are included in several available clinical screening tools. Some tools also guide the interview and evaluation process, to help clinicians find out more about specific occupational situations, and provide information that can guide individualized efforts to address these issues. We have identified seven representative approaches including the Örebro Musculoskeletal Pain Screening Questionnaire (ÖMPSQ) (Linton and Hallden 1998), the Psychosocial Risk for Occupational Disability Instrument (PRODI) (Schultz et al. 2005) the Back Disability Risk Questionnaire (BDRQ) (Shaw et al. 2005), the 'blue flags' screening process (Shaw et al. 2009), the Work Disability Diagnosis Interview (WoDDI) (Durand et al. 2002), the Obstacles to Return-to-work Questionnaire (ORQ) (Marhold et al. 2002), and the Participatory Ergonomics (PE) approach first described by Loisel and colleagues (Loisel et al. 2001a).

The approaches listed above differ in method, content, and specific objectives. Some were designed to provide a quantification of disability risk in research cohorts, whereas others were designed as practical tools to guide clinical interviewing. Although brief patient questionnaires and semi-structured clinical interviews have been the primary mode of screening patients for risk of chronic disabling LBP, detailed assessment can be more informative. The first three approaches are questionnaires exclusively based on patient self-report. The ÖMPSQ includes information on job physical demands and satisfaction, and expectations about RTW and the safety of RTW. It is the only one of these instruments that has been subjected to formal validation in multiple settings. The PRODI includes more occupational factors, such as skill discretion, decision authority, job security, co-worker/supervisor support, control, overall support, resources, RTW expectation, and employer response to LBP. The BDRQ was designed for early screening of acute LBP, and includes physical work demands, RTW expectations, availability of modified duty, delay in reporting the LBP problem, and negative supervisor responses.

The other methods collect more detail through interviews and other assessments. In 1997, Kendall and colleagues developed a system for early identification and management of clinical and occupational risk factors (termed Yellow Flags) for unnecessary/prolonged disability in LBP (Kendall 1999). This list of specific questions was designed to prompt healthcare practitioners to identify persons at high risk for prolonged disability and to explore these factors. This approach has been re-conceptualized into blue flags (worker perceptions of an adverse work environment) and black flags (objective measures of employment conditions, physical job demands, and insurance system characteristics) (Shaw et al. 2009; Main 2002). The ORQ includes questions on difficulties returning to work, physical workload and perceived harmfulness, social support, worries about sick leave, work satisfaction, and RTW expectations. The WoDDI includes both self-report and a semi-structured diagnostic interview to address job satisfaction, work history, occupation and industry type, prior attempts to RTW, absence duration, job demands, ergonomic risk factors, work schedule, job control, environmental conditions, diversity of work tasks, and working relationships. The participatory ergonomics approach advocated by Loisel incorporates the WoDDI as well as an on-site workplace evaluation by a physical therapist.

The choice of an ideal screening method for important workplace factors depends in part on the intended application. Unfortunately, data on predictive performance are available only for screening questionnaires. These can identify the probability of delayed RTW but by themselves may not be able to specify the issues unique to an individual case (Durand et al. 2002). The reliability, validity, and added value of a more detailed, in-depth but less structured interview are difficult to quantify, but this approach may be necessary to guide clinical and workplace interventions. We recommend a staged method of screening, involving multiple methods as needed (questionnaire, interview, worksite visit), as an effective and efficient approach to identifying obstacles to recovery in the workplace. Risk stratification questionnaires are more appropriate during an acute stage, to identify risk factors early on. More detailed methods can be used when screening is positive for workplace factors, or when there is a more prolonged absence from work (subacute or chronic back pain and disability). This approach is consistent with other screening methods in primary care that typically start with a patient self-report questionnaire (e.g. depression, sleeping disorders, irritable bowel syndrome) (Dejesus et al. 2007; Doghramji 2004).

## 19.4 **Intervention strategies based on workplace risk factors**

Several disciplines have contributed to the range of strategies now available to address workplace risk factors, including occupational, rehabilitation and behavioural medicine, clinical and occupational psychology, kinesiology, and occupational and physical therapy. Interventions have focused on employer efforts to improve support from supervisors and co-workers, or to reduce ergonomic exposure (Baril et al. 2003; Nicholas 2002; Shaw et al. 2006a). Acute care interventions include coordinating medical care with RTW efforts, managing the use of various treatments, modifying provider behaviour (Derebery et al. 2002; Loisel et al. 2005), and improving the readiness of patients to RTW through physical conditioning, education, and often formal or informal counselling (Gatchel et al. 2003; Linton and Nordin 2006). A recent review of workplace-based return-to-work interventions led reviewers to conclude moderate or strong evidence for five categories of intervention: (1) early contact by the workplace with the worker; (2) an offer of job accommodation; (3) contact between healthcare provider and workplace; (4) ergonomic work site visit; and (5) presence of a RTW coordinator (Franche et al. 2005). These findings emphasize the importance of communication among stakeholders and the need for job accommodations in order to facilitate a successful RTW process. Matching patients to early interventions for LBP based on individual risk factors may improve outcomes and the cost effectiveness of early intervention (Waddell 2004). Recent studies have shown preliminary evidence of patient clusters by risk factors in early stages of LBP (Boersma and Linton 2006; Shaw et al. 2009), providing further support for a risk factor-based approach to early intervention. We have categorized these factors into groups that connote different intervention strategies—some at an organizational level, others at an individual level. A risk factor-based intervention strategy could provide treatments that map directly onto measured risk factors for individual patients.

Workplace physical demands can be addressed through temporary work restrictions or modifications, and efforts to improve workplace ergonomics, ideally through an inclusive, participatory approach (Anema et al. 2003; Krause et al. 1998). In some instances, directed physical therapy and exercise can have a role in restoring work ability (Lindström et al. 1992; Cooper et al. 1997). Cognitive-behavioural strategies may help workers to cope with job strain. Social/managerial factors suggest interventions to improve relationships and communication between supervisors and workers, and the importance of flexibility in the workplace in the return to work process (Shaw, Robertson et al. 2006). Some interventions rely on an ergonomics approach as a process for safe reintegration, yet also include substantial efforts to improve communication and resolve conflicts in the workplace (Arnetz et al. 2003).

Personal perceptions that work is dissatisfying, dangerous, or likely to cause re-injury may be important mediators of back pain disability. These perceptions could result in part from a lack of support, a mismatch with job requirements, job stress, or an undesirable physical or psychosocial working environment. It's unclear whether interventions should attempt to modify these beliefs in the absence of other workplace modifications or coordination efforts. In most cases, these perceptions are likely to be well-established over time, based on a realistic appraisal, so psychological approaches to alter these beliefs would seem daunting and misguided. The optimal strategy would rectify the factors underlying these perceptions, guided by a more detailed and broad-based inquiry (van Duijn et al. 2004). Interventions that have addressed workplace risk factors (such as those featuring improved communication, accommodations, RTW policies, procedures, or support) may actually accomplish this, but studies have not evaluated the impact on workplace perceptions. Thus it's not clear whether a possible change in perceptions precedes improvement in disability outcomes, or whether this is a secondary consequence of intervention. Nevertheless, these perceptions might be of value to providers outside of the workplace. They can help to identify significant RTW barriers that might not be amenable to change. This could lead to more active efforts to secure safe accommodation, to alert the workplace for the need for more positive communication and support, or to open a dialogue to suggest that a worker may want to consider an alternative position or employer.

The factors that relate to the approach to health and disability in the workplace suggest the strategy of a coordinated, positive, supportive and consistent approach to work disability (Shrey and Hursh 1999). Elements can include encouraging early reporting of potentially disabling back problems, treatment with selected providers, improved communication between providers and employers, rapidly providing temporary accommodations if needed, and coordinating the return-to-work process, with positive incentives to return to work (Bernacki and Tsai 2003).

## 19.5 **Opportunities for future research and practice improvement**

Although screening for workplace risk factors offers some promising opportunities, there are considerable limitations in current knowledge and practice that limit application. Future research on risk factor identification, targeted intervention, and impacts on outcomes can significantly contribute to this field.

Improvement in theoretical rigour and consistency in risk factor research are two areas for further development. The selection of prognostic variables, assessment methods, and choice of outcome measures varies considerably. General acceptance of a framework that defines categories of workplace variables that can be routinely incorporated across studies would be an important advance. Several conceptual models of RTW have been advanced (Loisel et al. 2001b; Young et al. 2005; Schultz et al. 2007), but most risk factor studies rely on readily-available data, rather than choosing factors based on a conceptual model. Others have selected variables and conducted analyses based on various classifications—physical versus psychological (Steenstra et al. 2005; Loisel 2007), modifiable versus non-modifiable (Shaw, Linton et al. 2006), locus of control (worker, workplace, physician or insurer) (Loisel et al. 2001b), and individual-level versus workplace-wide factors (Sullivan et al. 2005). In the review by Hartvigsen and colleagues, grouping variables within four clusters (perception of work, organizational aspects, social support, and stress) diminished the associations with outcomes, and resulted in their finding of mostly negative or inconclusive results (Hartvigsen et al. 2004). Thus, retaining the specificity of prognostic variables seems important. Some of the variables that have been assessed in just one or two studies may actually be important, but lack wider support. Other problems include inconsistency in statistical modelling techniques, varying durations of follow-up, and inclusion of different covariates when testing the independent association of factors with outcomes (Pransky et al. 2001; Linton et al. 2005).

Theoretically, interventions that alleviate causal risk factors should lead to effective disability prevention, and risk factor screening should provide a reasonable basis for determining who is likely to benefit from a specific intervention. However, variables commonly referred to as risk factors for chronic LBP might be more appropriately labelled as 'risk indicators' or 'risk markers', as most have not been subjected to rigorous criteria for concluding causation (e.g. demonstrating dose-response relationships), and many variables overlap in their ability to predict outcomes. Furthermore, there is some debate as to whether prognostic studies of LBP have been plagued by significant measurement and confounding biases (Hayden and Cote 2006). While there is widespread agreement that an early RTW reduces long-term disability risk, strategies for facilitating an early RTW have varied considerably. The diversity of successful RTW interventions calls into question the mechanisms underlying their effect. The complexities of workplace and worker factors related to disability, the inevitability of significant changes over time at work, and the impossibility of identifying identical control situations have seriously hampered efforts to conduct randomized, controlled trials. Instead, return-to-work interventions are sometimes evaluated only with pre- and post-comparisons within single organizations, sometimes without the benefit of a comparison non-intervention group. Though less rigorous, these studies can nevertheless provide an understanding of the key processes that lead to various outcomes (Kristensen 2005).

Significant logistical challenges exist for screening patients and assigning relevant treatments based on prognostic factors, and there is little consensus as to which intervention strategies match specific risk factors. One approach is to intervene only for those deemed 'high risk' based on a summation of all empirical risk factors, including both modifiable and non-modifiable (e.g. demographic) variables (Gatchel et al. 2003). Another approach is to develop an intervention that targets a single risk factor, then screen patients for those high on that risk factor. For example, Von Korff and colleagues (Von Korff et al. 2005) developed a brief fear reduction and physical activation intervention for primary care patients with chronic LBP, then provided the intervention only to those patients reporting significant activity limitations. The results showed improvements in pain-related fear and activity limitations compared with a no-treatment control group over a 2-year follow-up. Such studies have not been conducted in the acute or subacute stages of LBP, when there may be even greater potential for reducing work absence.

One new idea in RTW workplace intervention trials is the possibility of bolstering informal support and accommodation processes that occur naturally in the workplace setting and supporting or enhancing the self-management efforts of workers with pain or other health concerns (Varekamp et al. 2009). Based on the high prevalence of chronic back pain (15–30%) reported by working-age adults (Hardt et al. 2008; Watkins et al. 2008), most workers apparently find ways to manage back pain on the job and obtain help from others without the need for any long sickness absences or formal administrative processes, and this effective use of workplace leeway has been described in qualitative studies (Durand et al. 2009). This variety of 'workplace intervention' is actually planned and executed by workers themselves, without the need for formal managerial or administrative processes that document and track an employer's decision to 'allow' individual job modifications. To promote these self-management processes, employers can designate 'coping contacts' within the workforce, encourage and support worker self-management strategies, and provide frontline supervisors and employees greater autonomy for organizing and modifying job tasks (Varekamp et al. 2008; Werner et al. 2007). While the results of early studies look promising (Werner et al. 2007), such workplace programs based on peer support and worker empowerment require further study.

Despite some positive research findings, the dissemination of these intervention strategies to clinical and workplace settings has been slow. Even among specialists in occupational medicine and rehabilitation, many obstacles exist for intervening in the workplace, including barriers to employer communication, limited information about job tasks and prospects for modifying work, and employers unwilling or unable to provide modified or transitional work (Costa-Black et al. 2007; Loisel et al. 2005; Pransky et al. 2004). Cost-effectiveness, an important factor in the adoption of such experimental interventions, may be improved if interventions are directed only to those with demonstrable need based on risk factor assessment. In particular, authors have emphasized the need to reduce the growing list of workplace variables to a manageable set of core factors, improve the accuracy and utility of patient screening, and develop effective and plausible intervention strategies to address workplace concerns (Cedraschi and Allaz 2005; Feldman 2004; Shaw et al. 2006b).

In summary, we know that workplace factors are of primary importance in determining chronic work disability outcomes, they can be identified early on in the course of LBP, and certain workplace interventions appear to be very successful at improving outcomes. Although methods to screen for workplace factors are still under development, there are several sets of available questionnaires and interview guides that can help clinicians identify and address these problems. A number of interventions have led to much better RTW outcomes, mostly targeting the response of the workplace to a report of a disabling back condition, and the process of communication and facilitation around RTW. Despite all of this knowledge, there is still much to be learned—how to best identify and explore workplace factors, how to effectively address these factors, how to overcome perceptions that workplace factors are unmodifiable, and how to bring along providers, employers and others to optimize the long-term outcomes of workers with LBP.

## References

Anema, J.R., Steenstra, I.A., Urlings, I.J., Bongers, P.M., de Vroome, E.M., and van Mechelen, W. (2003). Participatory ergonomics as a return-to-work intervention: a future challenge? *American Journal of Industrial Medicine*, **44**, 273–81.

Arnetz, B.B., Sjogren, B., Rydehn, B., and Meisel, R. (2003). Early workplace intervention for employees with musculoskeletal-related absenteeism: a prospective controlled intervention study. *Journal of Occupational and Environmental Medicine*, **45**, 499–506.

Baril, R., Clarke, J., Friesen, M., Stock, S., and Cole, D. (2003). Work-ready group. Management of return-to-work programs for workers with musculoskeletal disorders: a qualitative study in three Canadian provinces. *Social Science & Medicine*, **57**, 2101–14.

Bernacki, E.J. and Tsai, S.P. (2003). Ten years' experience using an integrated workers' compensation management system to control workers' compensation costs. *Journal of Occupational and Environmental Medicine*, **45**, 508–16.

Boersma, K. and Linton, S.J. (2006). Psychological processes underlying the development of a chronic pain problem: a prospective study of the relationship between profiles of psychological variables in the fear-avoidance model and disability. *Clinical Journal of Pain*, **22**, 160–6.

Brouwer, S., Krol, B., Reneman, M.F. *et al*. (2009). Behavioral determinants as predictors of return to work after long-term sickness absence: an application of the theory of planned behavior. *Journal of Occupational Rehabilitation*, **19**, 166–74.

Cats-Baril, W.L. and Frymoyer, J.W. (1991). The economics of spinal disorders. In J.W. Frymoyer (Ed.) *The Adult Spine*, pp. 85–106. New York: Raven.

Cedraschi, C. and Allaz, AF. (2005). How to identify patients with a poor prognosis in daily clinical practice. *Baillieres Best Practice and Research in Clinical Rheumatology*, **19**, 577–91.

Cooper, J.E., Tate, R., and Yassi, A. (1997). Work hardening in an early return to work program for nurses with back injury. *Work*, **8**, 149–56.

Costa-Black, K.M., Durand, M.J., Imbeau, D., Baril, R., and Loisel, P. (2007). Interdisciplinary team discussion on work environment issues related to low back disability: a multiple case study. *Work*, **28**, 249–65.

Crook, J., Milner, R., Schultz, I.Z., and Stringer, B. (2002). Determinants of occupational disability following a back injury: A critical review of the literature. *Journal of Occupational Rehabilitation*, **12**, 277–95.

Dejesus, R.S., Vickers, K.S., Melin, G.J., and Williams, M.D. (2007). A system-based approach to depression management in primary care using the Patient Health Questionnaire-9. *Mayo Clinic Proceedings*, **82**, 1395–402.

Derebery, V.J., Giang, G.M., Saracino, G., and Fogarty, W.T. (2002). Evaluation of the impact of a low back pain educational intervention on physicians' practice patterns and patients' outcomes. *Journal of Occupational and Environmental Medicine*, **44**, 977–84.

Devereux, J.J., Buckle, P.W., and Vlachonikolis, I.G. (1999). Interactions between physical and psychosocial risk factors at work increase the risk of back disorders; an epidemiological approach. *Occupational and Environmental Medicine*, **56**, 343–53.

Devereux, J.J., Vlachonikolis, I.G., and Buckle, P.W. (2002). Epidemiological study to investigate potential interaction between physical and psychosocial factors at work that may increase the risk of symptoms of musculoskeletal disorder of the neck and upper limb. *Occupational and Environmental Medicine*, **59**, 269–77.

Doghramji, P.P. (2004). Recognizing sleep disorders in a primary care setting. *Journal of Clinical Psychiatry*, **65**(Suppl 16), 23–6.

Durand, M.J., Loisel, P., Hong, Q.N., and Charpentier, N. (2002). Helping clinicians in work disability prevention: the work disability diagnosis interview. *Journal of Occupational Rehabilitation*, **12**(3), 191–204.

Durand, M.J., Vézina, N., Baril, R., Loisel, P., Richard, M.C., and Nogomo, S. (2009). Margin of manoeuvre indicators in the workplace during the rehabilitation process: a qualitative analysis. *Journal of Occupational Rehabilitation*, **19**, 194–202.

Feldman, J.B. (2004). The prevention of occupational low back pain disability: evidence-based reviews point in a new direction. *Journal of Surgical Orthopaedic Advances*, **13**, 1–14.

Franche, R.L., Cullen, K., Clarke, J. *et al*. (2005). Research Team. Workplace-based return-to-work interventions: a systematic review of the quantitative literature. *Journal of Occupational Rehabilitation*, **15**, 607–31.

Gatchel, R.J., Polatin, P.B., Noe, C., Gardea, M., Pulliam, C., and Thompson, J. (2003). Treatment and cost-effectiveness of early intervention for acute low-back pain patients: A one-year prospective study. *Journal of Occupational Rehabilitation*, **13**, 1–9.

Guo, H.R., Tanaka, S., and Cameron, L.L. (1995). Back pain among workers in the United States: national estimates and workers at high risk. *American Journal of Industrial Medicine*; **28**, 591–602.

Hardt, J., Jacobsen, C., Goldberg, J., Nickel, R., and Buchwald, D. (2008). Prevalence of chronic pain in a representative sample in the United States. *Pain Medicine*, **9**, 803–12.

Hartvigsen, J., Lings, S., Leboeuf-Yde, C., and Bakketeig, L. (2004). Psychosocial factors at work in relation to low back pain and consequences of low back pain; a systematic, critical review of prospective cohort studies. *Occupational and Environmental Medicine*, **61**, e2.

Hasenbring, M., Marienfeld, G., Kuhlendahl, D., and Soyka, D. (1994). Risk factors of chronicity in lumbar disc patients. A prospective investigation of biologic, psychologic, and social predictors of therapy outcome. *Spine*, **19**, 2759–65.

Hayden, J., Côté, P., and Bombardier, C. (2006). Evaluation of the quality of prognosis studies in systematic reviews. *Annals of Internal Medicine,* **144**, 427–37.

Hoogendoorn, W.E., van Poppel, M.N., Bongers, P.M., Koes, B.W., and Bouter, L.M. (2000). Systematic review of psychosocial factors at work and private life as risk factors for back pain. *Spine*, **25**, 2114–25.

Kendall, N.A. (1999). Psychosocial approaches to the prevention of chronic pain: the low back paradigm. *Baillieres Best Practice and Research in Clinical Rheumatology*, **13**, 545–54.

Krause, N., Dasinger, L.K., and Neuhauser, F. (1998). Modified work and return to work: a review of the literature. *Journal of Occupational Rehabilitation*, **8**, 113–19.

Kristensen, T.S. (2005). Intervention studies in occupational epidemiology. *Occupational and Environmental Medicine*, **62**, 205–10.

Lindström, I., Ohlund, C., Eek, C., Wallin, L., Peterson, L.E., and Nachemson, A. (1992). Mobility, strength, and fitness after a graded activity program for patients with subacute low back pain. A randomized prospective clinical study with a behavioral therapy approach. *Spine*, **17**, 641–52.

Linton, S.J. (2001). Occupational psychological factors increase the risk for back pain: A systematic review. *Journal of Occupational Rehabilitation*, **11**, 53–66.

Linton, S.J. and Hallden, K. (1998). Can we screen for problematic back pain? A screening questionnaire for predicting outcome in acute and subacute back pain. *Clinical Journal of Pain*, **14**, 209–15.

Linton, S.J. and Nordin, E. (2006). A 5-year follow-up evaluation of the health and economic consequences of an early cognitive behavioral intervention for back pain: A randomized, controlled trial. *Spine*, **31**, 853–8.

Linton, S.J., Gross, D., Schultz, I.Z. *et al.* (2005). Prognosis and the identification of workers risking disability: research issues and directions for future research. *Journal of Occupational Rehabilitation*, **15**, 459–74.

Loisel, P. (2007). Pain in the workplace, compensation, and disability management. In R.F. Schmidt & W.D. Willis (Eds.) *Encyclopedia of Pain*, pp. 1703–5. New York: Springer.

Loisel, P., Durand, M.J., Berthelette, D. *et al.* (2001). Disability prevention–new paradigm for the management of occupational back pain. *Disease Management and Health Outcomes*, **9**, 351–60.

Loisel, P., Gosselin, L., Durand, P., Lemaire, J., Poitras, S., and Abenhaim, L. (2001). Implementation of a participatory ergonomics program in the rehabilitation of workers suffering from subacute back pain. *Applied Ergonomics,* **32**, 53–60.

Loisel, P., Durand, M.J., Baril, R., Gervais, J., and Falardeau, M. (2005). Interorganizational collaboration in occupational rehabilitation: perceptions of an interdisciplinary rehabilitation team. *Journal of Occupational Rehabilitation*, **15**, 581–90.

Main, C.J. (2002). Concepts of treatment and prevention in musculoskeletal disorders. In S.J. Linton (Ed.) *New avenues for the prevention of chronic musculoskeletal pain and disability. Pain research and clinical management, vol.* 12, pp. 47–63. New York: Elsevier.

Marhold, C., Linton, S.J., and Melin, L. (2002). Identification of obstacles for chronic pain patients to return to work: evaluation of a questionnaire. *Journal of Occupational Rehabilitation*, **12**, 65–75.

Marras, W. S., Ferguson, S. A., Burr, D., Schabo, P. and Maronitis, A. (2007). Low back pain recurrence in occupational environments. *Spine*, **32**, 2387–97.

Nachemson, A., Waddell, G., and Norlund, A.I. (2000). Epidemiology of neck and low back pain, in A. Nachemson and E. Jonsson (eds.) *Neck and back pain: The scientific evidence of causes, diagnosis, and treatment*, pp. 165–87. Philadelphia, PA: Lippincott Williams & Wilkins.

Nicholas, M.K. (2002). Reducing disability in injured workers: The importance of collaborative management. In S.J. Linton (Ed.) *New avenues for the prevention of chronic musculoskeletal pain and disability. Pain research and clinical management, vol.* 12, pp. 33–46. New York: Elsevier.

Pransky, G., Shaw, W.S., and Fitzgerald, T.E. (2001). Prognosis in acute occupational low back pain: Methodologic and practical considerations. *Human and Ecological Risk Assessment*, 7, 1811–25.

Pransky, G., Shaw, W.S., Franche, R.L., and Clarke, A. (2004). Disability prevention and communication among workers, physicians, employers, and insurers–current models and opportunities for improvement. *Disability and Rehabilitation*, 26, 625–34.

Schultz, I.Z., Crook, J., Berkowitz, J., Milner, R., and Meloche, G.R. (2005). Predicting return to work after low back injury using the Psychosocial Risk for Occupational Disability Instrument: a validation study. *Journal of Occupational Rehabilitation*, 15, 365–76.

Schultz, I.Z., Stowell, A.W., Feuerstein, M., and Gatchel, R.J. (2007). Models of return to work for musculoskeletal disorders. *Journal of Occupational Rehabilitation*, 17, 327–52.

Shaw, W.S., Robertson, M.M., McLellan, R.K., Verma, S., and Pransky, G. (2006). A controlled case study of supervisor training to optimize response to injury in the food processing industry. *Work* 26, 107–14.

Shaw, W.S. and Huang, Y.H. (2005). Concerns and expectations about returning to work with low back pain: identifying themes from focus groups and semi-structured interviews. *Disability and Rehabilitation*, 27, 1269–81.

Shaw, W.S., Pransky, G., Fitzgerald, T.E. (2001). Early prognosis for low back disability: Intervention strategies for health care providers. *Disability Rehabilitation*, 23, 815–28.

Shaw, W.S., Pransky, G., Patterson, W., and Winters, T. (2005). Early disability risk factors for low back pain assessed at outpatient occupational health clinics. *Spine*, 30, 572–80.

Shaw, W.S., Robertson, M.M., Pransky, G., and McLellan, R.K. (2006a). Training to optimize the response of supervisors to work injuries–needs assessment, design, and evaluation. *American Association of Occupational Health Nurses Journal*, 54, 226–35.

Shaw, W.S., Linton, S.J., and Pransky, G. (2006b). Reducing sickness absence from work due to low back pain: How well do intervention strategies match modifiable risk factors? *Journal of Occupational Rehabilitation*, 16, 591–605.

Shaw, W.S., van der Windt, D.A., Main, C.J. *et al.* (2009). Early patient screening and Intervention to address individual-Level occupational factors ('blue flags') in back disability. *Journal of Occupational Rehabilitation*, 19, 64–80.

Shrey, De and Hursh, N.C. (1999). Workplace disability management: International trends and perspectives. *Journal of Occupational Rehabilitation*, 9, 45–59.

Steenstra, I.A., Verbeek, J.H., Heymans, M.W., and Bongers, P.M. (2005). Prognostic factors for duration of sick leave in patients sick listed with acute low back pain: a systematic review of the literature. *Occupational and Environmental Medicine*, 62, 851–60.

Sullivan, M.J., Feuerstein, M., Gatche,l R., Linton, S.J., and Pransky, G. (2005). Integrating psychosocial and behavioral interventions to achieve optimal rehabilitation outcomes. *Journal of Occupational Rehabilitation*, 15, 475–89.

van Duijn, M., Miedema, H., Elders, L., and Burdorf, A. (2004). Barriers for early return-to-work of workers with musculoskeletal disorders according to occupational health physicians and human resource managers. *Journal of Occupational Rehabilitation*, 14, 31–41.

van Tulder, M.W., Koes, B.W., and Bouter, L.M. (1995). A cost-of-illness study of back pain in The Netherlands. *Pain*, 62, 233–40.

Varekamp, I., de Vries, G., Heutink, A., and van Dijk, F.J.H. (2008). Empowering employees with chronic diseases; development of an intervention aimed at job retention and deisgn of a randomised controlled trial. *BMC Health Services Research*, 8, 224.

Varekamp, I., Heutink, A., Landman, S., Koning, C.E.M., de Vries, G., and van Dijk, F.J.H. (2009). Facilitating empowerment in employees with chronic disease: Qualitative analysis of the process of change. *Journal of Occupational Rehabilitation*, **19**, 398–408.

Volinn, E., La,i D., McKinney, S., *et al.* (1988). When back pain becomes disabling: A regional analysis. *Pain*, **33**, 33–9.

Von Korff, M., Balderson, B.H.K, Saunders, K., *et al.* (2005). A trial of an activating intervention for chronic back pain in primary care and physical therapy settings. *Pain*, **113**, 323–30.

Waddell, G., Aylward, M., and Sawney, P. (2002). *Back pain, incapacity for work and social security benefits: An international literature review and analysis*. London: The Royal Society of Medicine Press.

Waddell, G. (2004). *The Back Pain Revolution* (2nd edn., pp. 265–82. New York: Churchill-Livingstone.

Wasiak, R., Pransky, G., Verma, S., and Webster, B. (2003). Recurrence of low back pain: definition-sensitivity analysis using administrative data. *Spine*, **28**, (19), 2283–91.

Watkins, E.A., Wollan, P.C., Melton, L.J. 3rd, and Yawn, B.P. (2008). A population in pain: report from the Olmstead County health study. *Pain Medicine*, **9**, 166–74.

Weir, R. and Nielson, W.R. (2001). Interventions for disability management. *Clinical Journal of Pain*, **17** (4 Suppl), S128–32.

Werner, E.L., Laerum, E., Wormgoor, M.E., Lindh, E., and Indahl, A. (2007). Peer support in an occupational setting preventing LBP-related sick leave. *Occupational Medicine*, **57**, 590–5.

Westmorland, M.G., Williams, R.M., Amick, B.C. 3rd, Shannon, H., and Rasheed, F. (2005). Disability management practices in Ontario workplaces: employees' perceptions. *Disability and Rehabilitation*, **27**, 825–35.

Young, A.E., Roessler, R.T., Wasiak, R., McPherson, K.M., van Poppel, M.N.M., and Anema, J.R. (2005). A developmental conceptualization of return to work. *Journal of Occupational Rehabilitation*, **15**(4), 557–68.

Part 5

# **Practitioner's Role in the Process of Care**

Chapter 20

# The Physician as Disability Advisor for Back Pain Patients

James Rainville, Glenn S. Pransky, Sarah Gibson, and Pradeep Suri

## 20.1 Introduction

It is a proper and likely inescapable function of physicians to sanction disability in the course of treating illness (Sullivan and Loeser 1992). In acute or obvious illness, these dual roles result in little controversy, as recommending a temporary suspension of personal and occupational responsibilities may be beneficial to the process of healing. Moreover, significantly impaired body function often necessitates a period of convalescence—recognized by physicians, patients, and society as reasonable. On the other hand, for the problem of low back pain (LBP), where the pathology is less overt and where symptoms often endure beyond the expected time required for healing, physicians may be faced with a difficult dilemma. What level of disability is appropriate for the pathology, symptoms, and impaired function exhibited by a patient? Here inter-physician variation increases dramatically regarding the degree of work disablement endorsed, or restriction of activity recommended for a given set of complaints.

The variability in recommendations may have enormous consequences for patients with LBP, including an impact on the probability of transitioning from acute to chronic disability. It is recognized that inappropriate disability can lead to decreased quality of life due to inactivity, while prolonged absence from normal social roles (including work) is deleterious to physical and mental well-being (Shulman 1994; McGrail et al. 2002). Appropriate and early return to activities and work avoids the consequences of illness reinforcement: assumption of the sick role, deterioration in family dynamics, dependence on drugs, creation of secondary gain, learned disability, as well as other negative impacts (Derebery and Tullis 1983).

Do physicians' disability recommendations make a difference? For LBP, limited evidence suggests that they do. Several authors have noted that consistent, evidence-based physician recommendations about disability that encourage resumption of activity independent of pain status lead to improved disability outcomes in LBP and other disorders (Indahl et al. 1998; Hagen et al. 2002; Rainville et al. 2002) Of importance, physicians may influence patients' disability in the opposite direction—advising avoidance of activities to those with back pain. Though the magnitude of this effect on disability is unknown, it is probably of consequence. This is supported by the results from cross-sectional studies of general practitioners (GPs) and their patients with acute LBP and rheumatologist and their patient with subacute LBP. Both studies observed that high ratings of pain beliefs in physicians were associated with a higher rate of pain beliefs of their patients (Poiraudeau et al. 2006; Coudeyre et al. 2007).

Recently, researchers have begun to acknowledge the importance of physicians' disability recommendations. Not surprisingly, findings have revealed that a complex interaction of physician, patient, social, and political factors influence physician recommendations.

This chapter will explore current knowledge about physician disability recommendations for patients with LBP. It will also review results of attempts to influence these recommendations, and suggest areas where further research may be beneficial.

## 20.2 Magnitude of the physician role as disability advisor

Nearly all patient–physician encounters for musculoskeletal disorders include recommendations about the appropriate level of activity for the illness under treatment. These generally include advice about use and mobility of the injured body part for personal care, domestic, and recreational activities. Additionally, physicians are often asked or required to make recommendations about the ability of their patients to work. Many jurisdictions in the USA mandate such recommendations, when injury is alleged to result from vocational activities or exposures. In the UK and many other countries, the provision of sickness certification is mandated as part of the contractual services delivered by GPs.

The actual percentage of patient encounters during which physicians are asked to certify disability is substantial. Bollag et al. (2007) reported that 4% and Soler and Okkes (2004) reported that 11% of patient encounters for GPs resulted in the issuance of sickness certificates. Pransky et al. (2002) and Englund et al. (2000a) reported that primary care providers were asked to supply opinions concerning work ability in about 9% of all patient encounters. All studies found that musculoskeletal diagnoses dominated these requests (Englund and Svardsudd 2000). For this reason, practices specializing in musculoskeletal disorders also have a high number of patient encounters where definitions of 'work capacity' are required (Arrelov et al. 2007).

## 20.3 The content of physician recommendations

As activity and work recommendations are an essential part of many patient–physician encounters, it is worthwhile exploring the content of these recommendations. To date, most studies examining physicians' recommendations have substituted patient histories or vignettes for actual patient encounters, with recognized research limitation (Jones et al. 1990). The results demonstrate a striking lack of consistency in physicians' assessment of all types of disability. This includes disability assessment of common musculoskeletal disorders (Haldorsen et al. 1996; Patel et al. 2003), social security disability eligibility (Carey et al. 1988), and ill-health retirement determinations (Elder et al. 1994). Not surprisingly, studies limited to LBP-related disability have also demonstrated a lack of consensus among physicians (Chibnall et al. 2000; Rainville et al. 2000). When explored further however, despite high variability between physicians, individual physicians exhibited consistent patterns in their disability recommendations, ranging from lenient to strict (Getz and Westin 1995; Chibnall et al. 2000; Rainville et al. 2000). The detrimental implications of this inconsistency and inequality are obvious for both patients with LBP and disability systems they access. Clearly, the most negative impact is unnecessary disability with associated overall decline in economic well-being and health (Waddell et al. 2000). Additionally, the inconsistency of disability recommendation encourage 'doctor shopping' where patients search for physicians that support their position on disability. Consistent patterns of disability recommendation for individual physicians can establish medical reputations, leading to funnelling of patients to specific medical providers who will either refute or support disability claims. Ultimately, this variance in medical opinions probably consumes countless hours of debate as legal systems try to sort out conflicting physicians' disability recommendations.

## 20.4 **Physicians' characteristics that influence disability recommendations**

There are several possible explanations for the high level of observed variability in activity recommendations for LBP. One source of variability may result from differences in the depth of medical knowledge about LBP. To examine this, Rainville et al. (2000) compared chronic low back pain (CLBP) work and activity recommendations of family physicians and orthopaedic spine surgeons. They noted that orthopaedic spine surgeons were only slightly more permissive than family physicians with work restrictions and very similar with activity restrictions. These finding were corroborated by Englund et al. (2000a). Apparently, the level of expertise as reflected by medical specialty has a limited influence on disability recommendations.

A potential, but unexplored source of variability in physicians' disability recommendations may be differences in theories about the aetiology of spinal degeneration and CLBP. For decades, medical wisdom supported an injury model of LBP, where exposures of the spine to physical stresses were deemed responsible for spinal degeneration (Nachemson 1975). Indeed, the injury model spawned empirical recommendation about posture, lifting techniques, and back health, and inspired decades of ergonomic research. It is logical for physicians that are strong proponents of this model to advise patients against activities perceived to be harmful to the spine.

The injury model of LBP has been considerably weakened over the last two decades, in part by the failure of ergonomic interventions to reduce back injuries, but mainly from epidemiological, genetic, and neurobiological research that offered alternative explanations for low back disorders (Martimo et al. 2007). A fundamentally different model of spinal degeneration has emerged in which the aetiology of degeneration is explained by genetically encoded, age-activated degenerative processes (Ala-Kokko, 2002) As such, this model undermines the alleged role of physical exposure in spinal degeneration, and weakens the association between persistent pain complaints and ongoing damage or harm. Theoretically, physicians endorsing this model of LBP would more likely recommend that activity avoidance is medically unnecessary.

Another possible source of variation in disability recommendations may be inadequate medical education or poor preparation of physicians for determining disability (Sullivan and Loeser 1992). Indeed, a majority of surveyed physicians indicated that they have learned little about disability programmes from any source (Carey et al. 1987), do not feel confident in their ability to determine patient disability (Zinn and Furutani 1996), and felt burdened by participation in this task (Zinn and Furutani 1996). Furthermore, many physicians feel inadequately educated about work capabilities and risk for injury from occupation exposures (Pransky et al. 2002). Despite concerns about their role as disability advisors, the degree of physicians' dislike of this role or their feelings of inadequacy towards this process are not reflected in the duration of sickness certification for patients under their care (Tellness et al. 1990).

A related area of importance is the physician's ability to identify the small number of cases at high risk for progression from acute, self-limited injury to a chronically disabled state. These cases may benefit the most from interventions designed to avoid prolonged disability at an early stage. Unfortunately, physicians have little training in risk prediction for low back injury and are often unaware of specific advice or intervention that can alter the progression to disablement (W.S. Shaw et al. 2001; Haldorsen et al. 2002).

Perhaps reflecting these problems, patients did not view the physician as an active facilitator of return to work and activity in one study (Roberts-Yates 2003). These patients cited the physician's lack of experience, dissociation from the workplace, disinterest in workplace issues and needs, and failure to devote the necessary time as evidence of their ineffective role in this issue.

One could easily theorize that inherent beliefs, fears, and concerns that healthcare providers hold about pain and function should be strong determinants of their recommendations for activity and work after an injury. This association is supported by several studies. Utilizing the Healthcare Providers' Pain and Impairment Relationship Scale (Rainville et al. 1995), Rainville et al. (2000) discovered that pain attitudes and beliefs of physicians were the strongest predictor of their work/activity recommendations. Similarly, Houben et al. (2004) noted that physical therapists' work/activity recommendations were strongly predicted by the strength of their pain attitudes and beliefs as well. Poiraudeau et al. (2006) noted that rheumatologists with strong fear-avoidance pain beliefs were less likely to follow guidelines on prescribing physical and occupational activities for LBP. Linton et al. (2002) reported that physicians' recommendations for sick leave were strongly dependent on their own fear-avoidance beliefs with regard to back pain.

## 20.5 **Physician-patient relationship factors**

Despite this evidence of a connection between providers' beliefs and work recommendations, some studies suggest that other characteristics of physicians may override their personal beliefs. Gulbrandsen et al. (2007) grouped physicians into four groups based on combinations of characteristics including their perceived burden of sickness certification, doubt, permissiveness, personality, degree of paternalism, job satisfaction, opinion of sick certification as medical task, and sociopolitical attitudes. Despite prominent differences between groups, no association was found between group-level differences of physician traits and rates of sickness certification. Watson et al. (2008) found no relationship between physicians' pain attitudes and the frequency of issued illness certificate for non-specific LBP. Instead, they noted that sickness absences certification for LBP was predicted by the physicians' sickness certification behaviours for all medical illnesses in general.

The above findings suggest that there are other characteristics—besides physicians' pain attitudes and beliefs—that determine physicians' disability recommendation. Mounting evidence suggests that the physician recommendations may be largely determined by a seldom-studied factor—the physician-patient relationship.

Discordance is common between physicians and patients concerning the issue of LBP and work (Lofgren et al. 2007; von Knorring et al. 2008). Physicians and patients often differ in terms of expectation of the length of disability for LBP (Kapoor et al. 2006), especially as symptoms become more chronic (Reiso et al. 2004). Physicians tend to rely more heavily on clinical findings, whereas patients tend to assess job related factors such as stress and the physical strenuous nature of work (Reiso et al. 2000).

When differences of opinion occur, it seems that patients' opinions often win. Pransky et al. (2002) noted that primary care providers relied mainly on patient input for disability assessment. Englund and Svardsudd (2000) observed that in cases where primary care physicians could not medically justify 'sick-listing' certification, a certificate was issued anyway in 87% of cases. In a separate study, Englund and Dahlgren (2002) noted that the most important factor affecting 'sick-listing' was the patient's attitude to 'sick-listing', as those wishing 'sick-listing' were 'sick-listed' to a greater degree than those who were reluctant. Mayhew and Nordlund (1998) found that 41% of family physicians reported feeling pressured to write unwarranted work excuses and had a sense of being manipulated by their patients. Brook (1996) reported that hostile, demanding, threatening and malingering patients, frequently influenced physicians' completion of disability requests. Zinn and Furutani (1996) found that 40% of physicians reported a willingness to exaggerate clinical data for patients they felt deserving of disability.

The observations described above document that significant discordance exists between patients and physicians about the degree to which illness justifies limitation on activity and work.

For some physicians, the discordance may be trivial—they feel unable to judge the appropriateness of disability more accurately than their patients, and therefore rely upon their patient's 'better judgment'. It is also possible that in order to avoid this discordance, many physicians adapt rather neutral attitudes about pain and function (Rainville et al. 1995). These neutral attitudes may serve the physician well, as it allows the physician to easily acquiesce to the disability position adapted by their patients, and thus avoid conflict.

For many other physicians, this discordance is troubling. However, they still may acquiesce to the patient's requests. One important reason for this is suggested in the study by Zinn and Furutani (1996), where over 80% of physicians felt that refusing to fill out disability forms could adversely affect the doctor–patient relationship, and 62% felt that it reflected a conflict of interest. These findings suggest that most primary care physicians see their role as gatekeepers for compensation systems as subservient to their role as patient advocate, especially when their relationship is long term and includes care for all medical problems (Hussey et al. 2004). From a practical point of view, it may be much less time-consuming for physicians to simply acquiesce to patients demands and avoid conflict.

It appears that the interaction of patients' beliefs, behaviours, and demands, with internal physician characteristics of professionalism, social desirability, and negotiation strategies can profoundly influence disability recommendations (Monday et al. 1988). Research is needed on how physicians cope with their conflicting roles as patient advocate and gatekeeper to disability benefits, with the goal of identifying potential interventions that would improve their performance as disability advisors.

## 20.6 **Patients' perceptions of disability**

This discordance may in part result from patients perceiving the disabling effect of their problem differently than physicians do. For many chronic musculoskeletal disorders, physical factors actually play a relatively minor role in influencing disability outcomes. Indeed, it appears that patients with chronic musculoskeletal symptoms who continue to seek medical care may possess attitudes and beliefs about pain and function that are more restrictive and potential disability levels that are significantly higher than others in the general population with a similar malady (Szpalski et al. 1995; Waxman et al. 1998). Past research suggests that much of the observed variance in self-reported disability results from factors that are independent of the physical aspects of the musculoskeletal afflictions. Influential factors include coping abilities (Turner et al. 2000), affect and personality (Gatchel et al. 1993; Maxwell et al. 1998), fear-avoidance beliefs (Swinkels-Meewisse et al. 2006), educational level (Roth and Geisser 2002), work issues (Bigos et al. 1991), and concerns about benefit loss and secondary gain (Rainville et al. 1997; Klekamp et al. 1998). Though frank malingering is probably quite rare, somatization, distortion, and some exaggeration may be common (Ensalada 2000). These areas of non-medical distress can strongly influence patients' behaviours and magnify their perception of disability, especially as it relates to work.

Patients relating back pain to exposure to physical activities, fear of re-injury, and the belief that pain indicates harm are likely important factors influencing disability (Rainville et al. 1993; Waddell et al. 1993; Jensen et al. 1994; Symonds et al. 1996). People with a history of back pain, and those with blue-collar occupations more often attribute back pain to external factors such as physical activities and the work environment, though misconceptions about back pain are widespread, even in the group reporting no back pain (Linton and Wang 1993; Goubert et al. 2004). Patients may be reluctant to continue activities that are believed to have precipitated their back pain. With this in mind, a recommendation to remain active and return to work may be ineffective unless it's accompanied by information that resolves or addresses fears of re-injury. Physician-presented patient education, such as that reported by Indahl et al. (1998), that attempts to displace the injury model of spinal degeneration with a more benign hypothesis, and dissociates pain and function, may offer some encouraging results. This approach is clearly in need of further study.

## 20.7 Factors external to the physician-patient relationship that influence disability

Employers can also have an influence on physician behaviour regarding disability by engaging more cooperative physicians, communicating their return to work expectations and providing alternative duty (Habeck et al. 1991; Pransky et al. 2002; L. Shaw et al. 2002; W.S. Shaw 2003; van Duijn et al. 2004). Baril and Nordqvist (Baril et al. 2003; Nordqvist et al. 2003) conducted qualitative studies of return-to-work programmes, contrasting the perceptions of workers, employers, physicians, and others involved in the process. Although physicians focused on individual factors as the most important determinants of return-to-work outcome, workers and health and safety managers readily identified workplace-specific factors as the most important determinants for returning to work.

Yet another influence may be the healthcare system itself, including level of reimbursement for services related to caring for disabled workers, local market effects, and provider-induced utilization in work-related musculoskeletal disorders. Johnson et al. (1999) demonstrated that healthcare providers incur a benefit in the form of healthcare utilization in disabling work-related musculoskeletal disorders. For some providers who offer costly diagnostic and therapeutic procedures, a disincentive may exist to return patients quickly. The burden of salary replacement benefits may motivate some insurers to authorize expensive medical services, especially when the medical provider insists that return-to-work recommendations are contingent on performing a procedure or test. Even for clinics specializing in work-related musculoskeletal disorders that are established specifically to improve care, incentives to increase utilization can lead to a net increase in disability, as aptly demonstrated in a series of Ontario clinics by Sinclair et al. (1997).

Legal jurisdictional influences on physician behaviour in relation to disability are highly significant. This is a key factor in the profound differences across jurisdictions in mean lengths of disability for equivalent conditions—despite absence of differences in the nature and the severity of injury, and the availability return to work opportunities (Johnson et al. 1996).

In summary, the recommendations for work/activities made by physicians to patients with musculoskeletal complaints are the product of the complex interaction of many factors. In addition to the obvious factors of the medical condition itself, as well as idiosyncratic characteristics of the physician and patient, factors external to the physician-patient encounter also influence physicians' recommendations. These include the work place, medical systems, and legislation.

## 20.8 Efforts to influence physician recommendations

Interventions have attempted to improve the quality of physician recommendations about work resumption after injury, with varying degrees of success.

### 20.8.1 Medical educational efforts

Efforts to improve physicians' education about the impact of activity recommendations on disability have been sparse, and the results are unimpressive. Lie (2003) reported on an educational effort in Norway to decrease the length of sick leaves by augmenting the knowledge base of GPs. Participating physicians received education about common musculoskeletal disorders and financial compensation for spending extra time with patients with extended sick leaves. Unfortunately, no impact on sick listing practices or disability outcomes were noted.

Perhaps it is not the direct knowledge about musculoskeletal disorders that is most important, but instead the pain attitudes and beliefs of the practitioners that are most critical in disability recommendations. If so, efforts to directly alter these may be of some benefit. This issue has also received limited study. Latimer et al. (2004) reported on an educational project designed to change the attitudes and beliefs about pain and function of physical therapy students. Results indicated that substantial changes in favour of endorsing function occurred following the teaching module and these changes were maintained 1 year out.

From another perspective, training for physicians should focus on skills that directly address the findings that it is psychosocial and not medical issues that are the primary determinants of disability. This implies developing an ability to elicit and address the factors that may inhibit successful return to work and knowledge of how to effectively address these factors (L. Shaw et al. 2002). Related skills such as prognostic screening and selective referral to resources based on the specific barriers to return to work, may also be directly related to producing evidence-based return-to-work recommendations, inasmuch as these interventions are necessary to insure a high likelihood of compliance and success (W.S. Shaw et al. 2001; Haldorsen et al. 2002).

### 20.8.2 Guidelines

In the mid 1990s, leading researchers developed medical guidelines to address disability issues in musculoskeletal disorders, especially LBP, urging physicians to facilitate return to work (Frank et al. 1996; Canadian Medical Association 1997). The premise was that evidence-based guidelines, norms, and other 'scientific' material would lead to practice change once physicians were informed about them (Verbeek et al. 2002). In isolation, educational efforts appear to have minimal impact, especially in low back pain (Rao et al. 2002; Verbeek et al. 2002).

Direct efforts to mandate that physicians' work recommendations be based on clinical and not subjective criteria have shown some promise. In a case-controlled study, Hall et al. (1994) examined the impact of a mandate that all low back injured workers be released to unrestricted (versus restricted) work, unless objective medical contraindications were present. This mandate resulted in twice the number of patients returning to unrestricted work, without an adverse effect on the probability of successful return to those work activities. Similar finding were noted by Hiebert et al. (2003). Both studies were undertaken in private business settings where physicians were employees and modest control over physicians' actions could be elicited. As such the applicability of these findings to more traditional medical practice settings is questionable. This is demonstrated by a study in a less controlled setting by Scheel et al. (2002) which demonstrated that simply providing physicians with a mechanism to return patients to work sooner was insufficient, even though most physicians readily acknowledged the importance of improved return to work outcomes. In part, these results may reflect the highly skewed distribution of length of disability amongst a minority of patients, the inherent difficulty in engaging physicians, as well as the multitude of factors besides physician recommendations that shape outcomes (Scheel et al. 2002).

### 20.8.3 Systems efforts

Realizing the limitation of interventions that are aimed at medical providers alone, several recent projects have taken a broad-based, systemic approach, thereby acknowledging that physician behaviour occurs in a larger context that includes patient knowledge, expectations, and behaviours. As observed by Grimshaw, Deyo, and others, most successful approaches: (1) include some form of medical educational outreach with use of academic detailing by recognized leaders; (2) include changes in the processes that direct physicians to the desired behaviour; (3) include simultaneous education of patients; (4) include a high and sustained level of administrative and financial support; and (5) acknowledge that one technique may not be suitable for all (Oxman et al. 1995; Deyo et al. 2000; Grimshaw et al. 2001).

Community-wide interventions have been attempted in several countries. These interventions theorized that by simultaneously supplying both the public and medical providers with similar information about the benefits of activity and work, the discordance between physicians and patients could be lessened. One could argue that as the community is brought along, physician-patient dialogue might change and achieve concordance at a point consistent with evidence-based guidelines.

Buchbinder et al. (2001a, 2001b) initiated this type of intervention in Australia. The intervention used a multimedia campaign to disseminate information about the benefits of staying active with back pain, including work. The result was a large, significant improvement in back pain beliefs and less fear-avoidance regarding physical activity. This was paralleled by improvements in beliefs and practice intentions of physicians. Of equal importance, the researchers noted a clear decline in the number of claims for back pain, days of compensation and medical cost for claims during the campaign.

A similar system wide approach was taken for a public health initiative entitled 'Working Backs Scotland' (Waddell et al. 2007). The initiative utilized a combination of radio and a website to disseminate information targeting both people with back pain and employers. Concurrently, information supplied to medical providers advised *against* recommending bed rest, activity restrictions and issuing sickness certification for back pain. This initiative also demonstrated a shift in public beliefs away from rest to staying active, and a comparable shift in professional advice. However, no changes in work or compensation outcomes were noted. These results exposed a flaw in the 'Working Back Scotland' intervention—it avoided direct discussions of work The lack of changes in work-related factors suggests that work expectations during a back pain episode must be addressed directly for these interventions to be successful.

Smaller and more focused systemic changes can also impact physicians' behaviours and responses. Bernacki and Tsai (2003) described a successful workers' compensation management system at an employer-level that decreased lost time by 73% and the number of medical claims by 61% over a 10-year period. In this system, physicians' expectations for advising light duty and return to work are unambiguous; there are appreciable rewards for providers to work within the system, and employers will accommodate a returning injured worker. Similar programmes have reported comparable results (Green-McKenzie et al. 2002; McGrail et al. 2002). Eccleston and Yeager (1998) concluded that these types of programme generated savings of 9–54%, not by reducing medical costs, but by providing earlier and more effective return-to-work recommendations from treating physicians.

Some innovative approaches recognize that physicians are trained to perform within a medical model; to the extent that determinants of disability are primarily psychosocial, not medical, their training and orientation are poorly suited to effectively address issues of return to work (Hunt et al. 2002). Based on this presumption, one successful approach places physicians as a contributing member of a team that provides specific recommendations about return to work and facilitates the return to work process (Durand and Loisel 2001; Edlund and Dahlgren 2002). Another approach trains physicians to become more effective communicators about LBP, its prognosis, and the optimal approach for management (McGrail et al. 2002).

### 20.8.4 **Legislative efforts**

Clearly social systems that compensate individuals for illness and disability have a profound potential to influence human behaviours. As such, changes in these systems, especially changes that affect eligibility, should have the ability to change societal expectations and the financial burden of disability. The positive effects of altering eligibility criteria for financial compensation are demonstrated in studies by Cassidy et al. (2000) and Claussen (1998).

Even though changes in the public support of disability can be legislated, these may have limited impact on physicians' disability recommendation. Englund et al. (2000b) noted no change in the 'sick listing' practices of physicians collected before and after a legislative reform, other than they completed the forms more thoroughly after the reform. Legislative changes instituted in Sweden in 1995 aimed at reducing costs of sickness absence by mandating that physicians exclude non-medical criteria for sick-listing, recommend more part-time sick-listing, and pursue faster rehabilitation did not meet any of their goals. Indeed, a survey of physicians by Getz and Westin (1993) reported that a majority of physicians believed that legislation resulting in a higher percentage of refusals for disability applications would not bring many applicants back to employment, but would instead transfer the financial burden of disability to other public sources of support. Apparently, physicians' attitudes towards disability and their behaviours with patients requesting disability certification are not easily impacted by legislative efforts, most likely because they do not lessen the demands of patients for disability certification.

## 20.9 **Summary and conclusions**

When attending to patients with musculoskeletal complaints, physicians are required to give advice about the appropriate level of activities and work for the condition under treatment. Evidence suggests that this advice varies greatly between physicians. This variation results from multiple factors. From the perspective of physicians, differences in medical knowledge, attitudes and beliefs, negotiation abilities, and professionalism surrounding the doctor–patient relationship can all influence their recommendation. Patient, employer, and societal factors may also influence these recommendations.

Prolonged work avoidance has no identified therapeutic benefit and significant adverse effects on social well-being. Although some physicians recognize the impact of poor recommendations, most efforts to persuade physicians to discourage patients from sustained work absence have been unsuccessful. This may be in part due to an incomplete understanding by physicians of the processes whereby back pain-related disability becomes chronic (Guzman et al. 2002). Regardless, efforts to harmonize physicians' recommendations to promote full return to activity or work despite chronic musculoskeletal pain seem warranted. One-dimensional interventions such as physician education or implementation of evidence-based guidelines have had limited effect on disability recommendations. Based on the available evidence, significant changes in physician recommendations will require educating both physicians and patients, along with altering societal expectations about back pain and work (Aylward and Waddell 2002). Successful multidimensional efforts have included educational material to enhance physicians' knowledge combined with effective community-based efforts to influence patients' functional expectations before they enter the physicians' office. During the medical encounter, physicians should be motivated to address the issues where there is disagreement about disability, consistent with the standards of high quality doctor-patient communication. Accepting the input, and understanding the needs of employers and governmental organizations can aid the physician in providing appropriate medical input for these entities.

Thus, future research should concentrate on interventions that can change the attitudes and actions of key players in the disablement process, within the context of a particular sociopolitical environment. Even in the setting of expectations for prolonged disability, interventions that address all of the most significant factors underlying extended LBP-related work absence could be successful (Loisel et al. 2003). Our future challenge will be to generalize these findings in a way that will enable physicians, patients and employers to accept early, rapid, and safe return to activity and/or work as an expected outcome.

## Acknowledgements

Dr Suri is supported by the Rehabilitation Medicine Scientist Training K12 Program (RMSTP) and the National Institutes of Health (K12 HD 01097).

## References

Ala-Kokko, L. (2002). Genetic risk factors for lumbar disc disease. *Ann Med*, **34**, 42–7.

Arrelov, B., Alexanderson, K., Hagberg, J., Lofgren, A., Nilsson, G., Ponzer, S. (2007). Dealing with sickness certification—a survey of problems and strategies among general practitioners and orthopaedic surgeons. *BMC Public Health*, **7**, 273.

Aylward, M., Waddell, G. (2002) *Low back Pain, Incapacity, and Social Security*. London: Royal Society of Medicine Press.

Baril, R., Clarke, J., Friesen, M., *et al.* (2003). Work-Ready Group. Management of return-to-work programs for workers with musculoskeletal disorders: a qualitative study in three Canadian provinces. *Soc Sci Med*, **57**, 2101–14.

Bernacki, E.J., Tsai, S.P. (2003). Ten years' experience using an integrated workers' compensation management system to control workers' compensation costs. *J Occup Environ Med*, **45**, 508–16.

Bigos, S.J., Battie, M.C., Spengler, D.M., *et al.* (1991). A prospective study of work perceptions and psychosocial factors affecting the report of back injury. *Spine*, **16**, 1–6.

Bollag, U., Rajeswaran, A., Ruffieux, C., Burnand, B. (2007). Sickness certification in primary care - the physician's role. *Swiss Med Wkly*, **137**, 341–6.

Brook, T.R. (1996). How patients stress, con, and intimidate physicians to file dubious disability reports. *J Natl Med Assoc*, **88**, 300–4.

Buchbinder, R., Jolley, D., Wyatt, M. (2001). 2001 Volvo Award Winner in Clinical Studies: Effects of a media campaign on back pain beliefs and its potential influence on management of low back pain in general practice. *Spine*, **26**, 2535–42.

Buchbinder, R., Jolley, D., Wyatt, M. (2001). Population based intervention to change back pain beliefs and disability: three part evaluation. *BMJ*, **322**, 1516–20.

Canadian Medical Association (1997). The Physician's Role in Helping Patients Return to Work after an Illness or Injury. *Can Med Assoc* **156**, 680A–C.

Carey, T.S., Fletcher, S.W., Fletcher, R., *et al.* (1987). Social Security disability determinations. Knowledge and attitudes of consulting physicians. *Med Care*, **25**, 267–75.

Carey, T.S, , Hadler, H.M., Gillings, D., *et al.* (1988). Medical disability assessment of the back pain patient for the Social Security Administration: the weighting of presenting clinical features. *J Clin Edidemiol*, **41**, 691–7.

Cassidy, J.D., Carroll, L.J., Cote, P., *et al.* (2000). Effect of eliminating compensation for pain and suffering on the outcome of insurance claims for whiplash injury. *New Engl J Med*, **342**, 1179–86.

Chibnall, J.T., Dabney, A., Tait, R,C. (2000). Internist judgment of chronic low back pain. *Pain Med*, **3**, 231–6.

Claussen, B. (1998). Physicians as gatekeepers: will they contribute to restrict disability benefits? *Scand J Prim Health Care*, **16**, 199–203.

Coudeyre, E., Tubach, F., Rannou, F., *et al.* (2007). Fear-avoidance beliefs about back pain in patients with acute LBP. *C J Pain*, **23**, 720–5.

Derebery, V.J., Tullis, W.H. (1983). Delayed recovery in the patient with a work compensable injury. *J Occup Med*, **25**, 829–35.

Deyo, R.A., Schall, M., Berwick, D.M., *et al*. (2000). Continuous quality improvement for patients with back pain. *J Gen Intern Med*, **15**, 647–55.

Durand, M.J., Loisel, P. (2001). Therapeutic return to work: Rehabilitation in the workplace. *Work*, **17**, 57–63.

Eccleston, S.M., Yeager, C.M. (1998). *Managed care and medical costs in workers' compensation: a national inventory, 1997–1998*. Cambridge, MA: Workers Compensation Research Institute.

Edlund, C., Dahlgren, L. (2002). The physician's role in the vocational rehabilitation process. *Disabil Rehabil*, **24**, 727–33.

Elder, A.G., Symington, I.S., Symington, E.H. (1994). Do occupational physicians agree about ill-health retiral? A study of simulated retirement assessments. *Occup Med*, **44**, 231–5.

Englund, L., Svardsudd, K. (2000). Sick-listing habits among general practitioners in a Swedish county. *Scand J Prim Health Care*, **18**, 81–6.

Englund, L., Tibblin, G., Svardsudd, K. (2000a). Variations in sick-listing practice among male and female physicians of different specialties based on case vignettes. *Scand J Prim Health Care*, **18**, 48–52.

Englund, L., Tibblin, G., Svardsudd, K. (2000b). Effects on physicians' sick-listing practice of an administrative reform narrowing sick-listing benefits. *Scand J Prim Health Care*, **18**, 215–9.

Ensalada, L.H. (2000). The importance of illness behavior in disability management. *Occup Med*, **15**, 739–54.

Frank, J.W., Brooker, A.S., DeMaio, S.E., *et al*. (1996). Disability resulting from occupational low back pain. Part II: What do we know about secondary prevention? A review of the scientific evidence on prevention after disability begins. *Spine,* **21**, 2918–29.

Gatchel, R.J., Polatin, P.B., Mayer, T.G. (1993). The dominant role of psychosocial risk factors in the development of chronic low back pain disability. *Spine,* **20**, 2702–9.

Getz, L., Westin, S. (1993). Restrictions in connection with disability pensions–physicians' view on the revised legislation. *Tidsskr Nor Laegeforen*, **113**, 2133–6.

Getz, L., Westin, S. (1995). Assessment by consulting physicians and general practitioners about complex disability pension matters. *Tidsskr Nor Laegeforen*, **115**, 1748–53.

Green-McKenzie, J., Rainer, S., Behrman, A., *et al*. (2002). The effect of a health care management initiative on reducing workers' compensation costs. *J Occup Environ Med*, **44**, 100–5.

Goubert, L., Crombez, G., De Bourdeaudhuij, I. (2004). Low back pain, disability and back pain myths in a community sample: prevalence and interrelationships. *Eur J Pain*, **8**, 385–94.

Grimshaw, J.M., Shirran, L., Thomas, R., *et al*. (2001). Changing provider behavior: an overview of systematic reviews of interventions. *Med Care*, **39**(Suppl 2), II2–45.

Gulbrandsen, P., Hofoss, D., Nylenna, M., Saltyte-Benth, J., Aasland, O.G. (2007). General practitioners' relationship to sickness certification. *Scand J Prim Health Care*, **25**, 20–6.

Guzman, J., Yassi, A., Cooper, J.E., *et al*. (2002). Return to work after occupational injury. Family physicians' perspectives on soft-tissue injuries. *Can Fam Physician*, **48**, 1912–9.

Habeck, R.V., Leahy, M.J., Hunt, H.A., *et al*. (1991). Employer factors related to workers' compensation claims and disability management. *Rehab Counseling Bull*, **34**, 210.

Hagen, K.B., Hilde, G., Jamtvedt, G., Winnem, M.F. (2002). The Cochrane review of advice to stay active as a single treatment for low back pain and sciatica. *Spine,* **27**, 1736–41.

Haldorsen, E.M.H., Brage, S., Johannesem, T.S., *et al*. (1996). Musculoskeletal pain: concepts of disease, illness and sickness certification in health professionals in Norway. *Scan J Rheumatol*, **4**, 224–32.

Haldorsen, E.M., Grasdal, A.L., Skouen, J.S., *et al*. (2002). Is there a right treatment for a particular patient group? Comparison of ordinary treatment, light multidisciplinary treatment, and extensive multidisciplinary treatment for long-term sick-listed employees with musculoskeletal pain. *Pain*, **95**, 49–63.

Hall, H., McIntosh, G., Melles, T., *et al*. (1994). Effect of discharge recommendations on outcome. *Spine*, **19**, 2033–7.

Hiebert, R., Skovron, M.L., Nordin, M., Crane, M. (2003). Work restrictions and outcome of nonspecific low back pain. *Spine*, **28**, 722–8.

Houben, R.M.A., Vlaeyen, J.W.S., Peters, M., *et al.* (2004). Healthcare providers' attitudes and beliefs toward common low back pain. Factor structure and psychometric properties of the HC-PAIRS. *Clin J Pain*, **20**, 37–44.

Hunt, D.G., Zuberbier, O.A., Kozlowski, A.J., *et al.* (2002). Are components of a comprehensive medical assessment predictive of work disability after an episode of occupational low back trouble? *Spine*, **27**, 2715–9.

Hussey, S., Hoddinott, P., Wilson, P., Dowell, J., Bardour, R. (2004). Sickness certification system in the United Kingdom: qualitative study of views of general practitioners in Scotland. *BMJ*, **328**, 88.

Indahl, A., Haldorsen, E.H., Holm, S., Reikeras, O., Ursin, H. (1998). Five-year follow-up study of a controlled clinical trial using light mobilization and an informative approach to low back pain. *Spine*, **23**, 2625–30.

Jensen, M.P., Turner, J.A., Romano, J.M. (1994). Relationship of pain-specific beliefs to chronic pain adjustment. *Pain*, **57**, 301–9.

Johnson, W.G., Baldwin, M.L., Burton, J.F., Jr. (1996). Why is the treatment of work-related injuries so costly? New evidence from California. *Inquiry*, **33**, 53–65.

Johnson, W.G., Burton, J.F., Jr, Thornquist, L., *et al.* (1999). Why does workers' compensation pay more for health care? *Benefits Q*, **9**, 22–31.

Jones, T.V., Gerrity, M.S., Earp, J. (1990). Written case simulations: So they predict physicians' behaviors. *J Clin Epidemiol*, **43**, 805–15.

Kapoor, S., Shaw, W.S., Pransky, G., Patterson, W. (2006). Initial patient and clinician expectations of return to work after acute onset of work-related low back pain. *J Occup Environ Med*, **48**, 1173–80.

Klekamp, J., McCarty, E., Spengler, D.M. (1998). Results of elective lumbar discectomy for patients involved in the workers' compensation system. *J Spinal Disord,* **11**, 277–82.

Krause, N., Dasinger, L.K., Neuhauser, F. (1998). Modified work and return to work; a review of the literature. *J Occ Rehab*, **8**, 113–39.

Latimer, J., Maher, C., Refshauge, K. (2004). The attitudes and beliefs of physiotherapy students to chronic back pain. *Clin J Pain*, **20**, 45–50.

Lie, H. (2003). Could sick leaves be reduced by augmenting the knowledge of the general practitioner? *Tidsskr Nor Laegeforen*, **123**, 2068–71.

Linton, S.J., Vlaeyen, J., Ostelo, R. (2002). The back pain beliefs of health care providers: Are we fear-avoidant? *J Occup Rehabil*, **12**, 223–32.

Linton, S.J., Wang, L.E. (1993). Attributions (beliefs) and job satisfaction associated with back pain in an industrial setting. *Percept Mot Skills*, **76**, 51–62.

Lofgren, A., Hagberg, J., Arrelov, B., Ponzer, S., Alexanderson, K. (2007). Frequency and nature of problems associated with sickness certification tasks: a cross-sectional questionnaire study of 5455 physicians. Scand J Prim Health Care, **25**, 178–85.

Loisel, P., Durand, M.J., Diallok, B., *et al.* (2003). From evidence to community practice in work rehabilitation: the Quebec experience. *Clin J Pain,* **19**, 105–13.

Martimo, K.P., Verbeek, J., Karppinen, J., *et al.* (2007). Manual material handling advice and assistive devices for preventing and treating back pain in workers. *Cochrane Database Syst Rev*, **3**, CD005958.

Maxwell, T.D., Gatchel, R.J., Mayer, T.G. (1998). Cognitive predictors of depression in chronic low back pain: toward an inclusive model. *J Behav Med*, **21**, 131–43.

Mayhew, H.E., Nordlund, D.J. (1998). Absenteeism certification: the physician's role. *J Fam Pract*, **26**, 651–5.

McGrail, M.P., Jr., Calasanz, M., Christianson, J., *et al.* (2002). The Minnesota Health Partnership and Coordinated Health Care and Disability Prevention: the implementation of an integrated benefits and medical care model. *J Occup Rehabil*, **12**, 43–54.

Monday, J., Therrien, S., Duguay, M., *et al.* (1988). The Physician and disability certificates: preconceived attitudes and behaviors. *Can J Psychiatry*, **33**, 599–605.

Nachemson, A. (1975). Towards a better understanding of low-back pain: a review of the mechanics of the lumbar disc. *Rheumatol Rehabil*, **14**, 129–4.

Nordqvist, C., Holmqvist, C., Alexanderson, K. (2003). Views of laypersons on the role employers play in return to work when sick-listed. *J Occup Rehabil*, **13**, 11–20.

Oxman, A.D., Thomson, M.A, , Davis, D.A, , et al. (1995). No magic bullets: a systematic review of 102 trials of interventions to improve professional practice. *CMAJ*, **153**, 1423–31.

Patel, D., Buschbacker, R., Crawford, J. (2003). National variability in permanent partial impairment ratings. *Am J Phys Med Rehabil*, **82**, 302–6.

Poiraudeau, S., Rannou, F., Baron, G., *et al.* Fear-avoidance beliefs about back pain in patients with subacute low back pain. *Pain,* **124**, 305–11.

Poiraudeau, S., Rannou, F., Le Henanff, A., *et al.* (2006). Outcome of subacute low back pain: influence of patients' and rheumatologists' characteristics. *Rheumatology*, **45**, 718–23.

Pransky, G., Katz, J.N., Benjamin, K. (2002). Improving the physician role in evaluating work ability and managing disability: a survey of primary care practitioners. *Disabil Rehabil*, **24**, 867–74.

Pransky, G., Katz, J.N., Benjamin, K., Himmelstein, J. (2002). Improving the physician role in evaluating work ability and managing disability: a survey of primary care practitioners. *Disabil Rehabil*, **24**, 867–74.

Rainville, J., Ahern, D.K., Phalen, L. (1993). Altering beliefs about pain and function in a functionally oriented treatment program for chronic low back pain. *Clin J Pain*, **9**, 196–201.

Rainville, J., Bagnall, D., Phalen, L. (1995). Health care providers' attitudes and beliefs about functional impairments and chronic back pain. *Clin J Pain*, **11**, 287–95.

Rainville, J., Carlson, N., Polatin, P., Gatchel, R.J., Indahl, A. (2000). Exploration of physicians' recommendations for activities in chronic low back pain. *Spine*, **25**, 2210–7.

Rainville, J., Hartigan, C., Jouve, C., Martinez, E., Hipona, M., Limke, J. (2002). Does medical advice about pain and function influence patients with chronic low back pain. *International Society for Study of the Lumbar Spine*, Cleveland, OH, 15–18 May, 2002.

Rainville, J., Sobel, J.B., Hartigan, C., *et al.* (1997). The effect of compensation involvement on the reporting of pain and disability by patients referred for rehabilitation of chronic low back pain. *Spine*, **22**, 2016–24.

Rao, J.K., Kroenke, K., Mihaliak, K.A., *et al.* (2002). Can guidelines impact the ordering of magnetic resonance imaging studies by primary care providers for low back pain? *Am J Manag Care*, **8**, 27–35.

Reiso, H., Gulbrandsen, P., Brage, S. (2004). Doctors'prediction of certified sickness absence. *Fam Pract*, **21**, 192–9.

Reiso, H., Nygard, J.F., Frage, S., Gulbrandsen, P., Tellnes, G. (2000). Work ability assessment by patients and their GPs in new episodes of sickness certification. *Fam Pract*, **17**, 139–44.

Roberts-Yates, C. (2003). The concerns and issues of injured workers in relation to claims/injury management and rehabilitation: the need for new operational frameworks. *Disabil Rehabil*, **25**, 898–907.

Roth, R.S., Geisser, M.E. (2002). Educational achievement and chronic pain disability: mediating role of pain-related cognitions. *Clin J Pain*, **18**, 286–96.

Scheel, I.B., Hagen, K.B., Herrin, J., *et al.* (2002). Blind faith? The effects of promoting active sick leave for back pain patients: a cluster-randomized controlled trial. *Spine,* **27**, 2734–40.

Shaw, L., Segal, R., Polatajko, H., *et al.* (2002). Understanding return to work behaviors: promoting the importance of individual perceptions in the study of return to work. *Disabil Rehabil*, **24**, 185–95.

Shaw, W.S., Pransky, G., Fitzgerald, T.E. (2001). Early prognosis for low back disability: intervention strategies for health care providers. *Disabil Rehabil*, **23**, 815–28.

Shaw, W.S., Robertson, M.M., Pransky, G., *et al.* (2003). Employee perspectives on the role of supervisors to prevent workplace disability after injuries. *J Occup Rehabil*, **13**, 129–42.

Shulman, B.M. (1994). Worklessness and disability; expansion of the biopsychosocial perspective. *J Occ Rehabil*, **4**, 113–22.

Sinclair, S.J., Hogg-Johnson, S.H., Mondloch, M.V., *et al.* (1997). The effectiveness of an early active intervention program for workers with soft-tissue injuries. The Early Claimant Cohort Study. *Spine*, **22**, 2919–31.

Soler, J.K., Okkes, I.M. (2004). Sick leave certification: an unwelcome administrative burden for the family doctor? The role of sickness certification in Maltese family practice. *Eur J Gen Pract*, **10**, 50–5.

Sullivan, M.D., Loeser, J.D. (1992). The diagnosis of disability. Treating and rating disability in a pain clinic. *Arch Intern Med*, **152**, 1829–35.

Swinkels-Meewisse, I.E., Raelofs, J., Verbeek, A.L., *et al.* (2006). Fear-avoidance beliefs, disability, and participation in workers and non-workers with acute low back pain. *Clin J Pain*, **22**, 45–54.

Symonds, T.L., Burton, A.K., Tillotson, K.M., Main, C.J. (1996). Do attitudes and belief influence work loss due to low back trouble? *Occup Med*, **46**, 25–32.

Szpalski, M., Nordin, M., Skovron, M.L., *et al.* (1995). Health care utilization for low back pain in Belgium. Influence of socio-cultural factors and health beliefs. *Spine*, **20**, 431–42.

Tellness, G., Sandvik, L., Moum, T. (1990). Inter-doctor variation in sickness certification. *Scan J Prim Health Care*, **8**, 45–52.

Turner, J.A., Jensen, M.P., Romano, J.M. (2000). So beliefs, coping, and catastrophizing independently predict functioning in patients with chronic pain? *Pain*, **85**, 115–25.

van Duijn, M., Miedema, H., Elders, L., *et al.* (2004). Barriers for early return-to-work of workers with musculoskeletal disorders according to occupational health physicians and human resource managers. *J Occup Rehabil*, **14**, 31–41.

Verbeek, J.H., van Dijk, F.J., Malmivaara, A., *et al.* (2002). Evidence-based medicine for occupational health. *Scand J Work Environ Health*, **28**, 197–204.

von Knorring, M., Sundberg, L., Lofgren, A., Alexanderson, K. (2008). Problems in sickness certification of patients: a qualitative study on views of 26 physicians in Sweden. *Scand J Prim Health Care*, **26**, 22–8.

Waddell, G., Burton, K., Aylward, M. (2000). Work and common health problems. *J Insur Med*, **39**, 109–20.

Waddell, G., Newton, M., Henderson, I., *et al.* (1993). A Fear-Avoidance Beliefs Questionnaire (FABQ) and the role of fear- avoidance beliefs in chronic low back pain and disability. *Pain*, **52**, 157–68.

Waddell, G., O'Connor, M., Boorman, S., Torsney, B. (2007). Working Backs Scotland: a public and professional health education campaign for back pain. *Spine*, **33**, 2139–43.

Watson, P.J., Bowey, J., Purcell-Jones, G., Gales, T. (2008). General practitioner sickness absence certification for low back pain is not directly associated with beliefs about back pain. *Eur J Pain*, **12**, 314–20.

Waxman, R., Tennant, A., Helliwell, P. (1998). Community survey of factors associated with consultation for low back pain. *BMJ*, **317**, 1564–7.

Zinn, W., Furutani, N. (1996). Physician perspective on the ethical aspects of disability determination. *J Gen Intern Med*, **11**, 525–32.

# Chapter 21

# The Attitudes and Beliefs of Clinicians Treating Back Pain: Do They Affect Patients' Outcome?

Tamar Pincus, Rita Santos, and Steven Vogel

## 21.1 Introduction

Many common musculoskeletal disorders do not have clear pathophysiological explanations for pain. Classifications of clinical presentations often rely on broad-based descriptions of symptoms such as 'simple low back pain'. Even where guidelines exist, these often focus broadly on patient management issues rather than the detail of diagnosis and treatment. In the absence of detailed and specific best practice guidance, clinicians' interventions are likely to be informed by their individual beliefs and attitudes (Foster et al. 2003a). The word attitude is derived from Latin, meaning 'fit and ready for action'. Attitudes are affectively loaded constructs that precede behaviour and guide choices and decisions for action (Hogg and Vaughan 2005). Given the complexities of musculoskeletal conditions and the proposed role of attitudes and beliefs in informing treatment, it is important to consider patients and practitioners in the process of care (Foster et al. 2003b). Both attitudes and their associated beliefs are addressed in this chapter with a particular focus on clinicians working primarily with musculoskeletal conditions. Low back pain (LBP) has been most thoroughly studied and is used as an exemplar. In complement to the previous chapter, this chapter highlights differences between professional groups, further discusses which beliefs and attributions in clinicians relate to patient outcome, and reviews measurements of clinicians' beliefs.

Back pain and neck pain are directly and indirectly costly to society (Maniadakis and Gray 2000; Picavet and Schouten 2003). Direct costs are often estimated through healthcare utilization, while indirect costs include days off work etc. Most people who have had an episode of back pain will have another, but might not seek help (Croft et al. 1998). A significant minority of people experiencing back pain will progress to chronic and long-term disability. The development of prevention strategies are required to avoid the high levels of distress and personal impact for these individuals and to reduce the impact on service utilization and cost to society (Linton 2002). Risk factors for the development of persistent musculoskeletal pain have been identified, and some of them include patients' beliefs and behaviours (Croft et al. 2006). Unhelpful 'myths' about back pain have also been studied in the general population. A large study of Norwegian populations found that as many as 50% believed that radiography and imaging tests were needed and that back pain indicated an injury (Ihlebaek and Eriksen 2003).

Another large survey study in Norwegian populations (Werner et al. 2005) found that approximately 20% of respondents, regardless of previous or current experience of back pain, agreed with the statement 'Bed rest is the mainstay of therapy for back pain'. In addition, only a third of respondents agreed with the statement 'One recovers faster from back pain if one continues to work or returns as soon as possible'. Similarly, a postal study of over 1600 respondents from the general population in Belgium found that 77% believe that if one has back pain, wrong movements can lead to serious problems, and 35% believed that back pain required bed rest (Goubert et al. 2004). These findings suggest that there is still a long way to go in disseminating evidence and current ideas about recovery from back pain in the general population.

Such beliefs encourage avoiding normal activities during back pain episodes, and are in direct contradiction to current guidelines (Burton et al. 2004). These beliefs and behaviours are difficult to change once entrenched. Testing theories about their acquisition is important, in order to prevent the development of unhelpful beliefs and maladaptive behaviours in future patients. A much neglected area of research is the complex interaction between patients and clinicians, including passing on information and messages about the threat posed by back pain, and advice about protective behaviours which supposedly reduce this threat. This raises the question as to whether inappropriate advice from clinicians influences the transition from acute pain to chronic disability?

## 21.2 How could clinicians increase the risk of long-term problems?

There are several ways in which clinicians may impact on the long-term well-being of their patients with musculoskeletal pain in general and back pain specifically. Effects of specific treatment interventions, adverse effects of treatment, failure to diagnose, and practical problems about timely and correct referral are outside the scope of the current chapter. However, clinicians almost always offer advice to patients, and some of this advice might slow down recovery. Most practitioners do not advocate bed rest these days (Ihlebaek and Eriksen 2004; Werner et al. 2005; Buchbinder and Jolley 2007), suggesting that for the majority of clinicians, in the case of bed rest, evidence, beliefs, and behaviour are in consensus. However, as myths about back pain are still prevalent in the general population, the problem may lie in eliciting and identifying harmful beliefs held by patients, and in communicating more appropriate knowledge as part of an educational element during treatment.

There are several hypothetical routes by which clinicians' communications with patients could be influenced by their own misconceptions, and contribute to patients unhelpful beliefs about back pain. These in turn may influence behaviours in patients that impede recovery. Individual factors that have been identified in patients as obstacles to recovery include fear of movement and hypervigilance (Vlaeyen and Linton 2000), described in this volume in Chapters 14 and 16. Clinicians may inadvertently reinforce fearful beliefs. Suggestions such as 'listen carefully to your body', 'watch out for any signs of pain', and including minor bodily asymmetries (such as uneven leg length) in causal explanations of pain may enhance or promote hypervigilance and increase fear. Increased fear has been shown to result in avoidance, culminating in a vicious circle leading to increased disability and suffering (Crombez et al. 1999; reviewed in this volume in Chapter 16).

Another hypothetical route is a recommendation for rest from work, which may include formal sick certification. The evidence on the link between clinicians' beliefs and sick certification is reviewed below, and is far from conclusive. Our own studies, described in detail below, suggest that although sick certification is rare amongst musculoskeletal practitioners in the UK, many hold the belief that a short rest from work is necessary for the body to allow healing (Pincus et al. in preparation). Current guidelines recommend moderated work duties or work as normal during episodes of musculoskeletal back pain (Waddell and Burton 2001; Staal et al. 2003). However, to date, there is no evidence that directly evaluates the cost and benefit of short-term time off work accompanied with advice to stay active and avoid bed rest.

Clinicians may also offer subtle communications about perceived harm from work. Part of patient evaluation carried out by most clinicians includes a search for possible causal factors, and most musculoskeletal practitioners explore work-related factors routinely. While this is a useful part of the investigation, it may inadvertently convey a message that work is harmful and should be avoided. Similarly, communication of empathy with suffering, such as 'Oh yes, I can see that would really hurt' may unwittingly convey a message about perceived damage if communicated in a work-related context.

## 21.3 **Measuring clinicians' beliefs**

A systematic review of current measures of beliefs and attitudes towards back pain in healthcare practitioners (Bishop et al. 2007) examined the quality of each measure in terms of their conceptual model, reliability, validity, burden (respondent and administrative), alternative forms, and language adaptations. The authors concluded that the theoretical model for most of the measures lacked validity, as items were commonly adapted from those proposed for patients. The content, adapted from patient questionnaires, does not necessarily provide a comprehensive representation of clinicians' beliefs.

Some measures of clinicians' attitudes and beliefs are very specific. For example, the Fear Avoidance Beliefs Questionnaire for Health Care Practitioners (FABQ; Coudeyre et al. 2006), is an adaptation of the Fear Avoidance Beliefs Questionnaire, developed for patients (Waddell et al. 1993). The questionnaire includes two subscales, examining beliefs about physical exercise and beliefs about work. It has been criticized for wording items almost exclusively in reference to exercise, rather than daily activities (Pincus et al. 2006a). A longer questionnaire measuring fear avoidance beliefs in practitioners was developed by Linton and colleagues (Fear avoidance beliefs tool; Linton et al. 2002). This instrument combines questions from several questionnaires (including the TSK, the FABQ, and the PAIRS) and adds items reflecting beliefs about sick leave as a treatment for back pain, and items measuring information giving by practitioners. Given the complexity of the questionnaire and the lack of information about reliability and validity, findings are difficult to interpret.

A questionnaire with a related underlying model is the Health Care Providers Pain and Impairment Relationship Scale (HC-PAIRS; Rainville et al. 1995). The HC-PAIRS was adapted from the Pain and Impairment Relationship Scale (PAIRS; Riley et al. 1988), originally developed for patients with chronic LBP, to measure beliefs about the link between pain and movement and activities. The items were adapted directly, by changing the reference from 'I' to 'Back pain patients' (Rainville et al. 1995). There are several studies reporting good reliability and validity on this scale. However, subsequent research suggests that the original factor solution needs adjusting and some items were removed, resulting in a single-factor solution, which has been shown to be moderately linked to self-report of recommendations about work and activity in response to a vignette of a patient (Houben et al. 2004).

A more comprehensive approach, albeit still focused on fear avoidance beliefs in clinicians, was taken in the development of the PABS-PT (Ostelo et al. 2003). The PABS-PT was developed from existing questionnaires for patients with chronic low back pain, including the Tampa Scale for Kinesiophobia (TSK, Miller et al. 1991); the Pain Catastrophizing Scale (PCS, Sullivan et al. 1995); the Back Beliefs Questionnaire (BBQ, Symonds et al. 1996); the FABQ (Waddell et al. 1993), plus items that were deemed to have clinical value. The resulting questionnaire consists of two subscales, labelled 'biomedical orientation' and 'behavioural orientation'. Although the authors report acceptable clinimetric properties for the questionnaire, the subscale measuring behavioural orientation has not performed well in subsequent research (Watson et al. 2008).

The Attitudes to Back Pain Scale for Musculoskeletal Practitioners (ABPS-MP; Pincus et al. 2006b) is a comprehensive questionnaire that includes items measuring beliefs about long-term treatment of patients with back pain, beliefs associated with referring patients elsewhere, and clinicians' sense of being connected to a health network. Unlike other instruments, it was developed through qualitative interviews with clinicians, as opposed to be adapted from instruments designed for patients. In addition, it includes subcategories measuring factors similar to those measured in the HC-PAIRS and PABS-PT, such as beliefs in reactivation of patients, beliefs in a biomedical model, and attitudes to exploring psychological aspects of the patients' problems. Although the questionnaire has good reported clinimetric properties (Pincus et al. 2006b; Bishop et al. 2007) it has not yet been tested in reference to reported clinical decision-making.

In summary, there are a handful of published questionnaires available to measure clinicians' beliefs and attitudes about back pain, but research in this area is still in its infancy. Even the most studied questionnaires have only been used in small national cohorts, and there are limitations, notably in reference to clear underlying models and comprehensiveness. Still missing from current measurements are several important areas, including items: (1) reflecting beliefs about clinicians' role in returning/maintaining people at work during episodes of back pain; (2) reflecting beliefs about the use of analgesia; and (3) reflecting beliefs about the need for hands-on 'manual' treatment for back pain.

## 21.4 The effect of clinician's beliefs on clinical decisions and behaviour

Arguably, clinicians' beliefs drive their clinical decisions and behaviour, although the degree of the impact of beliefs compared to other influences remains unknown. It has been argued by researchers in this field that attitudes need to be *in situ* prior to behaviour (Evans et al. 2005), based on the theory of planned behaviour. Research that has attempted to link beliefs and behaviours in practitioners is often compromised because of the difficulties of measuring clinical decisions and behaviour in real-life situations. Most published research exploring these relationships employs self-report of behaviour, or reported putative clinical behaviour in response to vignettes of patients.

A general exploration of beliefs was carried out in a study of 187 physical therapy physicians in Sweden, which found that the majority held the belief that the patients' own resources and the relationship between the clinician and patient were more important to outcome than treatment techniques. They also endorsed the view that the whole person should be treated, rather than the site of pain (Stenmar and Nordholm 1994). In a study exploring common 'myths' about low back pain in Norwegian general practitioners (GPs) (n=436) and physiotherapists (n=311), seven statements were presented to practitioners, corresponding to common mistaken beliefs about back pain (Ihlebaek and Eriksen 2004). The vast majority of the practitioners did not endorse the beliefs that tests were useful, that back pain indicated injury or that bed rest was useful. Neither study explored how beliefs were linked to clinical decisions, recommendation, treatment, and advice.

Several cross-sectional studies have found a relationship between reported beliefs and reported practice. A cross-sectional questionnaire study carried out with 60 GPs and 71 physiotherapists in Sweden (Linton et al. 2002) findings suggested that clinicians high in 'fear-avoidance' beliefs were also more likely to believe that sick leave was a good treatment for back pain. The study is limited by the choice of measurement, which mixed items from several published scales. Some of the items are difficult to interpret in the context of fear-avoidance (e.g. giving information about which activities to do and which to avoid).

In an attempt to clarify the relationship between fear-avoidance beliefs in GPs and their clinical decisions, questionnaires including a version of the FABQ (Waddell et al. 1993) were sent to French GPs (Coudeyre et al. 2006). Sixteen per cent (n=139) of the total responders (n=864) scored above a cut-point indicating high fear-avoidance beliefs, and these were associated with self-report of giving less information about back pain and higher rates of recommending sick leave.

The belief that pain should result in reduced activity has also been studied in 142 orthopaedic surgeons and family practitioners in the USA (Rainville et al. 2000). Responses on the HC-PAIRS (Rainville 1995) were moderately correlated with responses to three vignettes, and accounted for around 22% of the variance of recommendations about work. Similarly, a study of 156 Dutch manual therapists measured beliefs about the perceived harmfulness of physical activity, using the HC-PAIRS, and correlating responses with responses to a vignette of a patient. Although the correlations between beliefs and reported recommendations for work and physical activities were low to moderate(ranging from 0.25–0.62), beliefs were the only significant predictor of these recommendations when controlling for gender, years of experience, and perceived severity of symptoms and pathology, albeit accounting for only 16% of the variance (Houben et al. 2004).

In a large study of general practitioners (n=442) and physiotherapists (n=580) in the UK (Bishop et al. 2008), beliefs were measured using the PABS-PT (Houben et al. 2005). Higher biomedical beliefs and lower behavioural beliefs were associated with reported advice to stay off work in responses to a vignette of a patient with LBP, although the amount of variance accounted for by these beliefs was not reported. The study demonstrated that the belief that LBP necessitates at least some avoidance of work was common in both groups (around 30%), but only a few believed that bed rest was beneficial (Bishop et al. 2008).

One of the only studies that attempted to link beliefs and clinical behaviour in practitioners, (rather than self-report of such behaviour) explored the correlation between beliefs measured on the PABS-PT and sick leave certification (SLC) in 83 GPs in the UK (Watson et al. 2008). Neither biomedical nor psychosocial beliefs predicted SLC, but the findings were compromised by poor measurement of beliefs. In addition, there is some evidence to suggest that a common reason for GPs for giving SLC to people with a physical problem is to maintain their interpersonal relationship (Campbell and Ogden 2006). This motivation is currently not measured in questionnaires about attitudes and beliefs in clinicians.

Long-term treatment of back pain patients might be considered as an obstacle to recovery, especially in the absence of clear improvement in terms of increased activity. This was studied in chiropractors, osteopaths, and physiotherapists in the UK using mixed methods (Pincus et al. 2006c). A screening survey was sent to 200 practitioners in each profession. All those who reported treating at least one patient more than eight times over 3 months with no improvement (n=30, around 10% of each profession) were interviewed. In addition, 12 practitioners were interviewed who reported that they never treat long term without improvement. The themes emerging from the interviews provided a clear rationale for long-term treatment. Across the professions, practitioners believed that ending treatment would result in a void of care for patients. They saw their role as much wider than dealing with back pain per se, but rather, as providers of counselling and psychological support, in addition to providing 'holistic' treatment, including education about health in general. Several questionable beliefs also emerged, including the belief that on and off manual treatment prevented worsening pain and damage, and the belief that a sufficiently exhaustive search would lead to a biomechanical cause for back pain. Above all, a strong belief was expressed in patients' right to decide about ending treatment. While the study raises promising possibilities about expanding the healthcare role of musculoskeletal practitioners, there is also a danger that long-term treatment fosters dependence and reduced self-management in patients.

Of note during the interviews it emerged that those practitioners, who reported never treating long-term without improvement, all recalled at least one patient where they did so. This suggests that the 10% rate of positive responses on the survey may be an underestimate.

Finally, a small qualitative study explored the beliefs of six physiotherapists, found a high degree of biomedical orientation towards back pain in the clinicians. This was particularly evident for chronic pain situations where complex psychosocial factors were relevant. Resultant attitudes divided patients into 'good' (active and motivated) and 'difficult' to treat patients (passive and non-participatory). There was some indication that there may be inequality of treatment towards the latter group and that the physiotherapists associated the difficult to treat group with being disheartened and frustrated (Daykin and Richardson 2004). A further qualitative study exploring clinical reasoning in musculoskeletal physiotherapists, suggested that clinicians took a dynamic approach to reasoning rather than using a single approach or orientation to treatment. Five categories of reasoning were identified: biomedical, psychosocial, pain mechanisms, chronicity, and severity/irritability (Smart and Doody 2007). Deconstructing the influence of treatment orientation and clinical reasoning strategies remains a challenge. Identifying the effectiveness of different strategies and approaches in particular situations would enhance patient care and could inform the education of clinicians.

In conclusion, the majority of research linking clinicians' beliefs about back pain to their clinical behaviour has focused on the belief that pain was related to disability and that in the presence of pain, activities should be reduced. This belief, conceptualized as fear-avoidance, has been shown to be moderately linked to reported recommendations for reduced activities and work in several studies, and across several national populations. However, the variance unaccounted for by beliefs far outweighs that explained by clinicians' beliefs, suggesting that research should explore other factors affecting clinical recommendations. In addition, the methodology employed is limited by failure to establish causal links, limited measurement of beliefs and above all, failure to measure behaviour, rather than reported or hypothetical behaviour.

## 21.5 Can practitioners' beliefs be changed, and if so, is the change reflected in clinical behaviour?

Campaigns have been carried out aimed at shifting practitioners' beliefs and increasing guideline adherent practice. A Norwegian campaign aimed at doctors, physiotherapists, and chiropractors carried out between 2002–2005, emphasized optimistic advice to stay active during back pain, and encourage early return to work (Werner et al. 2008). Practitioners' beliefs were measured in a questionnaire consisting of seven statements. Measures of behaviour included reported use of diagnostic imaging and referral patterns. Responses at baseline and post campaign were obtained only for 25% of those contacted, considerably limiting the value of the findings. The results supported a shift towards consensus with guidelines between 2002 and 2005, but this shift appeared independent of exposure to the campaign. However, despite this general shift and the focused intervention, over 20% of the practitioners failed to endorse an item suggesting that recovery from back pain is enhanced by early return to work. How such beliefs translate into advice to stay off work, and in sick certification for back pain is not known.

In contrast to the findings from the Norwegian campaign, a much more costly and high profile media campaign was carried out in Australia with significant results (Buchbinder et al. 2001). In addition to the general population, a survey of GPs was carried out before and after the campaign. Doctors reported awareness of the campaign (89%) and that it had changed their beliefs about back pain (32%). The survey suggested that doctors in the county in which the campaign was carried out were almost fourfold more likely to endorse the belief that people could return to work with back pain. They also were three times more likely to reject bed rest as treatment. These beliefs were maintained 3 and 4 years post intervention (Buchbinder and Jolly 2005; 2007). Most important, the changes to beliefs in the general population and in general practitioners corresponded to a reduction in claims for back problems.

In another large randomized control trial (RCT) aimed at musculoskeletal practitioners, the trial arm participants (n=876) were sent a printed information pack about guideline recommendations for the management of back pain (Evans et al. 2005). Responses to a vignette of a patient included questions about the practitioners' recommendations for activity, work, and bed rest, and these were categorized as consistent/inconsistent with guidelines. Practitioners' beliefs were also measured, using a modified version of the HC-PIRS (Rainville et al. 1995). The results indicated a shift in beliefs, albeit of a small order, indicating a reduction in the belief that back pain should affect daily function. In addition, in the trial arm, reported behaviour became significantly more guideline consistent in reference to advice about staying active and returning to work, suggesting that an educational package can affect both beliefs and clinical behaviour.

As part of two larger RCT's Vonk and colleagues (2004) describe a small exploratory investigation addressing the relationship between clinicians' orientation as measured by the PABS-PT and their professional group. The biomedical orientation subscale of the PABS-PT was reduced in those practitioners who received training (1.5 days) to deliver a behavioural graded activity programme. In a larger study of physiotherapy students in Australia exposure to a 16 hour unit of learning on chronic back pain changed some subscale scores on The HC-PAIRS at immediate and one year follow up (Vonk et al. 2004).

## 21.6 **Differences between professional groups**

As professional philosophy, training, settings, and practice vary between professional groups treating back pain, it is important to examine difference in the beliefs of such groups. Two studies set out to test such differences explicitly. In a large survey of Norwegian practitioners, Werner and colleagues (2005) found that although three-quarters of responding physicians (GPs) endorsed that statement 'Back pain recovers best by itself', none of the responding chiropractors agreed, and over 70% disagreed with the statement. Physiotherapists were mostly (40%) unsure about the statement, but 10% of the responders in this group endorsed bed rest as treatment for back pain, in contrast to the chiropractors, who unanimously rejected the statement. Such differences in beliefs, if communicated to patients in the course of seeking care from different practitioners, must cause confusion.

A study of musculoskeletal practitioners (chiropractors, osteopaths, and physiotherapists) in the UK found overall considerable consensus across the groups (Pincus et al. 2007) and has been seen elsewhere (Vonk et al. 2009). Endorsement across the groups of a psychosocial component of treatment, and the emphasis on reactivation was demonstrated (Pincus et al. 2007). There were small but significant differences between the groups on some of the subscales of the ABS-MP. Notably, physiotherapists most highly endorsed beliefs in the value of limiting the time span of treatment and chiropractors scored least highly on this factor. This finding held true even for a subgroup of physiotherapists who practised privately.

## 21.7 **Summary: current knowledge on clinicians' beliefs**

There is a rising interest in the treatment-extrinsic factors that may affect outcome in patients with back pain, and in the role that communication with clinicians might play to reduce or increase obstacles to recovery. Research in this area is still in its early stages. There are some methodological issues related to measuring clinicians' beliefs. In addition, since it is not clear which

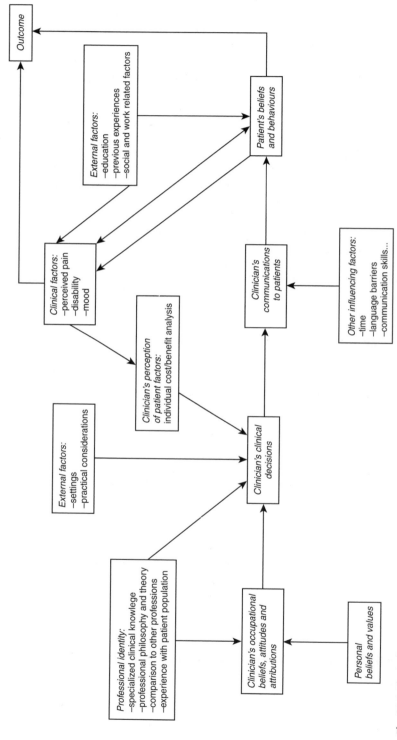

**Fig. 21.1** The indirect causal path from clinician's cognition to patient outcome.

clinicians' beliefs increase obstacles to recovery in patients, interventions have tended to focus on the messages communicated to patients, and have attempted to increase knowledge and awareness of guideline recommendations in clinicians. In general, such campaigns have been moderately successful, but results may be significantly improved if specific beliefs demonstrated to have a negative effect on patients were addressed directly.

Clinicians' education, the role of the clinical environment, habitual clinical behaviour, and practical considerations must also play a considerable role in clinical encounters. There is scope and a need to investigate these systematically. Most important is the link between non-treatment interventional behaviour and patient outcomes. This may represent an important component of the 'non-specific' aspects of care that seem to add to the effectiveness of specific interventions. The difficulty in establishing a clear causal path from clinicians' beliefs, through their behaviour, to affect patients' perceptions and behaviour and culminate in positive or negative outcome is illustrated in Figure 21.1 (informed by Evans 2007). There is to date no prospective study that examines the relationship between clinicians' beliefs and patients' outcome, along the causal route indicated in Figure 21.1. Clearly, the methodological complexity of such a study will be considerable. In addition, there is a need to clearly identify and measure factors extrinsic to beliefs that play a part in clinicians' clinical decisions and communication to patients.

## Conclusion

Beliefs in clinicians probably affect their behaviour, which in turn may affect the behaviour, perception of pain and self and ultimately, outcome in patients. Research is needed to improve measurement, so that beliefs/attitudes in clinicians can be measured and examined in RCTs and in prospective cohorts.

## References

Bishop, A., Foster, N.E., Thomas, E. and Hay, E.M. (2008). How does the self-reported clinical management of patients with low back pain relate to the attitudes and beliefs of health care practitioners? A survey of UK general practitioners and physiotherapists. *Pain*, 135, 187–95.

Bishop, A., Thomas, E. and Foster, N. (2007). Health care practitioners' attitudes and beliefs about low back pain: A systematic search and critical review of available measurement tools. *Pain*, 132, 91–101.

Buchbinder, R., Jolley, D. and Wyatt, M. (2001). Volvo Award Winner in Clinical Studies: Effects of a media campaign on back pain beliefs and its potential influence on management of low back pain in general practice. *Spine*, 26, 2535–42.

Buchbinder, R. and Jolley, D. (2005). Effects of a media campaign on back beliefs is sustained 3 years after its cessation. *Spine*, 30, 1323–30.

Buchbinder, R. and Jolley, D. (2007). Improvements in general practitioner beliefs and stated management of back pain persist 4.5 years after the cessation of a public health media campaign. *Spine*, 32, 156–62.

Burton, A.K., Balagué, F., Cardon, G., *et al.* (2006). Chapter 2. European guidelines for prevention in low back pain : November 2004. *Eur Spine J*, 15(Suppl 2), S136–68.

Campbell, A. and Ogden, J. (2006). Why do doctors issue sick notes? An experimental questionnaire study in primary care. *Family Practice*, 23, 125–30.

Coudeyre, E., Rannou, F., Tubach, F., *et al.* (2006). General practitioners' fear-avoidance beliefs influence their management of patients with low back pain. *Pain*, 124, 330–37.

Crombez, G., Vlaeyen, J.W., Heuts, P.H., and Lysens, R. (1999). Pain-related fear is more disabling than pain itself: evidence on the role of pain-related fear in chronic back pain disability. *Pain*, 80, 329–39.

Croft, P.R., Macfarlane, G.J., Papageorgiou, A.C., Thomas, E. and Silman, A.J. (1998). Outcome of low back pain in general practice: a prospective study. *British Medical Journal*, 316, 1356–9.

Croft, P.R., Dunn, K. and Raspe, H. (2006). Course and prognosis of back pain in primary care: The epidemiological perspective. *Pain*, **122**, 1–3.

Daykin, A.R. and Richardson, B. (2004). Physiotherapists' pain beliefs and their influence on the management of patients with chronic low back pain. *Spine*, **29**, 783–95.

Evans, D.W. (2007). 'Changing the practice of osteopaths, chiropractors and musculoskeletal physiotherapists, in relation to the management of back pain.' PhD Thesis. Keele University.

Evans, D.W., Foster, N.E., Underwood, M., Vogel, S., Breen, A.C. and Pincus, T. (2005). Testing the effectiveness of an innovative information package on practitioner reported behaviour and beliefs. The UK Chiropractors, Osteopaths and Musculoskeletal Physiotherapists Low Back Pain Management Trial. *BMC Musculoskeletal Disorders*, **6**, 41.

Foster, N.E., Pincus, T., Underwood, M., Vogel, S., Breen, A. and Harding, G. (2003a). Understanding the process of care for musculoskeletal conditions—why a biomedical approach is inadequate. *Rheumatology*, **42**, 401–4.

Foster, N.E., Pincus, T., Underwood, M., Vogel, S., Breen, A. and Harding, G. (2003b). Treatment and the process of care in musculoskeletal conditions: A multidisciplinary perspective and integration. *Orthopedic Clinics of North America*, **34**, 239–44.

Goubert, L., Crombez, G. and De Bourdeaudhuij, I. (2004). Low back pain, disability and back pain myths in a community sample: prevalence and interrelationships. *European Journal of Pain*, **8**, 385–94.

Hogg, M. and Vaughan, G. (2005). *Social Psychology*. London: Pearson Prentice Hall.

Houben, R.M.A., Vlaeyen, J.W.S., Peters, M., Ostelo, R.W.J.G., Wolters, P.M.J.C. and Stomp-van den Berg, S.G.M. (2004). Health care providers' attitudes and beliefs towards common low back pain: factor structure and psychometric properties of the HC-PAIRS. *Clinical Journal of Pain*, **20**, 37–44.

Houben, R.M.A., Ostelo, R.W.J.G., Vlaeyen, J.W.S., Wolters, P.M.J.C., Peters, M. and Stomp-van den Berg, S.G.M. (2005). Health care providers' orientations towards common low back pain predict perceived harmfulness of physical activities and recommendations regarding return to normal activity. *European Journal of Pain*, **9**, 173–83.

Ihlebaek, C. and Eriksen, H.R. (2003). Are the 'myths' of low back pain alive in the general Norwegian population? *Scandinavian Journal of Public Health*, **31**, 395–8.

Ihlebaek, C. and Eriksen, H.R. (2004). The 'myths' of low back pain: status quo in Norwegian general practitioners and physiotherapists. *Spine*, **29**, 1818–22.

Linton, S.J. (2002). New Avenues for the Prevention of Chronic Musculoskeletal Pain and Disability. *Pain Research and Clinical Management*. **12**. Amsterdam: Elsevier.

Linton, S.J., Vlaeyen, J. and Ostelo, R. (2002). The back pain beliefs of health care providers: are we fear-avoidant? *Journal of Occupational Rehabilitation*, **12**, 223–32.

Maniadakis, N. and Gray, A. (2000). The economic burden of back pain in the UK. *Pain*, **84**, 95–103.

Miller, R.P., Kori, S.H. and Todd, D.D. (1991). The Tampa Scale. Unpublished report, Tampa, FL.

Ostelo, R.W.J.G., Stomp-van den Berg, S.G.M., Vlaeyen, J.W.S., Wolters, P.M.J.C. and de Vet, H.H.W. (2003). Health care provider's attitudes and beliefs towards chronic low back pain: the development of a questionnaire. *Manual Therapy*, **8**, 214–22.

Picavet, H.S.J. and Schouten, J.S.A.G. (2003). Musculoskeletal pain in the Netherlands: Prevalences, consequences and risk groups, the DMC3-study. *Pain*, **102**, 167–78.

Pincus, T., Vogel, S., Burton, A.K., Santos, R. and Field, A.P. (2006a). Fear avoidance and prognosis in back pain: A systematic review and synthesis of current evidence. *Arthritis and Rheumatism*, **54**, 3999–4010.

Pincus, T., Vogel, S., Santos, R., Breen, A., Foster, N.E. and Underwood, M. (2006b). The attitudes to back pain scale in musculoskeletal practitioners (ABS-mp): The development and testing of a new questionnaire. *Clinical Journal of Pain*, **22**, 378–86.

Pincus, T., Vogel, S., Breen, A., Foster, N.E. and Underwood, M. (2006c). Persistent back pain - why do physical therapy clinicians continue treatment? A mixed methods study of chiropractors, osteopaths and physiotherapists. *European Journal of Pain*, **10**, 67–76.

Pincus, T., Foster, N.E., Vogel, S., Santos, R., Breen, A. and Underwood, M. (2007). Attitudes to back pain amongst musculoskeletal practitioners: A comparison of professional groups and practice settings using the ABS-mp. *Manual Therapy*, **12**, 167–75.

Rainville, J., Bagnall, D. and Phalen, L. (1995). Health care providers' attitudes and beliefs about functional impairments and chronic back pain. *Clinical Journal of Pain*, **11**, 287–95.

Rainville, J., Carlson, N., Polatin, P., Gatchel, R.J. and Indahl, A. (2000). Exploration of physicians' recommendations for activities in chronic low back pain. *Spine*, **25**, 2210–20.

Riley, J.F., Ahern, D.K. and Follick, M.J. (1988). Chronic pain and functional impairment: assessing beliefs about their relationship. *Archives of Physical Medicine and Rehabilitation*, **69**, 579–82.

Smart, K. and Doody, C. (2007). The clinical reasoning of pain by experienced musculoskeletal physiotherapists. *Manual Therapy*, **12**, 40–49.

Staal, J.B., Hlobil, H., van Tulder, M.W., Waddell, G., Burton, A.k., Koes, B.W., *et al.* (2003). Occupational health guidelines for the management of low back pain: an international comparison. *Occupational and Environmental Medicine*, **60**, 618–26.

Stenmar, L. and Nordholm, L.A. (1994). Swedish physical therapists' beliefs on what makes therapy work. *Physical Therapy*, **74**, 1034–39.

Sullivan, M.J.L., Bishop, S.R. and Pivik, J. (1995). The pain catastrophizing scale: development and validation. *Psychological Assessment*, **7**, 624–32.

Symonds, T.L., Burton, A.K., Tillotson, K.M. and Main, C.J. (1996). Do attitudes and beliefs influence work loss due to low back trouble? *Occupational Medicine*, **46**, 25–32.

Vlaeyen, J.W. and Linton, S.J. (2000). Fear-avoidance and its consequences in chronic musculoskeletal pain: A state of the art. *Pain*, **85**, 317–32.

Vonk, F., Verhagen, A.P., Geilen, M., Vos, C.J. and Koes, B.W. (2004). Effectiveness of behavioural graded activity compared with physiotherapy treatment in chronic neck pain: design of a randomised clinical trial. *BMC Musculoskeletal Disorders*, **5**, 34.

Vonk, F., Pool, J.J.M., Ostelo, R. and Verhagen, A. (2009). Physiotherapists' treatment approach towards neck pain and the influence of a behavioural graded activity training: An exploratory study. *Manual Therapy*, **14**, 131–7.

Waddell, G. and Burton, A.K. (2001). Occupational health guidelines for the management of low back pain at work: evidence review. *Occupational Medicine*, **51**, 124–35.

Waddell, G., Newton, M., Henderson, I., Somerville, D. and Main, C.J. (1993). A Fear-Avoidance Beliefs Questionnaire (FABQ) and the role of fear-avoidance beliefs in chronic low back pain and disability. *Pain*, **52**, 157–68.

Watson, P.J., Bowey, J., Purcell-Jones, G. and Gales, T. (2008). General practitioner sickness absence certification for low back pain is not directly associated with beliefs about back pain. *European Journal of Pain*, **12**, 314–20.

Werner, E.L., Ihlebaek, C., Skouen, J.S. and Laerum, E. (2005). Beliefs about low back pain in the Norwegian general population: are they related to pain experiences and health professionals? *Spine*, **30**, 1770–6.

Werner, E.L., Ihlebaek, C., Laerum, E., Wormgoor, M.E. and Indahl, A. (2008). Low back pain meia campaign: No effect on sickness behaviour. *Patient Education and Counseling*, **71**, 198–203.

# Part 6

# Clinical Implications: New Approaches to Diagnostics and Treatment

# Chapter 22

# International Guidelines for the Diagnostics and Treatment of Acute, Subacute, and Chronic Back Pain

## Maurits van Tulder and Bart Koes

## 22.1 Background

Evidence-based medicine has become increasingly more important over the past decade. The management of low back pain (LBP) has been positively affected by the availability of more scientific research and better use of critical appraisal techniques to evaluate and apply research findings (Chou 2005). A large number of systematic reviews are available within and outside the framework of the Cochrane Back Review Group that have evaluated the diagnostic and therapeutic interventions of LBP (Bombardier et al. 1997; Bouter et al. 2003). This large body of evidence has greatly improved our understanding of what does and does not work for LBP. However, in clinical practice this evidence should be integrated with the clinical expertise of the care provider and patient's preferences and expectations (Sackett 1996). Recently, the evidence from trials and reviews have formed the basis for clinical practice guidelines on the management of LBP that have been developed in various countries around the world (Koes et al. 2001). This chapter provides an overview of existing guidelines on LBP and discusses the challenges of implementation of these guidelines.

## 22.2 Guidelines

Since publication of the Quebec Task Force report in 1987, a number of clinical guidelines for the management of LBP in primary care have been developed in various countries worldwide. We have identified 26 clinical guidelines. We did not include guidelines that were not available in English, Dutch, and German; guidelines that were on prevention of back pain or occupational healthcare; and guidelines that were not officially approved. The final list of guidelines that we evaluated is:

1. Quebec Task Force on Spinal Disorders; Canada (Spitzer et al. 1987).

2. Agency for Health Care Policy and Research (AHCPR); United States (Bigos et al. 1994).

3. Dutch College of General Practitioners (NHG); the Netherlands (Faas et al. 1996), update (Chavannes et al. 2005).

4. Israeli Low back Pain Guideline Group; Israel (Reis & Lahad 2007).

5. Royal College of General Practitioners (RCGP); United Kingdom (Hutchinson et al. 1996; updates 1999, 2001).

6. National Advisory Committee on Health and Disability; New Zealand (National Health Committee 1997, update 2004; Kendall et al. 1997).

7. Finnish Medical Association (Duodecim); Finland (Malmivaara et al. 1999).

8. Swiss Medical Society (FMH); Switzerland (Keel et al. 1998).

9. Veterans Health Administration (VHA); United States, 1999.

10. Council on Technology Assessment in Health Care (SBU); Sweden (Nachemson & Johnson 2000).

11. Danish Institute for Health Technology Assessment; Denmark 2000.

12. Drug Committee of the German Medical Society; Germany 2000, update 2007.

13. Florida Agency for Health Care Administration & Department of Health; United States 1999, update 2000.

14. International Paris Task Force, France/Canada (Abenhaim et al. 2000).

15. Dutch Physiotherapy Guidelines (KNGF); the Netherlands (Bekkering et al. 2003).

16. Institute for Clinical Systems Improvement (ICSI); United States 2001, update 2005.

17. Philadelphia Panel; United States 2001.

18. COST B13 Working Group on Guidelines for the Management of Acute Low Back Pain in Primary Care (van Tulder et al. 2006).

19. COST B13 Working Group on Guidelines for Chronic Low Back Pain in Primary Care (Airaksinen et al. 2006).

20. American College of Physicians; American Pain Society Low Back Pain Guidelines Panel, United States (Chou et al. 2007).

21. Center of Excellence for Orthopaedic Pain Management Austria, (Friedrich & Likar 2007).

22. The Care and Research Institute (IRCCS), Italy (Negrini et al. 2006).

23. National Health and Medical Research Council, 2003, Australia.

24. Clinic on Low-Back Pain in Interdisciplinary Practice (Clip) Guidelines. Canada (Rossignol et al. 2007).

25. Royal Dutch Association for Physiotherapy; Manual Therapy Guidelines; the Netherlands 2005 (Heijmans et al. 2003).

26. Dutch Quality Institute for Healthcare; the Netherlands 2003.

## 22.3 Quality of guidelines

Since guidelines provide recommendations aimed at influencing or changing clinicians' behaviour, it is important for potential users to critically appraise the internal and external validity of these recommendations. The AGREE instrument is a helpful tool to help this process (The AGREE collaborative group 2000; www.agreecollaboration.org). The AGREE instrument consists of 23 items in six domains (Table 22.2): (1) scope and purpose of the guideline, (2) stakeholder involvement, (3) rigour of development, (4) clarity and presentation, (5) applicability, and (6) editorial independence. Each item is rated on a 4-point scale: 1= strongly disagree, 2 = disagree, 3 = agree, and 4 = strongly agree. Domain scores are calculated by dividing the difference between the obtained score and the minimum possible score by the difference between the maximum possible and minimum possible score. MacDermid et al. (2005) showed that the AGREE instrument is reliable and valid for assessing the quality of clinical guidelines relevant to physical therapy practice.

**Table 22.1** Domains and items of the AGREE instrument (www.agreecollaboration.org)

| AGREE domain | AGREE item |
|---|---|
| Scope and purpose | The overall objective of the guideline is specifically described |
| | The clinical question covered by the guideline is specifically described |
| | The patients to whom the guideline is meant to apply are specifically described |
| Stakeholder involvement | The guideline development group includes individuals from all the relevant professional groups |
| | The patients' views and preferences have been sought |
| | The target users of the guideline are clearly defined |
| | The guideline has been piloted among target users |
| Rigour of development | Systematic methods were used to search for evidence |
| | The criteria for selecting the evidence are clearly described |
| | The methods used for formulating the recommendations are clearly described |
| | The health benefits, side effects and risks have been considered in formulating the recommendations |
| | There is an explicit link between the recommendations and the supporting evidence |
| | The guideline has been externally reviewed by experts prior to its publication |
| | A procedure for updating the guideline is provided |
| Clarity and presentation | The recommendations are specific and unambiguous |
| | The different options for the management of the condition are clearly presented |
| | Key recommendations are easily identifiable |
| | The guideline is supported with tools for application |
| Applicability | The potential organizational barriers in applying the recommendations have been discussed |
| | The potential cost implications of applying the recommendations have been considered |
| | The guideline presents key review criteria for monitoring and/or audit purposes |
| Editorial independence | The guideline is editorially independent from the funding body |
| | Conflicts of interest of guideline development members have been recorded |

The AGREE group has stated that it is not yet possible to set a threshold score for the domain scores to make a distinction between 'good' and 'bad' guidelines. The AGREE instrument was developed through consensus among experts. There is little scientific evidence that the criteria included in the AGREE instrument, regardless of how logical and useful they may seem, are indeed associated with biased recommendations. Future research in this area may lead to a greater understanding of the relevance of each item.

In general, the quality of most guidelines was satisfactory (Table 22.2). The domains that were least often addressed by the guideline development committees were stakeholder involvement, applicability, and editorial independence, with mean AGREE scores of 52, 40, and 40, respectively. The guidelines scored best on the domains clarity and presentation (mean score 81) and scope and purpose (mean score 74). Many presented unambiguous recommendations, different

**Table 22.2** Scores on the AGREE domains

| Guidelines | Domains | | | | | |
|---|---|---|---|---|---|---|
| | Scope and purpose | Stakeholder involvement | Rigour of development | Clarity and presentation | Applicability | Editorial independence |
| 1. QTF (CAN) | 100 | 42 | 48 | 92 | 22 | 67 |
| 2. AHCPR (US) | 100 | 83 | 86 | 83 | 33 | 33 |
| 3. NHG (NL) | 78 | 83 | 48 | 75 | 33 | 33 |
| 4. ISR | 67 | 42 | 38 | 63 | 33 | 33 |
| 5. RCGP (UK) | 89 | 83 | 86 | 83 | 33 | 33 |
| 6. NZ | 81 | 58 | 88 | 100 | 44 | 42 |
| 7. FIN | 56 | 50 | 57 | 67 | 33 | 33 |
| 8. SUI | 67 | 50 | 38 | 63 | 33 | 33 |
| 9. VHA (US) | 100 | 33 | 48 | 92 | 11 | 17 |
| 10. SWE | 100 | 50 | 86 | 83 | 44 | 33 |
| 11. DK | 89 | 58 | 33 | 83 | 56 | 33 |
| 12. GER | 78 | 38 | 88 | 96 | 96 | 83 |
| 13. Florida (US) | 67 | 33 | 10 | 67 | 0 | 0 |
| 14. Paris | 78 | 42 | 62 | 75 | 44 | 33 |
| 15. KNGF (NL) | 44 | 50 | 38 | 42 | 0 | 0 |
| 16. ICSI (US) | 78 | 50 | 50 | 100 | 89 | 42 |
| 17. Philadelphia (US) | 89 | 75 | 76 | 83 | 33 | 50 |
| 18. COST B13 acute | 61 | 50 | 81 | 67 | 72 | 92 |
| 19 COST B13 chronic | 61 | 46 | 74 | 75 | 44 | 17 |
| 20. ACP (US) | 89 | 46 | 95 | 92 | 56 | 83 |
| 21. Austria | 67 | 54 | 48 | 46 | 11 | 8 |
| 22. Italy | 39 | 46 | 62 | 88 | 44 | 17 |
| 23. Australia | 61 | 79 | 98 | 92 | 56 | 50 |
| 24. CLIP (CAN) | 22 | 25 | 43 | 92 | 22 | 25 |
| 25. MT (NL) | 89 | 50 | 93 | 100 | 28 | 58 |
| 26. CBO (NL) | 61 | 75 | 76 | 100 | 61 | 33 |

1) Spitzer et al. 1987; 2) Bigos et al. 1994; 3) Faas et al. 1996, update Chavannes et al. 2005; 4) Reis and Lahad 2007; 5) Hutchinson et al. 1996; updates 1999, 2001; 6) National Health Committee 1997, update 2004; Kendall et al. 1997; 7) Malmivaara et al. 1999; 8) Keel et al. 1998; 9) Veterans Health Administration (VHA); United States, 1999; 10) Nachemson and Johnson 2000; 11) Danish Institute for Health Technology Assessment; Denmark 2000; 12) Drug Committee of the German Medical Society; Germany 2000, update 2007; 13) Florida Agency for Health Care Administration & Department of Health; United States 1999, update 2000; 14) Abenhaim et al. 2000; 15) Bekkering et al. 2003; 16) Institute for Clinical Systems Improvement (ICSI); United States 2001, update 2005; 17) Philadelphia Panel; United States 2001; 18) van Tulder et al. 2006; 19) Airaksinen et al. 2006; 20) Chou et al. 2007; 21) Friedrich & Likar 2007; 22) Negrini et al. 2006; 23) National Health and Medical Research Council, 2003, Australia; 24) Rossignol et al. 2007; 25) Heijmans et al. 2003; 26) Dutch Quality institute for Healthcare; the Netherlands 2003.

options for management and key recommendations were easily identifiable. Furthermore, almost every guideline had good scores on the domain of rigour of development (mean score 62).

Potential conflicts of interest were not explicitly described in most of the guidelines. Only the Quebec Task Force clearly reported that the editorial board was independent from the funding body, and the Danish and Philadelphia Panel guidelines gave the impression of editorial independence. As most guidelines were supported by either a professional association (for example, the Dutch guidelines by the College of General Practitioners in the Netherlands), a national organization (for example, the Danish guidelines by the National Institute of Health), or a commercial organization (for example, the Paris Task Force by Mayoly-Spindler Laboratories) it seems important to explicitly state whether the final recommendations were developed independently from the supporting agency. Also, other potential conflicts of interest (for example, financial support from pharmaceutical companies for research, advice, or travelling) should be disclosed as they may increase the potential risk of biased recommendations.

Few guidelines included tools to facilitate their application in clinical practice. Some included only one, such as a patient booklet in the UK guidelines, or a screening questionnaire in the New Zealand guidelines. Guidelines of the Agency for Health Care Policy and Research in the US provided a set of clinical decision algorithms, a patient booklet and a quick reference guide for clinicians, and the Dutch General Practitioners' guidelines included a summary document, a patient information letter, an 'expertise improvement package', and a programme for individual re-education. The Quebec Task Force included evaluation forms for diagnostic and therapeutic procedures, consultation, and ergonomic description of work, and matrices for diagnostic and therapeutic procedures.

In sum, many international guidelines for the management of LBP have been published and their quality of development and reporting seem to vary (van Tulder et al. 2004). At present, the AGREE instrument is probably more known among guideline developers than 10 years ago when the AGREE instrument was just published. The most recently published guidelines seem to meet more AGREE items compared with the older guidelines. However, there still is room for improvement. We have identified which AGREE items need special attention in future guidelines or updates of existing guidelines.

## 22.4 **Recommendations on diagnostics and treatment**

Although there are some differences between guidelines, most guidelines have similar recommendations for diagnostics and treatment of acute and chronic LBP. Below the recommendations of the European guidelines are presented, because this was a large initiative in which LBP experts from many European countries participated. It probably best reflects international consensus on the management of LBP.

## 22.5 **European guidelines**

To increase consistency in the management of non-specific LBP across countries in Europe, the European Commission approved a programme for the development of European guidelines for the management of low back pain, called 'COST B13'. The main objectives of this COST action were:

◆ Developing European guidelines for the prevention, diagnosis and treatment of non-specific LBP.

◆ Ensuring an evidence-based approach through the use of systematic reviews and existing clinical guidelines.

◆ Enabling a multidisciplinary approach; stimulating collaboration between primary healthcare providers and promoting consistency across providers and countries in Europe.

◆ Promoting implementation of these guidelines across Europe.

This project started in 1999 and the guidelines were finalized in 2004. To ensure an evidence-based approach, recommendations were based on Cochrane and other systematic reviews and on existing national guidelines. The European guidelines could be used as a basis for future national guidelines or future updates of existing national guidelines. The European guidelines could also help healthcare providers to make evidence-based decisions, improve the quality and outcome of healthcare, lead to a more rational and efficient use of resources, and identify gaps in the existing scientific evidence in order to prioritize future research.

The target population of the guidelines consists of healthcare providers who are reached through individuals or groups that are going to develop new guidelines or update existing guidelines, and their professional associations that will disseminate and implement these guidelines. Indirectly, these guidelines also aim to inform the general public, low back pain patients, and policy makers in Europe.

Four working groups have been initiated within this COST B13 action that produced the final guidelines on prevention, management of acute LBP, management of chronic low back pain, and management of pelvic girdle pain. The experts in the groups represented all countries that had issued guidelines for low back pain or were developing guidelines and all relevant health professions. The recommendations for the management of acute and chronic LBP are summarized in Boxes 22.1 and 22.2.

## 22.6 **Implementation of guidelines**

Development and dissemination of guidelines does not automatically mean that healthcare providers will read, understand, and use the guidelines. Passive dissemination of information is generally ineffective and specific implementation strategies are necessary to establish changes in practice. Systematic reviews have shown that a clear and strong evidence base, clear messages, consistent messages across professions, clear sense of ownership, communication with all relevant stakeholders, charismatic leadership, continuity of care, continuous education, and continuous evaluation are successful ingredients for implementation of guidelines (Grimshaw et al. 2001; Burgers et al. 2003). However, several barriers to implementation of guidelines have been identified. The practice behaviour of health professionals may be influenced by a lack of knowledge, a shortage of time, disagreement with the guideline content, or reluctance from colleagues to adhere to the guideline (Cabana et al. 1999; reviewed in this volume in Chapters 20 and 21). Furthermore, health professionals may get lost in the large number of different guidelines received.

Dissemination needs to be supplemented by active implementation strategies. Development of an implementation plan is an essential first step. It may be helpful to identify local champions for change, who are influential people that may motivate their peers to accept and start using the guideline. Setting clear, specific and realistic objectives, and identifying barriers to change behaviour of health professionals should have priority in getting evidence into clinical practice. Because there is not one single intervention that is clearly more effective than others, a multifaceted approach starting with strategies that are likely to have visible results is recommended. Recently, a number of trials have evaluated implementation strategies for low back pain guidelines (Rossignol et al. 2000; McGuirk et al. 2001; Bekkering et al. 2003; Dey et al. 2004; Engers et al. 2005). Four of these studies were randomized trials, one a non-randomized trial. All studies compared the implementation strategy with usual care by general practitioners or physiotherapists.

## Box 22.1 European guidelines on the management of acute low back pain

### Summary of recommendations for diagnosis of acute non-specific low back pain

◆ Case history and brief examination should be carried out.

◆ If history-taking indicates possible serious spinal pathology or nerve root syndrome, carry out more extensive physical examination including neurological screening when appropriate.

◆ Undertake diagnostic triage at the first assessment as basis for management decisions.

◆ Be aware of psychosocial factors, and review them in detail if there is no improvement.

◆ Diagnostic imaging tests (including X-rays, computed tomography [CT] and magnetic resonance imaging [MRI]) are not routinely indicated for non-specific LBP.

◆ Reassess those patients who are not resolving within a few weeks after the first visit, or those who are following a worsening course.

### Summary of recommendations for treatment of acute non-specific low back pain

◆ Give adequate information and reassure the patient.

◆ Do not prescribe bed rest as a treatment.

◆ Advise patients to stay active and continue normal daily activities including work if possible.

◆ Prescribe medication, if necessary for pain relief; preferably to be taken at regular intervals; first choice paracetamol, second choice non-steroidal anti-inflammatory drugs (NSAIDs).

◆ Consider adding a short course of muscle relaxants on its own or added to NSAIDs, if paracetamol or NSAIDs have failed to reduce pain.

◆ Consider (referral for) spinal manipulation for patients who are failing to return to normal activities.

◆ Multidisciplinary treatment programmes in occupational settings may be an option for workers with subacute LBP and sick leave for more than 4–8 weeks.

The three randomized trials reported some improvement on process outcomes (an increase in adherence to recommendations), but did not show any significant differences on patient outcomes.

Although guidelines are expected to improve patient outcomes, the evidence is sparse and not yet convincing. This is a bit disappointing, because one would expect that successful implementation of evidence-based guidelines is associated with improved patient outcomes. Failure to find positive results may be related to insufficient content and/or intensity of the implementation strategies. But the control groups may also have performed better that expected. General practitioners and physiotherapists who participated in the trials may have volunteered because they were interested in LBP, and they may have already been familiar with the latest evidence in this field. This limitation potentially decreased the contrast in guideline adherence between the implementation and control groups in the trials, and may be the most important reason for the lack of difference in patient outcomes between groups. It is also possible that general practitioners and physiotherapists in the control groups read the guidelines better than they would have done if they had not participated in these trials.

## Box 22.2 European guidelines on the management of chronic low back pain

### Summary of diagnosis in chronic low back pain

#### Patient assessment

◆ Physical examination and case history: the use of diagnostic triage, to exclude specific spinal pathology and nerve root pain, and the assessment of prognostic factors ('yellow flags') are recommended. We cannot recommend spinal palpatory tests, soft tissue tests and segmental range of motion, or straight leg raising tests (Laseque) in the diagnosis of non-specific chronic LBP.

◆ Imaging: we do not recommend imaging (plain radiography, CT or MRI), bone scanning, SPECT, discography or facet nerve blocks for the diagnosis of non-specific chronic low back pain unless a specific cause is strongly suspected.

◆ MRI is the best imaging procedure for use in diagnosing patients with radicular symptoms, or for those in whom discitis or neoplasm is suspected.

◆ Electromyography: we cannot recommend electromyography for the diagnosis of non-specific chronic low back pain.

#### Prognostic factors

Assessment of work-related factors, psychosocial distress, depressive mood, severity of pain and functional impact, prior episodes of LBP, extreme symptom reporting and patient expectations should be included in the diagnosis of patients with non-specific chronic low back pain.

### Summary of treatment of chronic low back pain

◆ *Conservative treatments:* cognitive-behavioural therapy, exercise therapy, brief educational interventions, and multidisciplinary (biopsychosocial) treatment can each be recommended for non-specific CLBP. Back schools and short courses of manipulation can also be considered. The use of physical therapy (TENS, heat/cold, traction, laser, ultrasound, short wave, interferential, massage, corsets) cannot be recommended.

◆ *Pharmacological treatments:* noradrenergic or noradrenergic-serotoninergic antidepressants, weak opioids, and the short term use of NSAIDs, muscle relaxants, and capsicum plasters can be recommended for pain relief; strong opioids can be considered in patients who do not respond to all other treatment modalities.

◆ *Invasive treatments:* acupuncture, epidural corticosteroids, intra-articular (facet) steroid injections, local facet nerve blocks, intradiscal injections, trigger point injections, botulinum toxin, prolotherapy, radiofrequency facet denervation, intradiscal radiofrequency lesioning, intradiscal electrothermal therapy, radiofrequency lesioning of the dorsal root ganglion, and spinal cord stimulation cannot be recommended for CLBP. Percutaneous electrical nerve stimulation (PENS) and neuroreflextherapy can be considered where available.

*Surgery* for non-specific CLBP cannot be recommended unless 2 years of all other recommended conservative treatment (inclusive multidisciplinary approaches with combined programmes of cognitive intervention and exercises) have failed, or such combined programmes are not available, and only then in carefully selected patients.

## 22.7 **Discussion**

Since the available evidence is international, one would expect that each country's guidelines would give more or less similar recommendations regarding diagnosis and treatment. Comparison of clinical guidelines for the management of LBP in primary care from 11 different countries showed that the content of the guidelines regarding the diagnostic classification (diagnostic triage) and the use of diagnostic and therapeutic interventions is quite similar. However, there were also some discrepancies in recommendations across guidelines (Koes et al. 2001). Differences in recommendations between guidelines may be due to the incompleteness of the evidence, different levels of evidence, magnitude of effects, side effects and costs, differences in healthcare systems (organization/financial), or differences in membership of guidelines committees. More recent guidelines may have included more recently published trials and, therefore, may end up with slightly different recommendations compared with older guidelines. Also, guidelines may have been based on systematic reviews that included trials in different languages; the majority of existing reviews have considered only studies published in a few languages, and several, only those published in English.

Recommendations in guidelines are not only based on scientific evidence, but also on consensus. Guideline committees may consider various arguments differently, such as the magnitude of the effects, potential side effects, cost-effectiveness, and current routine practice and available resources in their country. Especially as we know that effects in the field of LBP, if any, are usually small and short-term effects only (Keller et al. 2007), interpretation of effects may vary among guideline committees. Also, guideline committees may differently weigh other aspects such as side effects and costs. The constitution of the guideline committee and the professional bodies they represent, may introduce bias—either for or against a particular treatment. This does not necessarily mean that one guideline is better than the other or that one is right and the other is wrong. It merely shows that when translating the evidence into clinically relevant recommendations more aspects play a role, and that these aspects may vary locally or nationally.

However, most international guidelines on the management of LBP include similar recommendations in diagnostics and treatment. During the last 10–15 years, various guideline committees around the world have evaluated the available evidence, considered other aspects such as side effects, costs, patient preferences and expectations, and availability, and developed similar recommendations. So there seems to be consensus on optimal management for acute and chronic LBP. Changing the behaviour of care providers to result in less variation in practice and improved adherence to guideline recommendations is the biggest challenge for the next decade.

## References

Abenhaim, L., Rossignol, M., Valat, J.P. *et al.* (2000). The role of activity in the therapeutic management of back pain. Report of the International Paris Task Force on Back Pain. *Spine,* **25** (4 Suppl.), S1–33.

Airaksinen, O., Brox, J.I., Cedraschi, C. *et al.* On behalf of the COST B13 Working Group on Guidelines for Chronic Low Back Pain. (2006). Chapter 4. European guidelines for the management of chronic nonspecific low back pain. *European Spine Journal,* **15** (Suppl 2), S192–300.

Bekkering GE, Hendriks HJM, Koes BW, *et al.* National Practice Guideline for the physiotherapeutic management of patients with low back pain. *Physiotherapy* 2003; **89**:82–96 [first published in Dutch in 2001].

Bigos S, Bowyer O, Braen G. *Acute low back problems in Adults. Clinical Practice Guideline no. 14.* AHCPR Publication No. 95–0642. ed. Rockville, MD: Agency for Health Care Policy and Research, Public Health Service, U.S., Department of Health and Human Services, USA, 1994.

Bombardier C, Esmail R, Nachemson AL, Back Review Group Editorial Board. The Cochrane Collaboration Back Review Group for spinal disorders. *Spine* 1997; **22**:837–40.

Bouter LM, Pennick V, Bombardier C; The Editorial Board of the Back Review Group. Cochrane back review group. *Spine* 2003; **28**:1215–18.

Burgers JS, Grol RP, Zaat JO, Spies TH, van der Bij AK, Mokkink HG. Characteristics of effective clinical guidelines for general practice. *Br J Gen Pract* 2003; **53**:15–19.

Cabana MD, Rand CS, Powe NR, *et al*. Why don't physicians follow clinical practice guidelines? A framework for improvement. *JAMA* 1999; **282**:1458–65.

Chavannes AW, Mens JMA, Koes BW, *et al*. Dutch general practice guideline for non-specific low back pain [in Dutch] *Huisarts Wet* 2005; **48**:113–23.

Chou R. Evidence-based medicine and the challenge of low back pain: where are we now? *Pain Practice* 2005; **5**(3):153–78.

Chou R, Qaseem A, Snow V *et al*. Clinical Efficacy Assessment Subcommittee of the American College of Physicians; American College of Physicians; American Pain Society Low Back Pain Guidelines Panel. Diagnosis and treatment of low back pain: a joint clinical practice guideline from the American College of Physicians and the American Pain Society. *Ann Intern Med* 2007; **147**(7):478–91.

Danish Institute for Health Technology Assessment. Low back pain: frequency, management and prevention from a health technology perspective. Copenhagen: National Board of Health, 2000.

Dey P, Simpson CWR, Collins SI, *et al*. Implementation of RCGP guidelines for acute low back pain: a cluster randomized controlled trial. *Br J Gen Pract* 2004; **54**:33–7.

Drug Committee of the German Medical Society. *Recommendations for treatment of low back pain* [in German]. Köln: Drug Committee of the German Medical Society, 2000, update 2007.

Dutch Institute for Healthcare Improvement (CBO). *Clinical guideline for non-specific low back pain*, 2003 [in Dutch]. Amsterdam: CBO.

Engers AJ, Wensing M, van Tulder MW *et al*. Implementation of the Dutch low back pain guideline for general practitioners: a cluster randomized controlled trial. *Spine* 2005; **30**:559–600.

Faas A, Chavannes AW, Koes BW *et al*. NHG-Standaard 'Lage-Rugpijn' (in Dutch). *Huisarts Wet* 1996; **39**:18–31.

Florida Agency for Health Care Administration and the Department of Health. Universe of Florida patients with low back pain or injury: medical practice guidelines. Tallahassee, FL: Florida Agency for Health Care Administration and the Department of Health, 1999, update 2000.

Friedrich M, Likar R. Evidenz- und konsensusbasierte österreichische Leitlinien für das Management akuter und chronischer unspezifischer Kreuzschmerzen. *Wien Klin Wochenschr* 2007; **119**(5–6):189–97.

Grimshaw J, Shirran L, Thomas R. Changing provider behavior: an overview of systematic reviews of interventions. *Medical Care* 2001; **29**:II2–II45.

Heijmans M, Hendriks HJM, Koes BW *et al*. National Practice Guideline for manual therapy for patients with low back pain [in Dutch]. *Ned Tijdschr Fys* 2003; **113** (Suppl. 3):1–24.

Hutchinson A, Waddell G, Feder G, Breen A, Burton K, Sears C. *Clinical Guidelines for the Management of Acute Low Back Pain*. London: Royal College of General Practitioners, UK, 1996 (updated in 1999, 2001).

Institute for Clinical Systems Improvement (ICSI). *Adult low back pain*. Bloomington, MN: Institute for Clinical Systems Improvement (ICSI), 2005.

Keel P, Weber M, Roux E, Gauchat M-H, Schwarz H, Jochum H. *Kreuzschmerzen: Hintergründe, Prävention, Behandlung*. Bern: Verbindung der Schweizer Ärzte, FMH; Switzerland, 1998.

Keller A, Hayden J, Bombardier C, van Tulder M. Effect sizes of non-surgical treatments of non-specific low-back pain. *Eur Spine J* 2007; **16**:1776–88.

Kendall N, Linton S, and Main C. *Guide to Assessing Psychosocial Yellow Flags in Acute Low Back Pain: Risk Factors for Long-Term Disability and Work Loss*. Wellington: National Advisory Committee on Health and Disability, and ACC (Accident Rehabilitation and Compensation Insurance Corporation), 1997.

Koes BW, Van Tulder MW, Ostelo R, Kim BA, Waddell G. Clinical guidelines for the management of low back pain in primary care: an international comparison. *Spine* 2001; **26**:2504–13.

**Laerum E, Storheim K, Brox JL.** New clinical guidelines for low back pain. *Tidsskr Nor Laegeforen* 2007; **127**(20):2706.

**MacDermid JC, Brooks D, Solway S,** *et al.* Reliability and validity of the AGREE instrument used by physical therapists in assessment of clinical practice guidelines. *BMC Health Serv Res* 2005; **5**:18.

**Malmivaara A, Kotilainen E, Laasonen E, Poussa M, Rasmussen M.** *Clinical Practice Guidelines of the Finnish Medical Association Duodecim. Diseases of the low back.* Duodecim: The Finnish Medical Association 1999 (Finland) (available in English).

**McGuirk B, King W, Govind J, Lowry J, Bogduk N.** Safety, efficacy, and cost effectiveness of evidence-based guidelines for the management of acute low back pain in primary care. *Spine* 2001; **26**:2615–22.

**Nachemson AL, Jonsson E. (Eds.)** Neck and back pain: the scientific evidence of causes, diagnosis, and treatment. Philadelphia, PA: Lippincott Williams & Wilkins, 2000.

**National Health and Medical Research Council Australian Acute Musculoskeletal Pain Guidelines Group.** *Management of acute musculoskeletal pain.* Brisbane: National Library of Australia Cataloguing-in-Publication, 2003.

**National Health Committee. National Advisory Committee on Health and Disability, Accident Rehabilitation and Compensation Insurance Corporation.** *New Zealand Acute Low Back Pain Guide.* Wellington, New Zealand; 1997, update 2004.

**Negrini S, Giovannoni S, Minozzi S,** *et al.* Diagnostic therapeutic flow-charts for low back pain patients: the Italian clinical guidelines. *Euro Medicophys* 2006; **42**(2):151–70.

**Philadelphia panel.** Philadelphia panel evidence-based clinical practice guidelines on selected rehabilitation interventions for low back pain. *Phys Ther* 2001; **81**:1641–74.

**Reis S, Lahad A.** Clinical guidelines for diagnosis and treatment of acute low back pain. *Harefuah* 2007; **146**(8):631–5, 644.

**Rossignol M, Abenhaim L, Seguin P** *et al.* Coordination of primary health care for back pain. A randomized controlled trial. *Spine* 2000; **25**:251–9.

**Rossignol M, Arsenault B, Dionne C** *et al. Clinic on Low-Back Pain in Interdisciplinary Practice (Clip) Guidelines.* 2007. http://www.santpub-mtl.qc.ca/clip.

**Sackett DL, Rosenberg WM, Gray JA,** *et al.* Evidence based medicine: what it is and what it isn't. *BMJ* 1996; **312**:71–72.

**Spitzer WO, LeBlanc FE, Dupuis M** *et al.* Scientific approach to the assessment and management of activity-related spinal disorders. *Spine* 1987; **12**(Suppl. 7):S1–S59.

**The AGREE (Appraisal of Guidelines, Research, and Evaluation in Europe) Collaborative Group.** Guideline development in Europe. An international comparison. *Int J Technol Assess Health Care* 2000; **16**:1039–49.

**The Dutch Institute for Healthcare Improvement (CBO).** *Clinical guideline for non-specific low back pain,* 2003 [in Dutch].

**Van Tulder MW, Tuut M, Pennick V** *et al.* Quality of primary care guidelines for acute low back pain. *Spine* 2004; **29**(17):E357–62.

**Van Tulder MW, Becker A, Bekkering T** *et al.* European guidelines for the management of acute low back pain in primary care. *Eur Spine J* 2006; **15**(Suppl 2):S169–91.

**Veterans Health Administration, Department of Defense.** Clinical practice guideline for the management of low back pain or sciatica in the primary care setting. Washington (DC): Department of Veterans Affairs (US); 1999.

**Wong DA, Mayer T, Watters W,** *et al.* Unremitting low back pain: North American Spine Society Phase III Clinical Guidelines for multidisciplinary spine care specialists. La Grange, Ill.: *North American Spine Society,* 2000:**96**.

# Part 7

# Clinical Approaches for Patients with Acute and Subacute Low Back Pain

# Chapter 23

# Engaging Patients in their Own Care for Back Care: The Role of Education and Advice in the Prevention of Chronic Pain and Disability

Chris J. Main and Kim Burton

## 23.1 Introduction

There is a spectrum of views about the actual and potential role of education and advice in the prevention of chronic pain and disability. There is on the one hand an optimism bordering on the naïve that an essential feature of the problem of chronic low back pain (CLBP) and disability is a simple knowledge deficit (on the part of patients), the correction of which by provision of knowledge and advice will be sufficient to prevent chronic pain or disability. Then there is an opposing view that education and advice are valueless or that patients are uneducable. In attempting to find a middle way between these two extremes, we begin with a review of the evidence, viewed from a number of perspectives. In considering the role of education for patients we shall also consider the role of the healthcare professional (HCP). We shall then attempt to integrate the findings into an action plan, with suggestions for a refocusing of our educational efforts in secondary prevention in patients with recurrent or persistent pain in which our principal objective is the prevention of unnecessary disability or distress rather than the prevention of further pain per se which is unlikely to be achievable.

In n developing an analysis or our current state of knowledge we shall consider: (1) the educational process; (2) types of intervention; (3) effectiveness and sustainability; (4) influence of patient characteristics; and (5) the influence of health professionals, beliefs and treatment orientations. We shall then consider: (1) education content for LBP patients; (2) the educational context; and (3) the development of an educational strategy. Finally, we will then attempt to draw a number of conclusions.

We shall, where possible, draw specifically on education/advice in the context of LBP and other musculoskeletal conditions, in which the provision of education and advice has been examined. However, we will focus particularly on their role in tacking obstacles to recovery and optimal function in the context of secondary prevention.

Our primary focus will be on the prevention of unnecessary limitations in functioning and adverse effects on well-being rather than on the prevention of persistent pain per se. Finally, by way of introduction, we declare our own starting point, or biases. We view the provision of education and advice as a core element of clinical management; and we have attempted to be open-minded about the value of education and advice. Thus we begin with an evaluation of research findings. We suspect however that education and advice may be a necessary but not sufficient condition for producing effective behaviour change. We are mindful therefore, in the appraisal of effectiveness of educational strategies, to require consideration of the effect of knowledge in the context of overall clinical or self-directed management, rather than restrict our attention to the establishment of improved understanding of low back pain (LBP) and its effects, important though that is, in addressing obstacles to optimal function and well-being.

## 23.2 Current state of knowledge

### 23.2.1 The educational process

Any web-based search for information about LBP or advice on its management will yield an astonishing quantity and quality of material, ranging from unashamed commercial pitches, via thinly disguised pseudo-scientific studies promising miracle cures, to properly conducted scientific studies illustrating the limitations of our knowledge. Education and advice have, in fact, been included explicitly within the behaviourally-based approach to prevention and rehabilitation developed in the Back Schools, pioneered in companies such as Volvo in Sweden in the early 1970s. Backs schools offered a strategy for primary prevention, but subsequently became a therapeutic strategy in the management of LBP for those who had already developed LBP, and later became an educational 'vehicle' widely adopted in clinical treatment.

### General educational principles

Wensing and Grol (2005) describe the five different types of educational intervention highlighted by the Cochrane EPOC group (Thorsen and Makele, 1999): (1) provision of educational materials: (2) large-scale educational meetings: (3) small-scale educational meetings: (4) outreach visits; and (5) use of opinion leaders. They summarize the conclusions of 39 reviews of controlled trials and conclude that:

> the effects on professional behaviour and health outcomes of reading educational materials or attending courses are often limited. Small-scale and interactive education may be more effective, but little research evidence supports this. Factors that may increase the effectiveness of education include longer time period, an appropriate group compensation, needs assessment before the activity, active participation, individualisation and the use of local opinion leaders (p. 147).

Wensing and Grol offered, however, the further observation that 'Although the effects of education on behaviour may be limited, it is often a first necessary step in a process of implementation of innovations. Education is particularly valuable if it is part of a broader implementation strategy that includes other interventions as well' (p. 147). Although these reflections are directed particularly at the education of HCPs they illustrate the general principle that effective education needs to be embedded within targeted implementation strategies, and suggest that education of LBP patients similarly might need to be linked with specific behavioural change strategies.

### Researching the effectiveness of educational interventions

Hutchinson and Baker (1999) having noted that HCPs were often reluctant to value research into the effectiveness of educational interventions, and having identified a number of factors which might influence the effectiveness of intervention, stressed the need for 'rigorously designed research' as a priority in medical education and drew attention to the increase in behavioural complexity as the focus of the educational endeavour widened

### Education about the nature of LBP

Waddell (2004) offers a fascinating historical view of different ways in which LBP has been understood. These differing perspectives have in turn influenced our approach to patient education. There has been a plethora of educational materials developed about LBP, but traditionally,

LBP has been viewed from three distinct, but related, perspectives. Firstly, LBP has been viewed primarily as a structural problem and much educational material has reflected this. Typically, illustrations of the spine with its vertebrae, nerves and associated musculature are accompanied by illustrations of 'slipped discs', or other physical effects of trauma and disease. Underpinning this approach has been an attempt to provide reassurance about safe activity, but (arguably) presenting the back as a weak and vulnerable structure. Until relatively recently, this primarily 'orthopaedic view' of the origins of LBP was at the heart of most educational material, and although not inaccurate was unrepresentative of the much larger proportion of LBP for which no structural abnormality, physiological abnormality or disease can be identified. Secondly, the 'biomechanical view', locating the source of LBP in terms of misalignments of various sorts to be corrected by spinal manipulation and mobilization, has underpinned the manual therapies, and evident particularly in chiropractic and osteopathy. This is similar to the orthopaedic view in requiring some sort of passive treatment, delivered by an HCP as a corrective. Thirdly, and perhaps most common of all, has been the plethora of pharmacological approaches designed to abolish or ameliorate the pain signal itself, in which the 'educational' component is confined primarily to advice about dose and warnings about side-effects.

Considered together, the impact of these three general approaches has been a primary focus on 'abnormality' and promulgated the view that the back was 'fragile' and that every caution must be taken to avoid damaging it, but none of these general approaches has focused explicitly on the potential benefits of self-help or equipped patients to embark on more effective self-management.

## Education about the management of LBP

Waddell (2004) contrasts traditional biomedical education with some of the early attempts to address beliefs about fears of hurting and harming and offer simple messaging about positive adaptive coping as illustrated in the psychosocial leaflet developed by Symonds et al. (1995), and its later derivative *The Back Book* (Roland et al. 2002), an evidence based attempt to provide biopsychosocial information and advice.

In fact even the earliest pain management programmes advocated a fairly strict behavioural approach (Fordyce 1976), incorporated educational components on the nature of pain behaviour and strategies designed to restore function. The later development of cognitive-behavioural therapy (CBT) to problems of chronic pain (Turk et al. 1983) gave considerable impetus to the investigation of pain cognitions, with the development of a host of psychometric tools designed to capture patient beliefs and expectations. It had become evident to pain clinicians that unhelpful or mistaken beliefs were common features of patients presenting with chronic pain. Iatrogenic confusion and distress were frequently observed in patients attending pain management programmes (Main et al. 2008). An essential component in addressing such unhelpful beliefs (and maladaptive pain behaviours) was the provision of information about the nature of pain, pain mechanisms, the role of emotion and the relationship between pain and disability as a precursor to tackling these powerful psychological obstacles to improved function. Education and the provision of advice therefore have always been at the heart of pain management, but it has not been possible to disentangle their specific worth within such a complex type of therapeutic intervention.

## 23.2.2 **Types of intervention**

Engers et al. (2008) have defined patient education as 'any set of planned condition-specific educational activities in a one-to-one situation, designed to improve patients' health behaviours and health status in regard to the low back problem' (p. 21), a reasonable starting point perhaps, (apart from the exclusion of education delivered on a group basis), but potentially including a wide range of interventions ranging from a five minute oral information session to multidisciplinary 3-hour sessions, although they acknowledge a 'thin line between individual patient education lasting several hours, psycho-education and counselling'. For the purpose of this review we shall focus firstly on public health initiatives and secondly on initiatives directed at LBP consulters.

## Public health initiatives and media campaigns

Prior back trouble is a strong predictor of future recurrence (Burton and Tillotson 1991). This has led to the proposal that those who have survived previous episodes of back pain with little trouble are at reduced risk of future disability, compared with those who present for the first time or those who have had more severe prior episodes (Hazard et al. 1996, McIntosh et al. 2000). Therefore, interventions that aim to alter community views, targeted at populations as a whole, may be an effective way of improving outcomes from back pain. Population-based approaches clearly have potential benefits. Modifying the knowledge or attitudes of a large proportion of the community simultaneously, provides social support for behavioural change and maintenance of change over time (Redman et al. 1990); and, because of the ubiquitous nature of back pain, even small or modest impacts in those at low or medium risk are likely to deliver large improvements on a population-based scale (Rose, 1992). Importantly, shifting the whole distribution of population beliefs invariably alters the beliefs of those hard to identify high-risk individuals (Redman et al. 1990), and may prime the population for more targeted approaches

Several countries have performed mass media campaigns in an attempt to modify population beliefs about back pain, with varying degrees of success (Buchbinder et al. 2001; Waddell et al. 2007; Werner et al. 2008). The outcomes to date have shown concordant results with respect to shifting public attitudes and beliefs about back pain towards being more optimistic and proactive, yet have yielded mixed results with respect to actual behaviour change (Buchbinder et al. 2008). It would appear that more intensive and expensive media campaigns may be more effective than low-budget campaigns, television may be more effective than radio and print media, and that explicit recommendations regarding work may be needed if changes in work-related outcomes are wanted (Buchbinder et al. 2008). Furthermore, to ensure consistency and reinforcement of the messages of a media campaign, it is important to garner widespread support for the key messages from all the important stakeholders. Indeed social influences have also been shown to play a more important role than scientific influences in shaping the behaviours and medical decisions of physicians (Dixon 1990).

## Education and advice within a cognitive-behavioural approach

During the past two or three decades, however, there has been increasing recognition of the importance of cognitive factors and this has been reflected in the design of a range of research studies, particularly in the treatment of low back pain, which have included a focus to a greater or lesser extent on the modification of beliefs and behaviour, in the context of early intervention. Clearly all therapeutic encounters incorporate, at least to some extent, a focus on cognitions and behaviour, but CBT differs in that the *explicit* focus of intervention is on the modification of thoughts *and* behaviour, rather than medical or biomechanical abnormality. The psychosocial component within the cognitive-behavioural approach (CBA) is offered within a framework of reactivation and therefore should be viewed more as 'psychologically informed physiotherapy' rather than psychotherapy per se.

## Specific evaluations of educational interventions in LBP

An early randomized controlled trial (RCT) of *The Back Book* versus a traditional biomedical booklet (Burton et al. 1999) demonstrated a significant shift in inevitability of back problems with reduction of fear of physical activity in highly fearful LBP patients. Both Von Korff et al. (1998) and Moore et al. (2000) reduced back-related worries and fear-avoidance beliefs worry in RCTs of an educational approach that focused on self-management. Albaladejo et al. (2010), in a primary care RCT, found that the additional of a short education programme on active management to usual care led to a small but consistent improvement in disability, pain, and quality of life. In another RCT conducted in Spain, Kovacs et al. (2010) found in a group of institutionalized elderly subjects that *The Back Book* and a 20-min group talk improved disability 6 months later.

In the context of early interventions (usually in terms of secondary prevention) the derivation of simpler psychosocial interventions than 'full-blown CBT', containing a specific but narrower focus on pain- or disability-specific cognitions and behaviour, in patients with less entrenched disability, has offered an alternative to 'traditional' physiotherapy, based on manipulation or mobilization. Linton and Andersson (2000) conducted an interesting RCT compared a CBT programme of six 2-hour sessions with the Symonds et al. (1995) pamphlet (referenced above) and a conventional packet of 'biomedical' material. Although the CBT programme was more effective in reducing future sickness absence, all three groups improved in pain, fear-avoidance and catastrophizing. In such 'patient-centred' approaches, the role of education and advice is fundamental.

### Education and advice within psychologically informed re-activation.

Education and advice have been core ingredients in the development of CBA approaches to re-activation delivered in primary and secondary care. Many of the early educational approaches seemed to be based on assumption of a 'knowledge deficit' for which provision of adequate education was required. Stages in the development of the CBA are shown in Box 23.1.

The psychosocial intervention in the 'first-wave' studies included a fairly didactic educational approach. Thus in an early study comparing back school with an exercise intervention for patients

## Box 23.1 Stages in the development of the cognitive-behavioural approach

### Wave 1

- ◆ Educational approaches (e.g. back schools).
- ◆ Assumption of a knowledge deficit.
- ◆ Generic approach.
- ◆ No assessment of competency in cognitive-behavioural approach.

### Wave 2

- ◆ Specific cognitive and behavioural content.
- ◆ Generic approach.
- ◆ No specific training in yellow flag elicitation.

### Wave 3

- ◆ Specific yellow flag training.
- ◆ Competencies assumed.
- ◆ Individualized approach.

with chronic back pain, demonstrated that both approaches led to clinical improvement at 6-weeks follow-up (Klaber-Moffett et al. 1986). The back school patients continued to improve thereafter but the reasons were not fully explored. Education per se thus may be of value. Indeed in a later controlled study Frost et al. (2004) found that a simple discussion with a physiotherapist concerning the causes of back pain and advice on how to remain active was as successful in the long-term as routine physiotherapy, but the level of disability was low and although both groups improved, the improvements were modest, suggesting that the improvements may have been suboptimal.

In a second-wave study (including a more developed psychosocial 'CBT' component, Klaber-Moffett et al. 1999), the intervention consisted of a physiotherapist-led exercise class including strengthening exercises, stretching exercises, relaxation and 'brief education on back care'. The results demonstrated that, at 6- and 12-month follow-up, the changes in the intervention group were significantly greater than in the control group (and at no greater cost), despite the fact that their intervention was surprisingly brief—only eight 1-hour sessions over 4 weeks. Furthermore those participants who scored more highly on fear avoidance beliefs were more likely to benefit from the programme, suggesting that education about fear and avoidance may have been important (Klaber et al. 2004). Although it is not known whether such factors were in fact identified and targeted as such in the intervention group, and the physiotherapists involved seem to have been given only minimal training in cognitive-behavioural techniques. Nonetheless the study is one of the first explicitly to recognize the possible influence of cognitive factors on early community-based interventions for LBP.

George et al. (2003) compared a simple intervention for patients with acute low-back pain, designed to challenge fear-avoidance beliefs and promote early activation, with standard care. Although the intervention is described as 'Fear-Avoidance Physical Therapy' and would seem to be a prime candidate for psychologically enhanced physiotherapy, the intervention seems to have consisted essentially of an initial orientation with *The Back Book* (Roland et al 2002), followed by a behaviourally-focused approach to re-activation. Those in the treatment group demonstrated greater changes in fear-avoidance beliefs although it appears unlikely that there was any sort of systematic attempt to address cognitions, over and above the educational material. Finally, in the UK BEAM Trial (UK BEAM Trial Team 2004) exercise, manipulation and manipulation followed by exercise were compared with 'best care' in general practice (which included delivery of *The Back Book* and teaching all practice staff the active management approach. Change in patients' back beliefs in all three 'experimental' conditions at 3-month follow-up, with sustained but reduced change by 12 months suggests that an additional common 'educational component' may have been a feature of all three treatment conditions.

In one of the first third-wave studies, Hay et al. (2005) compared manual therapy with a simple, individualized CBT pain management approach provided by physiotherapists for patients presenting to their general practitioner (GP) with LBP of less than 12 weeks. A core part of the training for the physiotherapists included broadly-based training in pain management, with a specific educational focus on the nature of LBP, pain mechanisms, and the development of disability.

In a later trial, Johnson et al. (2007) compared an active treatment intervention consisting of a 6-week community-based group intervention programme based on active exercise and education using a CBT approach with a control arm comprising usual GP care supplemented with educational material. Each of the intervention sessions started with group discussion and ended with exercise, with the duration spent on exercise increasing throughout the course. Even though 'the therapists at times found it difficult to adopt the communication style characteristic of a CBT approach and some methods, including challenging patients' beliefs and fears were limited', the study showed nonetheless a beneficial influence of patient preference and recommended the targeting of interventions at subgroups. In the most recent such RCT (Lamb et al. 2010), a cognitive-behavioural intervention for LBP delivered to patients in groups was found to be superior to 'best practice advice', and the difference was sustained at 1yr. follow. The content of the training programme (Hansen et al. 2010) indicates a comprehensive educational package, but although more cost-effective, the actual clinical difference was relatively small and the research design did not permit determination of whether the difference was attributable to treatment content (CBT approach versus best practice advice) or to treatment delivery (group versus individualized treatment).

## Suggestions for a way forward (Wave 4)

Having reviewed the somewhat disappointing results (in terms of size of effect) of RCTs on early psychosocial interventions, van der Windt et al. (2008) concluded:

◆ The results of most randomized trials on the effectiveness of psychosocial interventions for back pain in primary care show only small differences in function or other outcome measures when compared with active control treatments.

◆ Possible explanations for these 'negative findings' include selection of heterogeneous patient populations; insufficient targeting of interventions on modifiable risk factors; insufficient competencies of care providers; insufficient intensity or duration of the intervention; inadequate adherence to treatment protocols; inadequate assessment of outcome.

In fact Hay et al. (2008) have designed a more individualized and focused approach to intervention linking the screening of patients with a specially developed subgrouping tool (Hill et al. 2008) designed to identify psychosocial risk factors, with specifically targeted therapeutic objectives for which the HCPs have been specifically trained. A variety of educational approaches (both didactic and experimental), including role play with simulated patients and clinical mentoring were employed. The outcome of this trial is imminent. If successful, it will be the first early intervention trial to have shown that training physiotherapists to identify and target yellow flags can influence patient outcome in patients at risk of developing chronicity.

## 23.3.3 **Effectiveness and sustainability**

Even assuming that an appropriate set of educational messages can be delivered, how effective are they in effecting desired behaviour change, and are the effects sustained? Engers et al. (2008) offered a review focusing on advice/information given by an HCP to improve patient understanding of LBP problems and what they should do about them. Unfortunately group education was excluded, as were studies comparing an educational intervention as part of an intervention programme with other non-educational interventions; such as trials on multidisciplinary treatment or a back school that included patient education compared to manual therapy. The reviewers were therefore able only to compare individual patient education with either no intervention or non-educational intervention on the one hand or different types of individual patient education on the other. Nonetheless given the perhaps over-restrictive methodological constraints, the authors felt able to draw a number of conclusions, shown in Box 23.2.

The authors further observe that 'it is very difficult to evaluate the effects or oral and written patient education' and that 'none of the papers explicitly described the theoretical model on which the intervention was based'. The recommendations for the design of educational material are shown in Box 23.3 would still seem to be relevant.

Giving information in the form of a booklet can help. *The Back Book* (Roland et al. 2002), a simple low-cost booklet which informs the patient on self-managing back pain and how to keep active and adopt an active lifestyle, can be used as an aspect of clinical management. The clinician

## Box 23.2 Major conclusions from Cochrane Review on individual patient education for LBP

For individual patients with acute or sub-acute LBP, a 2.5-hour individual patient education session was more effective than no intervention.

- However less intensive patient education did not seem to be more effective than no intervention.

- Individual education appeared to be equally effective to interventions like chiropractic manipulation and physiotherapy for patients with acute or subacute LBP.

- However, for patients with chronic LBP, individual education was less effective than more intensive treatment and the effectiveness of individual education is unclear.

- There is no difference between the effects of various types of individual patient education.

- That form of educational intervention is preferred and what content, intensity, and frequency are best remains unclear.

Adapted from Engers, A. J., Jellema, P., Wensing, M., van der Windt, D.A.W.M., Grol, R., & van Tulder, M.W. Individual patient education for low back pain (Review). 4. © 2008, The Cochrane Library: John Wiley and Sons Ltd, with permission.

must ensure, however, that the patients read and understand the information they have been given. In order to do this it is essential that the clinician is sure about what the patients already know and understand (or misunderstand) about their pain.

In their review, Burton and Waddell (2002) concluded:

Carefully selected and presented information and advice about back pain in line with current management guidelines can [their italics] have a positive effect on patients' beliefs and clinical outcomes. Written material is just one way of achieving this and, whilst its effect size may be small, its very low patient cost may render it highly cost effective. Nevertheless, there is considerable scope for refinement of the messages and their method of delivery within the whole scope of health care and the contribution of innovative educational interventions for back pain deserves further scientific investigation (p. 256).

## Box 23.3 Recommendations for the design of educational material

- Be clear about the core content of the message.
- Identify the targeted audience.
- Specify learning objectives.
- Address style and format as well as content of the material.
- Associate learning objectives with recommendations for behavioural change.
- Check comprehension and reinforce adherence.

Reprinted from Burton, A.K. & Waddell, G. (2002). Educational and informational approaches. In S.J. Linton (Ed). *New avenues for the prevention of chronic musculoskeletal pain and disability: Pain research and clinical management. Vol 12*, pp. 245–58. Copyright (2002) with permission from Elsevier.

23.3.4 **Influence of patient characteristics**

The relevance or worth of any approach to guiding self-management will be affected to an extent by the patient's 'starting-point'. Patient beliefs, preferences and expectations influence both treatment seeking and response to treatment. Professional training is predominantly biomedical or biomechanical in emphasis and, while addressing patient symptoms is at the core of the consultation, patient beliefs are seldom systematically identified or addressed. As potential obstacles to behavioural change, they need to be identified and, if necessary, addressed.

## The decision to consult

Patients' attitudes, perceptions, and beliefs about their back pain, its likely course, and the usefulness of specific treatments, may influence an individual's decision to seek healthcare. There is evidence from community surveys that about half of those who experience LBP in a 1-year period will consult a HCP, and that while pain severity influences consulting behaviour in the acute phase (<2 weeks), after this, those who consult are more likely to have externalized locus of control beliefs with regard to pain management (Waxman et al. 1998). An individual's attitudes and beliefs about the relationship between their pain and function appear to be associated with their level of disability (Poiraudeau et al. 2006). Thus those who believe more strongly that their pain means they should avoid physical activities and abandon normal roles, report higher levels of disability than those with opposite beliefs, and are thus more likely to consult, re-consult and use further healthcare resources.

## Influences of beliefs, expectations, and preferences on participation in treatment and on treatment outcome

Patients' beliefs, expectations, and preferences about treatments for back pain are likely to influence their engagement in and adherence to treatment plans, yet empirical data are lacking. However there is growing evidence from systematic reviews (Crow et al. 1999; Mondloch et al. 2001; Linde et al. 2007) across a wide range of health conditions that patients' expectations influence their health outcomes. Data from musculoskeletal pain studies, and in particular, back pain, demonstrate relationships between treatment preferences and expectations and patients' clinical and return-to-work outcomes (Heyman et al. 2006; Johnson et al. 2007; Preference Collaborative Group, 2008). Positive attitudes towards treatment and confidence in benefit from specific treatments have been shown to lead to between a twofold to fivefold greater likelihood of improvement (Kalauokalani et al. 2001; Linde et al. 2007), although this finding is not consistent across all studies (Klaber-Moffett et al. 1999; Cherkin et al. 2009).

In addition, general outcome and recovery expectations, irrespective of treatment, have been shown to influence both clinical outcome (Foster et al. 2008) and occupational outcomes (Turner et al. 2006, 2008). Nonetheless in evaluating this body of scientific evidence, a degree of caution is warranted. According to Main et al. (2010a), methodological problems include the challenge of capturing the beliefs, expectations, or preferences of patients who decline to participate in cohort studies or clinical trials; the study of these factors is usually a secondary objective, and thus, the statistical comparisons often lack power. In addition, few studies have measured beliefs, expectations, or preferences beyond the baseline measurement point and the effects of patients' treatment preferences and expectations may differ according to the nature, invasiveness, or unpleasantness of the interventions.

In conclusion, the evidence demonstrates the importance of patients' beliefs and expectations to treatment engagement, adherence, and outcome. However, as a precursor to the design of further interventions, we still require a clearer understanding of the nature of change and the underlying processes involved. Attempting to address such beliefs within a reactivation framework has become an integral part of new approaches to the prevention associated incapacity both in health-care settings (Hay et al. 2005) and in occupational of pain-associated settings (Shaw et al. 2009); but in addressing the secondary prevention agenda, and shifting our focus from distal outcomes to mediators of behavioural change, the role of education and advice in shifting core beliefs and expectations seems to be fundamental.

### 23.3.5 The influence of HCPs' beliefs and treatment orientations.

In attempting to evaluate the role of education within a self-management approach as a strategy for behaviour change, however, a further difficulty arises. Even assuming that we know what needs to be taught and what patient characteristics need to be addressed, there is clear evidence that HCPs' beliefs, preferences, and expectations influence both intervention delivery and patient outcomes and recently, more attention has been directed at these factors.

### The nature of HCPs' beliefs and treatment orientations

The characteristics of the HCP, such as their status as professionals, their therapeutic style, the words they use with patients, their beliefs about the problem, and their confidence or conviction in treatments have all been suggested as non-specific effects of treatment (Crow et al. 1999; Ernst 2001; Feinstein 2002). The beliefs, expectations, and preferences of HCPs therefore likely influence their choice of assessment methods, explanation to patients, and treatment approach.

There is evidence that HCPs, such as primary care doctors, physical therapists, and rheumatologists, hold a wide range of beliefs about pain that correlate with their recommendations to patients (Coudeyre et al. 2006; Poiraudeau et al. 2006). Studies have emphasized the predominance of biomedically (or structure) -orientated pain beliefs among HCPs (Ostelo et al. 2003; Daykin and Richardson 2004; Bishop and Foster 2005; Bishop et al. 2008). They have also shown that some HCP groups are more biomedical than others in their attitudes and their advice is characterized by advising patients to restrict activity, be vigilant about their backs and beliefs in a structural cause of back pain (Pincus et al. 2007).

### Influences on design/delivery of interventions and clinical outcomes

Several studies have shown that the attitudes, beliefs and treatment orientations of HCPs are associated with the advice they give to patients as well as the choice of interventions. Houben et al. (2004) showed that HCPs' pain attitudes and beliefs significantly correlated with, and were the strongest predictor of, their work and activity recommendations to patients. The same authors subsequently found that HCPs with a more biomedical treatment orientation viewed daily activities as more harmful for a LBP patient compared with those with a more behavioural orientation, and that biomedically-orientated therapists were more likely to advise patients to limit their activities and work (Houben et al. 2005). Bishop et al. (2008) found that these HCPs' pain attitudes and beliefs were significantly associated with their reported practice behaviour, such as the type of advice to patients about returning to work. Those with high biomedical orientations and low behavioural orientations were much more likely to advise continued work absence (44.9%), than those with high behavioural and low biomedical scores (11.9%). Other studies have demonstrated that advice to restrict work or daily physical activities is associated with higher fear avoidance beliefs of HCPs (Linton et al. 2002; Coudeyre et al. 2006; Poiraudeau et al. 2006;)

There is evidence that at the level of the individual back pain patient, HCPs find it difficult to be consistent in applying best evidence from guideline recommendations. In-depth qualitative interviews have highlighted that the use of diagnostic investigations may be influenced by patient demand, avoidance of risk or giving patients 'peace of mind' rather than being driven by clinical need (Corbett et al. 2009). In making decisions with individual patients, HCPs draw heavily on their own beliefs about the effectiveness of treatments, prior clinical experience and the pre-eminence of their relationship with the patient (Corbett et al. 2009).

Studies recently have started to incorporate measures of HCPs' attitudes and beliefs and to develop educational programmes that attempt to modify these (Jellema et al. 2005; Overmeer et al. 2009; Sieben et al. 2009). However, to date, few studies have measured HCPs' attitudes and beliefs in parallel with patients' outcomes. Jellema et al. showed that GPs' attitudes were modifiable by a short training session and that their back pain-related attitudes became less biomedical, but the trial showed no significant differences in patient outcomes. Overmeer et al. (2009) found that a university-based course of 8 days over 12 weeks resulted in a shift from a biomedical to a biopsychosocial orientation with a concomitant increase in their understanding of the nature of psychosocial factors. However, their patients perceived the therapists' behaviour before and after the education course as similar and were equally satisfied with their treatment and treatment outcome

Finally, this growing body of literature suggests that the attitudes, beliefs, and preferences of HCPs, might serve as barriers to optimal patient outcomes. However, the limitations of available studies include the frequent use of non-validated measurement tools or tools that have been adapted from patient measures for use with HCPs. Indeed a recent review highlighted that the number of tools available with which to measure HCPs' attitudes and beliefs about musculoskeletal pain is limited (Bishop et al. 2007), and that the development and testing of these tools is in its infancy.

## 23.4 From evidence to action: some suggestions for improving the effectiveness of educational strategies in secondary prevention

What do patients need to know? The central proposition underpinning this chapter is that for optimal self-management of LBP and its effects, knowledge per se is not what patients need, but rather they need information needed to develop, embed and maintain optimal pain coping strategies. In developing a strategy to achieve this however, patients need to understand the nature of their predicament, in this case the nature of LBP and its effects.

A number of key educational messages identified by Main et al. (2010a) are shown in Box 23.4. These key messages link across to a set of colloquial myths which act as obstacles to recovery and participation, and are summarized in Box 23.4. Surprisingly perhaps, the myths are not confined to patients: these beliefs are still held by some HCPs, irrespective of discipline.

### 23.4.1 Educational content

Patients need to be offered a plausible understanding of LBP, in language which they understand, which shifts the primary focus from structural mechanisms, pathology and disease, to an understanding of LBP in terms of central pain mechanisms and the development of persistent pain/disability within a biopsychosocial framework (Main et al. 2010b).

They may have unhelpful or mistaken beliefs about LBP and its relationship with pain-associated limitations and the suffering that accompanies persistent LBP. Main et al. (2010a) have highlighted three particularly important types of belief/expectations which need to be considered

#### Beliefs about the nature of pain

Pain researchers have identified a number of different types of belief or appraisal about the nature of pain. Beliefs about the extent to which pain can be controlled would appear to be one of the most powerful determinants of adjustment to pain and the development of incapacity, possibly

## Box 23.4 Key educational messages

- ◆ The perception of pain is a consequence of the interpretation of pain which is shaped by our memories and prior experience.
- ◆ Our response to pain is influenced both by our beliefs about it and the emotional significance we attribute to it.
- ◆ Back pain patients' beliefs, expectations, and preferences should be elicited and used in the clinical decision-making process to help select treatments that have the best chance of promoting patient recovery and return to work.
- ◆ Beliefs about the nature of pain, fears of hurting, harming, and further injury, and self-efficacy beliefs are the most important beliefs to consider.
- ◆ The attitudes and beliefs of healthcare practitioners are part of the dynamic interaction within back pain consultations, and are significantly associated with the advice and recommendations they give to patients and their treatment decisions.
- ◆ Societal influences play an important role in determining the outcome of back pain and development of disability.

mediating the influence of pain and depression. These core constructs can also be viewed as specific therapeutic targets. Correction of fundamental misunderstandings about the nature of pain, its effects and probable course are likely not only to facilitate optimal management but also prevent unnecessary iatrogenic misunderstandings and distress. An important stage in optimal adaptation to a chronic condition seems to depend upon patients' ability to come to terms with what they can and cannot control. This is turn may be affected by specific fears of hurting, harming, and further injury.

### Specific fears of hurting, harming, and further injury

Since the early-mid 1990s, there has been an increasing research focus on the role of fear and avoidance in the development and maintenance of disability, (Leeuw et al. 2007). Among people with chronic low back pain, pain-related fear has been found to be associated with reduced lumbar flexion (Geisser et al. 2004) and pain-related fear and pain catastrophizing have been found to be stronger predictors of overall disability than pain intensity. One study found that pain-related fear was also the strongest predictor of performance (van den Hout et al. 2001). However in acute low back pain only modest correlations between pain intensity, pain-related fear, avoidance behaviour and disability have been detected (Sieben et al. 2005) and more general perceptions about illness may also be influential (Foster et al. 2009).

### Self-efficacy beliefs

According to self-efficacy theory, once a situation has been perceived as involving harm, loss, threat, or challenge and individuals have considered a range of coping strategies open to them, what they do will be dependent on what they believe they can achieve (Bandura, 1977). Asghari and Nicholas (2001) have shown that pain self-efficacy beliefs are an important determinant of pain behaviours and disability associated with pain, over and above the effects of pain, distress, and personality variables. Taken together, clinical and experimental investigations suggest that perceived coping *inefficacy* may lead to preoccupation with distressing thoughts and concomitant physiological arousal, thereby increasing pain, decreasing pain tolerance and leading to increased use of medication, lower levels of functioning, poorer exercise tolerance, and increased invalidism.

Such beliefs therefore would seem to have considerable potential as targets within clinical management.

Self-efficacy has been found to account for the greatest proportion of variance in physical performance even after anticipated pain and re-injury have been excluded although pain intensity was also a significant (albeit limited) predictor of performance (Lackner et al. 1996). Thus expectancies of harm and pain catastrophizing, rather than being primary causal determinants of function, may be components of one's confidence of successful task performance (Nicholas 2007). Treatment recommendations derived from this interpretation emphasize the importance of goal and quota setting, and monitoring of pain and task performance as components of pain management and as such fit well within modern pain management and suggest further specific targets for advice and education.

### 23.4.2 **The educational context**

Communication is at the heart of the clinical consultation and one of the essential 'vehicles' by which information and advice is transmitted. Maguire and Pitceathley (2002) identified a number of key tasks in communication with pain patients. They are shown in Table 23.1 in which it can be seen that education and the provision of advice is not only a major component of HCP-patient communication, but that tailoring the information and ensuring patient understanding is fundamental.

### 23.4.3 **Developing an educational strategy**

#### Reconsideration of the role of education and advice in behaviour change

The importance of beliefs and expectations as influences on patient behaviour and clinical outcome has already been highlighted, and in the modification of beliefs and expectations, education clearly has a key role. It appears to be assumed often that change in beliefs and expectations will lead inevitably to a cascade of behaviour change and improved clinical outcome. However both

**Table 23.1** Common back pain myths

| Myth | Reality |
| --- | --- |
| ◆ Back pain means serious damage and injury | ◆ This is not always the case: pain can occur without injury. Even when specific tissues are affected, activity and work are not precluded. Temporary discomfort is often part of recovery |
| ◆ Work/activity is the cause: something must be damaged so work/activity will just make it worse | ◆ Normal work/activity can trigger symptoms, but is unlikely to cause substantial damage. The actual condition is usually not made worse by continuing work (assuming control of significant risks). Work/activity may be difficult or uncomfortable, but that doesn't mean it is doing harm |
| ◆ Medical treatment and tests are necessary | ◆ Most people, for most episodes of LBP problems, do not seek healthcare. Tests and imaging are generally unhelpful for LBP |
| ◆ Back problems must be rested | ◆ Quite the contrary—activity leads to faster and more sustained recovery and return to work. Temporary reduction of activity may be required, but long-term rest is detrimental |
| ◆ Sick leave is needed as part of the treatment | ◆ Often sick leave is not needed–staying at work is desirable, perhaps with some temporary modifications |
| ◆ No return to work/activity till 100% fit and pain free | ◆ This is clearly unrealistic and unhelpful—many workers can and do go back to work with ongoing symptoms, and they come to no harm |

Adapted from Kendall et al. (2009).

cross-sectional studies and longitudinal studies have consistently demonstrated that pain-associated disability has multiple determinants.

## Guidelines as a vehicle for education

The role of the HCP traditionally has been focused primarily on assessment, diagnosis, and treatment. Recognition of their specific role as educators is evident in the plethora of guidelines for all sorts of conditions which are now available, with several developed specifically for back pain (Burton et al. 2006; Waddell and Burton 2001; NICE 2010). Perhaps then we know what needs to be done; but we need to implement it.

That provision of information, although perhaps necessary is not sufficient, was illustrated by Grimshaw et al. (2004) in their systematic review of effectiveness and efficiency of guideline dissemination and implementation strategies. Included within the 235 relevant studies they identified, were 23 comparisons of multifaceted involving educational outreach, yielding modest to moderate improvements in care with a median absolute improvement in performance across interventions of 14.1% in 14 cluster randomized comparison of reminders, 8.1% in four cluster randomized comparison of dissemination of educational materials, 7.0% in five cluster randomized comparisons of audit and feedback, and 6.0% in 13 cluster randomized comparisons of multifaceted interventions involving educational outreach, with no relationship found between the number of component interventions and the effects of multifaceted interventions.

## The challenge of implementation

According to Michie et al. (2005), evidence-based guidelines are not implemented effectively, with the result that best health outcomes are not achieved and they suggest that this may be due to a lack of theoretical understanding of the processes involved in changing the behaviour of HCPs. There is now a burgeoning literature on linking theory and intervention and Michie et al. (2008) recommend the incorporation of psychological theory in developing evidence-based practice and the mapping of theoretically derived behavioural determinants to specific behaviour change techniques. The task therefore for education is to provide advice not only about the nature of the condition (e.g. LBP), but to understand the processes underpinning behaviour change and how to implement it. A number of theories such as the Social Cognitive Theory (Bandura 1977) and its core concept of self-efficacy; and the concept of illness representation embedded within the 'common-sense' model of self-regulation (Leventhal et al. 1980) are all illuminating, but in trying to 'deconstruct' the educational process, the theory of planned behaviour (Azjen 1991) perhaps has been most extensively researched. It appears to lend itself well to specify elements in communication that can be specifically targeted. If indeed it is appropriate to 'deconstruct' the communication process in order to enhance its effectiveness, the focus of education and advice needs to be not only on the nature of the condition (e.g. LBP) but how to gain mastery over it and understanding the processes underpinning behavioural change becomes fundamental. In a sense then education and advice becomes embedded within strategies for cognitive and behavioural change.

## Patient-mediated strategies

Of all the mediators of behavioural change, constructs, self-efficacy appears to have the most direct relevance in the context of guided self-management in that it can be mapped directly onto specific behavioural 'targets'. There remains the question however of whether patients can actually effect the necessary changes and appropriate education and advice would seem to be a key component of this process. Wensing et al. (2005) have reviewed the effectiveness of patient-mediated strategies in implementing healthcare innovations. As a precursor to their review they state 'Increasingly patients expect to be well-informed about treatment options and to be involved in making decisions' (p. 185). They appraise the effectiveness of four types of patient strategy: (1) health education or advertising through the mass media; (2) preparation for contact with care providers; (3) communication through single contacts or within episodes of care; and (4) feedback on healthcare received. They conclude 'some strategies to implement innovations through patients are promising, but our understanding of the effects on professional behaviour and processes of care is, as yet, limited' (p. 185). They do however find some evidence for effect of interventions to enhance self-management in the fields of asthma, cancer, and diabetes.

### 23.4.4 **Rolling out LBP education at a systems level: example of the flags framework**

Kendall et al. (1997) coined the term 'yellow flags' to encompass psychological and social-environmental risk factors for prolonged disability and failure to return to work as a consequence of musculoskeletal symptoms. The particular focus was on LBP. The psychological factors included fears about pain and injury and unhelpful beliefs about recovery, as well as emotional distress. The socio-environmental factors included the worker's perceptions that the workplace was unsupportive and overly supportive healthcare providers. The monograph provided a guide to the assessment of yellow flags that included a clinical interview and a psychosocial screening questionnaire. As with many such guidelines, their impact on clinical practice was unclear (Grol and Buchan 2006).

Following an international conference and think tank (*The Decade of the Flags, 2007*), the further research on flags was reviewed and the overall remit broadened, particularly in respect of occupational obstacles to recovery (blue flags) and system or contextual obstacles (black flags) and a completely revised monograph was produced (Kendall et al. 2009). Although this initiative has not as yet been fully evaluated, and indeed is still something of a 'work in progress', the authors have developed a 'tool box' of information and advice about flags as part of a website which is under continual development (http://www.tsoshop.co.uk/flags). The project has some interest from an educational point of view in that it represents a specific attempt to link provision of evidence-based information about the nature of the condition, with specific actions, and a range of implementation strategies at the levels of the individual, the workplace and the wider social context so that guided self-management is fully embedded into its biopsychosocial context.

### 23.5 **Conclusion**

Understanding chronic and recurrent LBP requires an understanding of the individual concerned in terms of attitudes and beliefs, emotional responses, and pain coping strategies. The role of education and advice is an essential component in the development of a self-management approach. We might usefully consider development of a range of evidence-based educational materials, using a range of 'vehicles' within an educational 'stepped care approach' such as recommended in the Flags monograph (Kendall et al. 2009), ranging from simple advice (e.g. *The Back Book*) with more sophisticated and detailed source material designed to enable the development of specific adaptive pain coping strategies. The further educational objectives might include enabling the identification and management of obstacles to recovery, identifying mediators of outcome in terms of modifiable risk factors and consideration of strategies to turn obstacles to recovery into opportunities for change. However to effect sustained impact we need to recognize the importance not only of the focus, content and format of our educational advice, but also develop effective implementation strategies. The challenge therefore for education in facilitating effective self-directed behaviour change is to develop the evidence base of the effectiveness of different behaviour change strategies, derived from a sharper theoretical understanding of behavioural change theories (Michie 2005) and evaluate their effectiveness in optimizing the clinical outcomes for our LBP patients. Our educational focus therefore has to move beyond knowledge about the nature of LBP and its effects, but to strategies designed to minimize its impact with the development of appropriate self-management strategies. The role of education and advice becomes less focused on provision of biomedical information to plug a knowledge deficit and more directed at illumination of ways in which to minimize the impact of LBP within a patient-centred approach (guided self-management) so that the role of the HCP becomes less of an educator and more of a coach.

## References

Albaladejo, C., Kovacs, F.M., Royuela, A., del Pino R., & Zamora, J. (2010). The efficacy of a short education program and a short physiotherapy program for treating low back pain in primary care. *Spine*, **35**, 483–96.

Asghari, A., & Nicholas, M.K. (2001). Pain self-efficacy beliefs and pain behaviour. A prospective study. *Pain*, **94**, 85–100.

Azjen, I. (1991). The theory of planned behaviour. *Organisation Behaviour and Human Decision Processes*, **50**, 179–211.

Bandura, A. (1977) Self-efficacy: Towards a unifying theory of behavioural change. *Psychological Review*, **84**, 191–215.

Bishop, A., & Foster, N.E. (2005) Do physical therapists in the United Kingdom recognize psychosocial factors in patients with acute low back pain? *Spine*, **30**, 1316–22.

Bishop, A., Thomas, E., & Foster, N.E. (2007) Health care practitioners' attitudes and beliefs about low back pain: A systematic search and critical review of available measurement tools. *Pain*, **132**, 91–101.

Bishop, A., Foster, N.E., Thomas, E., & Hay, E.M. (2008). How does the self-reported clinical management of patients with low back pain relate to the attitudes and beliefs of health care practitioners? A survey of UK general practitioners and physiotherapists. *Pain*, **35**, 187–95.

Buchbinder, R., Jolley, D., & Wyatt, M. (2001). Population based intervention to change back pain beliefs and disability: Three part evaluation. *British Medical Journal*, **322**, 1516–20.

Buchbinder, R., Gross, D., Werner, E., & Hayden, J. (2008). Understanding the characteristics of effective public health interventions for back pain and methodological challenges in evaluating their effects. *Spine*, **33**, 74–80

Burton, A.K., Balagué, F., Cardon, G., *et al.* on behalf of the COST B13 Working Group on Guidelines for Prevention in Low Back Pain. (2006). European guidelines for prevention in low back pain November 2004. *European Spine Journal*, **15**(Suppl. 2), S136–68

Burton, A.K., & Tillotson, K.M. (1991). Prediction of the clinical course of low-back trouble using multivariable models. *Spine*, **16**, 7–14.

Burton, A.K., & Waddell, G. (2002). Educational and informational approaches. In S.J.Linton (Ed). *New avenues for the prevention of chronic musculoskeletal pain and disability: Pain research and clinical management. Vol 12*, pp. 245–58. Amsterdam, Elsevier.

Burton, A.K., Waddell, G., Tillotson, K.M., & Summerton, N. (1999). Information and advice to patients with back pain can have a psositive effect: A randomized control trial of a novel educational booklet in primary care. *Spine*, **24**, 2484–91.

Cherkin, D., Sherman, K., Avins, A., *et al.* (2009). A randomised trial comparing acupuncture, simulated acupuncture and usual care for chronic low back pain. *Archives of Internal Medicine*, **169**, 858–66.

Corbett, M., Foster N.E., & Ong, B. (2009). GP attitudes and self-reported behaviour in primary care consultations for low back pain. *Family Practice*, **26**, 359–64.

Coudeyre, E, Rannou, F., Tubach, F., *et al.* (2006). General practitioners' fear-avoidance beliefs influence their management of patients with low back pain. *Pain*, **124**, 330–7.

Crow, R., Gage, H., & Hampson, S. (1999). The role of expectancies in the placebo effect and their use in the delivery of health care: A systematic review. *Health and Technology Assessment*, **3**, 3.

Daykin, A.R., & Richardson, B. (2004). Physiotherapists' pain beliefs and their influence on the management of patients with chronic low back pain. *Spine*, **29**, 783–95.

Dixon, A. (1990). The evolution of clinical policies. *Medical Care*, **28**, 201–20.

Engers, A. J., Jellema, P., Wensing, M., van der Windt, D.A.W.M., Grol, R., & van Tulder, M.W. (2008). *Individual patient education for low back pain (Review)*. 4. The Cochrane Library: John Wiley and Sons Ltd.

Ernst, E. (2001). Towards a scientific understanding of placebo effects. In: D. Peters (Ed.) *Understanding the Placebo Effect in Complementary Medicine: Theory, Practice and Research*, pp. 17–30. London: Churchill Livingstone.

Feinstein, A. (2002) Post-therapeutic response and therapeutic style: re-formulating the placebo effect. *Journal of Clinical Epidemiology*, **55**, 427–9.

Fordyce, W.E. (1976). *Behavioral Methods for Chronic Pain and Illness*. St. Louis, MO: Mosby.

Foster, N.E., Bishop, A., Thomas, E., *et al*. (2008). Illness perceptions of low back pain patients in primary care: What are they, do they change and are they associated with outcome? *Pain*, **136**, 177–87.

Foster, N.E., Thomas, E., Bishop A., Dunn K.M., & Main, C.J. (2009) Distinctiveness of psychological obstacles to recovery in low back pain patuents in primary care. *Pain,* **148**:398–406.

Frost, H., Lamb, S.E., Doll, H.A., Carver, P.T., & Stewart-Brown, S. (2004). Randomised control trial of physiotherapy compared with advice for low back pain. *British Medical Journal*, **328**, 798.

Geisser, M., Haig, A., & Wallborn, A. (2004) Pain relaed fear, lumbar flexion and dynamic EMG among persons with chronic musculoskeletal low back pain. *Clinical Journal of Pain*, **20**, 61–9.

George, S.Z., Fritz, J.M., Bialowsky, J., & Donald, D.A. (2003). The effect of a fear-avoidance-based therapy for patients with acute back pain: Results of a randomised clinical trial. *Spine,* **28**, 2551–60.

Grimshaw, J.M., Thomas, R.E., MacLennan, G., *et al*. (2004). Effectiveness and efficiency of guideline dissemination and implementation strategies. *Health Technology Assessment*, **8**, 6

Grol, R., & Buchan, H. (2006). Clinical guidelines: What can we do to increase their use? *Medical Journal of Australia*, **185**, 301–2

Hansen, Z., Daykin, A., & Lamb, S.E. (2010). A cognitive-behavioural programme for the management of low back pain in primary care: A description and justification of the intervention used in the Back Skills Training Trial. *Physiotherapy*, **96**, 87–94.

Hay, E.M., Mullis, R., Lewis, M., *et al*. (2005). Comparison of physical treatments versus a brief pain management programme for back pain in primary care: a randomised clinical trial in physiotherapy practice. *Lancet*, **365**, 2024–9.

Hay, E.M, Dunn, K.M, Hill, J.C., *et al*. (2008). A randomised clinical trial of subgrouping and targeted treatment for low back pain compared with best current care. The STarT Back Trial Study Protocol *BMC Musculoskeletal Disorders*, **9**, 58

Hazard, R., Haugh, L., Reid, S., Preble, J.B., & MacDonald, L. (1996). Early prediction of chronic disability after occupational low back injury. *Spine*, **21**, 945–51.

Heymans, M.W., de Vet, C.W., Knol, D L., Bongers, P.M., Koes B.W., & van Mechelen, W. (2006). Workers' beliefs and expectations affect return to work over 12 months. *Journal of Occupational Rehabilitation*, **16**, 685–95.

Hill, J.C., Dunn, K.M., Lewis, M., *et al*. (2008). A Primary Care Back Pain Screening Tool: Identifying patient subgroups for initial treatment. *Arthritis and Rheumatism*, **59**, 632–41.

Houben, R.M.A., Vlaeyen, J.W.S., Peters, M., *et al*. (2004). Health care providers' attitudes and beliefs towards common low back pain: Factor structure and psychometric properties of the HC-PAIRS. *Clinical Journal of Pain*, **20**, 37–44.

Houben, R.M.A, Ostelo, R.W.J.G., Vlaeyen, J.W.S, Wolters P., Peters M., & Stomp-van den Berg, S. (2005). Health care providers' orientations towards common low back pain predict perceived harmfulness of physical activities and recommendations regarding return to normal activity. *European Journal of Pain*, **9**, 173–83.

Hutchinson, A., & Baker, R. (1999). *Making Use of Guidelines in Clinical Practice*. Abingdon: Radcliffe Medical Press.

Jellema, P., van der Windt, D.A.W., van der Horst, H., Blankenstein, A., Bouter, L., & Stalman, W. (2005). Why is a treatment aimed at psychosocial factors not effective in patients with (sub)acute low back pain? *Pain*, **118**, 350–9.

Johnson, R.E., Jones, G.T., Wiles, N.J., *et al*. (2007). Active exercise, education, and cognitive behavioural therapy for persistent disabling low back pain: A randomised controlled trial. *Spine*, **32**, 1578–85

Kalauokalani, D, Cherkin, D.C., Sherman, K.J., Koepsell, T.D., & Deyo, R.A. (2001). Patients' preferences. Lessons from a trial of acupuncture and massage for low back pain: patient expectations and treatment effects. *Spine*, **26**, 1418–24.

Kendall, N.A.S., Linton, S.J., & Main C.J. (1997). *Guide to assessing psychosocial Yellow flags in acute low back pain: Risk factors for long-term disability and work loss*. Wellington: Accident Rehabilitation and Compensation Insurance Corporation of New Zealand and the National Health Committee.

Kendall, N.A.S., Burton, A.K., Main, C.J., & Watson, P.J. (2009). *Tackling musculoskeletal problems, a guide for the clinic and workplace: Identifying Obstacles using the Psychosocial Flags framework*. London: The Stationery Office.

Klaber-Moffett, J.A., Chase, S.M., Portek, I., & Ennis J.R. (1986). A controlled, prospective study to evaluate the effectiveness of a back school in the relief of chronic low back pain. *Spine,* **11**, 120–22.

Klaber-Moffett, J.A., Torgerson D., Bell-Syer, S., *et al*. (1999). A controlled, prospective study to evaluate the effectiveness of a back school in the relief of chronic low back pain. *British Medical Journal,* **319**, 279–83.

Klaber-Moffett, J., Carr, J., & Howarth, E. (2004). High fear-avoiders of physical activity benefit from an exercise program for patients with back pain. *Spine,* **29**, 1167–73.

Kovacs, F., Abraira, V., Santos, S., *et al*. (2010). A comparison of two short education programs for improving low back-related disability in the elderly. *Spine,* **32**, 1053–9.

Lackner, J.M., Carosella, A.M., & Feuerstein, M. (1996). Pain expectancies, pain, and functional self-efficacy expectancies as determinants of disability in patients with chronic low back disorders. *Journal of Consulting and Clinical Psychology*, **64**, 212–20.

Lamb, S.E., Hansen, S., Lall R., *et al*. (2010). Group cognitive behavioral treatment for low-back pain in primary care: a randomised controlled trial and cost-effectiveness analysis. *Lancet*, **375**, 916–23.

Leeuw, M, Goossens, M.E.J.B., Linton S.J., Crombez, G., Boersma, K., & Vlaeyen J.W.S. (2007). The fear avoidance model of musculoskeletal pain: Current state of scientific evidence. *Journal of Behavioural Medicine*, **30**, 77–94.

Leventhal, H., Meyer, D., & Nerenz, D. (1980). The common sense representation of illness danger. In: Rachman S, (Ed.) *Contributions to Medical Psychology*, pp. 42–65. New York: Pergamon.

Linde, K., Witt, C.M., Streng, A., *et al*. (2007). The impact of patient expectations on outcomes in four randomized controlled trials of acupuncture in patients with chronic pain. *Pain*, **128**, 264–71.

Linton, S., Vlaeyen, J., &Ostelo, R. (2002). The back pain beliefs of health care providers: are we fear-avoidant? *Journal of Occupational Rehabilitation*, **12**, 223–32.

Linton, S.J., & Andersson T. (2000). Can chronic disability be prevented? A randomised trial of a cognitive-behavioural intervention and two forms of information for patients with spinal pain. *Spine*, **25**, 2825–31.

McIntosh, G, Frank, J, Hogg-Johnson, S., Bombardier, C., & Hall, H. (2000). Prognostic factors for time receiving workers' compensation benefits in a cohort of patients with low back pain. *Spine*, **25**, 147–57.

Maguire, P., & Pitceathley, C. (2002). Key communication skills and how to acquire them. *British Medical Journal,* **325**, 697–700.

Main, C.J., Sullivan, M.J.L., & Watson, P.J. (2008) *Pain Management. Practical applications of the biopsychosocial approach in clinical and occupational settings*. Edinburgh:Churchill-Livingstone.

Main, C.J., Foster N., & Buchbinder, R. (2010a). How important are back beliefs and expectations for satisfactory recovery from back pain? *Best Practice and Research Clinical Rheumatology, 24,* 205–217.

Main, C.J., Buchbinder, R., Porcheret, M., & Foster, N. E. (2010b). Addressing patient beliefs and expectations in the consultation. *Best Practice and Research Clinical Rheumatology, 24,* 219–25.

Michie, S., Johnston, M., Abraham, C., Lawton, R., Parker, D., & Walker, A. (2005) making psychological theory useful for implementing evidence based practice: A consensus approach. *Quality and Safety in Health Care, 14,* 26–33.

Michie, S., Johnston, M., Francis, J., Hardeman, W., & Eccles M. (2008). From theory to Intervention: mapping theoretically derived behavioural determinants to behaviour change techniques. *Applied Psychology: An International Review, 57,* 660–80.

Mondloch, M., Cole, D., & Frank, J. (2001). Does how you do depend on how you think you'll do? A systematic review of the evidence for a relation between patients' recovery expectations and health outcomes. *Canadian Medical Association Journal, 165,* 174–9.

Moore, J.E., von Korff, M., Cherkin, D., Saunders, K., & Lorig, K. (2000). A randomised trial of a cognitive-behavioral program for enhancing back pain self-care in a primary care setting. *Pain, 88,* 145–53.

NICE (2010) Early management of persistent non-specific low back pain. London: National Institute for Health & Clinical Excellence.

Nicholas, M.K. (2007). The pain self-efficacy questionnaire: Taking pain into account. *European Journal of Pain, 11,* 153–63.

Ostelo, R.WJ.G., Stomp-van den Berg, S.G.M., Vlaeyen, J.W.S., Wolters, M.J.C., & de Vet H.C.W. (2003). Health care provider's attitudes and beliefs towards chronic low back pain: The development of a questionnaire. *Manual Therapy, 8,* 214–22.

Overmeer, T, Boersma, K, Main C.J., & Linton S. (2009) Do physical therapists change their beliefs, attitudes, knowledge, skills and behaviour after a biopsychosocially orientated university course? *Journal of Evaluation in Clinical Practice, 15,* 724–32.

Pincus, T, Foster N.E., Vogel, S., Santos R., Breen, A., & Underwood, M. (2007). Attitudes to back pain amongst musculoskeletal practitioners: a comparison of professional groups and practice settings using the ABS-mp. *Manual Therapy, 12,* 167–75.

Poiraudeau, S., Rannou, F., Baron, G., *et al.* (2006). Fear-avoidance beliefs about back pain in patients with subacute low back pain. *Pain, 124,* 305–11.

Preference Collaborative Review Group. (2008). Patients' preferences within randomised trials: systematic review and patient level meta-analysis. *British Medical Journal, 337,* a1864–64.

Redman, S., Spencer, E., & Sanson-Fisher, R. (1990). The role of mass media in changing health-related behaviour: a critical appraisal of two methods. *Health Promotion International, 5,* 85–101.

Roland, M., Waddell, G., Klaber-Moffett J., Burton, K., & Main, C.J. (2002). *The Back Book (2*nd *Edit.).* Norwich: The Stationery Office.

Rose, G. (1992). The strategy of preventive medicine. Oxford: Oxford University Press.

Shaw, W.S., van der Windt, D.A,Main C.J., Loisel, P., & Linton S.J., Decade of the Flags Working Group (2009). Early patient screening and intervention to address individual-level occupational factors ('blue flags') in back disability. *Journal of Occupational Rehabilitation. 19,* 64–80.

Sieben, J.M., Portegijs, P.J.M., Vlaeyen J.W.S., & Knottnerus, J.A. (2005). Pain-related fear at the start of a new low back pain episode. *European Journal of Pain, 9,* 635–41.

Sieben, J.M, Vlaeyen, J.W.S, Portegijs, P.J.M, *et al.* (2009). General practitioners' treatment orientations towards low back pain: Influence on treatment behaviour and patient outcome. *European Journal of Pain, 13,* 412–8.

Symonds, T.L., Burton, A.K., Tillotson K.M., & Main C.J. (1995). Absence resulting from low back trouble can be reduced by psychosocial intervention in the workplace. *Spine, 20,* 2738–45.

Thorsen T., & Makela, M. (1999). *Theory and Practice of Clinical Guidelines Implementation. DSI Rapport 99.05.* Copenhagen:DSI Danish Institute for Health Services Research and Development.

Turk, D.C., Meichenbaun, D, & Genest, M. (1983). *Pain and Behavioral Medicine. A cognitive-behavioral perspective.* New York: Guilford Press.

Turner, J.A., Franklin, G., Fulton-Kehoe, D., *et al.* (2006). Worker recovery expectations and fear-avoidance predict work disability in a population-based workers' compensation back pain sample. *Spine, 31*, 682–89.

Turner, J.A., Franklin, G., Fulton-Kehoe, D., *et al.* (2008). ISSLS prize winner: Early predictors of chronic work disability: A prospective, population-based study of workers with back injuries. *Spine, 33*, 2809–2818.

UK BEAM Trial team (2004). United Kingdom back pain and exercise (UK BEAM) randomised trial: effectiveness of physical treatment for back pain in primary care. *British Medical Journal, 329*, 1377

van den Hout, J.H., Vlaeyen, J.W.S., Houben, R.M.A., Soeters, A.P.M., & Peters, M.L. (2001). The effects of failure feedback and pain-related fear on pain report, pain tolerance, and pain avoidance in chronic low back pain patients. *Pain, 92*, 247–57.

van der Windt, D.A.W., Hay, E.M., Jellema, P., & Main, C.J. (2008). Psychosocial interventions for low back pain in primary care: Lessons learned from recent trials. *Spine, 33*, 81–9.

Von Korff, M., Moore J.E., Lorig, K., *et al.* (1998). A randomised trial of a lay person-led self-management group for back pain patients in primary care. *Spine, 23*, 2608–615.

Waddell G. (2004). *The Back Pain Revolution (2nd. Edn.)* Edinburgh, Churchill-Livingstone.

Waddell, G., & Burton, A.K. (2001). Occupational health guidelines for the management of low back pain at work: Evidence review. *Occupational Medicine, 51*, 124–35.

Waddell, G., O'Connor, M., Boorman, S., & Torsney, B. (2007). Working Backs Scotland. A Public and Professional Health Education Campaign for Back Pain. *Spine 32*, 2139–43.

Waxman, R, Tennant, A., & Helliwell, P. (1998). Community survey of factors associated with consultation for low back pain. *British Medical Journal, 317*, 1564–7.

Wensing, M., & Grol, R. (2005). Educational Interventions. In R. Grol, M. Wensing M., & M. Eccles (Eds.) *Improving Patient Care: The Implementation of Change in Clinical Practice,* pp. 147–57. Edinburgh: Elsevier.

Wensing, M., Elwyn, G., & Grol R. (2005). Patient-mediated strategies. In R. Grol, M. Wensing, & M. Eccles. (Eds.) *Improving Patient Care: The Implementation of Change in Clinical Practice* (pp 185–96). Elsevier: Edinburgh.

Werner, E.L., Ihlebaek, C., Laerum, E., Wormgoor, M., & Indahl, A. (2008). Low back pain media campaign: no effect on sickness behaviour. *Patient Education and Counselling, 71*, 198–203.

# Chapter 24

# Motivational Issues in Pain Management

Robert D. Kerns, Mark P. Jensen, and
Warren R. Nielson

Disease self-management has emerged as a dominant approach to keeping chronic illness under control, reducing its impact on physical health status and functioning, and improving coping with the psychosocial sequelae of the illness (Clark et al. 1991; Lorig et al. 1999; Newman et al. 2004). Consistent with this zeitgeist, as the field of pain medicine has matured, it has become increasingly apparent that an approach that emphasizes self-management may be key to control of acute pain and prevention of the progression to chronic pain (Damush et al. 2003) and to promoting optimal adjustment and adaptation to persistent pain conditions such as arthritis (Keefe et al. 2000), fibromyalgia (Okifuji and Hare 2011), and chronic back pain (Hoffman et al. 2007), among others. Given a growing body of research that documents important roles of psychological factors, including pain-related coping, as predictors of the development of chronic pain, it is intuitively appealing to predict that early efforts to promote use of adaptive pain coping or self-management skills among persons with acute pain can play a role in resolving pain and preventing the development of chronic pain. Adoption of adaptive pain self-management coping skills is predicted to contribute to positive adjustment and accommodation to acute pain and to facilitate resolution of the experience of pain and its potential negative impacts.

Optimal self-management involves numerous behaviour changes by persons with pain, including taking medications when indicated, physical exercise, undertaking preventive action, learning stress reduction strategies, moderating or pacing activities, and changing other aspects of their lifestyles. It is in this context that psychological interventions have been developed and promoted as important alternatives to more traditional medical and rehabilitation therapies (Turk and Gatchel 2002). Dominant among the numerous psychological therapies that have been applied to chronic pain management are those that assist individuals in developing a perspective of personal control and mastery and adoption of a range of adaptive cognitive and behavioural pain coping skills (Turk et al. 1983). Significant reductions in pain severity, disability, and affective distress, as well as reductions in healthcare resource utilization have been repeatedly documented. However, high rates of treatment refusal and treatment dropout continue to be reported (Turk and Rudy 1991). Equally problematic are reports that many patients fail to adhere to therapist recommendations related to cognitive and behavioural pain management skill acquisition and practice (Heapy et al. 2005). A variety of contributors to dropout and poor adherence have been suggested including a failure to take into account important individual differences in treatment planning, the overall complexity of therapist recommendations for skill development, and patient motivation for making changes (Jensen 2002; Kerns et al. 1998). After all, because the ability of patients to manage chronic pain depends much more on what they do than on what is done to them, motivation can be viewed as a primary issue in pain self-management.

Specific attention to motivation and factors that influence motivation may serve an important role in improving engagement and participation in pain self-management interventions, including interventions for persons experiencing acute pain (Kerns et al. 2006). Motivation for engaging in pain self-management has emerged as a particularly important focus of research in the past decade. Of great heuristic importance has been the development of a sound and integrative conceptual motivational model of pain self-management (Jensen et al. 2003) and tools for measuring the core constructs of the model, especially those designed to measure persons' 'pain readiness to change' (Kerns and Habib 2004; Nielson et al. 2003, 2008, 2009). In addition, Kerns (1994) has suggested that a prescriptive approach to pain treatment planning may be an important strategy for promoting engagement and participation in treatment and for improving outcomes. He calls for individual tailoring of training in new pain coping skills strategies by matching patients' preferences for a more limited number of specific treatment components. Jensen (2002) and Kerns and his colleagues (Kerns et al. 1998) have also suggested that the incorporation of specific motivational enhancement strategies may also promote engagement of a larger proportion of otherwise appropriate patients as well as adherence to therapist recommendations for skill acquisition and practice. Frantsve and Kerns (2007) have drawn attention to issues of patient–provider interactions and shared medical decision-making in pain management and their importance in considering patient motivation for engaging in pain self-management. These theoretical, clinical, and empirical developments have contributed to increased attention to issues of motivation in the field of pain management.

In this chapter we describe a motivational model of pain self-management and discuss its potential relevance in clinical situations. Briefly, according to the model, patients' readiness to engage in pain self-management at the time of acute injury or illness, or even in the context of the emergence of unexplained pain, is expected to influence their coping responses to pain, their efforts to acquire and use new adaptive pain coping strategies, and ultimately, the course of pain and the likelihood that pain will resolve. We also describe methods for assessing motivation and readiness to adopt a self-management approach to chronic pain, methods for promoting motivation for pain treatment and for learning and implementing adaptive pain-coping skills, and strategies for tailoring pain treatment to patient preferences, interests, and expectations for treatment. We conclude the chapter with a more explicit discussion of the implications of the motivational model and motivational issues for understanding and addressing the process of transitioning from acute to chronic pain, and for preventing this transition.

## 24.1 Models of motivation and a motivational model of pain self-management

Theories of motivation attempt to explain the initiation, direction, persistence, intensity, and termination of a particular behaviour (Landy and Becker 1987). Motivation can thus be viewed as a process that involves all of the factors that influence behaviour. Most theories and models of human behaviour, including a motivational model we are developing for understanding pain self-management, assume that behavioural change is influenced primarily by two factors: (1) the perceived importance of behaviour change and (2) the patient's belief that behaviour change is possible (i.e. self-efficacy) (Jensen et al. 2003). In fact, because of the high degree of overlap among the models, as well as the fact that it is often possible to explain changes in motivation or behaviour from the viewpoint of any one of the models, finding unequivocal support for one model over the others is quite difficult (Weinstein 1993).

On the other hand, the existence of significant areas of overlap among motivational models may be used to form a foundation for a general model of motivation for pain self-management.

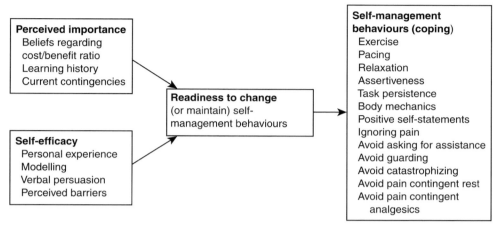

**Fig. 24.1** Motivational model of pain self-management. Reprinted from *The Journal of Pain*, 4(9), Mark P. Jensen, Warren R. Nielson, and Robert D. Kerns. Toward the development of a motivational model of pain self-management, pp. 477–92, Copyright (2003), with permission from Elsevier.

An initial version of such a model, the Motivational Model for Pain Self-Management, is presented in Figure 24.1. The primary outcome variable in this model is pain self-management coping behaviour, which may be defined by a set of behaviours and cognitions that are thought to reflect 'adaptive' pain management, and by avoidance of behaviours or cognitions that are thought to reflect 'maladaptive' pain management. The specific self-management coping behaviours listed in Figure 24.1 were drawn from the coping responses that clinicians and researchers have most closely associated with improved function and with positive outcomes in pain treatment (Jensen et al. 1994; Loeser and Turk 2001; Nielson et al. 2001), but the list is by no means exhaustive.

Self-management behaviour that is adaptive for one condition may, however, be ineffective or even harmful for another condition. For example, while patients with low back pain may benefit from maintaining a programme of regular aerobic exercise, the same exercises might cause further joint damage in patients with knee or hip arthritis. As more is learned about the relative importance of specific coping behaviours and cognitions and about the conditions under which these are adaptive, maladaptive, or neutral, the operational definition of pain self-management listed in Figure 24.1 should be updated.

The concept of readiness to self-manage pain (Prochaska and DiClemente 1984a; Kerns et al. 1997) is central to the Motivational Model for Pain Self-Management because it defines motivation. The model hypothesizes that patients will engage in specific pain self-management strategies dependent on their readiness, or motivation, to use these strategies. In the model, motivation is influenced by the two primary variables already mentioned, i.e. beliefs about the importance of engaging versus not engaging in pain self-management behaviours ('outcome expectancies', 'value', 'importance'), and beliefs about one's ability to engage in pain self-management behaviours ('self-efficacy', 'confidence'). Perceived importance is influenced by the value of expected outcomes, such as pain reduction, increased strength and activity tolerance, increased cognitive abilities, versus the perceived costs of pain self-management. The outcome expectancies are in turn affected by the patient's learning history, since a history of reinforcers or punishers for certain pain self-management behaviours will respectively increase or decrease the value placed on pain self-management.

Similarly, a number of factors can contribute to a patient's confidence in his or her ability to engage in a specific behavioural response. These include a history of successfully engaging in that response while undergoing treatments that elicit new behavioural responses to pain (Fordyce 1976; Fordyce et al. 1968), modelling of behaviour by others (Bandura 1986), effective persuasion (Miller and Rollnick 2002), and the removal of perceived barriers.

Although the Motivational Model for Pain Self-Management may appear static, with its final endpoint determined by the effects of perceived importance and self-efficacy on readiness to self-manage pain, we view the model as dynamic because of the many factors described above that influence motivation. The model provides what we hope is a frame of reference for understanding patient motivation for self-management, and, more importantly, for identifying ways to improve this motivation.

Moreover, preliminary evidence supports hypotheses based on this model. Molton and colleagues (Molton et al. 2008) obtained survey data from 130 adults with spinal cord injury (SCI) and chronic pain, that included: (1) measures of average pain intensity during the past week; (2) readiness to self-manage pain (assessed using the Multidimensional Pain Readiness to Change Questionnaire, see Nielson et al. 2003, and discussion of motivational measures in the next section); (3) and ratings of perceived importance, self-efficacy, and frequency of use of both (a) regular exercise and (b) task persistence as pain management strategies. Task persistence was used by too many of the sample to be able to test the mediation hypotheses of the Motivational Model of Pain Self-Management; however, the distribution of the amount of exercise reported by the sample had enough variance to test the model's hypotheses. Molton et al.'s findings supported the model. Specifically, patient self-efficacy for exercise, perceived importance of exercise, and motivation (readiness) were all significantly associated with reported exercise frequency. As predicted, they also found that the effects of self-efficacy and perceived importance were mediated by motivation. Thus, patient readiness to make changes in (or maintain) exercise behaviour is influenced by their perception of the importance of exercise and their perception of their own ability to exercise. In turn, patient readiness to exercise is a strong predictor of exercise behaviour.

## 24.2 **Measurement of motivation in pain self-management**

Central to the ability to test the validity of any theoretical or conceptual model is the ability to reliably measure its core constructs. Similarly, the foundation of effective theoretically-informed clinical intervention is assessment of the target of the intervention. For over a decade, the authors of this chapter have embarked on a programme of research designed to develop and test measures of the concept of pain readiness to change as described in the Motivational Model of Pain Self-Management described above.

In large measure, this measurement development effort has been informed by the Transtheoretical Model of Behaviour Change (TTM) of Prochaska and his colleagues (Prochaska and DiClemente 1984a; 1984b). The TTM incorporates the notion that behaviour modification involves two interrelated dimensions. *Stages of change* is based on the observation that individuals vary to the extent that they are 'prepared' or motivated to make changes in a specifically targeted behaviour. The second dimension, *processes of change*, focuses on activities and events that contribute to successful behaviour modification. A framework for considering 'stages of change' and the development of reliable strategies for assessing an individual's 'stage' has been pursued. Four or five stages have been identified across multiple studies in several areas of health behaviour change such as tobacco use, exercise, and diet (Prochaska et al. 1992). These are generally labelled 'precontemplation' referring to individuals who report a low interest in, or consideration of, changing their behaviour; 'contemplation' describing individuals who report thinking about behaviour changes, but appear unlikely to change in the near future; 'preparation' describing those who are actively considering attempts to change their behaviour and are likely to do so in the next month; 'action' referring to individuals currently engaged in behaviour change efforts; and finally, 'maintenance' describing individuals engaged in maintaining their already changed health behaviour. Identification of these groups of individuals has been shown to be valuable in predicting success in treatment designed to modify behaviour, as well as maintenance of treatment effects.

Informed by both a cognitive-behavioural perspective on chronic pain (Turk et al. 1983) and the TTM, Kerns and his colleagues propose that individuals with chronic pain similarly vary in their degree of readiness to adopt a self-management approach to their problem (Kerns et al. 1997). It is hypothesized that patients' degree of readiness to change may predict both engagement in self-management therapies, and outcomes. Based on integration of these models, it has been hypothesized that self-management interventions such as cognitive-behaviour therapy, through a process of reconceptualization, skill acquisition, and skill practice, may promote increased acceptance of a self-management approach. Conversely, increased acceptance of this perspective may be expected to enhance perceptions of personal control and responsibility for pain management, promote adherence to treatment recommendations for skill acquisition and practice, and contribute to improved outcomes.

Application of the pain readiness to change model begins with a consideration of the specific beliefs that may be held by persons in different 'stages' of readiness to adopt a pain self-management approach. Some persons hold strong beliefs that their pain problem is due to physical injury or disease that requires medical attention. Such persons often believe that personal responsibility for the condition or its solution rests with physicians and believe that self-management approaches are misguided and unlikely to yield benefits. Persons adhering to these beliefs are considered to be in a 'precontemplation' stage and are thought to be unlikely to be interested in engaging in self-management therapies for pain. Others may believe that there are limits to the utility of a medical approach and that learning self-management approaches may be useful. Such persons may actively consider the benefits of acquiring assistance in learning personal skills for improving pain control and reducing its negative impacts. 'Contemplation' is the term that has been used to characterize a state of emerging interest in engaging in self-management treatment. Within the model, the active learning of self-management strategies takes place in the 'action' stage, while persons who have already incorporated self-management into their overall approach to chronic pain are in the 'maintenance' stage.

The following sections describe ongoing efforts to develop psychometrically sound strategies for the measurement of these sets of beliefs consistent with the concept of pain readiness to change. Ultimately, the value of these tools is believed to be contingent on their ability to reliably predict engagement, adherence, and outcomes from pain self-management therapies and their utility in more extensive tests of the Motivational Model of Pain Self-Management described above.

## 24.2.1 **The Pain Stages of Change Questionnaire (PSOCQ)**

The PSOCQ (Kerns et al. 1997) was developed to provide a reliable measure of motivation or readiness to adopt a self-management approach to chronic pain and to assess the validity and utility of the pain readiness to change model. Published data largely support the reliability, factor structure, and criterion-related validity of the PSOCQ (Biller et al. 2000; Dijkstra et al. 2001; Jensen et al. 2000, 2004; Kerns et al. 1997, 2005; Maurischat et al. 2002, 2006). Four scales of the PSOCQ have been identified that are consistent with the four stages of the change process described above. Item examples from the scales that assess precontemplation, contemplation, action, and maintenance are 'All of this talk about how to cope better is a waste of time', 'Even if my pain doesn't go away, I am ready to start changing how I deal with it', 'I am developing new ways to cope with my pain', and 'I have learned some good ways to keep my pain problem from interfering with my life', respectively. The measure has now been used for research in several countries and has been translated into other languages including Dutch (Dijkstra et al. 2001), German (Maurischat et al. 2002), and Norwegian (Strand et al. 2007).

Classification of persons into one of the four stages of change has been most often been accomplished by labelling persons based on the highest score on the four PSOCQ scales. More recently, utilizing cluster analysis and discriminant function analysis, Kerns and his colleagues proposed a strategy for classification of five subgroups of persons in terms of readiness to change based on profiles of scores on the PSOCQ (Kerns et al. 2005). The subgroups were labelled as Precontemplation, Contemplation, Noncontemplative Action, Participation, and Ambivalent. It remains for future research to determine which classification strategy has the greatest utility.

Since the initial publication of the measure and its psychometric properties, numerous additional reports provide evidence of its predictive validity. Kerns and Rosenberg (2000) demonstrated that pretreatment scores on the PSOCQ reliably discriminated persons who completed a 10-session programme of cognitive-behavioural therapy for chronic pain. Furthermore, these investigators found that increased action and maintenance scale scores, inferred as evidence of 'forward stage movement,' i.e. enhanced motivation and commitment to a self-management approach, were correlated with improved outcomes on several key variables. These results have generally been confirmed (Jensen et al. 2004; Kerns et al. 2005), although concerns have arisen about the sensitivity and specificity of the PSOCQ in predicting treatment engagement and participation (Biller et al. 2000), as well as concerns about the validity of the measure (e.g. Habib et al. 2003; Strong et al. 2002). Most recently, Burns and his colleagues have demonstrated that early treatment increases in readiness predict subsequent improvements in outcomes, providing the strongest evidence to date of a role of enhanced motivation or readiness as a mediator of improved outcomes associated with self-management treatments (Burns et al. 2005; Glenn and Burns 2003).

## 24.2.2 The Multidimensional Pain Readiness to Change Questionnaire (MPRCQ)

### Rationale

In designing strategies to promote patient acquisition of pain-related coping skills, a key question is whether their readiness to change is best conceptualized as unidimensional or multidimensional. Perhaps the most parsimonious way to view pain-related readiness to change is as a single dimension that perfuses all aspects of pain-related coping. The PSOCQ provides an example of this approach as it captures the extent to which individuals are generally ready to adopt a self-management approach. As noted above, the PSOCQ has been extremely useful in understanding the role of motivation in psychological pain treatments. An alternative, complementary, approach would be to assume that considerable variation may exist in the extent to which an individual would be willing to adopt specific adaptive coping strategies and curtail maladaptive strategies. Multidisciplinary pain programmes encourage patients to acquire a broad spectrum of coping skills ranging from exercise to positive self-statements to avoiding pain behaviours. Anecdotally, it seems that patients may view these various skills quite differently and appear more motivated to utilize some skills rather than others. There are likely many reasons why such differences can occur such as previous lack of efficacy, fear, personal beliefs, values and perceived social implications.

For example, if an individual believes that asking others for assistance is necessary, dislikes discontinuing work on a task before it is complete (pacing), feels that use of cognitive restructuring techniques (avoid catastrophizing) implies that they are mentally ill, or has low self-efficacy for particular coping behaviours they may be less willing to learn or adopt these strategies. Moreover, it has been observed for some time (e.g. Turk and Rudy 1991), that not all patients appear to benefit equally from multidisciplinary treatment. Designing interventions to enhance readiness to change for specific coping behaviours that are associated with lower motivation has the potential to improve treatment outcomes and adherence. In order to target specific behaviours, they must be accurately and reliably identified.

## Initial development

Nielson, et al. (2003) began development of a MPRCQ (pronounced 'em-perk') to provide an instrument that would allow initial research into a multidimensional model. The items for this questionnaire were based on the self-management strategies often taught in multidisciplinary programmes as described in our motivational model. Initial item development included ten primary scales as well as five cognitive control content scales. During the item analyses one scale, 'Avoid Guarding' was dropped because of difficulties in obtaining adequate internal consistency. The resulting 46-item questionnaire had adequate internal reliability ($\alpha = 0.70$ to 0.93) and there was little or no effect of social desirability. The final nine primary scales assess readiness to engage in the coping strategies of (1) exercise, (2) task persistence, (3) relaxation, (4) cognitive control, (5) pacing, (6) avoiding pain-contingent rest, (7) avoiding asking for assistance, (8) assertive communication, and (9) proper body mechanics. The five cognitive control subscales are (1) diverting attention, (2) self-statements, (3) reinterpreting sensations, (4) avoiding catastrophizing, and (5) ignoring pain. Good concurrent validity for the PSOCQ scales was obtained in the form of moderate correlations with the PSOCQ, the Chronic Pain Coping Inventory (Jensen et al. 1995, 2008), a measure of pain coping and the Survey of Pain Attitudes (Jensen and Karoly 2008; Jensen et al. 1994), which measures attitudes regarding pain self-management.

Although these data were encouraging, there were a number of elements of the MPRCQ that we felt warranted improvement. In particular, it is difficult to convey the concept of being *ready to stop* engaging in a behaviour. The awkwardness of this concept, along with the combination of instructions and the wording of some items that created apparent double negatives, made some items more difficult for patients to understand. In addition, we had based the MPRCQ response options on the stages of change and felt that, psychometrically and theoretically, it made more sense to have these options reflect a readiness to change continuum rather than the discrete stages of change. Indeed, the concept of discrete stages of change has been challenged in the health behaviour change literature. For example, West (2005) has suggested that stages of change are arbitrary, oversimplified (stages contain multiple constructs such as time, intent and past attempts to change) and include only motivational elements of which the patient is consciously aware.

## 24.2.3 **The MPRCQ2**

A second version of the MPRCQ, the MPRCQ2 was developed in order to address some of these concerns (Nielson et al. 2008). The most significant revision was division of items into two categories. This modification was made to address the 'double negative' contained in items involving discontinuation of maladaptive behaviours. The first category included behaviours that multidisciplinary treatment programmes seek to increase (e.g. exercise) and the second category contained those behaviours that are discouraged (e.g. contingent rest). Separate sets of instructions were provided for each of these two sections to increase clarity for patients completing the questionnaire.

Thus, for items designed to measure increases in adaptive behaviours the following instructions and options were:

> Please circle the number that best indicates your intention to use each of the following methods of coping with or managing your pain by using the 1 to 7 rating scale below:
>
> 1 = I am not doing this now, and am not interested in ever doing it.
>
> 2 = I might do this someday but I have made no plans to do it.
>
> 3 = I will probably start doing this sometime (in the next 6 months).
>
> 4 = I have made plans to start doing this soon (within the next month).
>
> 5 = I have recently started doing this (within the past month).
>
> 6 = I have been doing this for a while (more than a month but less than 6 months).
>
> 7 = I have been doing this for a long time (at least 6 months).

Items that measure decreases in maladaptive behaviours were placed in a second section of the questionnaire and prefaced with the following instructions:

> The following questions are <u>slightly different</u> than those that you have already answered. For the remaining questions, please circle the number that best indicates your intention to <u>stop</u> using each of the methods of coping with or managing your pain by using the 1 to 7 rating scale below:
>
> 1 = I am doing this now and am not interested in ever stopping.
>
> 2 = I might stop this someday, but I have made no plans to stop doing it.
>
> 3 = I will probably stop doing this sometime (in the next six months).
>
> 4 = I have made plans to stop doing this soon (within the next month).
>
> 5 = I have recently stopped doing this (sometime in the past month).
>
> 6 = I have not done this for a while (more than a month but less than 6 months).
>
> 7 = I have not done this for a long time (at least 6 months).

The MPRCQ2 is also considerably longer than the MPRCQ (containing 69 items) and was constructed utilizing a broad sample of individuals with chronic pain (fibromyalgia, arthritis, spinal cord injury, acquired amputation). The MPRCQ2 is reliable ($\alpha = 0.77–0.94$) and shows adequate construct validity. Confirmatory factor analysis identified two overall factors contained in the MPRCQ2, which we labelled 'Active Coping' and 'Perseverance'. The former is composed of scales that tap readiness to actively participate in pain management behaviours (e.g. Pacing, Exercise, Relaxation Techniques, Assertiveness, Proper Body Mechanics, Cognitive Coping Techniques) whereas the latter contains scales that involve a readiness to persist in activity (Avoidance of Pain-Contingent Rest, Avoidance of Asking for Assistance and Task Persistence). Interestingly, in this model, the Task Persistence scale was the only scale to load on both factors, suggesting that readiness to persist at tasks may be embedded in both readiness to actively cope and to persevere. An interesting direction for future research would be to explore the differential roles of readiness for Active Coping versus Perseverance in treatment participation, adherence and outcomes.

In addition to these two factors, other aspects of our data strongly supported the multidimensional nature of pain-related readiness for change. The low correlations among the MPRCQ2 scales, significant correlations between these scales and their criterion scales, and high internal consistencies all support this contention. Our confidence in this view was strengthened inasmuch as these results replicated the pattern obtain in our construction and analysis of the original MPRCQ using different clinical samples.

We were somewhat disappointed that during the process of developing the MPRCQ2 we were unable to create a readiness to Avoid Guarding scale. We had not be able to create a psychometrically acceptable Avoid Guarding scale for the MPRCQ and in the current iteration we had hoped that including different additional items would have resulted in a reliable, valid scale. Our item analyses indicated that in the Acquired Amputation and Arthritis samples the items of this scale were not well intercorrelated, although they were adequate in the Fibromyalgia ($\alpha = 0.79$) and Spinal Cord Injured ($\alpha = 0.72$) samples. Also puzzling was a lack of association between MPRCQ2 Guarding scale and the CPCI Guarding scale, a criterion measure. Clearly our understanding of readiness to Avoid Guarding requires revision and further exploration.

### 24.2.4 **Brief versions of the MPRCQ2**

The last of our triad of studies on the MPRCQ investigated the feasibility of short versions of the MPRCQ2. The MPRCQ2 is relatively long and in some contexts (e.g. lengthy batteries or questionnaires, repeated assessment over short intervals) it may be prohibitively long. Excessive response demands can adversely influence instrument reliability and validity, not to mention study participation rates. Following the successful development brief versions of other pain-related psychological questionnaires (Jensen et al. 2003; Tan et al. 2006) we have also developed one and two-item per scale versions of the MPRCQ2 (Nielson, et al. 2009). Patients attending Arthritis and Fibromyalgia Day programmes in London, Ontario served as the sample for this study. For the single-item version, we identified items that were at least moderately correlated with their parent scale, were sensitive to pre-post treatment change and had at least a modest pattern of association with the PSOCQ scales (concurrent validity). Each author then reviewed the items that met these criteria and selected those that he or she felt best represented the underlying construct. Final selection was based upon consensus among the four authors that the item best met criteria. In the few instances where any disagreement existed, the item that was selected by the majority was chosen. For the two-items per scale version, in order to maximize validity, regression analyses were conducted in which parent scale variance was predicted first entering the item selected using the preceding methodology and then entering other items from the parent scale. The item that produced the largest additional contribution to the prediction of variance and was viewed by the investigators as reflecting the breadth of the parent scale was chosen. For both pre and post-treatment time points, all but one two-item scale (Relaxation, 0.78 at post-treatment) had a correlation of 0.80 or greater with the parent scale. Change indices indicated that both the one and two-item scales were sensitive to changes that occurred over the course of the treatment programmes. Most of the scales correlated well with the PSOCQ criterion measure, in a similar pattern to that obtained between the parent scales and the PSOCQ. As might be expected, the two-item versions tended to correlate more highly with the parent scales than the single item versions. The two versions did not differ in their sensitivity to change.

These 13- and 26-item versions should be especially useful in three circumstances: (1) when administered with a large number of other questionnaires; (2) in treatment process studies where frequent re-administration is required in order to access pain-related readiness to change, for example, as a predictor of adherence; and (3) in predicting success in multidisciplinary treatment programmes (i.e. treatment outcomes).

### 24.2.5 **Future research**

The MPRCQ, the MPRCQ2 and its brief versions provide valid, reliable tools with which to study motivational processes associated with adoption of, and adherence to, pain self-management strategies. Motivation to learn and utilize pain self-management strategies is a factor that is well known to clinicians working in programmes that teach such skills. Although we are not aware of any formal surveys asking clinicians about the role of motivation, based upon our experiences discussion with colleagues and the few references to the issue in the literature (e.g. Thomson 2008), there is essentially uniform acknowledgment of the importance of motivational issues. By definition, the success of self-management strategies is highly dependent upon the motivation of the individual to learn and apply them. Given the apparent importance of motivational factors, it is surprising that they have not been the focus of more research interest. An improved understanding of the motivational processes that influence these outcomes is perhaps long overdue. We hope that our motivational model will encourage research in this area and that the MPRCQ2 and PSOCQ will provide psychometric windows into the processes involved in pain self-management.

One approach to research using these scales is to examine the variations in readiness to acquire or discontinue pain coping skills within and between patient groups. Figure 24.2, illustrates the variation in MPRCQ scale scores among patients seen at St Joseph's Health Care, London, Ontario. The MPRCQ profiles of those seen prior to entering the Fibromyalgia Day programme demonstrated lower scores on some MPRCQ scales compared a sample of rheumatology outpatients (inflammatory arthritis). It is worth noting that this type of inter-scale variation occurred even though overall readinesses to change scores are similar (in this case 4.6 for the arthritis sample and 4.3 for the FM sample). In addition, variation among MPRCQ scale scores appears to exist across scales for both groups such that, for example, in both groups patients were more willing to change their tendency to persist at tasks but less willing to avoid pain-contingent rest. Thus, a multidimensional measurement perspective also fits well with our motivational model of pain self-management (Figure 24.1) inasmuch as there appears to be variation among responses to different MPRCQ scales within a single group. Obviously, lack of variation would have provided some disconfirmatory evidence with regard to a multidimensional approach. There may also be different levels of perceived importance and self-efficacy associated with each self-management content area as well. That is, it would be expected that scales representing specific pain self-management content areas would also reflect underlying differences in perceived importance and/or self-efficacy. At least theoretically, higher MPRCQ scale scores should be associated with greater self-efficacy, greater perceived importance or both (see Molton et al. 2008).

The ability of the MPRCQ and MPRCQ2 to predict treatment outcomes is not yet established, but as research in this area progresses, the measure may be used to identify appropriate treatments or to suggest targets for motivational interviewing of patients. Research will also determine whether the multidimensional MPRCQ/MPRCQ2 represent an improvement over the more widely used, stage-based, unidimensional indices of motivation such as the PSOCQ. More generally, whether stage assignment versus simpler continuum-based readiness to change scores offers any predictive advantage and whether assessment modality-specific readiness offers advantages over assessment of general readiness to self-manage pain are important issues both theoretically and practically. The MPRCQ and MPRCQ2 reflect the specific behavioural targets within our Motivational Model of Pain Self-Management and, in this sense, these instruments are perhaps ideally suited for future efforts to evaluate that model. However, it is possible that a more trait-like readiness to change factor, accounting for the majority of variance in readiness to change individual coping behaviours will provide a more parsimonious account of changes in self-management behaviours. The specificity of that aspect of our model depends upon which of these possibilities is borne out by future research. In practice, clinical implications are whether interventions such as Motivational Interviewing should be directed toward individual self-management behaviours or are more efficiently applied to the broader adoptions of pain self-management skills as a whole (e.g. tailored vs. general Motivational Interviewing).

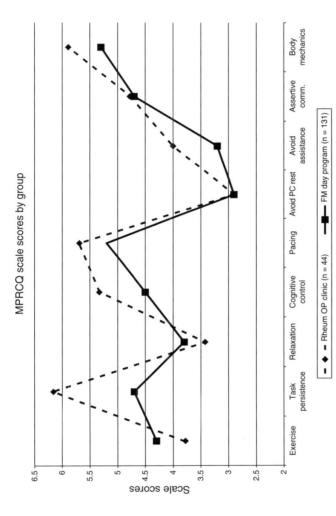

**Fig. 24.2** MPRCQ scale scores by group. Reprinted from *The Journal of Pain*, **4**(9), Mark P. Jensen, Warren R. Nielson, and Robert D. Kerns. Toward the development of a motivational model of pain self-management, pp. 477–92, Copyright (2003), with permission from Elsevier.

## 24.3 **Clinical and research implications**

### 24.3.1 **Motivational Interviewing**

As indicated previously, we view motivation for pain self-management as a state that can be altered by a number of factors, many of which can be influenced by clinician responses to patient behaviours. To enhance patient perceptions of the importance of pain self-management, clinicians can encourage positive outcome expectancies and outline the costs of not engaging in self-management strategies; they can help patients identify and incorporate into their lives positive contingencies (reinforcers) for self-management coping behaviours; and they can praise patients for making gradual changes in the direction of pain self-management (i.e. 'shaping'). To increase self-efficacy, the clinician can: encourage the patient to practice self-management strategies; provide the patient with opportunities to observe other patients engaging in pain self-management strategies; gently challenge 'distorted' cognitions, providing directed active listening to encourage and support self-efficacy beliefs; and help the patient develop a plan to address any perceived or real barriers to pain self-management.

Many of these suggestions have been incorporated into a set of therapeutic strategies called Motivational Interviewing (Miller and Rollnick 2002), which was designed specifically to increase motivation for positive change. Motivational interviewing is both a general approach and a set of specific therapeutic strategies designed to address ambivalence about adaptive change (e.g. adaptive pain management and return to work).

In terms of the general approach, Motivational Interviewing is patient-centred (Douaihy et al. 2005), thus what the patient says and does during a motivational interaction guides clinician responses. Motivational clinicians should seek to assess and address the patient's worries and concerns, build and enhance rapport and a collaborative relationship, provide information that the clinician knows or believes the patient is truly ready to hear, alter the focus of interventions from making treatment recommendations (the expert model) to supporting and enhancing patient self-care practices (the coaching model), and foster greater control of decision making and responsibility for self-care. To help facilitate an atmosphere of positive change and to build rapport, the single most important clinician response is listening to the patient, especially in a reflective way, rephrasing the thoughts and feelings that the patient is trying to communicate.

While skilled reflective listening might be considered the foundation of Motivational Interviewing, other specific responses are involved, including developing discrepancy, avoiding argumentation, rolling with resistance, and supporting self-efficacy (Miller and Rollnick 2002). Clinicians help patients see discrepancies by encouraging them to talk about the problem, listening specifically for discrepancies between their goals and their behaviours, and then reflecting back those discrepancies that are consistent with adaptive pain management. Arguments with patients are to be avoided because they could provide patients with an opportunity to talk themselves out of positive change. The concept of rolling with resistance refers to a strategy of avoiding confrontation, and in fact seeking to identify and reflect some adaptive component of any resistant comments a patient might make. Supporting self-efficacy refers to a set of clinician responses that elicit and reinforce positive patient statements about their capabilities.

When applied to pain self-management, the goal of Motivational Interviewing is to increase the probability that patients will make adaptive decisions concerning their response to chronic pain (Jensen 2002). Based on our Motivational Model for Pain Self-Management, to be most effective, Motivational Interviewing and other strategies should specifically target self-efficacy beliefs and the perceived importance of change, so as to alter a patient's readiness or motivation to change or maintain self-management behaviour, leading to subsequent changes in these behaviours.

## 24.4 **Implications of the motivational model and motivational issues for understanding and addressing the process from acute to chronic pain**

The Motivational Model assumes that a key factor in adjustment to chronic pain is pain coping behaviour; adaptive coping is thought to contribute to positive adjustment (minimal pain, minimal pain impact, and maximum functioning) and maladaptive coping is thought to contribute to poor adjustment and maladaptation. Along these lines, and according to the Motivational Model, an individual's readiness to self-manage pain at the time of acute injury would be expected to influence his or her coping responses to that pain, and ultimately contribute to the course of that pain and its influence.

While a number of studies have been performed to determine the predictors of movement from acute to chronic pain, and psychosocial factors are often identified as the factors most strongly associated with the development of chronic pain (cf. Schultz et al. 2004), coping responses, and self-efficacy and importance for adaptive coping, are rarely studied. When coping is studied, it consistently emerges as a significant predictor of future functioning in patients with acute pain (e.g. Potter and Jones 1992; Prkachin et al. 2007). We hypothesize that the ability to predict the development of chronic pain in individuals with acute or (sub)acute pain would be enhanced if researchers assessed a broader range of coping responses, self-efficacy for pain self-management, and the importance of pain self-management as the predictors in their model, and readiness to learn new coping strategies.

Similarly, in order to minimize the development of chronic pain, it would be useful to consider methods for maximizing adaptive coping and for encouraging the development of perceptions of self-efficacy for pain self-management and beliefs in the importance of pain self-management very early (or even before) the development of acute pain. For example, general education programmes provided to the population, through television and radio (public service) announcements, concerning the importance of remaining active following an acute injury (Liddle et al. 2007), and provided that this is supported following an appropriate medical evaluation, might decrease the incidence of the development of chronic pain in populations of individuals.

In health care settings, physicians and other health care providers who see patients who have been recently injured should strive to assess the patients' coping responses, and use interventions, as appropriate, to increase patient self-efficacy for and perceptions of the importance of adaptive responding (e.g. activity), in order to increase the changes that the patient will actually respond to the acute pain in an adaptive way. For these reasons, we view skills in Motivation Interviewing (briefly described above) as a key skill for health care providers who work with patients with both acute and chronic pain. In support of this idea, one recent study investigated primary care providers who were trained to utilize Motivational Interviewing and patient-centred counselling to increase the likelihood that patients would accept a referral to a multidisciplinary pain treatment programme (Heapy et al. 2005). In this study, pretreatment PSOCQ scores on the contemplation scale significantly predicted adherence to the therapist's recommendations for inter-session practice of pain-coping skills (e.g. relaxation, activity pacing). Furthermore, inter-session adherence was correlated with forward stage movement and behavioural goal accomplishment.

In a study in progress at the VA Connecticut Healthcare System, we are currently evaluating the efficacy of a modified cognitive-behavioural therapy approach that explicitly incorporates patient preferences, perceived importance, and expectancies of effectiveness for learning specific pain-coping skills, using a modified version of the MPRCQ and motivational interviewing in an effort to enhance forward stage movement and adherence. The treatment, labelled Tailored Cognitive-Behavioural Therapy, is informed by the Motivational Model of Pain Self-Management and by observations of the inherent flexibility in cognitive-behavioural therapy that allows for prescriptive treatment planning. The model also encourages the development of alternative strategies that attempt to match patients' apparent degree of readiness to change with specific interventions. Preliminary results have begun to help tease apart processes of change during the delivery of this pain self-management intervention (Burns et al. 2008a, 2008b; Kerns et al. 2008). These results further highlight the potential value of specifically targeting the beliefs and attitudes emphasized in the Motivational Model of Pain Self-Management.

It seems reasonable to conclude that theory driven research in the area of motivation has already proven useful in advancing our understanding of mechanisms and processes of change in persons adoption of adaptive pain self-management. Central to this work is the availability of reliable measures of core constructs of the model and the use of these measures in the context of trials of self-management treatment programmes in order to better understand these processes. Continued efforts to apply and study the model in this area appear to have the potential to enhance the effectiveness of self-management treatment and to promote the engagement and participation of a larger proportion of persons with chronic pain who may benefit from the interventions. The model similarly appears to have relevance for understanding the transition from acute to chronic pain, at least among persons who are vulnerable to this transition. It is intuitive that interventions informed by the Motivational Model and research designed to complement the provision of reassurance by providers when confronted with persons experiencing acute pain may have utility in promoting an adaptive response to acute pain and in reducing the likelihood of persistent pain and disability. Research informed by this interesting possibility is encouraged. Ultimately, we believe that a greater clinical and research focus on motivational issues will result in more adaptive adjustment to acute and chronic pain overall, and therefore contribute to less suffering.

## References

Bandura, A. (1986). *Social Foundations of Thought and Action: A Social Cognitive Theory*. Englewood Cliffs, NJ: Prentice Hall.

Biller, N., Arnstein, P., Caudill, M, Federman, C., Guberman, C. (2000). Predicting completion of cognitive-behavioral pain management program by initial measurement of chronic pain patients' readiness to change. *Clinical Journal of Pain*, **16**, 352–9.

Burns, J.W., Glenn, B., Lofland, K., Bruehl, S., Harden, R.N. (2005). Stages of change in readiness to adopt a self-management approach to chronic pain: the moderating role of early-treatment stage progression in predicting outcome. *Pain*, **115**, 322–31.

Burns, J., Rosenberger, P., Heapy, A, Shulman, M., Kerns, R. (2008a). Tailored versus Standard Cognitive-Behavioral Treatment for chronic pain: Differential effects of 'dose'. *Annual meeting of the Society for Behavioral Medicine*, San Diego, CA, 26–29 March.

Burns, J., Rosenberger, P., Heapy, A., Shulman, M., Kerns, R. (2008b). Effects of early-treatment changes in attitudes toward self-management of pain on treatment outcomes. *Annual meeting of the Society for Behavioral Medicine*, San Diego, CA, 26–29 March.

Clark, N.M., Becker, M.H., Janz, N.K., Lorig, K., *et al.* (1991). Self-management of chronic disease by older adults: a review and questions for research. *Journal of Aging and Health*, **3**, 3–27.

Damush, T.M., Weinberger, M., Perkins, S.M., *et al.* (2003). The long-term effects of a self-management program for inner-city primary care patients with acute low back pain. *Archives of Internal Medicine*, **163**, 2632–8.

Dijkstra, A., Vlayen, J., Rinjen, H., Nielson, W. (2001). Readiness to adopt the self-management approach to cope with chronic pain in fibromyalgic patients. *Pain*, **90**, 37–45.

Douaihy, A., Jensen, M.P., Jou, R.J. (2005). Motivating behavior change in persons with chronic pain. In B. McCarberg and S. Passik (Eds.) *Expert Guide to Pain Management*, pp. 217–32. Philadelphia, PA: American College of Physicians.

Fordyce, W. (1976). *Behavioral Methods for Chronic Pain and Illness.* Saint Louis, MO: Mosby.

Fordyce, W., Fowler, R., DeLateur, B. (1968). An application of behavior modification technique to a problem of chronic pain. *Behaviour Research and Therapy*, **6**, 105–7.

Frantsve, L. M., Kerns, R. D. (2007). Patient-provider interactions in the management of chronic pain: current findings within the context of shared medical decision making. *Pain Medicine*, **8**(1), 25–35.

Glenn, B., Burns, J.W. (2003). Pain self-management in the process and outcome of multidisciplinary treatment of chronic pain: evaluation of a stage of change model. *Journal of Behavioural Medicine*, **26**, 417–33.

Habib, S., Morrisey, S.A., Helmes, E. (2003). Readiness to adopt a self-management approach to pain: evaluation of the pain stage of change model in a non-clinic sample. *Pain*, **22**, 283–90.

Heapy, A., Otis, J., Marcus, K.S., *et al.* (2005). Intersession coping skill practice mediates the relationship between readiness for self-management treatment and treatment outcome. *Pain*, **118**, 360–8.

Hoffman, B.M., Papas, R.K., Chatkoff, D.K., Kerns, R.D. (2007). Meta-analysis of psychological interventions for chronic low back pain. *Health Psychol*, **26**(1), 1–9.

Jensen, M.P. (2002). Enhancing motivation to change in pain treatment. In D.C. Turk, and R.J. Gatchel (Eds.) *Psychological Treatment for Pain: A Practitioner's Handbook,* 2nd ed., pp. 71–93, New York: Guilford Publications.

Jensen, M.P., Karoly, P. (2008). *Survey of Pain Attitudes: Professional Manual.* Lutz, FL: Psychological Assessment Resources.

Jensen, M.P., Turner, J.A., Romano, J.M., Lawler, B.K. (1994). Relationship of pain-specific beliefs to chronic pain adjustment. *Pain*, **57**, 301–9.

Jensen, M.P., Turner, J.A., Romano, J.M., Strom, S.E. (1995). The Chronic Pain Coping Inventory: development and preliminary evaluation. *Pain*, **60**, 203–16.

Jensen, M.P., Nielson, W.R., Romano, J.M., Hill, M.L., Turner, J.A. (2000). Further evaluation of the pain stages of change questionnaire: is the transtheoretical model of change useful for patients with chronic pain? *Pain*, **86**, 255–64.

Jensen, M.P., Keefe, F.J., Lefebvre, J.C., Romano, J.M., & Turner, J.A. (2003). One- and two-item measures of pain beliefs and coping strategies. *Pain*, **104**, 453–69.

Jensen, M.P., Nielson, W.R., Turner, J.A., Romano, J.M., Hill, M.L. (2004). Changes in readiness to self-manage pain are associated with improvement in multidisciplinary pain treatment and pain coping. *Pain*, **111**, 84–95.

Jensen, M.P., Turner, J.A., Romano, J.M., Nielson, W.R. (2008). *Chronic Pain Coping Inventory: Professional Manual.* Lutz, FL: Psychological Assessment Resources.

Keefe, F.J., Lefebvre, J.C., Kerns, R.D., *et al.* (2000). Understanding the adoption of arthritis self-management: stages of change profiles among arthritis patients. *Pain*, **87**, 303–13.

Kerns, R.D., Habib, S. (2004). A critical review of the pain readiness to change model. *Pain*, **5**, 357–67.

Kerns, R., Rosenberg, R. (2000). Predicting responses to self-management treatments for chronic pain: application of the pain stages of change model. *Pain*, **84**, 49–55.

Kerns, R.D., Rosenberg, R., Jacob, M.C. (1994). Anger expression and chronic pain. *Journal of Behavioural Medicine*, 17, 57–67.

Kerns, R., Rosenberg, R., Jamison, R., Caudill, M., Haythornthwaite, J. (1997). Readiness to adopt a self-management approach to chronic pain: the Pain Stages of Change Questionnaire (PSOCQ). *Pain*, **72**, 227–34.

Kerns, R.D., Bayer, L.A., Findley, J.C. (1998). Motivation and adherence in the management of chronic pain. In A.R. Block, E.F. Kremer, and E. Fernandez (Eds.) *Handbook of Pain Syndromes: A Biopsychosocial Perspective*, pp. 99–121. Mahwah, NJ: Lawrence Erlbaum.

Kerns, R., Wagner, J., Rosenberg, R., Haythornthwaite, J., Caudill-Slosberg, M. (2005). Identification of subgroups of persons with chronic pain based on profiles on the pain stages of change questionnaire. *Pain*, **116**, 302–10.

Kerns, R.D., Jensen, M.P., Nielson, W.R. (2006). Motivational issues in pain self-management. In H. Flor, E. Kalso, and J.O. Dostrovsky (Eds.) *Proceedings of the 11th World Congress on Pain*, pp. 555–66. Seattle, WA: IASP Press.

Kerns, R.D., Rosenberger, P., Shulman, M., Heapy, A., Burns, J.W. (2008). Tailored CBT versus Standard CBT for treatment of chronic pain: Early treatment stage change in attitudes toward pain self-management and the working alliance. *Annual meeting of the American Pain Society*, Tampa, FL, May 8–10, 2008.

Landy, F., Becker, W. (1987). Motivation theory reconsidered. *Research on Organizational Behavior*, **9**, 1–38.

Liddle, S.D., Gracey, J.H., Baxter, G.D. (2007). Advice for the management of low back pain: a systematic review of randomised controlled trials. *Manual Therapies*, **12**(4), 310–27.

Loeser, J., Turk, D. (2001). Multidisciplinary pain management. In J. Loeser, S. Butler, C. Chapman, and D. Turk (Eds.) *Bonica's Management of Pain*, pp. 2069–79, Philadelphia, PA: Lippincott Williams & Wilkins.

Lorig, K.R., Sobel, D.S., Stewart, A.L, *et al.* (1999). Evidence suggesting that a chronic disease self-management program can improve health status while reducing hospitalization. *Medical Care*, **37**, 5–14.

Maurischat, C., Harter, M., Ayclair, P., Kerns, R.D., Bengel, J. (2002). Preliminary validation of a German version of the pain stages of change questionnaire. *European Journal of Pain*, **6**, 43–8.

Maurischat, C., Härter, M., Kerns, R.D., Bengel, J. (2006). Further support for the Pain Stages of Change Questionnaire: Suggestions for improved measurement. *European Journal of Pain*, **10**, 41–9.

Miller, W., Rollnick, S. (2002). *Motivational Interviewing: Preparing People to Change*, 2nd ed. New York: Guilford Press.

Molton, I.R., Jensen, M.P., Nielson, W., Cardenas, D., Ehde, D.M. (2008). A preliminary evaluation of the motivational model of pain self-management in persons with spinal cord injury related pain. *Journal of Pain*, **9**, 606–12.

Newman, S., Steed, L., Mulligan, K. (2004). Self management interventions for chronic illness. *Lancet*, **364**, 1523–37.

Nielson, W.R., Armstrong, J.M., Jensen, M.P., Kerns, R.D. (2009). Two brief versions of the Multidimensional Pain Readiness to Change Questionnaire (MPRCQ2). *Clinical Journal of Pain*, **25**, 48–57.

Nielson, W.R., Jensen, M.P., Hill, M.L. (2001). An activity pacing subscale for the Chronic Pain Coping Inventory: development in a sample of patients with fibromyalgia syndrome. *Pain*, **89**, 111–115.

Nielson, W.R., Jensen, M.P., Kerns, R.D. (2003). The Multidimensional Pain Readiness to Change Questionnaire (MPRCQ): initial development and validation. *Journal of Pain*, **4**,149–59.

Nielson, W.R., Jensen, M.P., Ehde, D.M., Kerns, R.D., Molton, I.R. (2008). Further development of the Multidimensional Pain Readiness to Change Questionnaire: the MPRCQ2. *Journal of Pain*, **9**, 552–65.

Okifuji, A., Hare, B.D. (2011). Management of musculoskeletal pain. In M.H. Ebert and R.D. Kerns (Eds.) *Behavioral and Psychopharmacologic Pain Management*, pp. 286–306. Cambridge: Cambridge University Press.

Potter, R.G., Jones, J.M. (1992). The evolution of chronic pain among patients with musculoskeletal problems: a pilot study in primary care. *British Journal of General Practice*, **364**, 462–4.

Prkachin, K.M., Schultz, I.Z., Hughes, E. (2007). Pain behavior and the development of pain-related disability: the importance of guarding. *Clinical Journal of Pain*, **23**(3), 270–7.

Prochaska, J., DiClemente, C. (1984a). *The Transtheoretical Approach: Crossing Traditional Boundaries of Therapy*. Homewood, IL: Dow Jones Irwin.

Prochaska, J. O., DiClemente, C. C. (1984b). Self change processes, self efficacy and decisional balance across five stages of smoking cessation. *Progress in Clinical Biological Research*, **156**, 131–40.

Prochaska, J. O., DiClemente, C. C., & Norcross, J. C. (1992). In search of how people change. Applications to addictive behaviors. *American Psychologist*, **47**, 1102–14.

Schultz, I.Z., Crook, J., Meloche, G.R., *et al.* (2004). Psychosocial factors predictive of occupational low back disability: towards development of a return-to-work model. *Pain*, **107**(1–2), 77–85.

Strand, E.B., Kerns, R.D., Christie, A., Haavik-Nilsen, K., Klokkerud, M., Finset, A. (2007). Higher levels of pain readiness to change and more positive affect reduce pain reports–a weekly study of arthritis patients. *Pain*, **127**, 204–13

Strong, J., Westbury, K., Smith, G., Mckenzie, I., Ryan, W. (2002). Treatment outcome in individuals with chronic pain: is the Pain Stages of Change Questionnaire (PSOCQ) a useful tool? *Pain*, **97**, 65–73.

Tan, G., Nguyen, Q., Cardin, S.A., Jensen, M.P. (2006). Validating the use of two-item measures of pain beliefs and coping strategies for a veteran population. *J Pain*, **7**, 252–60.

Thomson, D. (2008). An ethnographic study of physiotherapists' perceptions of their interactions with patients on a chronic pain unit. *Physiotherapy: Theory and Practice*, **24**, 408–22.

Turk, D.C., Gatchel, R.J. (Eds.) (2002). *Psychological Treatment for Pain: A Practitioner's Handbook,* 2nd edn. New York: Guilford Publications.

Turk, D.C., Rudy, T.E. (1991). Neglected topics in the treatment of chronic pain patients—relapse, noncompliance, and adherence enhancement. *Pain,* **44**, 5–28.

Turk, D., Meichenbaum, D., Genest, M. (1983). *Pain and Behavioral Medicine: A Cognitive-Behavioral Perspective*. New York: Guilford Press.

Weinstein, N. (1993). Testing four competing theories of health-protective behavior. *Health Psychology*, **12**, 324–33.

West, R. (2005). Time for a change: putting the Transtheoretical (Stages of Change) model to rest. *Addiction*, **100**, 1036–9.

# Chapter 25

# Pharmacotherapy of Low Back Pain

Kay Brune and Bertold Renner

## 25.1 Introduction

Acute low back pain (ALBP) is known to almost every human being aged above 50. Chronic low back pain (CLBP) is one of the major health problems in Western industrialized nations (Chou and Huffman 2007). The patients have often been suffering for years, lost their jobs and social ties. The costs to the healthcare systems are enormous. Consequently, drug research has attempted to find better remedies, regrettably with limited success (Deshpande et al. 2007; Chou et al. 2009; Jones and Lamdin 2010; Kuijpers et al. 2010; Roelofs et al. 2008a, 2008b; Staal et al 2008; Van Tulder et al. 2003, 2006a, 2006b). Other therapeutic attempts (not drug-based) were found to be even less effective (Deshpande et al. 2007; Staal et al. 2008; Furlan et al. 2009; Dowswell et al. 2009; Choi et al. 2010; Cui et al. 2010; Haroutiunian et al. 2010; Henschke et al. 2010; Oesch et al. 2010; Peterson and Hodler 2010; Rubinstein et al. 2010; Van Middelkoop et al 2010). The available armamentarium is insufficient and should be regarded as a mere walking stick to facilitate at least temporarily rehabilitation or reduction of pain to an acceptable level, but not as a cure.

To cope with CLBP, the use of drugs has to be integrated in a more complex treatment system, including physical therapy and psychotherapy as major pillars.

The complexity of the CLBP and the low effectiveness of its drug therapy result from several components. Among those are (compare Figure 25.1):

- The human spine is inadequately engineered for a long life and a predominantly sedentary lifestyle. Both further the loss of musculature and the decrease of bone density with age.

- Chronic structural remodelling of the human spine, often initiated by minor trauma and perpetuated by degeneration of the small intervertebral joints (zygapophysial joints), leads to narrowing of the intervertebral foramina, spasticity of the intervertebral muscles, overexposure of the intervertebral ligaments to tear stress, and—possibly most importantly—damage to the lumbar nerves and their meninges (Figure 25.1). These nerves and their meningeal sheaths are particularly vulnerable when leaving the spinal cord and encountering the degenerative and at times inflammatory environment at the intervertebral foramina which narrows with advancing age (see Chapter 4, this volume).

- Chronic nociceptor activation at the zygapophysial joints and progressing nerve damage (neurogenic pain) will lead to changes in the pain perception and emotional tinting in the central nervous system—a phenomenon which may be the major culprit of chronification of LBP (see Chapter 15).

- The fine structures of the zygapophysial joints allow for acute nociceptor activation in different anatomical structures. Additional meningeal and neuronal damage furthers chronic neuropathic pain and thus chronification.

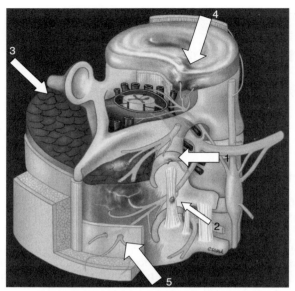

**Fig. 25.1** (See also Colour Plate 12) Schematic drawing of the lumbar intervertebral joints (zygapophysial joints), indicating the site of increased nociception in LBP (1–5). Note (outlined in light blue) cartilage and synovialis of the intervertebral joints, painful when irritated and inflamed; (red) intervertebral musculature which may—in order to immobilize the joint—become painfully spastic; the lumbar nerves (yellow) squeezing through the narrow intervertebral foramen, nerve damage and irritation of the meninges, causing nociceptor activation; the intervertebral disc—when damaged—leads to invasion of nerves and activation of nociception (pink in the (blue) intervertebral disk). Pathophysiological "sources" of low back pain: (1) Arthrosis of the vertebral joints (2) Damaged (extended) intervertebral ligaments (3) Spasticity of the deep intervertebral muscles (4) Raptured disc with secondary capillarisation and innervation (5) Damaged (irritated) neuronal fibers and sheaths due to degeneration and deformation of the lumbar spine and inflammatory processes in the meninges. Image by Christiane Wittek. Reproduced from Kubik, S.: FortbildK. Rheumatol., Bd.6, pp. 1-29 © Karger, Basel, 1981, with permission.

It is obvious that in acute and even more in CLBP, the complete therapeutic armamentarium has to be considered and the drugs to be used have to be selected carefully on the basis of the process (inflammatory or alternatively predominantly neuropathic) as well as on the basis of the risk factors innate to the individual patients who, in most instances, are elderly and often multimorbid.

## 25.2 **Strategies for drug therapy**

LBP often starts acutely. A trauma to the small joints of the lumbar spine causes an inflamed synovium. This inflammation may be furthered by a protruding, ruptured annulus fibrosus of the intervertebral disc of the lumbar joint which irritates the fine meninges surrounding and covering the lumbar nerves (Figure 25.1). Both tissues produce prostaglandins which in turn further nociceptor activation (wind up), hyperalgesia, and pain (Chapter 4, this volume). Hyperalgesia provokes spasticity of the local muscles (musculi intervertebrales and others), immobilizing the painful joint, but adding to the local nociceptor circuitry (Fitzgerald 2005). Under these conditions cyclo-oxygenase (COX) inhibitors often provide short-term relief which permits resuming physical activity and, as consequence, disappearance of the local spasticity. A COX inhibitor (selective

**Table 25.1** Effects of pharmacological interventions in chronic LBP (only drugs with proven effect alone[1])

| Drug classes | No. of studies | No. of participants | Statistical method | Effect size |
|---|---|---|---|---|
| **NSAID** | | | | |
| *Comparison NSAID vs. placebo for chronic, non-specific LBP, follow up ≤ 12 weeks* | | | | |
| Change in pain intensity from baseline on 100 mm VAS | 4 | 1020 | Weighted mean difference (fixed) 95% CI | −12.4 |
| Adverse events | 4 | 1034 | relative risk (fixed) 95% CI | 1.24 |
| **Antidepressants[2]** | | | | |
| *Comparison antidepressants vs. placebo for chronic, non-specific LBP* | | | | |
| Pain | 4 | 292 | Standardized mean difference (random) 95% CI | −0.02 |
| adverse effects | 2 | 157 | Relative risk (fixed) 95% CI | 0.93 |
| *Comparison SSRI vs. placebo* | | | | |
| Pain | 3 | 199 | Standardized mean difference (random) 95% CI | 0.11 |
| **Opioids** | | | | |
| *Comparison opioids (all types) vs. placebo for chronic LBP* | | | | |
| Pain | 7 | 2350 | Standardized mean difference (fixed) 95% CI | −0.54 |
| Adverse effects | 4 | 1176 | Relative risk (fixed) 95% CI | 1.28 |

With kind permission from Springer Science+Business Media: *European Spine Journal*, A systematic review on the effectiveness of complementary and alternative medicine for chronic non-specific low-back pain, **19**(8), 2010, Sidney M. Rubinstein.

[1] There is no reliable evidence of effectiveness for muscle relaxants (van Tulder 2003, 2006), antiepileptics, APAP (Davies 2008; Williams 2010), flupirtin (Li 2008, Worz 1996),tapentadol (Etropolski 2010, Wade 2009), topical NSAID (Haroutiunian 2010), glucosamine (Wilkens 2010), herbal remedies (Cui 2010) or other alternative medicines (Rubinstein 2010).

[2] For review see also Urquhart (2008).

or non-selective) will lessen pain, facilitate return to mobility, and give relief of muscle spasticity. The appropriate drug should be chosen on the basis of individual risk factors for each patient as well as on the risks inherent to the individual drug (Table 25.1; see also 25.4).

If acute low back pain (ALBP) does not resolve within a time period of few weeks, chronification is threatening. It may result from damage to the lumbar nerves, including the fine nerves, innervating the meninges and the relicts of the disrupted intervertebral discs (Freemont et al. 1997; Edgar 2007; Takahashi et al. 2008). These changes in the pain pathology are reflected in the observation that COX inhibitors tend to lose their effectiveness after a few weeks of use (Figure 25.2). The loss of pain relief often results in a desperate search for alternative therapeutic treatment options which, as outlined before, do not help, but cause unwanted drug effects (UDEs).

In some countries of Europe, flupirtine is believed to be effective under these conditions (Li et al. 2008). It is a potassium channel opener which might reduce spasticity and/or pain perception. However, RCT demonstrating reliable effects are lacking (Table 25.2). Flupirtine may cause liver damage (Arzneimittelkommission der Deutschen Ärzteschaft 2007).

In this (later) phase, three therapeutic options may be explored (Table 25.2):

♦ The use of opioids. They have a limited, but measurable effect even in neuropathic pain (Table 25.2).

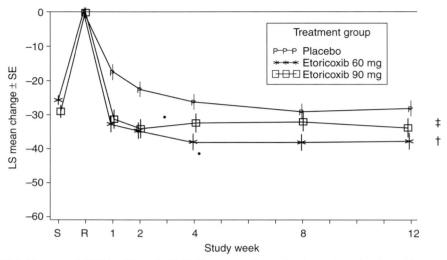

**Fig. 25.2** The use of COX inhibitors in ALBP (flare period) may lead to pain reduction with decreasing prevalence with time. Low back pain intensity scale (0 to 100-mm VAS). Least-squares mean change (mm) from baseline (flare/randomization visit) over the 12-week treatment period (all-patients-treated approach). Screening (S) to baseline (R) is the washout period from previous analgesics. Data points for each treatment group were shifted along the x-axis to maximize legibility at each time point. (Abbreviation: SE, standard error.) *P <0 .001 time weighted average versus placebo. †P=0.001 time weighted average versus placebo. ‡P=0.018 time weighted average versus placebo. Adapted from Birbara et al. (2003).

- ◆ Co-administration of antiepileptic drugs, as gabapentin and pregabalin, with opioids is frequent. However, there is only limited evidence that these compounds, often claimed to be effective in neuropathic pain, do work in CLBP (Table 25.3).
- ◆ Other types of combinations are also explored, e.g. opioids with muscle relaxants or antidepressants (Table 25.3). Again, strong evidence supporting clinical relevant effects of one or the other combination is lacking.

If LBP continues, the central nervous system becomes a major player. Indeed, evidence from functional magnetic resonance imaging (see, e.g. Kobayashi et al. 2009; also Chapter 6) indicates that the emotional tinting of the pain as well as its intensity changes with time. Constant pain perception dominates the day, and the patient may become depressive (Urquhart et al. 2008). Employing antidepressants (adrenalin/serotonin reuptake inhibitors [SSRIs]) may then be warranted—however, success is not guaranteed, and scientific evidence is scarce (Table 25.3).

It may be added that the infiltration of the small vertebral joints, ligaments, and muscles is often exercised (Henschke et al. 2010; Peterson and Hodler 2010). Administering local anaesthetics, steroids, and hyaluronic acid to these critical structures is not supported by evidence from randomized controlled trials (RCTs) (Manchikanti et al. 2010). The local injection into the complex tissues around lumbar joints may go along with infections, including intrathecal bacterial dissemination with deleterious consequences, as lasting impairment of the ability to walk and work. Herbal medicines (Cui et al. 2010), glucosamine (Wilkens et al. 2010), and homeopathic medicines are not of documented clinical value. Acupuncture has been tried, but the interpretation of the effects seen is controversial (Berman et al. 2010).

**Table 25.2** Evidence of therapeutic success in LBP from RCT

| Drug/class | Chronic LBP | p ≤ | Reference |
|---|---|---|---|
| **NSAID (non-selective)[1]** | | | |
| Diclofenac | – | – | Dreiser 2003 |
| Aceclofenac | – | – | Roeloffs 2008 |
| Naproxen | + | 0.01 | Berry 1982 |
| **NSAID (selective)** | | | |
| Celecoxib | – | 0.01 | Roelofs 2008 |
| Etoricoxib | + | 0.01 | Pallay 2004; Zerbini 2005; Birbara 2003 |
| Acetaminophen | – | – | Davies 2008; Williams 2010 |
| Glucocorticoids | – | – | Chou 2007 |
| **Opiods** | | | |
| Oxycodon | + | 0.01 | Webster 2006 |
| Oxymorphon | + | 0.01 | Katz 2007 |
| Tramadol | + | 0.001 | Schnitzer 2000; Deshpande 2007 |
| **Muscle relaxants** | | | |
| Benzodiazepines | – | – | van Tulder 2003, 2006 |
| Anticholinergic drugs | – | – | Kuijpers 2010 |
| Flupirtine | (+)[2] | 0.01 | Worz 1996; Li 2008[3] |

[1] Effective in ALBP (Roelofs et al 2008a; Dreiser et al 2003).
[2] Design questionable.
[3] Underpowered, no active controls, no placebo (comp. flupirtine vs. tramadol: no difference, no test of equality, under-powered).

**Table 25.3** Effect of combining drugs in LBP

| Drug combination | Study type | Acute/chronic LBP | Outcome | Reference |
|---|---|---|---|---|
| NSAID + opioid vs. NSAID alone (naproxen/oxycodon) | RCT | Chronic LBP (washout) | Combination sig. better p ≤ 0.001 | Jamison 1998 |
| NSAID + muscle relaxant | RCT | Acute LBP | Combination better p ≤ 0.01 | van Tulder 2003 |
| aceclofenac + tizanidin | RCT | Acute LBP | combination better p ≤ 0.01 | Pareek 2009 |
| NSAID + antiepileptic (celecoxib + pregabalin) | RCT | Acute LBP | Combination better p ≤ 0.01 | Romano 2009 |
| NSAID + opioid (APAR + tramadol) | RCT | Chronic LBP | Combination better p ≤ 0.01 | Ruoff 2003 |
| NSAID + opioid (APAP + tramadol) | RCT | Chronic LBP | Combination better p ≤ 0.001 | Peloso 2004 |

No randomized controlled trials (RCT) were done using opioids + muscle relaxants, opioids + antiepileptics or opioids + antidepressants (van Tulder et al, 2006a,b).

## 25.3 **COX inhibitors: drugs with proven effectiveness in ALBP**

The COX inhibitors are by far the most widely used drugs in ALBP. They divide into four subgroups:

- The non-acidic, non-COX-2 selective inhibitors, namely APAP (paracetamol), phenazone derivatives (propyphenazone, dipyrone).
- Acidic, non-selective COX-2 inhibitors, as, e.g. diclofenac, ibuprofen, meloxicame, naproxen, and piroxicam.
- Selective COX-2 inhibitors, namely celecoxib and etoricoxib.
- Selective and acidic COX-2 inhibitors. Lumiracoxib is the only member of the forth still group available in South America.

There is ample evidence that all COX inhibitors, given at adequate doses and in meaningful galenic formulations, reduce ALBP and facilitate mobilization. Hard evidence from RCTs is available for diclofenac and naproxen, but lacking for phenazone derivatives and APAP, despite the recommendation of the latter as first-line drug in many LBP guidelines (Davies et al. 2008). CLBP is less amenable to COX inhibitor treatment. RCTs exist only for etoricoxib (Birbara et al. 2003; Pallay et al. 2004; Zerbini et al. 2005), diclofenac, and naproxen (Berry et al. 1982; Jamison et al. 1998; Dreiser et al. 2003), but others are likely to be effective, too.

As shown in Figure 25.2, the few published, long-term evaluations of COX inhibitors indicate that there is a loss of effectiveness with time (cf. Pallay et al. 2004). This may be taken as an indication for an increasing contribution of neuropathic pain components (Chapter 4). Neuropathic pain is not amenable to COX inhibitors.

The COX inhibitors differ in their pharmacokinetic characteristics and potency (dosage) as well as in their typical side effects. It is accepted that all COX inhibitors increase the blood pressure (Johnson 1997) and the long-term risk of cardiovascular (CV) events, including cardiac infarction, thromboembolic events, and stroke (Cannon et al. 2006; Dajani and Islam 2008; Chang et al. 2010). The same risk exists for the long term-use of APAP (Sudano et al. 2010; for review see Brune et al. 2009). Given a similar mode of action, proof of the contention that selective COX-2 inhibitors go along with a higher CV risk is still lacking (Dajani and Islam 2008). Etoricoxib caused as many CV-events as diclofenac in a long-term study (Cannon et al. 2006). In any case, it appears meaningful to use these drugs at relatively low doses (Hinz and Brune 2008). On the other hand, the traditional, acidic COX inhibitors diclofenac, ibuprofen, meloxicame, naproxen, and piroxicam are more likely to cause gastrointestinal (GI) tract bleeds and perforations as compared to either non-selective, non-acidic or selective COX-2 inhibitors (Rahme and Nedjar 2007; Rahme and Bernatsky 2010). It appears meaningful to select the drug in CLBP according to the risk factors presented by the individual patient and the pharmacokinetic/pharmacodynamic characteristics of the drugs, i.e. otherwise healthy, aging patients could use all prototypes; elderly patients with serious CV-risks might be served best with naproxen, and those with GI-bleeds in their history may resort to COX-2-inhibitors, eventually in combination with proton pump inhibitors (PPI) (Table 25.4).

A few drug-specific, clinically relevant aspects should be kept in mind:

- Diclofenac is often overdosed. Twice daily 50mg or once 75mg (retardation) is often a sufficient dose and should not be exceeded as diclofenac causes liver damage, a dose-dependant phenomenon (Boelsterli 2003).
- Etoricoxib, naproxen, and piroxicam are eliminated slowly from the human organism. Consequently, giving the same dose daily leads to drug accumulation which may be the reason for the relatively high toxicity of piroxicam. Also, since naproxen is a non-selective inhibitor

**Table 25.4** Pharmacokinetic characteristics of oral COX inhibitors

**NSAID/COX inhibitors[e]**

| $t_{50}\%$ | Acidic | | | Non-acidic | | |
|---|---|---|---|---|---|---|
| | Short (~1 h) | Medium (~12 h) | Long (≥24 h) | Short (~1 h) | Medium (~12 h) | Long (≥24 h) |
| **Nonselective** | Ibuprofen[a] | Lornoxicam | – | Propyphenazone | Metamizol (dipyrone)[d] | – |
| $t_{50}\%$ (h) | 1–2 | 4–10 | | ~1–4 | >4 (MMA) | |
| $t_{max}$ (h)* | ~1* | ~1* | | ~1 | ~0.5–1 | |
| $F_O$ (%) | >80 | ~100 | | ~100[1] | ~100* | |
| $V_d$ (l/kg) | ~0.15 | ~0.15 | | ~1 | ~1 | |
| **Nonselective** | Ketoprofen[b] | Naproxen[‡,§,b] | Piroxicam[‡,b] | – | – | – |
| $t_{50}\%$ (h) | 1–2 | 12–15 | 34–60 | | | |
| $t_{max}$ (h) | 0.5–1* | 2–3* | 0.5–2* | | | |
| $F_O$ (%) | ~100 | ~100 | >90 | | | |
| $V_d$ (l/kg) | ~0.15 | ~0.15 | ~0.15 | | | |
| **Preferential‖** | Diclofenac[c] | – | Meloxicam[3] | APAP[c] | Celecoxib[¶] | – |
| $t_{50}\%$ (h) | 1–2 | | 18–24 | 1.5–2.5 | 4–12 | |
| $t_{max}$ (h) | 0.5–1* | | ~1* | 0.5–1 | 2–4 | |
| $F_O$ (%) | ~60 | | ~90 | ~80 | 20–40 | |
| $V_d$ (l/kg) | ~0.15 | | ~0.15 | ~1 | >>1 | |
| **Selective** | Lumiracoxib[c] | – | – | – | Rofecoxib[§] | Etoricoxib |
| $t_{50}\%$ (h) | 2–4 | | | | 17 | ~24 |
| $t_{max}$ (h) | 1–2 | | | | ~3 | 0.5–1 |
| $F_O$ (%) | ~100 | | | | ~100 | ~100 |
| $V_d$ (L/kg) | ~0.15 | | | | >1.5 | ~2 |

* depending on the galenic formulation; ‡ enterohepatic circulation; § drug accumulation; ‖ indicates inhibition of COX2 > COX1, as contrasted with selective inhibitors (COX2 inhibition >> COX1; i. e. lack of COX1 inhibition at therapeutic doses); ¶ depending on CYP2C9 status. Abbreviations: t50%, plasma elimination half life; tmax, time to maximal plasma concentration; FO, oral bioavailability; Vd, volume of distribution (comp. Brune et al. 2010; Brune et al. 2009).
[a] Interferes with platelet activity of ASA.
[b] High GI-toxicity, inhibits platelets for days.
[c] Hepatotoxicity.
[d] Agranulocytosis (rare).
[e] CV-risks in long-term use.

equally effective on COX-1 (which regulates platelet aggregation), an increased propensity for bleeds, including GI bleeds, may be the consequence (Rahme and Nedjar 2007). This risk may be antagonized partially by the co-administration of PPI (not effective in the low GI-tract) (Chan et al. 2010).

◆ Ibuprofen is generally seen as relatively harmless. However, administering too high doses, i.e. >1.2g/day, may increase its toxicity. Moreover, ibuprofen interferes with the effects of low-dose acetylic salicylic acid (ASA) on platelet aggregation. Therefore, higher doses (>1.2g/day) should be avoided and ibuprofen should not be given within one hour after the intake of ASA.

## 25.4 Opioids: drugs with moderate effect in CLBP

Opioids should not be used in ALBP: the effect is small, but UDEs are frequent. There are several RCTs assessing the effectiveness of opioids in CLBP. The data available indicate that oxycodon, oxymorphone, and tramadol may have therapeutic effects in CLBP (see Table 25.2). These opioids should be used. Others, as buprenorphine, fentanyl, or morphine, appear less suited. All of them display limited and variable bioavailability. Therefore, fentanyl is often administered as a patch. The fact that the absorption is slow and not reliable is often not realized. Peak plasma concentrations are achieved only about 2 days after the application of the patch. In addition, effective fentanyl concentrations persist for days after the removal of the patch.

The limited effect is counterbalanced by a relatively high rate of UDEs leading to high (~50%) dropout rates (Kuijpers et al. 2010; Machado et al. 2009). The therapeutic effect of the three opioids mentioned is seen as statistically significant, but of minor clinical importance (compare the effect size of Table 25.1). Consequently, opioids are often combined with other drugs which have no proven effectiveness of their own in CLBP, but may increase the effect of opioids as well as UDEs (see Table 25.3).

The risk of addiction going along with the use of opioids in CLBP appears to be low (Fishbain et al. 2008). Serious side effects are rare. The use of opioids together with other drugs in CLBP is common practice. But RCTs to document effects are still rare (Table 25.3). A pharmacological derivative of tramadol is tapentadol which is claimed to combine the opioid effect with noradrenaline/serotonin reuptake inhibition (Wade and Spruill 2009; Etropolski et al. 2010). The proof of superiority of this combined effect of tapentadol is not documented by a RCT.

## 25.5 Muscle relaxants may enhance the effect of analgesics

Muscle relaxants alone do not appear to be useful therapeutic agents in either ALBP or CLBP (Kuijpers et al. 2010). They are claimed, however, to be useful in combination with either NSAID in ALBP or with opioids in CLBP (Table 25.3). The culprit of the muscle relaxants is that they are heavily burdened with UDEs. The anticholinergic agents, as methocarbamol, orphenadrine, or tizanidine, go along with drowsiness, headaches, and typical anticholinergic effects, as increase of intraocular pressure, problems of voiding urine, and changes of the GI-tract motility. Alternatively, benzodiazepines, including diazepam and tetrazepam, may be used. They also increase sedation, tiredness, and drowsiness. They have no anticholinergic effects, but often induce drug abuse and drug dependency. Worldwide, there is a dramatic overuse of benzodiazepines in elderly people which gives rise to many fractures resulting of drowsiness and instability, particularly at night (Pariente et al. 2008).

Taken together, muscle relaxants may be used for short periods of time only. Benzodiazepines often induce abuse and cause fractures in elderly. In several European countries, flupirtine is used in ALBP. It is claimed to have a spasmolytic effect due to opening potassium channels. The effect of flupirtine in ALBP is not well documented (Li et al. 2008; Williams et al. 2010). Flupirtine should not be used in specific or CLBP as it may cause liver toxicity (Arzneimittelkommission der Deutschen Ärzteschaft 2007).

## 25.6 Antidepressants: sometimes useful as co-therapeutics in CLBP

Antidepressants, in particular SSRIs, have no place in ALBP. In CLBP, their effect, when given alone, is not different from placebo (Urquhart et al. 2008). One RCT claims effectiveness (Skljarevski et al. 2010). They appear to be beneficial in selected cases of CLBP when given in combination with opioids (Chou and Huffman 2007). It is still an unsettled question if this effect is due to the depressive mood of many patients with CLBP or whether it is based on an independent mechanism. Fluoxetine and duloxetine are used, but have as yet no proven indication in CLBP (Staal et al. 2008).

## 25.7 **Conclusion**

It becomes clear that LBP is and will remain a major health problem. There is little proven evidence of the therapeutic effects of many drugs and other treatments (Bouwmeester et al. 2009). In ALBP, only COX inhibitors, used cautiously, may help to regain mobility and social functions (Kroenke et al. 2009) which in turn allows for exercise that furthers recovery (Oesch et al. 2010).

As COX inhibitors lose effectiveness with time, opioids may step in. Their effect may be enhanced by co-medication with either muscle relaxants or antiepileptics. However, opioids + muscle relaxants or antidepressants show a high rate of UDEs. Most patients find these side effects intolerable which leads to a dropout-rate (in studies) around 50% (Kuijpers et al. 2010).

Obviously, the treatment of CLBP requires therapeutic planning and long-term therapy, including psychotherapy and physiotherapy as main pillars whilst the different drugs may be regarded as auxiliary.

The biggest problem is the inability of many patients to cope and wait. Some resort to remedies of unproven or even disproven value (effect), as herbal medicines, local steroids, topical non-steroidals, acupuncture, an injection therapy using steroids, etc., and surgical interventions. Whilst the former are unlikely to harm the patient seriously, attempts to inject into the fine zygapophysial joints and surgical interventions in patients who have no hard indication (nerve decay and paralysis) may add to the negative long-term outcomes of LBP.

## References

**Arzneimittelkommission der Deutschen Ärzteschaft.** 2007. 'Mitteilungen: Aus der UAW-Datenbank': Leberschäden unter Flupirtin. *Deutsches Ärzteblatt,* **104,** A 3200.

**Berman, B. M., Langevin, H. M., Witt, C. M. & Dubner, R.** 2010. Acupuncture for chronic low back pain. *N Engl J Med,* **363,** 454–61.

**Berry, H., Bloom, B., Hamilton, E. B. & Swinson, D. R.** 1982. Naproxen sodium, diflunisal, and placebo in the treatment of chronic back pain. *Ann Rheum Dis,* **41,** 129–32.

**Birbara, C. A., Puopolo, A. D., Munoz, D. R., et al.** 2003. Treatment of chronic low back pain with etoricoxib, a new cyclo-oxygenase-2 selective inhibitor: improvement in pain and disability—a randomized, placebo-controlled, 3-month trial. *J Pain,* **4,** 307–15.

**Boelsterli, U. A.** 2003. Diclofenac-induced liver injury: a paradigm of idiosyncratic drug toxicity. *Toxicol Appl Pharmacol,* **192,** 307–22.

**Bouwmeester, W., Van Enst, A. & Van Tulder, M.** 2009. Quality of low back pain guidelines improved. *Spine,* **34,** 2562–7.

**Brune, K. & Hinz, B.** 2004. Selective cyclooxygenase-2 inhibitors: similarities and differences. *Scand J Rheumatol,* **33,** 1–6.

**Brune, K., Hinz, B. & Otterness, I.** 2009. Aspirin and acetaminophen: should they be available over the counter? *Curr Rheumatol Rep,* **11,** 36–40.

**Brune, K., Renner, B. & Hinz, B.** 2010. Using pharmacokinetic principles to optimize pain therapy. *Nat Rev Rheumatol,* **6,** 589–98.

**Cannon, C. P., Curtis, S. P., Fitzgerald, G. A., et al.** 2006. Cardiovascular outcomes with etoricoxib and diclofenac in patients with osteoarthritis and rheumatoid arthritis in the Multinational Etoricoxib and Diclofenac Arthritis Long-term (MEDAL) programme: a randomised comparison. *Lancet,* **368,** 1771–81.

Chan, F. K., Lanas, A., Scheiman, J., Berger, M. F., Nguyen, H. & Goldstein, J. L. 2010. Celecoxib versus omeprazole and diclofenac in patients with osteoarthritis and rheumatoid arthritis (CONDOR): a randomised trial. *Lancet,* **376**, 173–9.

Chang, C. H., Shau, W. Y., Kuo, C. W., Chen, S. T. & Lai, M. S. 2010. Increased risk of stroke associated with nonsteroidal anti-inflammatory drugs: a nationwide case-crossover study. *Stroke,* **41**, 1884–90.

Choi, B. K., Verbeek, J. H., Tam, W. W. & Jiang, J. Y. 2010. Exercises for prevention of recurrences of low-back pain. *Cochrane Database Syst Rev,* CD006555.

Chou, R., Baisden, J., Carragee, E. J., Resnick, D. K., Shaffer, W. O. & Loeser, J. D. 2009. Surgery for low back pain: a review of the evidence for an American Pain Society Clinical Practice Guideline. *Spine,* **34**, 1094–109.

Chou, R. & Huffman, L. H. 2007. Medications for acute and chronic low back pain: a review of the evidence for an American Pain Society/American College of Physicians clinical practice guideline. *Ann Intern Med,* **147**, 505–14.

Cui, X., Trinh, K. & Wang, Y. J. 2010. Chinese herbal medicine for chronic neck pain due to cervical degenerative disc disease. *Cochrane Database Syst Rev,* CD006556.

Dajani, E. Z. & Islam, K. 2008. Cardiovascular and gastrointestinal toxicity of selective cyclo-oxygenase-2 inhibitors in man. *J Physiol Pharmacol,* **59** Suppl 2, 117–33.

Davies, R. A., Maher, C. G. & Hancock, M. J. 2008. A systematic review of paracetamol for non-specific low back pain. *Eur Spine J,* **17**, 1423–30.

Deshpande, A., Furlan, A., Mailis-Gagnon, A., Atlas, S. & Turk, D. 2007. Opioids for chronic low-back pain. *Cochrane Database Syst Rev,* CD004959.

Dowswell, T., Bedwell, C., Lavender, T. & Neilson, J. P. 2009. Transcutaneous electrical nerve stimulation (TENS) for pain relief in labour. *Cochrane Database Syst Rev,* CD007214.

Dreiser, R. L., Marty, M., Ionescu, E., Gold, M. & Liu, J. H. 2003. Relief of acute low back pain with diclofenac-K 12.5 mg tablets: a flexible dose, ibuprofen 200 mg and placebo-controlled clinical trial. *Int J Clin Pharmacol Ther,* **41**, 375–85.

Edgar, M. A. 2007. The nerve supply of the lumbar intervertebral disc. *J Bone Joint Surg Br,* **89**, 1135–9.

Etropolski, M. S., Okamoto, A., Shapiro, D. Y. & Rauschkolb, C. 2010. Dose conversion between tapentadol immediate and extended release for low back pain. *Pain Physician,* **13**, 61–70.

Fishbain, D. A., Cole, B., Lewis, J., Rosomoff, H. L. & Rosomoff, R. S. 2008. What percentage of chronic nonmalignant pain patients exposed to chronic opioid analgesic therapy develop abuse/addiction and/or aberrant drug-related behaviors? A structured evidence-based review. *Pain Med,* **9**, 444–59.

Fitzgerald, M. 2005. The development of nociceptive circuits. *Nat Rev Neurosci,* **6**, 507–20.

Freemont, A. J., Peacock, T. E., Goupille, P., Hoyland, J. A., O'Brien, J. & Jayson, M. I. 1997. Nerve ingrowth into diseased intervertebral disc in chronic back pain. *Lancet,* **350**, 178–81.

Furlan, A. D., Imamura, M., Dryden, T. & Irvin, E. 2009. Massage for low back pain: an updated systematic review within the framework of the Cochrane Back Review Group. *Spine,* **34**, 1669–84.

Haroutiunian, S., Drennan, D. A. & Lipman, A. G. 2010. Topical NSAID therapy for musculoskeletal pain. *Pain Med,* **11**, 535–49.

Henschke, N., Kuijpers, T., Rubinstein, S. M., et al. 2010. Injection therapy and denervation procedures for chronic low-back pain: a systematic review. *Eur Spine J,* **19**, 1425–49.

Hinz, B. & Brune, K. 2008. Can drug removals involving cyclooxygenase-2 inhibitors be avoided? A plea for human pharmacology. *Trends Pharmacol Sci,* **29**, 391–7.

Jamison, R. N., Raymond, S. A., Slawsby, E. A., Nedeljkovic, S. S. & Katz, N. P. 1998. Opioid therapy for chronic noncancer back pain. A randomized prospective study. *Spine,* **23**, 2591–600.

Johnson, A. G. 1997. NSAIDs and increased blood pressure. What is the clinical significance? *Drug Saf,* **17**, 277–89.

Jones, P. & Lamdin, R. 2010. Oral cyclo-oxygenase 2 inhibitors versus other oral analgesics for acute soft tissue injury: systematic review and meta-analysis. *Clin Drug Investig,* **30**, 419–37.

Katz, N., Rauck, R., Ahdieh, H., et al. 2007. A 12-week, randomized, placebo-controlled trial assessing the safety and efficacy of oxymorphone extended release for opioid-naive patients with chronic low back pain. *Curr Med Res Opin*, **23**, 117–28.

Kobayashi, Y., Kurata, J., Sekiguchi, M., et al. 2009. Augmented cerebral activation by lumbar mechanical stimulus in chronic low back pain patients: an FMRI study. *Spine (Phila Pa 1976)*, **34**, 2431–6.

Kroenke, K., Krebs, E. E. & Bair, M. J. 2009. Pharmacotherapy of chronic pain: a synthesis of recommendations from systematic reviews. *Gen Hosp Psychiatry*, **31**, 206–19.

Kuijpers, T., Van Middelkoop, M., Rubinstein, S. M., et al. 2010. A systematic review on the effectiveness of pharmacological interventions for chronic non-specific low-back pain. *Eur Spine J*.

Li, C., Ni, J., Wang, Z., LI, M., Gasparic, M., Terhaag, B. & Uberall, M. A. 2008. Analgesic efficacy and tolerability of flupirtine vs. tramadol in patients with subacute low back pain: a double-blind multicentre trial. *Curr Med Res Opin*, **24**, 3523–30.

Machado, L. A., Kamper, S. J., Herbert, R. D., Maher, C. G. & Mcauley, J. H. 2009. Analgesic effects of treatments for non-specific low back pain: a meta-analysis of placebo-controlled randomized trials. *Rheumatology (Oxford)*, **48**, 520–7.

Manchikanti, L., Singh, V., Falco, F. J., Cash, K. A. & Pampati, V. 2010. Evaluation of lumbar facet joint nerve blocks in managing chronic low back pain: a randomized, double-blind, controlled trial with a 2-year follow-up. *Int J Med Sci*, **7**, 124–35.

Oesch, P., Kool, J., Hagen, K. B. & Bachmann, S. 2010. Effectiveness of exercise on work disability in patients with non-acute non-specific low back pain: Systematic review and meta-analysis of randomised controlled trials. *J Rehabil Med*, **42**, 193–205.

Pallay, R. M., Seger, W., Adler, J. L., et al. 2004. Etoricoxib reduced pain and disability and improved quality of life in patients with chronic low back pain: a 3 month, randomized, controlled trial. *Scand J Rheumatol*, **33**, 257–66.

Pareek, A., Chandurkar, N., Chandanwale, A. S., Ambade, R., Gupta, A. & Bartakke, G. 2009. Aceclofenac-tizanidine in the treatment of acute low back pain: a double-blind, double-dummy, randomized, multicentric, comparative study against aceclofenac alone. *Eur Spine J*, **18**, 1836–42.

Pariente, A., Dartigues, J. F., Benichou, J., Letenneur, L., Moore, N. & Fourrier-Reglat, A. 2008. Benzodiazepines and injurious falls in community dwelling elders. *Drugs Aging*, **25**, 61–70.

Peloso, P. M., Fortin, L., Beaulieu, A., Kamin, M. & Rosenthal, N. 2004. Analgesic efficacy and safety of tramadol/ acetaminophen combination tablets (Ultracet) in treatment of chronic low back pain: a multicenter, outpatient, randomized, double blind, placebo controlled trial. *J Rheumatol*, **31**, 2454–63.

Peterson, C. & Hodler, J. 2010. Evidence-based radiology (part 1): Is there sufficient research to support the use of therapeutic injections for the spine and sacroiliac joints? *Skeletal Radiol*, **39**, 5–9.

Rahme, E. & Bernatsky, S. 2010. NSAIDs and risk of lower gastrointestinal bleeding. *Lancet*, **376**, 146–8.

Rahme, E. & Nedjar, H. 2007. Risks and benefits of COX-2 inhibitors vs non-selective NSAIDs: does their cardiovascular risk exceed their gastrointestinal benefit? A retrospective cohort study. *Rheumatology (Oxford)*, **46**, 435–8.

Roelofs, P. D., Deyo, R. A., Koes, B. W., Scholten, R. J. & Van Tulder, M. W. 2008a. Non-steroidal anti-inflammatory drugs for low back pain. *Cochrane Database Syst Rev*, CD000396.

Roelofs, P. D., Deyo, R. A., Koes, B. W., Scholten, R. J. & Van Tulder, M. W. 2008b. Nonsteroidal anti-inflammatory drugs for low back pain: an updated Cochrane review. *Spine (Phila Pa 1976)*, **33**, 1766–74.

Romano, C. L., Romano, D., Bonora, C. & Mineo, G. 2009. Pregabalin, celecoxib, and their combination for treatment of chronic low-back pain. *J Orthop Traumatol*, **10**, 185–91.

Rubinstein, S. M., Van Middelkoop, M., Kuijpers, T., et al. 2010. A systematic review on the effectiveness of complementary and alternative medicine for chronic non-specific low-back pain. *Eur Spine J*, **19**, 1213–28.

Ruoff, G. E., Rosenthal, N., Jordan, D., Karim, R. & Kamin, M. 2003. Tramadol/acetaminophen combination tablets for the treatment of chronic lower back pain: a multicenter, randomized, double-blind, placebo-controlled outpatient study. *Clin Ther*, **25**, 1123–41.

Schnitzer, T. J., Gray, W. L., Paster, R. Z. & Kamin, M. 2000. Efficacy of tramadol in treatment of chronic low back pain. *J Rheumatol,* **27,** 772–8.

Skljarevski, V., Zhang, S., Desaiah, D., Alaka, K. J., Palacios, S., Miazgowski, T. & Patrick, K. 2010. Duloxetine versus placebo in patients with chronic low back pain: a 12-week, fixed-dose, randomized, double-blind trial. *J Pain,* **11**(12), 1282–90.

Staal, J. B., De Bie, R., De Vet, H. C., Hildebrandt, J. & Nelemans, P. 2008. Injection therapy for subacute and chronic low-back pain. *Cochrane Database Syst Rev,* CD001824.

Staal, J. B., De Bie, R. A., De Vet, H. C., Hildebrandt, J. & Nelemans, P. 2009. Injection therapy for subacute and chronic low back pain: an updated Cochrane review. *Spine (Phila Pa 1976),* **34,** 49–59.

Sudano, I., Flammer, A. J., Periat, D., et al. 2010. Acetaminophen increases blood pressure in patients with coronary artery disease. *Circulation,* **122,** 1789–96.

Takahashi, K., Aoki, Y. & Ohtori, S. 2008. Resolving discogenic pain. *Eur Spine J,* **17** Suppl 4, 428–31.

Urquhart, D. M., Hoving, J. L., Assendelft, W. W., Roland, M. & VAN Tulder, M. W. 2008. Antidepressants for non-specific low back pain. *Cochrane Database Syst Rev,* CD001703.

Van Middelkoop, M., Rubinstein, S. M., Kuijpers, T., et al. 2010. A systematic review on the effectiveness of physical and rehabilitation interventions for chronic non-specific low back pain. *Eur Spine J.*

Van Tulder, M. W., Koes, B. & Malmivaara, A. 2006a. Outcome of non-invasive treatment modalities on back pain: an evidence-based review. *Eur Spine J,* **15** Suppl 1, S64–81.

Van Tulder, M. W., Koes, B., Seitsalo, S. & Malmivaara, A. 2006b. Outcome of invasive treatment modalities on back pain and sciatica: an evidence-based review. *Eur Spine J,* **15** Suppl 1, S82–92.

Van Tulder, M. W., Touray, T., Furlan, A. D., Solway, S. & Bouter, L. M. 2003. Muscle relaxants for non-specific low back pain. *Cochrane Database Syst Rev,* CD004252.

Wade, W. E. & Spruill, W. J. 2009. Tapentadol hydrochloride: a centrally acting oral analgesic. *Clin Ther,* **31,** 2804–18.

Webster, L. R., Butera, P. G., Moran, L. V., Wu, N., Burns, L. H. & Friedmann, N. 2006. Oxytrex minimizes physical dependence while providing effective analgesia: a randomized controlled trial in low back pain. *J Pain,* **7,** 937–46.

Wilkens, P., Scheel, I. B., Grundnes, O., Hellum, C. & Storheim, K. 2010. Effect of glucosamine on pain-related disability in patients with chronic low back pain and degenerative lumbar osteoarthritis: a randomized controlled trial. *JAMA,* **304,** 45–52.

Williams, C. M., Latimer, J., Maher, C. G., et al. 2010. PACE—the first placebo controlled trial of paracetamol for acute low back pain: design of a randomised controlled trial. *BMC Musculoskelet Disord,* **11,** 169.

Worz, R., Bolten, W., Heller, B., Krainick, J. U. & Pergande, G. 1996. [Flupirtine in comparison with chlormezanone in chronic musculoskeletal back pain. Results of a multicenter randomized double-blind study]. *Fortschr Med,* **114,** 500–4.

Zerbini, C., Ozturk, Z. E., Grifka, J., Maini, M., Nilganuwong, S., Morales, R., Hupli, M., Shivaprakash, M. & Giezek, H. 2005. Efficacy of etoricoxib 60 mg/day and diclofenac 150 mg/day in reduction of pain and disability in patients with chronic low back pain: results of a 4-week, multinational, randomized, double-blind study. *Curr Med Res Opin,* **21,** 2037–49.

# Part 8

# Subgroup-Specific Approaches for Patients at Risk For or With Chronic Pain

Chapter 26

# Reviewing the Concept of Subgroups in Subacute and Chronic Pain and the Potential of Customizing Treatments

Adina C. Rusu, Katja Boersma, and Dennis C. Turk

## 26.1 The conundrum of pain

The tradition in medicine is to make a differential diagnosis of patients on the basis of the presence of a set of signs and symptoms that meet the defining criteria for a specific disease and that are inconsistent with alternative diagnoses that may have some similarities. Once a patient receives a diagnosis a specific treatment or set of treatments will be prescribed preferably to cure the disease or at least to alleviate some if not all of the symptoms. However, not all patients exposed to the same pathogens or traumas meeting criteria for the same disease will present to the healthcare provider in the same way if they seek treatment at all and they may not respond to the same treatment in the same way. For example, only a small percentage exposed to an ankle fracture will develop complex regional pain syndrome, similarly a minority of people exposed to motor vehicle collision develop fibromyalgia but some do. Moreover, although a percentage of people who have amputations will develop phantom limb pain many do not.

In many pain syndromes (e.g. fibromyalgia syndrome (FM), chronic headache, low back pain (LBP), temporomandibular disorders (TMDs)), the definitive identification of causative agents is rare and physical findings are only minimally related to patient-reported symptomatology (e.g. pain severity). Even for pain syndromes with relatively clear-cut causative lesions or processes (e.g. osteoarthritis, postherpetic neuralgia, chronic postsurgical pain), the severity of the insult often bears only a modest relationship to the probability or intensity of pain report. For example, the presence of a severe zoster rash, or a unilateral mastectomy, or a near-complete loss of cartilage in the knee joint may produce no pain at all in one individual and severe chronic pain in another, indicting the presence of substantial individual differences in the processing of information related to noxious stimulation. Even when they receive identical treatments for the same diagnosis, responses are variable. In clinical trials, the emphasis tends to be on mean results with much less attention given to the variability in responses. Why do not all individuals exposed to the same insult demonstrate the same physical and psychological responses to the disease or trauma and how can the variability in response to treatment be explained?

## 26.2 Contributions to individual differences

### 26.2.1 Genotype

The traditional biomedical approach, however, loses sight of the fact that patients have unique genotypes and the phenotypic manifestation of an insult (i.e. disease or trauma). Mogil et al. (1999) demonstrated marked variability in the responses of different inbred genetic strains of mice. Since some of these strains were bred to have an absence of certain genes they implicate the role of genetic factors in the variability. The demonstration of individual genetic variability of rodents can reasonably be extrapolated to humans. Assume normal distribution in both pain sensitivity (thresholds) and endogenous pain control the combination of both being lower may place some individuals at risk (Edwards 2005). Human genetic studies suggest that single-nucleotide polymorphisms of specific genes contribute significantly to basal pain sensitivity. Single-nucleotide polymorphisms of the δ-opioid receptor gene (Kim et al. 2004) and the catechol-O-methyltransferease (*COMT*) gene (Zubieta et al. 2003) are associated with pain ratings in response to noxious stimuli and pain-induced μ-opioid receptor binding in the CNS (Zubieta et al. 2003). Polymorphisms of μ-opioid receptor gene (*OPRM1*), specifically the single nucleotide polymorphisms 118 A>G (substitution) have been shown to influence the efficacy of intravenous morphine (Chou et al. 2006; Landau et al. 2008; for more information see also Chapter 3). Thus, any two individuals with different polymorphisms of this gene may respond with wide variability to the same treatment for the same traumatic event-type of surgery. Response to the insult and response to treatment will be influenced by genetic characteristics.

### 26.2.2 Prior learning histories and psychological variations

In addition to individual uniqueness attributable to genotype, prior to symptom onset, patients have extensive life experiences and learning histories that that shape their personalities and ways of coping with trauma, injury, symptoms and that will influence their symptom presentation and response to both the treatment and the insult. Pain intensity is influenced by a range of psychosocial processes such as catastrophizing, which is associated with lower pain thresholds (Sullivan et al. 2001) and enhanced CNS processing (Gracely et al. 2004).

There has been a growing awareness of and empirical support for the importance of psychological factors in reports of pain, suffering, and disability (e.g. Gatchel and Turk 1999). For example, Flor and Turk (1988) found that physical factors in LBP and rheumatoid arthritis patients did not predict pain severity, life interference, or physician visits; whereas cognitive appraisals of helplessness and hopelessness were predictive of both self-report of pain impact and behavior in response to pain. Similarly, studies provide evidence in support of the role of variables other than medical diagnoses and identified physical pathology in treatment outcome (Jensen et al. 2001; Burns et al. 2003). They found that perceptions of control over pain and decreased beliefs about being disabled, and catastrophizing were associated with reductions in pain intensity, depression, number of physician visits, and physical disability.

Over the past two decades there has been growing interest in the presence of individual differences in endogenous pain modulation. Psychological factors may interact with physiological and genetic ones. People with chronic pain may demonstrate central augmentation (CA), key features of which are increased vigilance to noxious stimuli, facilitation of such stimuli, and impaired inhibition of them (Clauw 2010). CA can be manifested by *reduced* ability to *inhibit* noxious stimuli (frequently assessed via conditioned pain modulation, CPM) and by *facilitation* of noxious input (frequently assessed via temporal summation, TS).

CA has been evaluated in a variety of chronic pain populations, and although results have not been entirely consistent (Leffler et al. 2002; Staud et al. 2003; Sutton et al. 2008); increased CA has been identified in patients with various pain conditions, e.g. FM (Lautenbacher and Rollman 1997) and LBP (Peters and Schmidt 1992). It is not clear whether CA should be viewed as a catalyst for the development of chronic pain or a result of chronic pain. However at least one study demonstrated that impaired CA predicted postoperative pain severity and persistence up to 6 months among patients undergoing thoracotomy (Yarnitsky et al. 2008). Greater basal pain sensitivity and decreased pain-inhibitory capacity may serve as a diathesis for the development of chronic pain (Edwards et al. 2003).

If CA is a *risk factor* for the development of chronic pain, what is the association between CA and other risk factors? Since pain processing involves complex cerebral-spinal-peripheral connections, CA is likely to be associated with psychological risk factors. Although research on associations between indices of CA and psychological measures is in its infancy, there is some evidence for an association between CA and anxiety (Granot et al. 2008) and catastrophizing (Edwards et al. 2003; Edwards 2005; Granot et al. 2008; Goodin et al. 2009).

Studies of healthy, pain-free individuals reveal intact diffuse noxious inhibitory control (DNIC) functioning: the application of one noxious stimulus inhibits the perception of pain produced by the application of a second noxious stimulus (Edwards et al. 2003). However, studies of patients with chronic pain conditions (e.g. FM, chronic back pain, irritable bowel syndrome), suggest that they have either a diminished or non-existent DNIC response, and thus, experience increased pain intensity (Staud et al. 2003; Wilder-Smith et al. 2004). DNIC has also been demonstrated to predict who is likely to develop chronic pain following a specific trauma such as surgery (Yarnitsky et al. 2008). Thus it appears that efficiency in the DNIC response may explain individual variation in response to objectively comparable noxious stimulation and be a potential risk factor for chronic pain.

### 26.2.3 Environmental contributions

To complicate things further, people with specific diseases live in social environments not in isolation and responses from significant others contribute to the identified patient's response to symptoms, impact of symptoms the patients' lives, treatments prescribed and initiated, and response to treatments prescribed and self-initiated. Thus, the symptoms do not just occur in isolated body parts or body systems but in a unique individual. The individual differences present may explain the variation in how patients manifest, respond to, and adapt to their symptoms and disease as well as their compliance with and response to treatment. These individual differences are masked in the presentation of group averages in responses to treatment. Environmental influences exert profound effects on basal pain sensitivity with early exposure (Taddio et al. 1995; Anand et al. 1999; Taddio et al. 2002) and trauma (Scarini et al. 1994) altering subsequent pain sensitivity and placing individuals at risk for actue (Fillingim, Wilkinson, and Powell 1999) and chronic pain (Aaron et al. 1997; Lampe et al. 2003).

Consider the role of contextual factors on pain perception and response. Back pain may have been initiated by a trauma working in the garden or a trauma at work, a similar cause but a different context and with different meaning may lead to different responses such as how to treat, whether to treat, from whom to seek treatment, and appropriate actions to take. The context in which the symptoms began, at least to some extent, guide the response.

Now consider a man who awakens one morning with a severe headache. His first thought may be to question why does he have this headache. It is possible that his interpretation of the cause and the meaning of the symptoms may influence his level of emotional arousal and behaviours related to treatment. If he recalls that his father, who died of a brain aneurism, described a severe headache before his death and believes that his own headache is similar to that described by his father, it is likely that his emotional arousal will greatly increase, potentially exacerbating the headache, and he may rush to the emergency department at a local hospital. An alternative scenario may lead to very different responses to the same symptom, headache. If instead of relating the headache to his father's death but rather relates it to having had too much alcohol to drink the previous night, his level of emotional arousal might be significantly less elevated. He may decide to take an over-the-counter analgesic and lie down for a while. Here the same symptom, severe headache, was interpreted differently and resulted in different responses—levels of emotional arousal and treatment behaviours. Thus, variations observed may be related to premorbid individual differences. Response to treatments and adaptation to the disease are quite variable. This variation is lost when mean differences are reported.

## 26.3 **A diathesis–stress–environment conceptualization**

Based on the brief overview, a number of explanations might account for the differences in evolution of diseases, maintenance, and exacerbation of symptoms, and response to the pathology and to treatment as well. There is likely to be a normal distribution of sensory sensitivity, such that individuals will vary in their detection thresholds, and perception of noxious stimuli, this distribution is likely to be determined by individuals' genotypes. People also have unique learning histories that will also guide their beliefs, attitudes, and expectation regarding symptoms and treatments. Treatments are filtered through individual lens comprised of individual, pathophysiological, and environmental factors that result in differential experiences, responses, and beliefs and expectations. Thus, these factors—genotype, phenotype, environment, and learning—interact in such a way that considering them in isolation will provide an inadequate understanding. A more comprehensive perspective that we might consider is a complex diathesis–stress–environment model (Turk and Wilson 2010, see Figure 26.1). Individuals may be predisposed to the development of pain based on genetics, prior learning history and culture (diatheses). Initiation of a disease, trauma, or noxious sensory input (stresses) is filtered through the lens of this diathesis producing differential experiences, responses, and beliefs and expectations. The experience and responses to the stresses occur in a social content (environment) which can both directly and indirectly impact on diatheses and stresses altering the subsequent experience, beliefs and expectations. This model takes a longitudinal rather than cross-sectional perspective. Regardless of the causes of individual variations—genetics, prior learning history, environmental factors, one size most

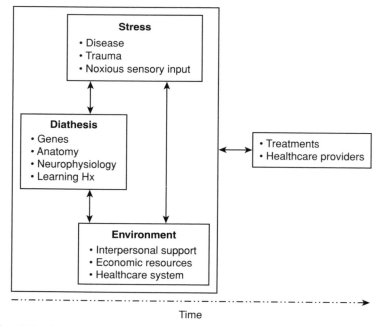

**Fig. 26.1** The diathesis–stress–environment model.

assuredly does not fit all when it comes to treating people with chronic pain even if they have the same diagnosis.

There are a number of subacute and chronic pain syndromes that are diagnosed in a large number of patients based on ill-defined criteria often without any clear understanding of the underlying mechanisms. For example, it is estimated that 3–6 million American seek treatment for FM each year (Wolfe et al. 1997). The current criteria for diagnosing FM consist of: (1) widespread pain of at least 3 months' duration and (2) pain present upon palpation of at least 11 of 18 specific locations, hence tender points (Wolfe et al. 1990). The two most common types of chronic headache are migraine and tension-type and for both the pathogenesis are unclear. Historically, migraines were attributed to abnormal vascular activity and the mechanism for tension-type headaches was assumed to be muscle contraction. However, studies have demonstrated that the muscle tension levels of people with migraine were actually higher than recorded in tension-type headaches leading some to suggest that these two types of headaches should be viewed along a continuum of severity rather than be viewed as categorically different (Marcus 1992).

Subacute and chronic pain syndromes create a great deal of distress and disability; yet, despite being prevalent, the aetiology and pathophysiology have remained elusive. Although no pathophysiological factors have been identified, it is not for lack of trying. Various biological and psychological factors have been investigated, but no definitive associations have been consistently demonstrated. However, to date, these syndromes remain recalcitrant to treatment. In fact the lack of understanding of the aetiology and maintaining factors has served as the impetus for the diversity of interventions that have been used. What seems apparent is that the treatment of these chronic pain syndromes has been based on the traditional model where the intervention is matched to medical diagnoses even when crudely defined. Prescribing treatment based on diagnoses is appropriate when there is a known aetiology but this approach has little basis when the cause is unknown. When there is no consensus regarding what treatment should be prescribed the choice becomes empirical, delivered on a trial-and-error basis depending on healthcare providers' predilections and experience. The lack of universal success may explain why so many treatments have been prescribed for these patients (Turk, 2002).

Lack of knowledge of the underlying mechanisms of the vague chronic pain syndromes has not inhibited efforts to treat these patients with diverse modalities. There are a range of treatments for subacute and chronic pain diagnosis. For example, there are over 50 pharmacological and more than 50 additional non-pharmacological treatments for fibromyalgia syndrome (Turk 2004). These treatments range from various classes of drugs (e.g. anticonvulsants, antidepressants, opioids) to very diverse somatic and psychological therapy exercise, spa therapy, magnetized mattresses, written emotional disclosure, and nerve blocks. Published studies of these disparate treatment approaches reveal that on average 30–40% of patients obtain 20–50% improvement in some symptoms (Turk 2004). This is a perplexing state of affairs, how could such a range of varied treatments produce similar effects for patients with the same diagnosis?

## 26.4 **Patient uniformity myth**

The absence of empirical data linking pathophysiology or patients' characteristics to successful outcome has impeded the design of individual treatment plans. Consequently chronic pain patients have tended to be treated as a homogeneous group based either on the medical diagnosis or the vaguely defined—'chronic pain syndrome'—for whom the same treatment is appropriate. For example patients with TMDs have been treated with a variety of intraoral appliances, biofeedback, oral surgery, and so forth, depending upon the conceptualization of the cause of the symptoms and the practitioner's training and experience (Turk et al. 1995). Chronic LBP patients have been treated with steroid injections, physical therapy modalities, chiropractic manipulations, and in multidisciplinary pain clinics with varying emphases ranging from relatively pure programmes based on operant conditioning (Vlaeyen et al. 1996) to those with heavy emphasis on physical conditioning (e.g. Mayer et al. 1987).

If the rationale for a treatment is that it addresses some underlying pathology—the 'pain generator'—then there should be some evidence implicating the source of the symptoms. For example, the basis for prescribing non-steroidal anti-inflammatory drugs (NSAIDS) is that an inflammatory process plays a causal role in the symptoms; consequently, these drugs should only be prescribed in the presence of inflammation. If the rationale for treating tension-type headaches with biofeedback is related to the presence of maladaptive muscular activity, then in would seem that biofeedback should only be offered to patients who demonstrate some level of excessively high muscular activity. If the use of operant conditioning treatment is predicated on alteration of maladaptive environmental contingencies reinforcing pain behaviours, then some effort should be made to offer this form of treatment only to those patients in whom such reinforcement contingencies have been demonstrated (Fordyce 1976). Few attempts, however, have been made to customize treatments to the mechanisms involved for specific patients. In short, we have adopted the patient uniformity myth—all patients with the same diagnosis, no matter how vague, are treated in a similar fashion as if they were a homogeneous group.

It is common to see patients with a wide range of diagnoses and locations of pain, not to mention demographics and individual differences, treated within the same rehabilitation programme with largely the same components (e.g. somatic, neuropathic, visceral, and psychogenic localized in extremities, back, head, abdominal, thoracic and rectal; Becker et al. 2000). Many pain rehabilitation treatment outcome studies even fail to mention the composition of the patient sample but simply refer to 'consecutively referred patients' or patients with 'non-malignant pain' or 'musculoskeletal disorders' (e.g. Becker et al. 1998; Cipher et al. 2001).

An implicit assumption of pain treatment facilities seems to be that providing multicomponent treatments to all chronic pain patients is appropriate since some component(s) will prove effective, and perhaps different ones for patients with different characteristics. Thus, a pain centre may include physical exercise, education in body mechanics, assertion training, systematic medication reduction, stress management, biofeedback, family counselling, the use of transcutaneous nerve stimulation, nerve blocks, and so forth. This is like treating a set of patients with a range of vitamin deficiencies with multivitamins with the hope that each patient will derive benefits from the appropriate vitamin contained within the collection comprising the multivitamin regimen rather than prescribing specific vitamin therapy based on individual patient needs.

Recent data suggest that greater attention should be given to identifying the characteristics of patients who improve and those who fail to improve when treated with the same intervention. Treatment should be prescribed only for those patients who are likely to derive significant benefit. The ability to predict improvement should be more efficient producing improved outcomes and reduction in costs. Furthermore, the ability to identify characteristics of patients who do not benefit from specific treatment should facilitate the development of treatment approaches tailored to the needs of those patients.

There has been a growing recognition that pain is a complex perceptual experience influenced by a wide range of psychosocial factors, including emotions, social and environmental context, sociocultural background, beliefs, attitudes, and expectations, as well as biological factors. Pain that persists for months and years, chronic pain, will influence all aspects of a person's functioning: emotional, interpersonal, avocational, and physical. Consequently, successfully treating chronic pain patients requires attention not only to the organic basic of the symptom but also to a range of factors that modulate nociception and moderate the pain experience and related disability.

It would be impossible to review the research on all of the attempts to identifying individual differences in patients with persistent along with there responses to different sets of treatments. We have narrowed the focus of the remainder of this chapter to several areas that we feel are representative of the developments over the past decade and that we believe have promise for the future evolution of understanding pain sufferers and treatment processes. In accordance with the aims of this volume, we focus on chronic non-cancer pain in adults, with a special interest on back pain.

Despite major advances in medical and surgical treatment, the incidence of low back pain disability continues to escalate (Waddell 1998). Several recent studies support the efficacy of rehabilitation programmes that incorporate psychological interventions for chronic back pain. For instance, in a study designed to evaluate psychological treatments in the prevention of chronicity in patients with sciatic pain, Hasenbring et al. (1999) compared two psychological treatments (biofeedback vs. cognitive-behavioural therapy, CBT) for patients at risk for chronicity with usual care and treatment refusers. One of the best predictors of disability was refusal of treatment. These results lend support to the notion that efficacy will be enhanced if cognitive-behavioural treatments are initiated earlier in the course of treatment and scheduled in accordance with individual psychological patterns of coping (Turk 1990a).

## 26.5 **Identification of patient subgroups**

Chronic pain syndromes are made up of heterogeneous groups of people even if they have the identical medical diagnosis. A common pitfall in clinical research and practice is the assumption of patient homogeneity. Inclusion of a diverse group of patients into the same category simply because they present a common set of symptoms may result in inconsistent research results. Several attempts have been made to identify groups of patients who differ on important variables and to evaluate differential treatment responses (e.g. Turk et al. 1996; Thieme et al. 2006; Verra et al. 2009). A significant problem with rehabilitation-oriented treatments is that: (1) a large number of patients refuse treatments offered; (2) a large number of patients drop out of treatment; and (3) the rates of relapse are relatively high (Richmond and Carmody 1999; Turk and Rudy 1990a).

A number of studies have focused on empirically identifying patient subgroups based on psychological characteristics and psychopathology. Numerous attempts to identify subgroups have relied on the use of traditional psychological measures such as the Minnesota Multiphasic Personality Inventory (MMPI) and the Symptom Checklist-90R (Swimmer et al. 1992; Hutten et al. 2001). Others have tried to identify subgroups of patients based on behavioural communications of pain—'pain behaviours' (Keefe et al. 1990), physical performance (Hutten et al. 2001), patient perceived aetiology (Waylonis and Perkins 1994), and psychophysiological response profiles (Thieme et al. 2006). Up to this point, the attempts to identify subgroups of patients with chronic pain reviewed have focused on single factors. Outcomes, however, are likely to be determined by the interactive effects of multiple factors, as single factors may not account for a statistically significant or clinically meaningful proportion of the variance in outcome. Several studies that included measures of both physical and psychological functioning have reported interactive effects of biopsychosocial factors on the outcomes (Mayer et al. 1987). Some authors have proposed that multidimensional rather than unidimensional classifications should be attempted for a problem as complex as chronic pain (Turk and Rudy 1988; Dworkin and LeResche 1992).

## 26.6 **Empirically-derived classification of patients with pain**

A number of studies have identified subgroups of patients according to psychosocial and behavioural characteristics (e.g. Turk and Rudy 1988; 1990a,b; Turk et al. 1998a; Johansson and

Lindberg 2000). Several studies found that patients classified into different subgroups on the basis of their psychosocial and behavioural responses responded differently to identical treatments (Dahlstrom et al. 1997; Thieme et al. 2006; Verra et al. 2009). Subgroups of chronic pain patients characterized by a number of psychosocial and behavioural characteristics seem to be fairly consistently observed across different pain syndromes (e.g. LBP, FM, TMD, headaches, cancer, spinal cord injuries, whiplash associated disorders; Turk et al. 1998b; Turk and Rudy 1990b; Soderlund and Denison 2006; Widerström-Noga et al. 2007; see Table 26.1) suggesting the independence of psychosocial factors from the physical pathology. Distinctiveness of the psychosocial profiling implies that patients in different subgroups may exhibit differential responses to treatment, which has been demonstrated in several outcome studies.

Turk and Rudy (1988) performed a cluster analysis on patients' responses to the West Haven-Yale Multidimensional Pain Inventory (MPI, Kerns et al. 1985), a frequently used measure in the chronic pain literature (Piotrowski 2007) that has been shown to be reliable, valid, and sensitive to change (Lousberg et al. 1999; Bergström et al. 2001). The MPI consists of a set of empirically-derived scales designed to assess the perceptions of: (1) pain severity; (2) interference with family and marital functioning, work, and social and recreational activities; (3) support received from significant others; (4) life control incorporating perceived ability to solve problems and feelings of personal mastery and competence; (5) affective distress; and (6) performance of activities.

Turk and Rudy (1988) identified three relatively homogenous groups and labelled one subgroup characterized by severe pain, compromised life activities and enjoyment, reduced sense of control, and high level of emotional distress as 'dysfunctional' (DYS). Another subgroup, also marked with relatively high degrees of pain and affective distress but further characterized by low levels of perceived support from significant others, was labelled 'interpersonally distressed' (ID). The third group consisted of chronic pain patients who appeared to be coping relatively well despite their long-standing pain. This group, which experienced low levels of pain, functional limitations, and emotional distress, was labelled 'adaptive copers' (AC). Reliable, external scales supported the uniqueness of each of the three subgroups of patients. The subgroups have been replicated in several studies conducted in Sweden (Bergström et al. 2001, Hellström and Jansson 2001), Finland (Talo et al. 2001), the Netherlands (Lousberg et al. 1997), and Germany (Flor et al. 1990) and using different measures of the constructs assessed by the MPI (e.g. Jamison et al. 1994).

## 26.7 **Subgrouping on the basis of the MPI**

To ascertain whether the three MPI subgroups differ only in the areas in which they are supposed (discriminant validity), a series of analyses were performed on physical functioning, pain severity, depressive mood, and perceived functional limitation (Turk and Rudy 1988). Interestingly, the

**Table 26.1** Distributions of the MPI profiles in various disorders

| Profiles | MPI FMS[1] | LB[2] | HA[2] | TMD[2] | Regional/local Cancer[3] | Metastatic Cancer[3] |
|---|---|---|---|---|---|---|
| | (91)* | (200) | (245) | (200) | (47) | (137) |
| DYS | 26% | 62% | 44% | 46% | 44% | 64% |
| ID | 39% | 18% | 26% | 22% | 18% | 5% |
| AC | 35% | 20% | 30% | 32% | 35% | 18% |

* numbers in parentheses = sample size
[1] Turk et al. (1996);
[2] Turk & Rudy (1990);
[3] Turk et al. (1998)

three subgroups did not differ in physical functioning (e.g. lumbar flexion, straight leg raise, and cervical range of motion). Similarly, Bergstrom et al. (2001) found that the subgroups did not differ on spinal and neck mobility, impaired reflexes, or Lasègue sign. These results reinforce the suggestion that psychosocial dimension of chronic pain syndromes may be independent of physical pathology. The independence of the psychologically based classification from medical diagnosis is particularly important, as it would be plausible to assume that patients with greater physical pathology have more to cope with and thus are more likely to be dysfunctional, whereas those who have less pathology would have less to cope with and therefore would more likely be adaptive copers. The abovementioned studies refute this possibility and support the notion that medical and psychosocial classifications are independent.

Using external measures of relevant constructs, Turk and Rudy (1988) found that: (1) the DYS patients reported significantly higher levels of pain than AC patients; (2) the DYS and ID groups reported significantly higher levels of depressed mood and perceived disability; and (3) the ID patients rated their interpersonal relationships with significant others to be significantly lower in quality compared with the DYS and AC patients. These data provide convergent validity for the three subgroups.

Comparing the taxonomic structure and profiles of distinct chronic pain groups can help to establish the generalizability of the MPI taxonomy. The three MPI subgroups have been replicated with a number of different pain populations. Turk and Rudy (1990b) directly compared the power and stability of the MPI taxonomy by studying samples of patients with chronic low back pain (CLBP), headache (HA), and temporomandibular disorders (TMD). The scale interrelationships for the three diagnostic groups were equivalent. All three syndrome groups were represented in each of the subgroups (see Table 26.1). Thus, it is possible that patients with CLBP, HA, and TMD who are classified within the same subgroup may be psychologically more similar to each other than patients with the same diagnosis but who are classified within different subgroups (see Table 26.1).

Similarly in another study, Turk et al. (1998) examined the covariance structures among the MPI scales (profile patterns) of three very different patient groups: chronic pain, FMS, and cancer patients. They discovered that the covariance structures were remarkably consistent among the three MPI profiles. Based on the results of these studies it appears that CP, FMS and cancer patients who are classified within the same MPI profile may be more similar to each other in subjective experience and response to symptoms than patients with the same diagnosis but who are classified to a different MPI profile (see Figure 26.2). These results suggest that although different physical diagnostic groups may require common biomechanical treatment targeting the pathophysiological mechanisms underlying each disorder, they may also benefit from specific psychosocial interventions tailored to their psychosocial-behavioural characteristics based on the MPI profiles.

Studies comparing the MPI subgroups have yielded evidence supporting differential response to the same intervention (e.g. Dahlstrom et al. 1997; Epker and Gatchel 2000; Rudy et al. 1995; Verra et al. 2009). For instance, when a rehabilitation pain management programme for FMS patients was tested, the DYS group improved in most areas, whereas the ID patients, who reported levels of pain and disability comparable to the DYS group, failed to respond to the treatment (Turk et al. 1998). There was little change in the AC patients, owing possibly to a floor effect. Strategier et al. (1997) reported similar results with a sample of patients with low back pain. Both these studies found that the AC group improvements were intermediate between the DYS and ID. The results further support the need for different treatments targeting characteristics of subgroups and suggest that psychosocial characteristics of patients with chronic pain are important predictors of treatment responses and may be used to customize treatment. For example, DYS

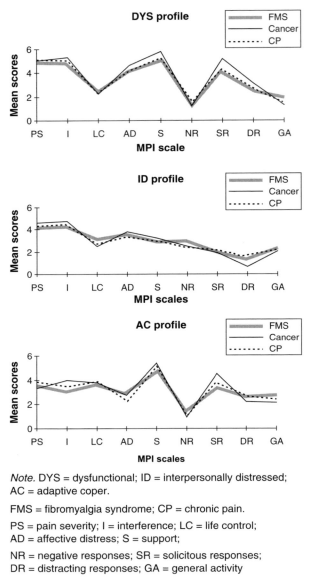

**Fig. 26.2** Mean MPI scale scores in three groups of patients with pain by MPI profile.

patients are characterized by high levels of emotional distress, feelings of little control, and high levels of inactivity and may warrant treatment with the focus on cognitive factors associated with their maladaptive beliefs (e.g. cognitive restructuring), whereas the ID patients may require additional treatment components addressing clinical needs specific to this group (e.g. interpersonal skills) and some components of the standard interdisciplinary treatment may not be essential for the AC patients.

Patient attrition is a major problem in pain rehabilitation programmes. It is possible that patients who receive a treatment that does not match with their specific needs (patterns of coping and adapting) would be more likely to terminate treatment. In one small-scale treatment study, Carmody (2001) observed that ID (47%) and DYS (33%) patients were significantly more likely to drop-out of group rehabilitation treatments than the AC group (11%). Data such as these reinforce the idea that treatments that are prescribed need to be congruent with patient characteristics. If patients are not satisfied with the treatment they are receiving and do not believe that the treatment components are addressing their particular concerns, especially when rehabilitation treatments can be very demanding, they will not be committed to the treatment. Clinicians will need to spend time developing tailored interventions to match patient needs and expectations. Moreover, they will need to expend extra effort motivating patients by educating them regarding the relevance of the components of the treatments being offered (see also Chapter 24).

The results described above implicate the importance of matching patients' characteristics to treatment. By specifically addressing patients' psychological needs, clinicians are likely to be able to enhance both the cost-effectiveness and the clinical effectiveness of interventions. Additionally, early identification of patients' modes of adapting to subacute pain may lead to the development of interventions that can prevent chronicity and long-term disability (Gatchel and Epker 1999; Johansson and Lindberg 2000).

Research by Vlaeyen et al. (1995) has emphasized the prominent role played by fear of injury and pain in patients with chronic pain. The presence of high levels of fear avoidance might serve as a target for treatment. The presence of other patient characteristics (e.g. endurance responses, catastrophizing, negative affectivity) might also serve as foci of treatment. The essential point is that they can target important patient differences. Psychosocial subgroups on the basis of pain-related fear and endurance will be reviewed in the following.

## 26.8 Subgrouping on the basis of pain-related fear and emotional distress

Although numerous studies underscore the importance of psychological factors in the development and perpetuation of pain problems, most do not explicitly propose any mechanisms of how these variables might interact. For example, a large range of cross-sectional, experimental, and prospective studies show that pain-related fear (e.g. catastrophizing, fear of movement) and more general emotional distress (e.g. depressed mood, anxiety) are related to pain and disability (Pincus et al. 2002; Leeuw et al. 2007). Yet, we have only just begun to understand how these and other important variables may interrelate within individuals as well as how these variables relate sequentially across time (Boersma and Linton 2006; Wideman et al. 2009). Understanding how risk factors interact within individuals is important because these variables might operate differently for different people, an assumption that is not being made within traditional correlational designs (Von Eye and Bergman 2003). For example, Clyde and Williams (2002) suggest in an overview of depression in chronic pain, that there is a need to take into account that there may be several pathways by which pain and depression co-occur, possibly resulting in different subtypes. They suggest that there is a need to take into account both vulnerability to depression, and the nature of the experience of pain as a stressor. In line with this, there could, for example, be a subgroup that has a general vulnerability for negative cognitive processing while, for another subgroup, depressive symptoms could be a mere consequence of the prolonged exposure to pain and of its interference with valued life goals. Related to this second possibility is the role that depressed mood has been assigned within the fear avoidance model (Vlaeyen et al. 1995). Here, depression is largely seen as a consequence of disability and subsequent lack of positive reinforcement, even though it is incorporated in the model that general vulnerability factors may influence and fuel pain catastrophizing. Even though the continuous development of theoretical models that propose interrelationships between risk factors is pivotal for furthering our understanding, there is also a need for empirical studies that focus on the interrelationships between, for example, depressive mood and pain-related fear within individuals and across time.

Studies that focus on discovering subpopulations could give important information of possible differential pathways by which pain, depression and pain-related fear co-occur in the process towards prolonged disability. In a line of studies investigating the interrelationship between pain-related fear variables and emotional distress, we consistently found that pain-related fear, and emotional distress can appear in isolation within individuals as well as they can appear in combination. Individuals with a combination of pain-related fear and emotional distress show by far the highest levels of disability, and these psychological patterns appear to be relatively stable over time (Boersma and Linton 2005, 2006a; Westman et al. 2011). For example, we used primary care patient's ratings of pain intensity, fear of movement, function, and depressed mood to distinguish possible patterns (Boersma and Linton 2005). We found four distinct profiles: a group of patients characterized by high pain, fear of movement and dysfunction, a group that was similar but in addition suffered from low mood, a group that was mostly characterized by low mood only, and a group that was characterized by relatively low scores on all variables. These four subgroups had clearly distinct outcomes at follow up with the subgroups characterized by fear of movement alone and fear of movement plus low mood developing the highest levels of sick leave. To replicate and extend the findings of this study, we performed another study where the aim was to identify possible distinctive patterns based only on psychological process variables (fear of movement, catastrophizing and depressed mood) and to test whether these patterns are in fact related to the development of disability (Boersma and Linton 2006a). In this study five meaningful subgroups were extracted that display differential profiles on measures of disability cross sectional as well as prospective.

These clusters, graphically displayed in Figure 26.3, largely replicated the results from the previous study (Boersma and Linton 2005) and give support to the fear avoidance model as there are strong relations between fear of movement and catastrophizing. However, as can be seen, the exact pattern in which these factors are organized varies between subgroups. Further, fear of movement and catastrophizing can be (cluster 2) but are not necessarily (cluster 1) accompanied by signs of depressed mood. Signs of depressed mood on the other hand, do not have to be accompanied by fear of movement and catastrophizing (cluster 4). In summary, in both these studies profiles emerged that were characterized by pain-related fear with- and without depressed mood, by low pain-related fear and no depressed mood ('low risk') and by depressed mood alone.

A recent study replicated and extended these findings by following a sample of 110 primary care patients with spinal pain over a period of 3 years (Westman et al. submitted). Three separate subgrouping analyses were performed at baseline, 1-year follow-up and 3-year follow-up. The results replicated the existence of subgroups characterized by emotional distress only, pain-related fear only, and emotional distress in combination with pain-related fear. Moreover, the results showed that these risk profiles displayed significant stability across the 3-year period, and showed increasingly distinct patterns of disability. In fact, individuals with an initial profile of pain-related fear and distress were three times more likely to remain fearful and distressed across the 3-year time period. Furthermore, the results showed that individuals displaying one of the three risk profiles at baseline had significantly worse recovery on all outcome variables (pain, function and sick leave) at 1 year, as well as 3-year follow-up, compared to individuals not displaying one of these risk profiles.

The results of these studies are in line with previous research that focuses on classifying pain patients in homogeneous subgroups based on their adjustment to pain, such as the studies using the MPI (Kerns et al. 1985; Turk and Rudy 1988; Bergström et al. 2001). As mentioned above,

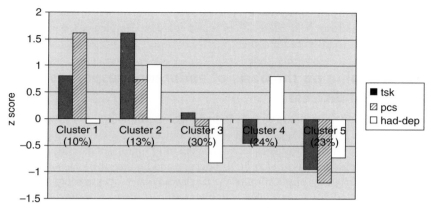

**Fig. 26.3** Subgroups based on fear of movement (TSK), catastrophizing (PCS), and depression (HADS-depression scale).

these studies report on three different subgroups: DYS, ID, and AC. When comparing the level of disability, the DYS group and the AC group from the MPI show some similarities with respectively the pain-related fear with and without depression and the 'low score profile' groups. The studies that have investigated pain-related fear within the three MPI subgroups support this idea; in these studies the DYS group had significantly more pain-related fear than the AC group (Asmundson et al. 1997; McCracken et al. 1999). Thus it appears that results from these studies converge on one another, and that where classifications derived from the MPI are made on the basis of maladjustment on a broad range of variables (pain-related, functional as well as psychosocial) the studies discussed above employ a more narrow theoretical framework with a sole psychological focus.

In summary, these studies elucidate the variations in the variable relationships between subgroups. These variations may have considerable implications for intervention, as the unfavourable outcome in relation to function and sick-leave for the risk profile groups suggests that the received healthcare is not helping. It is possible that the important underlying psychological processes are not dealt with in a sufficient way. An approach that would include a focus on pain-related fear on the one hand and more general emotional distress on the other hand could greatly improve patient functioning and enhance the secondary prevention of chronic disability including sick leave. Specific as well as more general cognitive-behavioural interventions have proven to be of use in rehabilitation as well as in preventive intervention (Linton and Andersson 2000; Sullivan and Stanish 2003; van den Hout et al. 2003; Woods and Asmundson 2008). However, since CBT is a collection of a wide range of techniques, knowledge on the existence of subgroups may further inform which components within CBT are most effective for whom. For example, it is possible that individuals characterized by mood disturbances that is not merely a consequence of pain-related fear, may not be helped by an intervention merely focused on, for example, *in vivo* exposure to feared and avoided movements. Indeed, even though exposure based treatments have shown effect for individuals with high levels of fear of movement, they also show that some patients respond better to exposure than others (Leeuw et al. 2008; Linton et al. 2008; Woods and Asmundson, 2008).

In a recent study, we analysed the individual differences between those with successful and non-successful outcome of an exposure based intervention for high pain-related fear (Flink et al. 2010). The results showed that individuals with a non-successful outcome where characterized by high levels of catastrophizing. Possibly, the exposure treatment was hindered by, or merely did not sufficiently address, pain related distress and could be complemented with other mood regulation techniques to improve outcome.

## 26.9 Subgrouping on the basis of endurance-responses and emotional distress

A number of prospective studies have shown that ongoing pain and disability are mediated by psychosocial factors (Linton 2000; Shaw et al. 2001; Pincus et al. 2002). As mentioned above, depression and fear-avoidance variables seem to be the most important psychosocial risk factors of chronic pain and disability (Fritz et al. 2001; Boersma and Linton 2006). However, researchers have noted limitations in the application of the fear-avoidance model to subgroups of patients where pain-related disability is associated with high task performance or overuse (Vlaeyen and Morley 2004). In particular, there is evidence for the role of endurance-related responses as predictors of chronic pain in patients (Hasenbring 1993; Hasenbring et al. 1994; Grebner et al. 1999). The avoidance-endurance model (AEM; described in more detail in Chapter 15) provides testable hypotheses about subgroups of patients with endurance-related responses and will therefore be briefly summarized in the following. The avoidance-endurance model of pain postulates opposite pathways into chronic pain: one via pain-related fear-avoidance responses (FAR), and at least another one other via endurance-related responses (ER). FAR including misinterpreting pain as a sign of serious injury, increasing fear, hypervigilance and avoidance behaviour may lead to physical deconditioning and disability (Smeets et al. 2007). ER behaviour despite severe pain is suggested to lead to chronic pain by physical overload of physical structures (Hasenbring et al. 2006; Hasenbring et al. 2009). Thought suppression (TS) represents a cognitive ER where patients suppress the perception of pain or the interruption of daily activities normally demanded by pain (e.g. Eccleston and Crombez 1999). A rebound effect was suggested which leads to more frequently occurring pain-related thoughts accompanied by the perception of failure and increased depression.

In order to identify pain patients at risk for developing chronic pain and disability at an early stage and to develop individually targeted treatments, it is important to identify specific subgroups of patients with homogenous and highly rigid responses pattern to pain. In a first study in chronic back pain patients, we investigated whether ER play a significant role in the phenomenology of the MPI subgroups (Rusu and Hasenbring 2008). Although it is assumed that the DYS group is associated with dysfunctional coping (Turk and Rudy 1988), only a few studies have investigated the relationship between DYS group and FAR. These studies have consistently shown that the DYS group reported significantly more catastrophizing, pain-related anxiety, avoidance, less control, and positive future thinking (Geisser et al. 1994; Asmundson et al. 1997; Hellström et al. 2000). However, little is known about the interrelation of the DYS group, ER and pain communication. It can be suggested that identification of maladaptive pain-related coping strategies strongly associated with MPI subgroups is important for their modification in treatment. Investigating the interrelationships between the MPI subgroups with regard to pain-related FAR, ER and pain communication, we found that, even after control for pain intensity and depression, patients classified as DYS reported more anxiety/depression, help-/hopelessness, and catastrophizing than did those classified as AC (Rusu and Hasenbring 2008). Furthermore, the DYS group showed more thought suppression compared to AC; however, subgroups did not differ significantly with regard to avoidance of social and physical activity, and endurance behaviour. In line with our expectations, DYS as well as ID patients showed more non-verbal pain behaviour compared to AC, which refers to the special role of operant conditioning.

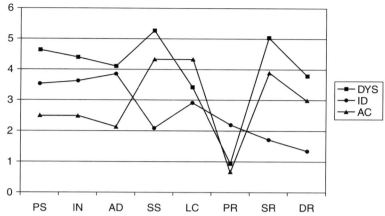

**Fig. 26.4** MPI-D scale scores for the DYS, ID, and AC profile (Rusu and Hasenbring, 2008). PS = Pain severity; IN = Interference; AD = Affective distress; SS = Social support; LC = Life control; PR = Punishing responses; SR = Solicitous responses; and DR = Distracting responses. This figure has been reproduced with permission of the International Association for the Study of Pain® (IASP®). The figure may not be reproduced for any other purpose without permission.

The results provided further verification of the ability of the MPI classification system (Turk and Rudy 1988; Rudy 2004) to successfully identify subgroups of patients. Only 11.6% of patients were not classified into primary subgroups. However, the distribution of profiles differed from previous studies. That is, studies of chronic pain patients consistently showed that the DYS profile described the largest proportion of patients (mean across study samples = 39%), the AC profile described approximately 38% of patients, and the ID profile described the smallest proportion of patients (24%). However, we found that the AC profile classified 61.7% and the DYS profile only 15.8% of patients in our sample. These differences may be related to varying study designs and methods, for instance, we collected data from general practices with a number of pre-determined selection criteria. Conversely, the majority of previous studies, in which DYS patients represented the largest group, took place in secondary care settings (Jamison et al. 1994; McCracken et al. 1999).

As indicated in Figure 26.4, DYS patients reported higher levels of pain severity and pain-related interference than the other two subgroups. In comparison to AC patients, DYS patients had higher levels of affective distress and perceived less ability to control their lives. The ID patients were distinguishable from the other two patient profiles by their marked differences on the social support scale and significant other response scales. These patients perceived their family members not to be very supportive of them and their pain problem.

A more focused examination revealed that the MPI subgroups were associated with distinct pattern of FAR and ER. The DYS group displayed more affective distress as well as more maladaptive pain-related cognitions; however, we found no differences in avoidance of physical and avoidance of social activities, in our sample. Again, this might be related to varying measures. For instance, the Kiel Pain Inventory (KPI; Hasenbring 1994) avoidance scales consider more general every-day behaviours related to avoidance behaviour, whereas measures like the Pain Anxiety Symptoms Scale (PASS; McCracken et al. 1992) or the Tampa Scale of Kinesiophobia (TSK; Vlaeyen et al. 1995; Clark et al. 1996) assess more specific escape/avoidance behaviours. Consequently, patients in our sample may have endorsed the KPI avoidance scales more, irrespective of the subgroup characteristics, due to the larger behavioural units considered by the KPI. As mentioned above, DYS patients exhibited more thought suppression, which is in line with recent experimental studies showing that thought suppression produced shorter tolerance time, more pain, and distress in a cold pressor test compared to acceptance based thoughts (Masedo and Esteve 2007). The results suggest that the application of techniques specifically geared toward the reduction of automatic and frequent thought suppression may be an important component in the treatment of DYS patients. Evidence from a randomized controlled intervention study for patients with acute sciatic pain has shown that a risk factor-based cognitive-behavioural intervention (RCBT; more information can be found in Chapter 27), which was aimed to specifically target dysfunctional endurance responses, was more effective compared to a standardized treatment (Hasenbring et al 1999). Alternatively, it might be useful to apply acceptance-based approaches to the treatment of the DYS group to reduce thought suppression. Both approaches might help patients to realize that their natural response to escape or avoid by suppressing the pain experience cognitively has been ineffective and may increase the urge for strategies of pain control, which undermines the understanding that pain reduction in the long-term is in most cases not achievable (Hasenbring et al. 1999; McCracken et al. 1999; Nicholas et al. 2003). Acceptance and RCBT might lead patients from pain reduction attempts (thought suppression as one of them) to acceptance of pain for the foreseeable future and satisfying lives despite the pain (McCracken et al. 1999; McCracken, 2005). Future research will be necessary to evaluate the additional contribution of these specific treatment possibilities to standardized protocols.

Contrary to our expectations, the MPI group differences in endurance behaviour were found to be insignificant. The AEM delineates the role of endurance responses, and particularly endurance behaviour plays in the transition from acute to chronic pain. We know from prospective studies of patients with acute sciatic pain that endurance behaviour and positive mood in spite of severe pain are important risk factors for the development of chronic pain (Hasenbring et al. 1994). However, the generalizability of these results in acute and subacute patients to populations of chronic pain patients is potentially questionable due to different conditions (acute and subacute versus persistent pain and primary care versus secondary care) applied. Seeing that the AC group displayed significantly higher scores on positive mood compared to both other subgroups could lead to the assumption that endurance behaviour in conjunction with positive mood may be helpful for adjustment to chronic pain. New treatment and assessment approaches emphasize the positive association between positive mood, acceptance, and adjustment (McCracken and Eccleston 2003; Pincus et al. 2004). However, further replication studies are needed to investigate the contribution of thought suppression and endurance behaviour within the MPI subgroups and to test the usefulness of the avoidance-endurance model in chronic pain populations.

In our previous studies we reported evidence for the prospective validity of AEM-based subgroups for back pain, assessed by a short screening instrument including depression, thought suppression and behavioural endurance (Risk Screening for Back Pain, RISC-BP; Hasenbring 1993; Grebner et al. 1999; Hallner and Hasenbring 2004). Besides a FAR subgroup, which showed high fear and avoidance, patients of the ER subgroup responded with thought suppression, depression and endurance behaviour (distress-endurance pattern DER), while a second ER subgroup showed endurance behaviour, minimization and positive mood in spite of pain (eustress-endurance pattern EER). A fourth subgroup was found (adaptive responses to pain AR) which was low on depression, thought suppression and behavioural endurance.

Hasenbring (1993) investigated in a prospective study these four subgroups and found that the DER as well as the EER subgroup reported higher pain intensity at the 6-month follow-up, less return to work and a higher rate of application for early retirement compared to the adaptive group. Consistent results were also reported by Grebner and colleagues (1999) in 82 patients undergoing lumbar disc surgery, showing that EER and FAR subgroups had a higher rate of early retirement at the 6-month follow-up compared to the adaptive group, and against their expectations also compared to the DER group.

In a recent study replicating and extending these findings, 162 primary care patients with subacute non-specific back pain were investigated at the start of medical treatment and at a 6-months follow-up (Hasenbring et al. submitted). Back pain patients were classified into the four AEM-based subgroups using RISC-BP and pre-defined cut-off points. Results revealed that both ER subgroups showed higher pain intensity at the 6-month follow-up compared to the adaptive subgroup. In contrast, subgroup analyses revealed that the adaptive group showed prospectively less pain chronicity compared to all other groups and less disability compared to FAR and DER subgroups. Preliminary support for the hypothesis that ER patients reveal a higher level of physical activity and a higher rate of static strain postures indicated by physical overload was found in a cross-sectional study measuring overt physical activity using accelerometry in patients 6 months after lumber disc surgery (Hasenbring et al. 2006). Additionally, Chapter 15 gives a comprehensive overview of further studies investigating AEM-based subgroups using different methodological approaches.

The purpose of another recent study in chronic back pain patients was to further test the content validity of the AEM subgroups and to elucidate the variations in the relationships between AEM-based subgroups and MPI scales; fear-avoidance and endurance responses (Rusu et al. submitted). Looking back at the MPI scales, the results revealed that the adaptive group scored lowest on the MPI scales *pain severity*, *interference*, and *affective distress*, while the FAR group showed by far the highest scores on these scales. DER patients reported significantly more pain intensity and disability (as assessed by the Graded Chronic Pain Scale; Von Korff et al. 1992) compared to the EER group and the adaptive group. When an independent measure of depression was used to assess depressive symptomatology (Beck Depression Inventory; Beck et al. 1961), as expected both subgroups with a depressive component, DER and FAR patients had significantly higher depression scores compared to the EER group, and DER patients scored significantly higher compared to the adaptive group. Multivariate analyses of variance further indicated that groups differed significantly for pain-related fear-avoidance and endurance responses, even after control of pain intensity and depression.

With regard to fear-avoidance responses, FAR and DER patients revealed significantly higher scores on the majority of fear-avoidance associated scales (e.g. helplessness, hopelessness, catastrophizing, and avoiding of social and physical activity) compared to the other two subgroups. EER patients differed significantly with regard to endurance variables (positive mood, thought suppression, minimizing thoughts, and behavioural endurance) compared to FAR patients even after control for depression and pain intensity. DER patients differed as well from FAR patients with regard to more thought suppression, minimization and behavioural endurance.

In summary, the studies reviewed in this section have advanced one way of assessing psychological subgroups based on the AEM and it clearly requires replication. In conclusion, the results of the studies reported indicate that AEM-based subgroups are useful for the identification of fear-avoidance as well as endurance-related responses to pain, underline the notion that the differentiation between the two endurance-related subgroups is pivotal and that new therapeutic strategies are strongly needed for patients with endurance-related coping, especially for those with an EER pattern. Future prospective studies should investigate the AEM subgroups in the prediction of long-term adjustment to pain using different outcomes, which are independent from the KPI and may better elucidate the conditions under which endurance-related responses may become adaptive or maladaptive. Finding further evidence for differences in psychosocial subgroups, whether classified by the MPI or other clinically relevant psychological measures, may improve treatment evaluation as well as the process of patient-therapy matching.

## 26. 10 Future directions and conclusion

We have attempted to provide an overview of areas that contribute to our understanding of the person with chronic pain and psychological variables that have implications for improvements in treatment. We noted that clinical outcomes tend to support addressing cognitive, affective, and behavioural contributors to the experience of and response to chronic pain. We now consider future directions beyond what we have already suggested.

### 26.10.1 Dual-diagnostic approach

Several authors have proposed the use of a dual-diagnostic approach, whereby two diagnoses are assigned concurrently, a biomedical and a psychosocial diagnosis (e.g. Turk 1990; Dworkin and LeResche 1992; Scharff et al. 1995). Treatment could then be directed toward both simultaneously. A patient diagnosed with LBP who was also classified on the MPI as DYS might require a different set of treatments than a patient with back pain who was classified on the MPI as being ID. Both patients with back pain would benefit from physical therapy, but the former might require attention to their perceptions of low self-efficacy and control as well as beliefs about being disabled, whereas the latter might benefit from interpersonal problem solving (Jensen et al. 1994; Jensen et al. 2001). On the other hand, two patients diagnosed with different medical syndromes, for example, FMS and TMD both of whom were classified as ID, might have very different physical treatments but might benefit from a similar psychological intervention (e.g. interpersonal problem solving, assertion training, and social support). Adopting a dual-diagnostic approach would serve the valuable function of encouraging clinicians as well as researchers to think concurrently in terms of these two different biomedical and psychosocial-behavioural but complementary diagnostic systems. Empirical studies would be needed to evaluate the efficacy of individualized treatments based on the dual-diagnostic approach.

### 26.10.2 Customizing treatments to patients' needs

Multiple studies, using a broad range of assessment instruments, have identified subgroups of patients with chronic pain. To date, there have been none that have customized treatment to the psychosocial and behavioural characteristics of patients with pain and particularly none of back pain patients. The studies that have been conducted have used retrospective methods rather than looking prospectively at differential response to the same treatment (e.g. Moore et al. 1986). A handful of studies, described above, support the potential value of treatment matching, although the results are not uniformly consistent. There is a critical need to make use of these results in designing treatments and evaluating their differential efficacy. Clinical investigations should be conducted to determine the relative utility of different treatment modalities based on the match of treatment to patient characteristics and classification to predict which patients are most likely to benefit from what combination of therapeutic modalities. The field might be advanced by asking a set of questions, namely, 'What treatment, by whom, is most effective for this individual, with that specific problem, under which set of circumstances?' (Paul 1967).

Treatments might be provided in a modular fashion, where there are separate components that are woven together into an overall treatment regimen based on individual patient characteristics.

All patients with back pain may require physical therapy and psychological support and encouragement; however, as indicated by the results reported above, some may need additional modules such as treatment of depression (Ingram et al. 1990) or the treatment of rigid endurance behaviour (Hasenbring et al. 1999). The combination of physical treatments, pharmacological treatments, and specific psychological interventions may provide unique and complementary advantages in addressing different symptoms.

It is important to acknowledge that the identification of subgroups, regardless of the methods used, does not mean that the resulting classification will incorporate all features of patients. Subgroups should be viewed as prototypes with significant room for individual variability. Thus, treatments matched to subgroup characteristics will also need to consider and address unique characteristics of the individual patient. It is noteworthy to mention that the transparent items contained in the MPI may facilitate denial of problems by patients classified as AC. Patients in the subgroups should be examined more carefully before assuming that they are truly adapting in a specific manner (e.g. Rusu and Hasenbring 2008). The MPI might be viewed as a screening instrument, and based on patient subgroup, the clinician would follow-up with additional assessment measures and procedures. The subgroup customization fits somewhere between the exclusively idiographic approach evaluated by single case treatment designs and the generic 'pain patient homogeneity' approach that has characterized much of the pain treatment outcome studies.

### 26.10.3 The transition from acute to chronic pain: secondary prevention

The vast majority of people who are injured recover in a reasonable amount of time and do not develop chronic disorders. Similarly, a significant number of people who develop chronic disorders associated with pain do not become physically and emotionally disabled. As noted previously, a number of efforts have been made to identify the predictors of disability among these groups (e.g. Hasenbring et al. 1994; Linton and Hallden 1997; Gatchel and Epker 1999; Johansson and Lindberg 2000 Riipinen et al. 2005; Jellema et al. 2007). There are, however, few longitudinal studies, and replications are the exception rather than the rule (Turner et al. 2000).

As noted earlier, a number of studies have begun to identify predictors of disability for injured workers with acute pain states and also predictors of response to treatment. Solely, identifying predictors is insufficient. The next step is to determine whether knowledge of predictors can guide treatment design and the development of strategies for improving outcome. Prevention and earlier interventions hold promise for reduction in the extent of disability (for more information see Chapters 11 and 30). The average person treated at a multidisciplinary pain centre has had symptoms of pain for an average of 7 years (Flor et al. 1992). By this time, patients have become so disabled that rehabilitation becomes a very difficult task, the outcomes, although reasonably good, could have been improved if implemented at an earlier stage. Linton and Bradley (1996) have reviewed a number of studies that may be viewed as secondary prevention, namely, treatments used with those who have already had a first pain episode and designed to prevent long-term disability. Given the natural history of many musculoskeletal pain disorders, it is important that early interventions are reasonably inexpensive. Providing expensive interventions for groups with high rates of natural recovery is inefficient and costly (Von Korff 1999). Efforts to prevent, or at least minimize, the consequences of exacerbations and relapse may be particularly cost-effective. The effects of early interventions are currently mixed (Jellema et al. 2005; Van der Windt et al. 2008), but the costs of chronicity are so extreme that research in this area is definitely warranted.

## 26.10.4 Overgeneralization based on pain clinic samples

Minimal attention has been given to those people who recover spontaneously or who make adequate and often exceptional accommodations to their conditions regardless of physical impairments and limitations. Much of what is known about chronic pain syndromes is based on people who seek treatment. These individuals are not a representative group, therefore it is likely that people will seek treatment when they have an exacerbation of their symptoms (e.g. Bradley et al. 1994). As a result, almost any treatment will appear reasonably successful. It is essential that research extends beyond the clinical population to community samples that are not seeking care.

## 26.10.5 Chronic pain should be treated like other chronic diseases

Even when successful, pain rehabilitation does not cure pain but emphasizes self-control and self-management of symptoms. Examination of the results of long-term opioid therapy reveals significant residual pain; similarly, the majority of people who have surgery or have spinal cord stimulators or drug delivery systems implanted continue to report substantial pain (Turk and Okifuji 1998). Because these pain sufferers are not cured, they require regular care and follow-up. We have tended to view chronic pain more as an acute condition that will resolve following treatment, but this is patently not the case. If we view chronic pain as a lifelong disease, then, as with other chronic diseases such as diabetes, we should expect treatment to be ongoing, requiring regular check-up and continuing care. From this perspective, treatment is not over after a few sessions or a 3–4 weeks rehabilitation programme. Instead, we should expect and plan for the need to include booster sessions (Lanes et al. 1995; Bendix et al. 1998). We need to give attention to the development and evaluation of treatments of pain as a chronic disease that is not cured but requires maintenance-enhancement strategies.

In conclusion, we noted the importance of considering a range of factors that contribute to individual differences, and posed a diathesis–stress–environment heuristic model. We focused on psychosocial factors to illustrate the importance of understanding meaningful groups of patients. Similar analyses focusing on genetics, pathophysiology, and environmental variables are also relevant and a need to be considered when developing a treatment plan. At this point, whether treatment tailoring will produce greater effects than providing completely idiographic or generic treatments can only be viewed as a reasonable hypothesis. The fact that a significant proportion of patients with chronic pain are not successfully treated by current general approaches and the identification of various subgroups of patients makes investigation of treatment matching of particular importance.

## References

Aaron, L.A., Bradley, L.A., Alarcon, G.S. *et al.* (1997). Perceived physical and emotional trauma as precipitating events in fibromyalgia. Associations with health care seeking and disability status but not pain severity. *Arthritis and Rheumatism,* **40**, 453–60.

Anand K.S., Coskun V., Thrivikraman K.V., Nemeroff C.B., Plotsky P.M. (1999). Long-term behavioral effects of repetitive pain inneonatal rat pups. *Physiology and Behavior,* **66**, 627–37.

Asmundson, G.J., Norton, G.R. and Allerdings, M.D. (1997). Fear and avoidance in dysfunctional chronic back pain patients. *Pain,* **69**, 231–6.

Beck, A.T., Ward, C.H., Mendelson, M., Mock, J. and Erbaugh, J. (1961). An inventory for measuring depression. *Archives of General Psychiatry,* **4**, 561–71.

Becker, N., Hojsted, J., Sjogren, P. and Eriksen J. (1998). Sociodemographic predictors of treatment outcome in chronic non-malignant pain patients. Do patients receiving or applying for disability pension benefit from multidisciplinary pain treatment? *Pain, 77*, 279–87.

Becker, N., Sjogren, P., Bech, P. *et al.* (2000). Treatment outcome of chronic non-malignant pain patients managed in a Danish multidisciplinary pain center compared to general practice: A randomised controlled trial. *Pain, 84*, 203–11.

Bendix, A.F., Bendix, T., Haestrup, C. and Busch, E. (1998). A prospective, randomized 5-year follow-up study of functional restoration in chronic low back pain patients. *European Spine Journal, 7*, 111–19.

Bergström, G., Bodin, L., Jensen, I.B., Linton, S.J. and Nygren, A. L. (2001). Long-term, non-specific spinal pain: reliable and valid subgroups of patients. *Behaviour Research and Therapy, 39*, 75–87.

Bradley, L.A., Alarcon, F.S., Triana, M. *et al.* (1994). Health care seeking behavior in fibromyalgia: Association with pain thresholds, symptom severity, and psychiatric morbidity. *Journal of Musculoskeletal Pain, 2*, 79–87.

Boersma, K. and Linton, S.J. (2005). Screening to identify patients at risk: profiles of psychological risk factors for early intervention. *Clinical Journal of Pain, 21*, 38–43.

Boersma, K. and Linton, S.J. (2006a). Psychological processes underlying the development of a chronic pain problem: a prospective study of the relationship between profiles of psychological variables in the fear-avoidance model and disability. *Clinical Journal of Pain, 22*, 160–6.

Boersma, K. and Linton, S.J. (2006b). Expectancy, fear and pain in the prediction of chronic pain and disability: A prospective analysis. *European Journal of Pain, 10*, 551–7.

Burns, J.W., Glenn, B., Bruehl S, Harden, R.N. and Lofland, K. (2003). Cognitive factors influence outcome following multidisciplinary chronic pain treatment: a replication and extension of a cross-lagged panel analysis. *Behaviour Research and Therapy, 41*, 1163–82.

Carmody, T.P. (2001). Psychosocial subgroups, coping, and chronic low-back pain. *Journal of Clinical Psychology in Medical Settings, 8*, 137–48.

Chou, W.Y., Wang, C.H., Liu, P.H., Liu, C.C., Tseng, C.C. and Jawan, B. (2006). Humanopioid receptor A118G polymorphism affects intravenous patient-controlled analgesia consumption after abdominal hysterectomy. *Anesthesiology, 5*, 334–37.

Cipher, D.J., Fernandez, E. and Clifford, P.A. (2001). Cost-effectiveness and health care utilization in a multidisciplinary pain center: Comparison of three treatment groups. *Journal of Clinical Psychology in Medical Settings, 8*, 237–44.

Clark, M.E., Kori, S.H. and Brockel, J. (1996). Kinesiophobia and chronic pain: psychometric characteristics and factor analysis of the Tampa Scale. *American Pain Society Abstracts, 77*.

Clauw, D. (2010). Fibromyalgia. In Ballantyne JC, Rathmell JP and Fishman SM. (Eds). *Bonica's Management of Pain, 4th ed.* Philadelphia, PA: Lippincott Williams & Wilkins.

Clyde, Z. and Williams, A. (2002). Depression and mood. In S. J. Linton (Ed.) *New avenues for the prevention of chronic musculoskeletal pain and disability* (Vol. 12, pp. 105–21). Amsterdam: Elsevier.

Dahlstrom, L., Widmark, G. and Carlsson, S. G. (1997). Cognitive-behavioral profiles among different categories of orofacial pain patients: diagnostic and treatment implications. *European Journal of Oral Science, 105*, 377–83.

Dworkin, S.F. and LeResche, L. (1992). Research diagnostic criteria for temporomandibular disorders: review, criteria, examination and specifications, critique. *Journal of Craniomandibular Disorders, 6*, 301–55.

Eccleston, C. and Crombez, G. (1999). Pain demands attention: a cognitive-affective model of the interruptive function of pain. *Psychological Bulletin, 125*, 356–66.

Edwards, R.R. (2005). Individual differences in endogenous pain modulation as a risk factor for chronic pain. *Neurology, 65*, 437–43.

Edwards, R.R., Fillingim, R.B. and Ness, T.J. (2003). Age-related differences in endogenous pain modulation: a comparision of diffuse noxious inhibitory controls in healthy older and younger adults. *Pain*, **101**, 155–65.

Edwards, R.R., Ness, T.J., Weigent, D.A. *et al.* (2003). Individual differences in diffuse noxious inhibitory controls (DNIC): association with clinical variables. *Pain*, **106**, 427–37.

Epker, J. and Gatchel, R.J. (2000). Coping profile differences in the biopsychosocial functioning of patients with temporomandibular disorders. *Psychosomatic Medicine*, **62**, 69–75.

Fillingim, R.B., Wilkinson, C.S. and Powell T. (1999). Self-reported abuse history and pain complaints among young adults. *Clinical Journal of Pain*, **15**, 85–91.

Flink, I., Boersma, K. and Linton, S. J. (2010). Catastrophizing moderates the effect of exposure in vivo for back pain patients with pain-related fear. *European Journal of Pain* **14**(8), 887–92.

Flor, H., Rudy, T.E. and Birbaumer, N. (1990). Zur Anwendbarkeit des West Haven-Yale Multidimensional Pain Inventory im deutschen Sprachraum. *Schmerz*, **4**, 82–87.

Flor, H., Fydrich, T. and Turk, D.C. (1992). Efficacy of multidisciplinary pain treatment centers: A meta-analytic review. *Pain*, **49**, 221–30.

Flor, H. and Turk DC. (1988). Chronic back pain and rheumatoid arthritis: predicting pain and disability from cognitive variables. *Journal of Behavioral Medicine*, **11**, 251–65.

Fordyce W. E. (1976). *Behavioral Methods for Chronic Pain and Illness*. St. Louis, MO: Mosby.

Fritz, J.M., George, S.Z. and Delitto, A. (2001). The role of fear-avoidance beliefs in acute low back pain: relationships with current and future disability and work status. *Pain*, **94**, 7–15.

Gatchel, R.J. and Epker, J. (1999). Psychosocial predictors of chronic pain and response to treatment. In R.J. Gatchel and D.C. Turk (Eds.) *Psychosocial factors in pain: Critical perspectives*, pp. 412–34. New York: Guilford Press.

Gatchel, R.J. and Turk, D.C., Eds. (1999). *Psychosocial Factors in Pain: Critical Perspectives*. New York: Guilford Press.

Geisser, M.E., Robinson, M.E. and Henson, C.D. (1994). The Coping Strategies Questionnaire and chronic pain adjustment: a conceptual and empirical reanalysis. *Clinical Journal of Pain*, **10**, 98–106.

Goodin, B.R., McGuire L., Allshouse M. *et al.* (2009). Associations between catastrophizing and endogenous pain-inhibitory processes: sex differences. *Journal of Pain*, **10**, 180–90.

Gracely, R.H., Geisser, M.E., Giesecke, T. *et al.* (2004). Pain catastrophizing and neural responses to pain among persons with fibromyalgia. *Brain*, **127**, 835–43.

Granot, M., Weissman-Fogel, I., Crispel, Y. *et al.* (2008). Determinants of endogenous analgesia magnitude in a diffuse noxious inhibitory control (DNIC) paradigm: do conditioning stimulus painfulness, gender and personality variables matter? *Pain*, **136**, 142–9.

Grebner, M., Breme, K., Rothoerl, R., Woertgen, C., Hartmann, A and Thomé, C. (1999). Coping and convalescence course after lumbar disk operations. Der *Schmerz*, **13**, 19–30.

Hallner, D. and Hasenbring, M. (2004). Classification of psychosocial risk factors (yellow flags) for the development of chronic low back and leg pain using artificial neural network. *Neuroscience Letters*, **361**, 151–4.

Hasenbring, M. (1993). Endurance strategies–a neglected phenomenon in the research and therapy of chronic pain? Der *Schmerz*, **7**, 304–13.

Hasenbring, M. (1994). *The Kiel Pain Inventory–Manual. Three questionnaire scales for assessment of pain-related cognitions, emotions and coping strategies*. Bern: Huber.

Hasenbring, M.I., Hallner, D. and Rusu, A.C. (2009). Fear-avoidance- and endurance-related responses to pain: development and validation of the Avoidance-Endurance Questionnaire (AEQ). *European Journal of Pain*, **13**, 620–8.

Hasenbring, M., Marienfeld, G., Kuhlendahl, D. and Soyka, D. (1994). Risk factors of chronicity in lumbar disc patients. A prospective investigation of biologic, psychologic, and social predictors of therapy outcome. *Spine*, **19**, 2759–65.

Hasenbring, M., Ulrich, H. W., Hartmann, M. and Soyka, D. (1999). The efficacy of a risk factor-based cognitive behavioral intervention and electromyographic biofeedback in patients with acute sciatic pain. An attempt to prevent chronicity. *Spine, 24,* 2525–35.

Hasenbring, M. I., Plaas, H., Fischbein, B. and Willburger, R. (2006). The relationship between activity and pain in patients 6 months after lumbar disc surgery: do pain-related coping modes act as moderator variables? *European Journal of Pain, 10,* 701–9.

Hasenbring, M. I., Hallner, D., Klasen, B., Streitlein-Böhme, I., Willburger, R. and Rusche, H. (submitted). Pain-related fear-avoidance and endurance responses versus response pattern in the prediction of future pain and disability: validation of the Risc Screening for Back Pain (RISC-BP).

Hellström, C. and Jansson, B. (2001). Psychological distress and adaptation to chronic pain: symptomatology in dysfunctional, interpersonally distressed and adaptive copers. *Journal of Musculoskeletal Pain, 9,* 51–67.

Hellström, C., Jansson, B. and Carlsson, S.G. (2000). Perceived future in chronic pain: the relationship between outlook on future and empirically derived psychological patient profiles. *European Journal of Pain, 4,* 283–90.

Hutten, M.M.R., Hermens, H.J. and Zilvold, G. (2001). Differences in treatment outcome between subgroups of patients with chronic low back pain using lumbar dynamometry and psychological aspects. *Clinical Rehabilitation, 15,* 479–88.

Ingram, R.E., Atkinson, J.H., Slater, M.A., Saccuzzo, D.P. and Garfin, S.R. (1990). Negative and positive cognition in depressed and non-depressed chronic pain patients. *Health Psychology, 9,* 300–14.

Jamison, R.N., Rudy, T.E., Penzien, D.B. and Mosley, T.H., Jr. (1994). Cognitive-behavioral classifications of chronic pain: Replication and extension of empirically derived patient profiles. *Pain, 57,* 277–92.

Jellema, P., van der Windt, D.A.W.M., van der Horst, H.E., Blankenstein, A., Bouter, L.M. and Stalman, W.A.B. (2005). Why is a treatment aimed at psychosocial factors not effective in patients with (sub)acute low back pain? *Pain, 118,* 350–59.

Jellema, P. van der Windt, D.A.W.M., van der Horst, H.E., Stalman, W.A.B., and Bouter, L.M. (2007). Prediction of an unfavourable course of low back pain in general practice: Comparison of four instruments. *British Journal of General Practice, 57,* 15–22.

Jensen, M.P., Turner, J.A. and Romano, J.M. (1994). Correlates of improvements in multidisciplinary treatment of chronic pain. *Journal of Consulting and Clinical Psychology, 62,* 172–79.

Jensen, M.P., Turner, J.A. and Romano, J.M. (2001). Changes in beliefs, catastrophizing, and coping are associated with improvements in multidisciplinary pain treatment. *Journal of Consulting and Clinical Psychology, 69,* 655–62.

Johansson, E. and Lindberg, P. (2000). Low back pain patients in primary care: Subgroups based on the Multidimensional Pain Inventory. *International Journal of Behavioral Medicine, 7,* 340–52.

Keefe, F.J., Bradley, L.A. and Crisson, J.E. (1990). Behavioral assessment of low back pain: identification of pain behavior subgroups. *Pain, 40,* 153–60.

Kerns, R.D., Turk, D.C. and Rudy, T.E. (1985). The West Haven-Yale Multidimensional Pain Inventory (WHYMPI). *Pain, 23,* 345–56.

Kim, H., Neubert, J.K., San Miguel, A. *et al.* (2004). Genetic influence on variability in human acute experimental pain sensitivity associated with gender, ethnicity and psychological temperament. *Pain, 109,* 488–96.

Lampe, A., Doering, S., Rumpold, G. *et al.* (2003). Chronic pain syndromes and their relationship to childhood abuse and stressful live events. *Journal of Psychosomatic Research, 54,* 361–7.

Landau, R., Kern, C., Columb, M.O., Smiley, R.M. and Blouin, J.L. (2008). Genetic variability of the μ-opioid receptor influences intrathecal fentanyl analgesia reqluirements in laboring women. *Pain, 139,* 5–14.

Lanes, T.C., Gauron, E.F., Spratt, K.F., Wernimont, T.J., Found, E.M. and Weinstein, J.N. (1995). Long-term follow-up of patients with chronic back pain treated in a multidisciplinary rehabilitation program. *Spine, 20,* 801–6.

**Lautenbacher, S. and Rollman, G.B.** (1997). Possible deficiencies of pain modulation in fibromyalgia. *Clinical Journal of Pain,* **13**, 189–96.

**Leeuw, M., Goossens, M.E.J.B., Linton, S.J., Crombez, G., Boersma, K. and Vlaeyen, J.W.** (2007). The fear-avoidance model of musculoskeletal pain: current state of scientific evidence *Journal of Behavioral Medicine,* **30**, 77–94.

**Leeuw, M., Goossens, M.E.J.B., van Breukelen, G.J.** *et al.* (2008). Exposure in vivo versus operant graded activity in chronic low back pain patients: results of a randomized controlled trial. *Pain,* **138**(1), 192–207.

**Leffler, A.S., Hansson, P. and Kosek, E.** (2002). Somatosensory perception in a remote pain-free area and function of diffuse noxious inhibitory controls (DNIC) in patients suffering from long-term trapezius myalgia. *European Journal of Pain,* **6**, 149–59.

**Linton, S.J.** (2000). A review of psychological risk factors in back and neck pain. *Spine,* **25** (9), 1148–56.

**Linton, S.J. and Bradley, L.A.** (1996). Strategies for the prevention of chronic pain. In R.J. Gatchel and D.C. Turk (Eds.), *Psychological approaches to pain management: A practitioner's handbook,* pp. 458–285. New York: Guilford Press.

**Linton, S.J. and Hallden, K.** (1997). Risk factors and the natural course of acute and recurrent musculoskeletal pain: Developing a screening instrument. In T.S. Jensen, J.A. Turner, and Z. Wiesenfeld-Hallin (Eds.) *Proceedings of the Eighth World Congress on Pain,* pp. 527–36. Seattle, WA: IASP Press.

**Linton, S. J. and Andersson, T.** (2000). Can chronic disability be prevented? A randomized trial of a cognitive-behavior intervention and two forms of information for patients with spinal pain. *Spine,* **25**, 2825–31.

**Linton, S. J., Boersma, K., Jansson, M., Overmeer, T., Lindblom, K. and Vlaeyen, J. W.** (2008). A randomized controlled trial of exposure in vivo for patients with spinal pain reporting fear of work-related activities. *European Journal of Pain,* **12**(6), 722–30.

**Lousberg, R., Schmidt, A.J., Groenman, N.H.** *et al.* (1997). Validating the MPI-DLV using experience sampling data. *J Behav Med,* **20**, 195–206.

**Lousberg, R., Van Breukelen, G.JP., Schmidt, A.J.M.** *et al.* (1999). Psychometric properties of the Multidimensional Pain Inventory, Dutch Language version (MPI-DLV). *Behavior Research and Therapy,* **7**, 167–82.

**Marcus, D.A.** (1992). Migraine and tension-type headaches: the questionable validity of current classification systems. *Clinical Journal of Pain,* **8**, 28–36.

**Masedo, A. and Esteve, M.R.** (2007). Effects of suppression, acceptance and spontaneous coping on pain tolerance, pain intensity and distress. *Behavior Research and Therapy,* **45**, 199–209.

**Mayer, T.G., Gatchel, R.J., Mayer, H.** *et al.* (1987). A prospective two-year study of functional restauration in industrial low back injury. *JAMA,* **258**, 1763–7.

**McCracken, L.M.** (2005). *Contextual cognitive-behavioral therapy for chronic pain. Progress in pain research and management, Vol. 33.* Seattle, WA: IASP Press.

**McCracken, L.M. and Eccleston, C.** (2003). Coping or acceptance: what to do about chronic pain? *Pain,* **105**, 197–204.

**McCracken, L.M., Zayfert, C. and Gross, R.T.** (1992). The pain anxiety symptoms scale: Development and validation of a scale to measure fear of pain. *Pain,* **50**, 67–73.

**McCracken, L.M., Spertus, I.L., Janeck, A.S., Sinclair, D. and Wetzel, F.T.** (1999). Behavioral dimensions of adjustment in persons with chronic pain: pain-related anxiety and acceptance. *Pain,* **80**, 283–9.

**Mogil, J.S., Wilson, S.G., Bon, K.** *et al.* (1999). Heritability of nociception I: responses of 11 inbred mouse strains on 12 measures of nociception. *Pain,* **80**, 67–82.

**Moore, J.F., Armentrout, D.P., Parker, J.C. and Kivlahan, D. R.** (1986). Empirically derived pain-patients MMPI subgroups: prediction of treatment outcome. *J Behav Med,* **9**, 51–63.

**Nicholas, M., Molloy, A., Tonkin, L. and Beeston, L.** (2003). *Manage your pain: practical and positive ways of adapting to chronic pain.* London: Souvenir Press.

Paul, G.L. (1967). Outcome research in psychotherapy. *Journal of Consulting and Clinical Psychology*, **31**, 109–18.

Peters, M.L. and Schmidt, A.J. (1992). Differences in pain perception and sensory discrimination between chronic low back pain patients and healthy controls. *Journal of Psychosomatic Research*, **36**, 47–53.

Pincus, T., Burton, K. Vogel, S. and Field, A. (2002). A systematic review of psychological factors as predictors of chronicity/disability in prospective cohorts of low back pain. *Spine*, **27**, 109–20.

Pincus, T., Williams, A., Vogel, S. and Field, A. (2004). The development and testing of the depression, anxiety and positive outlook scale (DAPOS). *Pain*, **109**, 181–8.

Piotrowski, C. (2007). Review of the psychological literature on assessment instruments used with pain patients. *North American Journal of Psychology*, **9**, 303–6.

Richmond, R.L. and Carmody, T.P. (1999). Dropout from treatment for chronic low back pain. *Professional Psychology*, **30**, 51–5.

Riipinen, M., Niemisto, L., Lindgren, K.-A., and Hurri, H. (2005). Psychosocial differences as predictors for recovery from chronic low back pain following manipulation, stabilizing exercises and physician consultation or physician consultation alone. *Journal of Rehabilitation Medicine*, **37**, 152–8.

Rudy, T.E. (2004). *Multiaxial assessment of pain: Multidimensional pain Inventory computer program user's manual*. Version 3.0. Pittsburgh, PA. University of Pittsburgh.

Rudy, T.E., Turk, D.C., Kubinski, J.A. and Zaki, H.S. (1995). Differential treatment responses of TMD patients as a function of psychological characteristics. *Pain*, **61**, 103–12.

Rusu, A.C. and Hasenbring, M. (2008). Multidimensional Pain Inventory derived classifications of chronic pain: Evidence for maladaptive pain-related coping within the dysfunctional group. *Pain*, **134**, 80–90.

Rusu, A.C., Scholich, S.L., Harenbrock, S. and Hasenbring, M. (submitted). Psychological factors discriminate clinical groups of chronic back pain patients: The role of endurance and fear-avoidance responses for distress and disability.

Scarinci, I.C., McDonald Haile, J., Bradley, L.A. and Richter, J.E. (1994). Altered pain perception and psychosocial features among women with gastrointestinal disorders and history of abuse: a preliminary model. *American Journal of Medicine*, **97**, 108–18.

Scharff, L., Turk, D.C. and Marcus, D.A. (1995). Psychosocial and behavioral characteristics in chronic headache patients: support for a continuum and dual-diagnostic approach. *Cephalagia*, **15**, 216–23.

Shaw, W.S, Pransky, G. and Fitzgerald, T.E. (2001). Early prognosis for low back disability: Interventions strategies for health care providers. *Disability and Rehabilitation*, **23**, 815–28.

Smeets, R.J.E.M. and Wittink, H. (2007). The deconditioning paradigm for chronic low back pain unmasked? *Pain*, **130**, 201–2.

Soderlund, A. and Denison, E. (2006). Classification of patients with whiplash associated disorders (WAD): Reliable and valid subgroups based on the Multidimensional Pain Inventory (MPI-S). *European Journal of Pain*, **10**, 113–19.

Staud, R., Robinson, M.E., Vierck, C.J. Jr. *et al.* (2003). Diffuse noxious inhibitory controls (DNIC) attenuate temporal summation of second pain in normal males but not in normal females or fibromyalgia patients. *Pain*, **101**, 167–74.

Strategier, L.D., Chwalisz, K., Altmaier, E.M. *et al.* (1997). Multidimensional assessment of chronic low back pain: predicting treatment outcomes. *Journal of Clinical Psychology in Medical Settings*, **4**, 91–110.

Sullivan, M.J.L. and Stanish, W.D. (2003). Psychologically based occupational rehabilitation: the pain-disability prevention program. *Clinical Journal of Pain*, **19**, 97–104.

Sullivan, M.J., Thorn, B., Haythornthwaite, J.A. *et al.* (2001). Theoretical perspectives on the relation between catastrophizing and pain. *Clinical Journal of Pain*, **17**, 52–64.

Sutton, J.T., Bachmann, G.A., Arnold, L.D. *et al.* (2008). Assessment of vulvodynia symptoms in a sample of U.S. women: a follow-up national incidence survey. *Journal of Women's Health*, **17**, 1285–92.

Swimmer, G.I., Robinson, M.E. and Geisser, M.E. (1992). Relationship of MMPI cluster types, pain coping strategy, and treatment outcome. *Clinical Journal of Pain*, **8**, 131–7.

Taddio, A., Goldbach, M., Ipp, M., Stevens, B. and Koren G. (1995). Effect of neonatal circumcision on pain response during vaccination in boys. *Lancet,* **345,** 291–2.

Taddio, A., Shah, V., Gilbert-MacLeod, C. and Katz J. (2002). Conditioning and hyperalgesia in newborns exposed to repeated heel lances. *Journal of the American Medical Association,* **288,** 857–61.

Talo, S., Forssell, H., Jeikkonen, S. *et al.* (2001). Integrative group therapy outcome related to psychosocial characteristics in patients with chronic pain. *International Journal of Rehabilitation Research,* **24,** 25–33.

Thieme K., Flor H. and Turk D.C. (2006). Psychological treatment in fibromyalgia syndrome: efficacy of operant behavioural and cognitive behavioural treatments. *Arthritis Research and Therapy,* 8, R121.

Thieme K., Rose U., Pinkpank T., Spies C., Turk D.C. and Flor H. (2006). Psychophysiological responses in patients with fibromyalgia syndrome. *Journal of Psychosomatic Research,* **61,** 671–80.

Turk, D.C. (1990). Customizing treatments for chronic pain patients; who, what, and why. *Clinical Journal of Pain,* **6,** 255–70.

Turk DC. (2002). Clinical effectiveness and cost effectiveness of treatments for chronic pain patients. *Clinical Journal of Pain,* **18,** 355–65.

Turk, D.C. (2004). Fibromyalgia: a patient-oriented perspective. In Dworkin, R.H., Breitbart, W.S. (Eds). *Psychosocial and Psychiatric Aspects of Pain: A Handbook for Health Care Providers,* pp. 309–38. Seattle, WA: IASP Press.

Turk, D.C. and Rudy, T.E (1988). Toward an empirically derived taxonomy of chronic pain patients: Integration of psychological assessment data. *Journal of Consulting and Clinical Psychology,* 56, 233–38.

Turk, D.C. and Rudy, T. E. (1990a). Neglected factors in chronic pain treatment outcome studies–Referral patterns, failure to enter treatment, and attrition. *Pain,* **43,** 7–25.

Turk, D.C. and Rudy, T. E. (1990b). The robustness of an empirically derived taxonomy of chronic pain patients. *Pain,* **42,** 27–35.

Turk, D.C. and Okifuji, A. (1998). Treatment of chronic pain patients: Clinical outcome, cost-effectiveness, and cost-benefits. *Critical Reviews in Physical Medicine & Rehabilitation,* **10,** 181–208.

Turk, D. C. and Wilson, H. D. (2010). Fear of activity as a prognostic factor in patients with chronic pain: conceptual models, assessment, and treatment implications. *Current Pain and Headache Reports,* **14,** 88–95.

Turk, D.C., Penzien, D.B. and Rains, J.C. (1995). Temporomandibular disorders. In Goreczny, ed. *Handbook of Recent Advances in Behavioral Medicine.* New York, NY: Plenum Press (pp. 55–77).

Turk, D.C., Okifuji, A., Sinclair, J.D. *et al.* (1996). Pain, disability, and physical functioning in subgroups of fibromyalgia patients. *Journal of Rheumatology,* **23,** 1255–62.

Turk, D.C., Okifuji, A., Sinclair, J.D. *et al.* (1998a). Differential responses by psychosocial subgroups of fibromyalgia syndrome patients to an interdisciplinary treatment. *Arthritis Care Research,* **11,** 397–404.

Turk, D.C., Sist, T.C., Okifuji, A. *et al.* (1998b). Adaptation to metastatic cancer pain, regional/local cancer pain, and non-cancer pain: role of psychological and behavioral factors. *Pain,* **74,** 247–56.

Turk, D.C., Okifuji, A., Sinclair, J.D. and Starz, T.W. (1998). Interdisciplinary treatment for fibromyalgia syndrome: clinical and statistical significance. *Arthritis Care & Research,* **11,** 186–95.

Turner, J.A., Franklin, G. and Turk, D.C. (2000). Predictors of long-term disability in injured workers: A systematic literature synthesis. *American Journal of Industrial Medicine,* **38,** 707–22.

Van den Hout, J.H., Vlaeyen, J., Heuts, P.H., Zijlema, J.H. and Wijnen, J.A. (2003). Secondary prevention of work-related disability in non-specific low back pain: does problem-solving therapy help? A randomized clinical trial. *Clinical Journal of Pain,* **19,** 87–96.

Van der Windt, D., Hay, E., Jellema, P. and Main, C. (2008). Psychosocial interventions for low back pain in primary care: Lessons learned from recent trials. *Spine,* **33,** 81–9.

Verra, M.L., Angst, F., Brioschi, R., *et al.* (2009). Does classification of persons with fibromyalgia into Multidimensional Pain Inventory subgroups detect differences inoutcome after a standard chronic pain management program? *Pain Research & Management,* **14,** 445–53.

Vlaeyen, J.W.S. and Morley, S. (2004). Active despite pain: the putative role of stop-rules and current mood. *Pain,* **110**, 512–16.

Vlaeyen, J.W.S., Kole-Snijders, A.M.J., Boeren, R.G.B. and van Eek, H. (1995). Fear of movement/(re) injury in chronic low back pain and its relation to behavioral performance. *Pain,* **62**, 363–72.

Vlaeyen, J.W.S., Haazen, I.W.C.J., Kole-Snijders, A.M.J. *et al.* (1996). Behavioural rehabilitation of chronic low back pain: Comparison of an operant treatment, and operant cognitive treatment and an operant respondent treatment. *British Journal of Clinical Psychology,* **34**, 95–118.

Von Eye, A. and Bergman, L.R. (2003). Research strategies in developmental psychopathology: dimensional identity and the person oriented approach. *Development and Psychopathology,* **15**, 553–80.

Von Korff, M. (1999). Pain management in primary care: An individualized stepped-care approach. In R.J. Gatchel and D.C. Turk (Eds.), *Psychosocial factors in pain: Critical perspectives* (pp. 360–73). New York: Guilford Press.

Von Korff, M., Ormel, J., Keefe, F.J. and Dworkin, S. F. (1992). Grading the severity of chronic pain. *Pain,* **50**, 133–49.

Waddell, G. (1998). *The back pain revolution.* Edinburgh: Churchill Livingstone.

Waylonis, G.W. and Perkins, R.H. (1994). Post-traumatic fibromyalgia. A long-term follow-up. *Am J Phys Med Rehabil,* **73**, 403–12.

Westman, A., Boersma, K., Leppert, J. and Linton, S.J. (2011). Fear-avoidance beliefs, catastrophizing, and distress: a longitudinal subgroup analysis on patients with musculoskeletal pain. *Clin J Pain,* **7**, 567–77.

Wideman, T.H., Adams, H.E. and Sullivan, M.J.L. (2009). A prospective sequential analysis of the fear-avoidance model of pain. *Pain,* **145**(1–2), 45–51.

Widerström-Noga, E.G., Felix, E.R., Cruz-Almeida, Y. and Turk. D.C. (2007). Psychosocial subgroups in persons with spinal cord injuries and chronic pain. *Archives of Physical Medicine and Rehabilitation,* **88**, 1628–35.

Wilder-Smith, C.H., Schindler, D., Lovblad, K., Redmond, S.M. and Nirkko, A. (2004). Brain functional magnetic resonance imaging of rectal pain and activation of endogenous inhibitory mechanisms in irritable bowel syndrome patient subgroups and healthy controls. *Gut,* **53**, 1595–601.

Wolfe, F., Smythe, H.A., Yunus, M.B. *et al.* (1990). The American College of Rheumatology 1990 criteria for the classification of fibromyalgia: report of the multicenter criteria committee. *Arthritis & Rheumatism,* **36**, 160–72.

Wolfe, F., Russell, I.J., Vipraio, G. *et al.* (1997). Serotonin levels, pain threshold, and fibromyalgia symptoms in the general population. *J Rheumatology,* **24**, 555–9.

Woods, M.P. and Asmundson, G.J. (2008). Evaluating the efficacy of graded in vivo exposure for the treatment of fear in patients with chronic back pain: a randomized controlled clinical trial. *Pain,* **136**, 271–80.

Yarnitsky, D., Crispel, Y., Eisenberg, E., Granovsky, Y., Ben-Nun, A., Sprecher, E., Best, L.A. and Granot M. (2008). Prediction of chronic post-operative pain: Pre-operative DNIC testing identifies patients at risk. *Pain,* **138**, 22–8.

Zubieta, J.K., Heitzeg, M.M., Smith, Y.R. *et al.* (2003). COMT val158met genotype affects mu-opioid neurotransmitter responses to a pain stressor. *Science,* **299**, 1240–43.

Chapter 27

# Risk Factor-Based Cognitive-Behavioural Therapy for Acute and Subacute Back Pain

## Monika I. Hasenbring, Bernhard W. Klasen, and Adina C. Rusu

## 27.1 Introduction

There is substantial evidence that treatment of patients with chronic back pain reveals limited success. Although several multimodal approaches including pharmacological, physiotherapeutical, and psychological features lead to statistical significant reduction of pain, pain-related disability, and work absenteeism, effect sizes are only small to moderate. Effects concerning clinical significance are rather marginal (Van der Windt et al. 2008). A number of systematic reviews concluded that offering patients multimodal treatment only when pain and disability had evolved into a chronic state and offering treatment in the same manner to each patient represent two of the central problems in treatment allocation (Morley et al. 1999; van Tulder et al. 2001; Hoffmann et al. 2007; Henschke et al. 2010). Turner and colleagues (1996) recommended the implementation of early educational and cognitive-behavioural interventions in the phase of subacute pain, when patients are still in primary care as well as more interventions targeted to the individual needs of the patients. Treating low back pain (LBP) patients not as a homogeneous group and identifying specifiable subgroups due to clinical, psychological, neurophysiological, and perhaps genetic risk variables represents an important topic for research (Turk 2005; Brennan et al. 2006; see Chapter 26). In line with this, Haldorsen (2003) pointed out that there is a challenge to find 'the right treatment to the right patient at the right time'.

In this chapter, we will present some basic considerations concerning: (1) the choice of an 'optimal' time point, starting with more comprehensive, multimodal treatment approaches at a cost-effective level; (2) potential criteria defining features of patients with back pain that may describe appropriate patients; and (3) finding the right treatment for a specific patient. A qualitative review of empirical evidence improving efficacy and effectiveness of current attempts in early, risk factor-based psychosocial interventions in the treatment of subacute back pain will follow. In the third section of this chapter, we will provide an illustrative description of current treatment options. Finally, we will try to draw some conclusions towards the need for future research and clinical practice.

## 27.2 Preliminary considerations

### 27.2.1 Finding the right time point for treatment

Bearing in mind that although a substantial number of acute low back pain (ALBP) patients will recover with little or no medical care, close to one-third of these patients tend to develop continuous or recurrent pain one year after an initial episode (Waddell 2004). As the duration of pain is one of the most important predictors of the development of severely chronic pain states, this leads to the conclusion that an effective treatment should start as early as possible. One of the first interventional strategies that focused on primary prevention was aimed at the prevention of the occurrence of back pain in healthy people at the workplace, since a number of risk factors for the occurrence of LBP have been shown to be work-related (see Chapter 19). However, despite the reduction of several ergonomic stressors at the workplace, the effects of these interventions on the development of pain and disability in healthy workers remained more than marginal (Shaw et al. 2006). The concept of secondary prevention—starting treatment in a phase of acute LBP with a duration of not more than 4 weeks—should be more cost-effective, because interventions are offered to fewer patients with a potentially greater effect. Within this context, it is less likely that a person who is healthy and who may have no risk of developing LBP or chronic states will receive an intervention that causes no effect but does cause costs. As described in more detail in the second section of this chapter, a number of randomized trials have been published during the past 10 years which aimed at secondary prevention of a recurrence of pain, pain-related disability, and work-related issues, conducted at the workplace, within primary care, and also on a population-based level. Although the results of these trials indicate that acute and subacute LBP is an optimal time point for starting multidisciplinary treatment, we recognize that there is substantial room for improvement of treatment offers.

### 27.2.2 Finding the right patient

Up to 60% of the patients, with ALBP will recover spontaneously with only little or no medical treatment. Therefore, a useful strategy is to optimize treatments by identifying those patients whose symptoms are likely to persist. Indeed, with the increasing knowledge about risk factors and mechanisms that may be indicative of the development of chronic back pain conditions, investigators and clinicians seek to develop new and even more effective treatment strategies early, in an effort to prevent chronicity and in as cost-effective a manner as possible.

As several chapters of this volume have shown, there is no doubt that psychosocial risk factors make a substantial contribution to the prediction of chronic pain, disability, and inability to work. This is true for variables such as depression and distress at work. Maladaptive responses to pain including catastrophizing about pain, fear of pain-related activities, more generalized fear-avoidance beliefs, and endurance-related responses such as thought suppression and task persistence behaviour despite severe pain all appear to contribute to disability (see chapters of Part 4 for further details). As most of these factors are related to each other, we are left with the question of their independent contribution (Foster et al. 2010). Additional important questions concern the difficulty of modifying proven risk factors and which risk factors will yield a maximum effect if modified successfully. For instance, it might be easier to modify the tendency of catastrophizing pain experiences by informing a patient in an acute or subacute pain episode about the harmless character of his pain condition than to reach a reduction of distress at work arising from long-lasting conflicts between the patient and his colleagues. Answering such questions will require intervention studies targeting specified psychological risk factors.

A pre-condition of an individually targeted treatment is the identification of psychosocial risk factors that are assessed with high reliability and predictive validity. Although it is desirable that a screening tool reveals adequate sensitivity and specificity, most of the currently available psychosocial screening measures reveal either high sensitivity and moderate specificity, or vice versa (see Chapter 11). Consequently, whether a screening tool should show higher specificity or sensitivity depends on costs. In the case of high-cost treatments, greater specificity is necessary in order not to treat patients that did not require this treatment. If more low-cost interventions are available, using an assessment measure or procedure with high sensitivity but only moderate specificity may be justifiable.

### 27.2.3 **Finding the right treatment**

The next step after identifying the relevant psychological risk factors indicating the development of ongoing or recurrent pain and increasing disability, is finding the right treatment approaches. Intervention-based psychological pain research over the past decades seems to follow a continuous alternation of deductive, theory driven, and inductive designs. In the 1960s, Fordyce (1976) extended the operant condition model conceptualizing functional mechanisms leading to the maintenance of so-called *'pain behaviours'*. For instance, facial expression of acute pain, caused by a sudden damage of physical structures, may come under environmental control. A decade later, stimulated by an extensive laboratory experimental research on attention and pain (Ahles et al. 1983; McCaul and Mallot 1984), Turk and colleagues (1983) developed a cognitive-behavioural model of pain emphasizing the role of dysfunctional cognitions, such as maladaptive attributions and perceptions of low self-efficacy. This model stimulated the cognitive-behavioural perspective and the application of a range of cognitive and behavioural techniques for the treatment of patients with persistent pain (Turk and Rudy 1986; Turk 1998). This perspective served as an important stimulant for numerous experimental and clinical studies searching for specific maladaptive cognitions, such as catastrophizing, fear of injury/re-injury, and fear-avoidance beliefs, leading to a more specific theoretical model of psychological mediators of pain, the fear-avoidance model (FAM; Vlaeyen and Linton 2000). New cognitive-behavioural treatment approaches, such as guided exposure, were developed, specifically treating patients suffering from high fear of pain, pain-related activities, and avoidance behaviour (e.g. Vlaeyen et al 2001; George et al. 2008). Recently, the avoidance-endurance model of pain was developed, focusing on additional cognitive, affective, and behavioural responses to pain that seem to act as risk factors for subsequent pain and disability. Pain-related fear may not only be followed by avoidance behaviour but also by a pattern of pain persistence with cognitions of thought suppression and marked endurance behaviour shown despite severe pain conditions. Moreover, there seems to be a subgroup of back pain patients impressing by very low fear, positive mood despite pain, and elevated endurance behaviour that also has a high probability to developing chronic pain conditions (Hasenbring et al. 2001, Hasenbring and Verbunt 2010, see Chapter 15 for more details). These high-risk patterns might optimally benefit from individually tailored cognitive-behavioural therapy (CBT) approaches that incorporate different kinds of activity pacing interventions.

## 27.3 **Early psychosocial interventions for LBP patients in primary care**

During the past decade, a number of randomized intervention trials in primary care settings have been conducted, in which psychological treatments were offered to LBP patients who had back pain of less than 12 weeks' duration. While duration and content of the psychological interventions differed between group discussions based on cognitive-behavioural principles (e.g. Linton and Andersson 2000; Hay et al. 2005), and guided exposure sessions developed to decreasing high fear of pain-related activities, most trials revealed significant reduction of pain, disability, and catastrophizing (George et al. 2008; Linton et al. 2008). However, no or only small differences between these psychological interventions and active control treatments have been reported. Although a number of reasons may be responsible for these results (Van der Windt et al. 2008), the most critical issue seems to be offering these interventions to a large proportion of patients who might not need them. These patients show few psychosocial risk factors and they will develop a high rate of spontaneous recovering, mirrored by the significant time effects. Subanalyses in some of these secondary prevention studies revealed low levels of psychological distress (e.g. Hay et al. 2005) and baseline disability (George et al. 2008), supporting this hypothesis. Therefore, it will be important to improve the indication of psychosocial interventions, for instance by focusing only on patients who show signs of psychosocial risk factors.

Jellema and co-workers (2005) performed a cluster-randomized trial (41 practices of general medicine) of 143 patients with LBP of less than 12 weeks' duration. Patients received a minimal interventions strategy, carried out by general practitioners (GPs), aimed at the assessment and modification of psychosocial prognostic factors compared to patients receiving usual care (N=171). The GPs received two training sessions of 2.5 hours each, provided by a GP with expertise in psychosocial interventions. The training consisted of theory, role-playing, and feedback on the practised skills. The minimal intervention arm consisted of a 20-minute session with the patient including three phases: exploration, information, and self-care. The authors designed this session to identify and modify psychosocial risk factors. That means risk factors are assessed after randomization and only in the intervention group. Consistent with our previous suggestion, the results of this trial, revealed significant reduction of disability, pain intensity, and sick leave due to back pain in both groups with no significant group difference. Within 6–13 weeks, 60–70% of the patients' symptoms had been resolved, which very likely mirrors the high rate of spontaneous recovering in patients with acute and subacute back pain in general. Since all patients in the minimal intervention group received the psychosocial interventions irrespective of the results of the physicians' rating, this trial covers a large number of low-risk patients known to showing a high rate of spontaneous recovering. Therefore, despite relative large sample sizes, those trials will be underpowered showing a significant group difference.

Another study conducted by the authors (Jellema et al. 2005) showed that, despite physician training, the risk assessment based on global physician ratings, are of doubtful reliability and low prospective validity (see also Streitlein-Böhme et al. 2008).

### 27.3.1 Risk factor-based cognitive-behavioural interventions (RCBIs)

RCBIs are guided by assessment of psychosocial risk factors. Randomized-controlled trials (RCTs) usually assess risk factors before randomization. The procedures published to date, differ in how the assessment of psychosocial risk factors ('yellow flags', see also Chapter 11) was handled. Some studies used a patient or physician rating of the perceived risk for the development of chronic pain, while other approaches used an independent, standardized assessment of psychosocial risk factors known to be reliable and valid. RCBI were allocated randomly only to high-risk patients. Low-risk patients were used for further comparison.

### RCBI guided by a global self-rating of individual risk for chronicity

Linton and colleagues published a number of early intervention studies in order to prevent work disability and they are leading in the development of psychosocial risk factor diagnostics (see Chapter 11). In 2000, they reported first results of a randomized trial with a 5-year follow-up published in 2006 (Linton and Andersson 2000; Linton and Nordin 2006). Although not explicitly named as a risk factor-based trial, it is, to our knowledge, one of the first early intervention studies that has targeted only high-risk patients. The authors used a global self-rating of their patients evaluating their personal risk for the development of chronic pain.

In the first study (Linton and Andersson 2000), 272 patients who fulfilled the inclusion criterion of less than 3 months of cumulated sick leave due to back pain were randomly allocated to three interventions groups (pamphlet, information-package, and CBT). Patients were recruited from local primary care facilities and via an advertisement in a local newspaper. Primary outcomes (all self-reported) were long-term sick-leave, healthcare use, and the self-perceived risk for developing long-term pain. The investigators included pain variables and different psychosocial characteristics, assessed with standardized questionnaires as secondary outcomes. In the pamphlet group participants received short written information based on the fear-avoidance model recommending positive thinking and remaining active and confronting with pain rather avoiding pain-related activities. In the information package group participants received more conservative written information presented once a week for 6 weeks with relatively broad and general information. Investigators typically conduct RCBI using a 6-session structured programme with a 2-hour session once a week and 6–10 patients per group. Certified behaviour therapists provided a treatment based on a written manual. The six sessions were concerned with the following topics: (1) causes of pain and prevention of chronic problems with information about pain, learning problem-solving skills and applied relaxation; (2) managing pain with activity scheduling and maintaining activities; (3) promoting good health and controlling stress at home and at work, with detecting warning signals and considering health beliefs; (4) adapting for leisure and work, with communication skills and assertiveness training in risk situations; (5) controlling flare-ups; and (6) maintaining and improving results making plans for adherence. Each of the sessions included initial information for a maximum of 15 minutes, structured exercises, and individually-tailored homework assignments. Results demonstrated significant group differences concerning sick absenteeism between CBT and the pamphlet group, using an intention-to-treat analysis. Both information groups showed an increase in the number of sick days from baseline to the 1-year follow-up, whereas CBT participants showed a slight decrease. The difference between CBT and pamphlet was still significant after 1 year. Regarding the number of visits to the physician and physical therapist per year, CBT patients showed a significant decrease, whereas both information groups showed an increase. The third main outcome, self-rated perception of long-term disability, revealed a significant decrease in CBT and a stable level in both information groups, although group differences at the follow-up were not significant. Furthermore, no group differences were found at follow-up concerning pain intensity, activity level, depression, and the fear-avoidance variables such as catastrophizing, fear-avoidance beliefs, or fear of pain/injury. Overall, the sample of this study has shown relatively mild problems at baseline level, perhaps due to the specific selection procedure of patients. However, the investigators reported a significant time effect with a decrease of scores in the fear-avoidance beliefs in all groups and a decrease in catastrophizing in both information groups, while the level of fear of pain/injury remained stable over time in all groups. The results on general anxiety and depression were comparable.

In a 5-year follow-up of the 2000 sample, Linton and Nordin (2006) conducted a reassessment by now comparing the CBT group with the combined information group due to the fact that in most variables there had been no differences between the pamphlet and the information package group. At this long-term follow-up, the CBT group was superior to the information group in most of the outcomes, specifically with respect to pain intensity, activities of daily living, quality of life, and medication use. A detailed cost analysis revealed lower pain and disability-related costs for the CBT group compared to the information group. Although the CBI sessions were six times more expensive than the information approach, the total costs were lower due to higher productivity (fewer days of sick leave) and a lower rate of healthcare costs due to fewer healthcare visits in the CBT group.

## RCBI guided by the results of a comprehensive psychosocial risk assessment

During the past decade, only a few studies have conducted a standardized and validated assessment of psychosocial risk factors in order to guide the indication of psychosocial interventions. For instance, Gatchel and colleagues (Gatchel et al. 2003; Whitfill et al. 2010) evaluated the efficacy of CBI as part of a multimodal functional restoration programme in patients suffering from acute low back pain. Hasenbring et al. (1999) investigated risk factor-based CBI in a sample of subacute sciatic pain patients who were offered (in addition to conservative medical treatment such as pain medication), relaxation and physiotherapy. In a recent RCT, Hasenbring et al. (submitted) compared a short physician-delivered counselling based on risk screening with group therapy interventions and treatment as usual in a sample of subacute non-specific LBP from different primary care practices. In all approaches, the investigators allocated patients with high psychosocial risk factors in the previous screening, randomly to targeted interventions and compared them with treatment as usual groups or with different standardized active treatments. Furthermore, both approaches used the low-risk group, matched carefully by gender, age, and diagnosis, as a further comparison group. We will describe these in more detail in the next section (see 'RCBI guided by a short theory-based screening of psychosocial risk factors').

Gatchel and co-workers (Gatchel et al. 2003) used a comprehensive assessment, consisting of two pain and disability visual analogue scales, Scale 3 ('Hysteria') of the Minnesota Multiphasic Personality Inventory (MMPI), and the fact of existing workers compensation in identifying patients showing a high psychosocial risk of not returning to work at a 12-month follow-up. In a prospective, longitudinal study of 421 patients with acute LBP (less than 10 weeks duration) this risk assessment yielded a correct classification of more than 90% of the cases, who did not return to work at the follow-up (Gatchel et al. 1995). In a second validation study using a number of standardized measurements of psychopathological disorders, coping styles, and specific traits in the domain of personality disorders, Pulliam et al. (2001) showed that high- and low-risk patients could be classified with 80% sensitivity and 81.5% specificity. High-risk patients were low on positive temperament and showed more workaholic tendencies measured with the Schedule for Nonadaptive and Adaptive Personality (SNAP, Clark 1993). High scorers on this scale are characterized by their placing work above leisure time and neglecting social contact such as friends and family in favour of work. They indicate that they do not finish a job until it is perfect, and they will drive themselves until exhausted. This pattern of pain-related cognitions, emotions and behaviour is comparable to the endurance pattern, described within the avoidance-endurance model of pain (Hasenbring and Verbunt 2010; see also Chapter 15 of this volume), and the concept of a maladaptive 'work style', described by Feuerstein and colleagues (2005).

Based on this psychosocial risk assessment, conducted within a number of orthopaedic practices, high-risk patients, randomized into the interventions group (HR-I), Gatchel and colleagues (2003) offered an early interdisciplinary intervention programme consisting of psychological components, physical therapy, occupational therapy, and case management. The protocol consisted of three physician and one physical therapy evaluation, nine physical therapy sessions of 15 minutes' individual training, nine physical therapy group sessions of 30 minutes' duration, nine 30-minute biofeedback/pain management sessions, nine group didactic lesions each lasting 45 minutes, nine case manager/occupational therapy sessions lasting 30 minutes each, and three interdisciplinary team conferences. Trained and licensed therapists administered all treatments. All sessions were ideally spaced over a 3-week period; however most patients did not need all sessions. The outcome assessed by structured telephone interviews at 3-, 6-, 9-, and 12-month follow-up, included return-to-work status, number of healthcare visits in general and related to LBP, number of disability days, pain intensity, and medication use. In all variables, the 22 HR-I patients showed a highly significant better outcome compared to high-risk patients without this interdisciplinary treatment (HR-NI, N=48). HR-I patients delivered a similar positive outcome as the low-risk patients at the 1-year follow-up on pain intensity and return to work. In a rough cost-comparison analysis, the authors reported significantly lower costs ($12,721 in HR-I compared to $21,843 in HR-NI) despite the costs for this early intervention programme (Gatchel et al. 2003).

In a recent RCT, this kind of early intervention programme was as effective as a new protocol that consisted of these interventions given in addition to a specific work-transition module (Whitfill et al. 2010).

## RCBI guided by a short theory-based screening of psychosocial risk factors

During the past two decades, Hasenbring and colleagues developed pain risk screening-based cognitive-behavioural approaches (PARIS-CBA) that were evaluated within two RCTs (Hasenbring et al. 1999, submitted). PARIS-CBA contains of different kinds of cognitive-behavioural interventions, such as short counselling sessions (PARIS-CBC), group therapy (PARIS-CBGT), and individual therapy interventions (PARIS-CBIT). A previous 'yellow-flag' screening that is based on the avoidance-endurance model (AEM) of pain (see Chapters 15 for the AEM and 11 for the screening RISC-BP) guides all approaches. The investigators developed standardized modules aimed at the modification of AEM-based dysfunctional pain response pattern, such as fear-avoidance-, distress-, or eustress-endurance pattern.

In the following, we will outline some basic principles of PARIS-CBA and different steps of interventions and modules, referencing the kind of intervention to which it is relevant. We recommend that these interventions be administered within a stepped-care programme due to limited financial resources. This ranges from short physician and/or physiotherapist counselling (15 minutes' duration) as a first step to cognitive-behavioural group therapy (6–12 weekly sessions of 100 minutes each) and cognitive-behavioural individual therapy (25–45 or more weekly sessions of 50 minutes each) as further steps. We consider the reliable and valid indication of the need to these more extensive approaches. Finally, we report on the results of two RCTs conducted in two different settings of medical care.

**Basic principles of PARIS-CBA** Irrespective of the kind of CBA, several principles guide the different procedures as well as the relationship between patient and CBA-provider. These include: (1) all interventions and modules will follow an individually tailored schedule; (2) the relationship between patient and CBA provider is based on principles of shared decision-making that have been shown to increase patient satisfaction and adherence (Joosten et al. 2008); and (3) all interventions are based on 'third wave' cognitive-behavioural methods, including learning principles, dysfunctional cognitions perspective, supporting individual resources including an increase of acceptance as well as interpersonal approaches.

The *principles of individualization* and *shared decision-making* are realized within several steps of PARIS-CBA interventions. The primary concern to: (1) the personal risk profile of a patient; (2) the patients' illness model; (3) the patients' individual treatment goals; and (4) the patients' level of motivation for behavioural changes, following the trans-theoretical model of behavioural change (Norcross et al. 2011; Prochaska et al. 2001). At first, the AEM-based yellow-flag screening (RIsc SCreening for Back Pain, RISC-BP) informs a patient whether screening data reveal a high-risk pattern for the development of chronic back pain and second, which precise pattern of high-risk behaviour is present—a fear-avoidance pattern or a distress or eustress-endurance-pattern. An important question for the provider is to reconfirm as to whether patients will recognize themselves when informed about their risk profile or which part of the risk behaviour will be familiar to them. We tailor this reinsurance to the individual model of illness representation that may be more somatic in some cases or more psychosocial in others. Our clinical impressions reveal that many patients with subacute pain report substantial psychosocial stress (e.g. conflicts with their partner or with colleagues at work) but they do not recognize a relation between these stressors and their pain problem. Further, a number of patients do recognize aspects of a distress-endurance pain pattern and they can imagine that this is a dysfunctional way to respond to pain but they do not know how to change this pattern.

We extend the principle of individualization and shared-decision-making in the development of treatment goals. CBA providers will propose different treatment goals to their patients and encouraging them to develop their own way. Furthermore, providers will continuously harmonize their own perspectives with the ideas, goals and wishes of their patients.

In addition to consideration of *learning principles* and modification of *dysfunctional pain-related cognitions and behaviour*, PARIS-CBA aims to promote the individual *awareness* of physical signs and individual needs, especially when pain increase will be only slight, as well as to increase the *acceptance* of the need for an individual balancing of physical needs and external demands. As a great number of individual pain situations will occur within an interpersonal context (e.g. with relatives, friends, or colleagues at work), *interpersonal approaches* including methods of social competence training will be included.

**PARIS-CBA: procedure and steps of intervention**  In the following, standardized procedures of the PARIS-CBA stepped-care programme will be presented, beginning with instructions concerning a preliminary provision of the patient with a biopsychosocial perspective in further diagnostics, yellow-flag assessment, individual goal assessment, and finally an overview of endurance-related interventions.

*Step 1: providing the patient with a biopsychosocial model of pain*  PARIS-CBA aimed at a harmonization of the illness models of different healthcare providers acting at the different settings of a stepped care model. As it is proposed to offer a yellow-flag screening by physicians in primary care, presenting such an illness model in a standardized manner should be part of the introduction of the screening procedure. PARIS-CBA proposes the following instruction the physician may give to his patient: 'During the past weeks your pain did not respond (enough) to the treatment I had proposed to you. Our careful diagnostics ruled out any serious illness. Therefore, we have to look for further potential influences that can cause or maintain back pain. *First*, it could be that biomechanical stress (e.g. long-lasting and/or recurrent dysfunctional body postures) may cause or maintain back pain via an increase of muscular load and muscular tension. Daily psychological stress, such as conflicts with colleagues or superiors at work may also increase muscular tension. Furthermore, if someone has to care for an ill or elderly relative, biomechanical (physical) and psychological stress may act simultaneously. *Second*, when pain does not respond to medical treatment as we would expect and when it lasts longer than anticipated, it very often leads to sleep disturbances, leading to increased fatigue during the day and increasing effort to maintain daily activities in spite of fatigue. This, in the long-term, may cause additional muscular tension and more and more depressive mood, leading to a vicious circle, which influences pain and disability. *Third*, how we do respond to pain emotionally is important, in our spontaneous automatic cognitions and concerning our behaviour, there are more functional and dysfunctional ways to respond to pain.' As a first step, we might ask patients to complete a short screening questionnaire and tell them that their responses will be used as a basis for discussion of further treatment options.

The physician may observe the reactions of his patients towards these potential pain factors and pathways. One patient will quickly respond positively when exploring psychological stress, for instance when he is suffering from some kind of stress. Another patient will look highly sceptical when mentioning psychological stress, but respond by nodding his head when mentioning sleep disturbances and depression as a consequence of pain or dysfunctional coping. This is one of the first steps in which the physician may explore the personal illness model of his patient. As all directions of a potential vicious circle are involved, the probability that patients may accept one aspect of the illness model is high.

*Step 2: Yellow-flag assessment and counselling* PARIS-CBA offers different kinds of presentation modes for the yellow-flag screening RISC-BP—such as a paper-and-pencil form or in a computer-based form, which might be conducted within a primary care practice or via Internet to be filled in at home (Hasenbring and Hallner, 1999). In the latter form, patients will receive a specific identification number and be asked to bring this to their physicians after answering the RISC-BP via computer at home. The physician has access to the results, will explain these to his patient, and will discuss the further steps of treatment with him. It is important to initially train physicians on how to explain screening results to the patient by using standardized instructions, which may be individually adapted to each patient.

In the following, we provide an example of these suggested instructions for the classification as high risk of development of chronic pain via the 'distress-endurance response' (DER) pattern: 'The screening revealed high scores in negative, depressive mood together with a tendency for thought suppression. This means that you mostly try to suppress pain and all thoughts about pain, in order not to interrupt your daily activities. The depression score is not on pathological level and many people do respond with automatic thoughts trying to suppress thoughts about pain sensations, but in most cases, this is not very successful. Unwanted thoughts will persist thoroughly and your mood might become more and more irritated and depressed. In your behaviour, you are scoring high on endurance behaviour, which might mean that you try to finish all activities of daily life despite your severe pain. On the one hand, being able to show endurance behaviour despite pain or other unwanted negative feelings is an important strength at times with a lot of daily stress. However, if we do chronically respond with thought suppression and endurance behaviour and are not able to realize short breaks during daily activities in order to relax, these responses will lead to long-term overload or overuse of muscles, discs and other physical structures, causing or maintaining your current pain. Is there anything you recognize and you may agree with?'

*Step 3: Individual goal assessment* Goal assessment differs between short physician counselling, group treatment, and individual treatment with respect to the increasing degree of individualization and further concerning the extent of potential changes in patients' dysfunctional cognitions and behaviour that may be possible. However, potential causes of dysfunctional pain pattern, such as motivational factors (Van Damme et al. 2010) or the kind of learning history are still a matter of research, which is just beginning. Motivational factors of persistent dysfunctional pain pattern may vary from more situational influences, such as short-term occupational pressure, to more individual factors. The latter may result, for example, from kinds of self-discrepancies (Kindermans et al. 2011) and long-term learning mechanisms. It is further a matter of research whether the resulting dysfunctional pattern are easy to change (e.g. merely by a short education or whether motivation, learning history, and other possible causes will afford more intense treatment methods in order to reach an adaptive modification). It seems to be plausible, that offering screening and counselling in the very early phases of subacute LBP will increase the probability of more situational influences of dysfunctional pain response pattern and that these will be more easily changeable by low-dose interventions. Before the physician decides to provide the patient with solutions, he should ask his patient whether he has ideas how to change his situation the next time it occurs. By this procedure, the physician may get a first impression of the level of motivation for behaviour change the patient may represent.

Following a first physician counselling, primary care providers may make one or two more appointments with their patients in order to evaluate their level of motivation for behaviour change. Providers should attempt to determine which among the transtheoretical levels of: (1) precontemplation in which there is no intention to change behaviour; (2) contemplation, in

---

### Box 27.1 Guiding principles of 'graded balancing'

1. Interruption of pain-related endurance should be realized very early, when pain increases from 3 to 4 (in case of an 11-numeric self-rating ranging from 0 to 10). Only in the case of early breaks, relaxation has a chance to be successful.
2. Only short breaks of current activity should be realized, finding an individual alternative leading to muscular and mental relaxation.
3. Automatically occurring thoughts as obstacles for balancing should be observed as a primary hindrance.
4. Individual motivation background and learning history of thought suppression and endurance behaviour has to be explored.

---

which patients are aware that a problem exists but have not yet made a commitment to take action; (3) preparation, in which patients are intending to take action and reporting some small behavioural changes; (4) action, in which they modify their behaviour or environment to overcome their problems; and (5) maintenance, in which patients work to prevent relapse and maintain the gains attained during action (Prochaska et al. 2001) is best applied to each patient. When level 2 or 3 are recognizable but the patient signals persistent failure to reach behavioural changes by his own effort, when psychological risk factors indeed persist, and when also pain persists for a couple of weeks, the next step of a CBA group intervention should be considered.

*Step 4: Endurance-related interventions following the principle of 'graded balancing'* In the case of a marked fear-avoidance-related pain response pattern, treatment strategies derived by the principles of *'graded exposure'* will be offering to the patient. Vancleef and co-workers describe this kind of treatment in more detail in Chapter 14 of this volume. Furthermore, this chapter will present some essential parts of the principle of *'graded balancing'* offered to patients with marked endurance-related pain response pattern (see Box 27.1).

Within the *short physician counselling* of 15 minutes' duration, only a few minutes are available for discussing alternatives of the individual dysfunctional pain pattern. 'Graded balancing' encourages the patient to have short breaks for relaxation when pain increases above an acceptable level and to observe automatic thoughts that normally occur when pain threatens to interrupt a current activity, thoughts that can be labelled as obstacles for realizing an effective short break. For example: 'I do not have time for a break right now', 'You can have a break later on, when you have finished your work', 'If you have a break right now, you will never finish your work'. The guiding principle is to find a balance between an acceptable degree of endurance (maintaining a current pain-irrelevant activity) and an increase of relaxation-inducing activities (e.g. interruption of current activities for physical activity in case of long-term sitting at work). In principle, *graded balancing* seems to be related to the concept of 'activity pacing', which has been described by other authors (e.g. Nicholas et al. 2003; McCracken 2005). The kind of relaxation-inducing activities depends on the mode of current activity. When pain increases following a long-term phase of sitting at work (e.g. in a forward bend position as a biomechanical strain position), a short break lying down (only for a few minutes) and later cycling or walking for a while may represent the situation-specific kind of relaxation. An important add-on of the physician counselling is a back book describing dysfunctional pain response pattern as well as alternative responses in the sense of 'graded balancing', based on the avoidance-endurance-model of pain.

Within six or more sessions of *PARIS-CBA group treatment*, more time is available for: (1) a more intense discussion of illness- versus health-related cognition and behaviour; (2) exercises for the detection of individual maladaptive automatic cognitions and behaviour; and (3) exercises, for example, role plays, for the modification of maladaptive automatic cognitions and behaviour. However, within a six-session PARIS-CBA group treatment including seven or eight patients, each patient will have two or three times the opportunity for individual exercises during these sessions.

In the case of a long learning history of maladaptive endurance coping and of additional psychosocial risk factors such as depression due to unsolved emotional problems, a *PARIS-CBA individual treatment* may be appropriate. Using a 25-session short-term therapy, there is time for analysis and change of persistent and stubborn kinds of meta-cognitions (e.g. 'If I continue with this therapy, my whole household will be in a mess'). These cognitions may act as powerful obstacles against adaptive cognitions (e.g. 'I will have a short break and relax for a little while before I continue with my activities').

**Empirical evidence for PARIS-CBA** In a first RCT, Hasenbring and colleagues (1999) evaluated the efficacy of a PARIS-CB individual therapy trial conducted in a sample of subacute sciatic pain patients during an inpatient hospital stay for conservative medical treatment. At the time of admission all patients underwent the RISC-BP psychosocial screening consisting of the Beck Depression Inventory (BDI) depression score and two subscales of the Kiel Pain Inventory, embedded in a more comprehensive psychosocial assessment. The evaluation of increased psychosocial risk as well as the classification of high-risk patients as individuals showing fear-avoidance responses (FARs), distress-endurance responses (DERs) or eustress-endurance responses (EERs) to pain followed the procedure published by Hasenbring (1993, see also Chapter 11 in this volume). The purpose of this intervention study was to evaluate the efficacy of a risk factor-based cognitive-behavioural regimen (in this study labelled as RCBT) in comparison with another active treatment and with a third group that only received treatment as usual, therefore conservative medical treatment (group HRIS). The second active treatment consisted of electromyographic biofeedback (BFB), a standardized behavioural treatment in patients with chronic pain, shown as effective in previous studies (Flor and Birbaumer 1993). These three groups were compared with a self-selected group of low-risk patients (LRIS) undergoing treatment as usual. The investigators hypothesized that both behavioural interventions, in addition to conservative medical treatment, would be more effective in the prevention of chronic pain than medical treatment without psychological intervention. Further, that high-risk patients who attended the behavioural interventions would demonstrate an improvement similar to that of low-risk patients, and finally, an individually scheduled risk factor-based cognitive behavioural treatment would be more effective than a standardized biofeedback regimen. The study provided follow-up assessments at 3, 6, 12, and 18 months after baseline. Results of repeated measurement ANOVAs have shown that according to the first hypothesis both active treatments (RCBT and BFB) revealed greater improvement in pain intensity than HRIS, while furthermore, RCBT exhibited greater pain reduction than BFB (see Figures 27.1–27.3).

Only the RCBT group revealed significantly better outcomes than HRIS patients; the BFB group scored as insignificant between RCBT and HRIS on the secondary outcomes of disability, depression, medication intake, and application for early retirement. A strength of this study was the calculation of different measures of clinical significance following the suggestions by Jacobson et al. (1984). For example, the group of low-risk patients, known to show a good outcome from previous studies (e.g. Hasenbring et al. 1994), was treated as a functional reference group and the percentage of high-risk patients showing an improvement within the range of LRIS for each experimental condition was assessed. The authors defined as two standard deviations of the mean within that functional group. At the time of discharge from the hospital, 83% of the RCBT

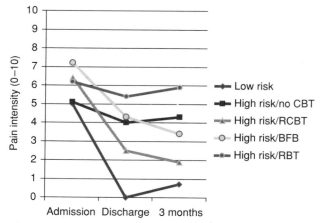

**Fig. 27.1** Pain intensity over time in different treatment and control groups from the time of admission to the hospital, discharge, and the 3-month follow-up. Reproduced from Hasenbring, M., Ulrich, H.W., Hartmann, M. & Soyka, D. The efficacy of a risk factor based cognitive behavioral intervention and EMG-biofeedback in patients with acute sciatic pain: an attempt to prevent chronicity. *Spine*, **24**, pp.2525–35 © 1999 Lippincott, Williams, and Wilkins with permission.

patients showed a decline of pain intensity that fulfilled this criterion in contrast to 18% in BFB and 0% in HRIS. At the 6 month follow-up, 63% in both RCBT and BFB groups fulfilled this criterion compared to 8% in HRIS. However, 66% in RCBT showed a clinically significant reduction in depression compared to 33% in BFB and 25% in HRIS. The investigators calculated the reliability of change index (RC; Jacobson et al. 1984) as a second measure of clinical significance. Values of RC exceeding 1.96 are unlikely to occur (p <0.05) unless an actual change in scores (of at least two standard deviations) occurs between pre-treatment and follow-up assessments. At the 6-month follow-up, 91% of the RCBT group showed a RC improvement in pain intensity compared to 78% in BFB, and 33% in HRIS. No patient in RCBT revealed a RC deterioration compared

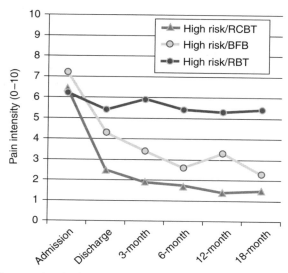

**Fig. 27.2** Pain intensity over time in the two treatment groups and the comparison group from the time of admission to the hospital, discharge, and the 3-, 6-, 12-, and 18-month follow-ups.

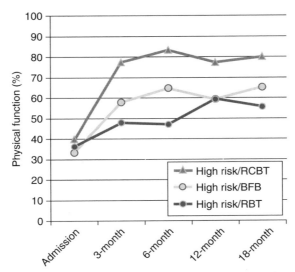

**Fig. 27.3** Physical function (%) over time in the two treatment groups and the comparison group from the time of admission to the hospital, discharge, and the 3-, 6-, 12-, and 18-month follow-ups.

to 8%, 22% and 33% at the long-term follow-ups in the BFB group. Finally, a self-selected group of patients who had refused an additional BT (RBT) showed no improvement over time, comparable to HRIS.

## 27.4 **Conclusion and future directions**

The recommendations not to treat LBP patients as a homogenous group of patients had a stimulating impact on the development of specific clinical, psychological, and neurobiological features that serve as a basis for subgrouping patients and targeting treatments more individually. Especially in the phase of acute and subacute back pain, a number of psychological features are identifiable as high-risk factors ('yellow flags') indicating a high probability of developing chronic pain and pain-related disability. Recent advances in the further development of approaches directed more and more towards subgroups of patients showing specific psychosocial risk profiles. However, controlled randomized trials, based on a preliminary reliable and valid yellow flag screening and offering CBT only to subgroups of patients who indeed show high psychosocial risk factors, are still rare. This research design would increase the probability that not too many patients receive CBT who would not need this kind of intervention. Systematic comparisons with the short- and long-term follow-up of low-risk patients, who have a high probability of good recovery and may serve as a functional reference group, should be conducted. Functional reference groups deliver norms of psychosocial functioning and should act as a further approach testing the clinical significance of a trial. Cognitive-behavioural interventions conducted as risk factor-based treatments, should draw on validated theoretical models, as recommended once again by several authors (e.g. Michie et al. 2008).

## References

Ahles, T.A., Blanchard, E.B. & Leventhal, H. (1983). Cognitive control of pain: attention to the sensory aspects of cold-pressor stimulus. *Cogn Res Ther*, 7, 159–78.

Brennan, G.P., Fritz, J.M. & Hunter, J. (2006). Identifying subgroups of patients with acute/subacute 'nonspecific' low back pain. Results of a randomized clinical trial. *Spine*, 31(6), 623–31.

Clark, L. (1993). *Schedule for Nonadaptive and Adaptive Personality (SNAP)*. Minneapolis, MN: University of Minneapolis Press.

Feuerstein, M., Nicholas, R.A., Huang, G.D., Haufler, A.J., Pransky, G. & Robertson, M. (2005). Workstyle: development of a measure of response to work in those with upper extremity pain. *J Occup Rehabil*, **15**, 87–104.

Flor, H. & Birbaumer, N. (1993). Comparison of the efficacy of electromyographic biofeedback, cognitive-behavioral therapy, and conservative medical interventions in the treatment of chronic musculoskeletal pain. *J Consult Clin Psychol*, **61**, 653–8.

Fordyce, W.E. (1976). *Behavioral methods for chronic pain and illness*. St. Louis, MO: Mosby.

Foster, N.E., Thoams, E., Bishop, A., Dunn, K.M., & Main, C.J. (2010). Distinctiveness of psychological obstacles to recovery in low back pain patients in primary care. *Pain*, **148**, 398–406.

Gatchel, R.J., Polatin, P. & Mayer, T. (1995). The dominant role of psychosocial risk factors in the development of chronic low back pain disability. *Spine*, **20**(24), 2702–9.

Gatchel, R.J., Polatin, P.B., Noe, C., Gardea, M., Pulliam, C. & Thompson, J. (2003). Treatment- and cost-effectiveness of early intervention for acute low-back pain patients: a one-year prospective study. *J Occup Rehabil*, **13**(1), 1–9.

George, S. Z., Zeppieri, G. Jr., Cere, A.L., *et al.* (2008). A randomized trial of behavioral physical therapy interventions for acute and sub-acute low back pain. *Pain*, **140**(1), 145–57.

Haldorsen, E.M.H. (2003). The right treatment to the right patient at the right time. *Occupational Environmental Medicine*, **60**, 235–6.

Hasenbring, M. (1993). Endurance strategies - a neglected phenomenon in the research and therapy of chronic pain? *Der Schmerz*, **7**, 304–13.

Hasenbring, M. & Hallner, D. (1999). Telemedizinisches Patienten-Diagnose-System. *Deutsches Ärzteblatt/ Praxis Computer*, **6**, 49–50.

Hasenbring, M.I. & Verbunt, J.A. (2010). Fear-avoidance and endurance-related responses to pain: new models of behaviour and their consequences for clinical practice. *Clin J Pain*, **26**, 747–53.

Hasenbring, M., Marienfeld, G., Kuhlendahl, D. & Soyka, D. (1994). Risk factors of chronicity in lumbar disc patients. A prospective investigation of biologic, psychologic, and social predictors of therapy outcome. *Spine*, **19**, 2759–65.

Hasenbring, M., Ulrich, H.W., Hartmann, M. & Soyka, D. (1999). The efficacy of a risk factor based cognitive behavioral intervention and EMG-biofeedback in patients with acute sciatic pain: an attempt to prevent chronicity. *Spine*, **24**, 2525–35.

Hasenbring, M., Hallner, D. & Klasen, B. (2001). Psychological mechanisms in the transition from acute to chronic pain: over- or underrated? *Schmerz*, **15**(6), 442–7.

Hasenbring, M.I., Klasen, B.W., Streitlein-Böhme, I. & Rusche, H. Risk-factor based cognitive-behavioural approaches in sub-acute low back pain patients: first results of a randomized, controlled trial (submitted).

Hay, E.M., Mullis, R., Lewis, M., *et al.* (2005). Comparison of physical treatments versus a brief pain management programme for back pain in primary care: a randomised clinical trial in physiotherapy practice. *Lancet*, **365**, 2024–29.

Henschke, N., Ostelo, R.W., van Tulder, *et al.* (2010). Behavioral treatment for chronic low back pain. *Cochrane Database Syst Rev*, **7**, CD002014.

Hoffmann, B.M., Papas, R.K., Chatkoff, D.K. & Kerns, R.D. (2007). Meta-analysis of psychological interventions for chronic low back pain. *Health Psychol*, **26**, 1–9.

Jacobson, N.S., Follette, W.C. & Revensdorf, D. (1984). Psychotherapy outcome research: Methods for reporting variability and evaluating clinical significance. *Behav Ther*, **15**, 336–52.

Jellema, P., van der Windt, D.A.W.M., van der Horst, H.E., *et al.* (2005). Should treatment of (sub)acute low back pain be aimed at psychosocial prognostic factors? Cluster randomised clinical trial in general practice. *BMJ*, **331**, 84.

Joosten, E.A.G., DeFuentes-Merillas, L., DeWeert, G.H., Sensky, T., vander Staak, C.P.F. & deJong, C.A.J. (2008). Systematic review of the effects of shared-decision making on patient satisfaction, treatment adherence and health status. *Psychotherapy and Psychosomatics 77*, 219–26.

Kindermans, H.P., Huijnen, I.P., Goossens, M.E., Roelofs, J., Verbunt, J.A. & Vlaeyen, J.W. (2011). 'Being' in pain: the role of self-discrepancies in the emotional experience and activity patterns of patients with chronic low back pain. *Pain, 152*(2), 403–9.

Linton, S.J. & Andersson, T. (2000). Can chronic disability be prevented? A randomised trial of a cognitive-behavioural intervention and two forms of information for patients with spinal pain. *Spine, 25*, 2825–31.

Linton, S.J. & Nordin, E. (2006) A 5-year follow-up evaluation of the health and economic consequences of an early cognitive behavioral intervention for back pain: a randomized, controlled trial. *Spine, 31*, 853–8.

Linton, S.J., Boersma, K., Jansson, M., Overmeer, T., Lindblom, K. & Vlaeyen, J.W. (2008). A randomized controlled trial of exposure in vivo for patients with spinal pain reporting fear of work-related activities. *Eur J Pain, 12*, 722–30.

McCaul, K.D. & Malott, J. (1984). Distraction and coping with pain. *Psychol Bull, 95*, 516–33.

McCracken, L.M. (2005). *Contextual cognitive-behavioral therapy for chronic pain* (Progress in pain research and management, vol. 33). Seattle, WA: IASP Press.

Michie, S., Johnston, M., Francis, J., Hardeman W. & Eccles, M. (2008). From theory to intervention: Mapping theoretically derived behavioural determinants to behaviour change techniques. *Applied Psychology, 57*, 660–80.

Morley, S., Eccleston, C. & Williams A. (1999). Systematic review and meta-analysis of randomized controlled trials of cognitive behaviour therapy and behaviour therapy for chronic pain in adults, excluding headache. *Pain, 80*, 1–13.

Nicholas, M., Molloy, A., Tonkin, L. & Beeston, L. (2003). *Manage your pain: practical and positive ways of adapting to chronic pain*. London: Souvenir Press.

Norcross, J.C., Krebs, P.M. & Prochaska, J.O. (2011). Stages of change. *J Clin Psychol, 67*, 143–54.

Prochaska, J.O., Redding, C.A. & Evers, K. (2001). The transtheoretical model and stages of change. In K. Glanz, F.M. Lewis, & B.K. Rimer (Eds.), *Health behavior and health education* (3rd edn.), pp. 60–84. San Francisco, CA: Jossey-Bass.

Pulliam, C.B., Gatchel, R.J. & Gardea, M.A. (2001). Psychosocial differences in high risk versus low risk acute low-back pain patients. *J Occup Rehabil, 11*(1), 43–52

Shaw, W.S., Linton, S.J. & Pransky, G. (2006). Reducing sickness absence from work due to low back pain: how well do intervention strategies match modifiable risk factors? *J Occup Rehab, 16*, 591–605.

Streitlein-Böhme, I., Hasenbring, M., Hallner, D. & Rusche H. (2008). Do psychosocial risk factors ('yellow flags') influence the diagnosis and therapy of acute and subacute low back pain in the general practitioner (GP) practice? *Z Allg Med, 84*, 538–42.

Sullivan, M.J.L., Bishop, S.R. & Pivik, J. (1995). The pain catastrophizing scale: development and validation. *Psychol Assess, 7*, 524–32.

Turk, D.C. (1998). Cognitive factors and persistent pain: A glimpse into Pandora's box. Presented at the 'Pain Management '98: Failed Back Surgery Syndrome Conference', Rotterdam, The Netherlands, 12 November, 1998.

Turk, D.C. (2005). The potential of treatment matching for subgroups of patients with chronic pain: lumping versus splitting. *Clin J Pain, 21*, 44–55.

Turk, D.C. & Rudy, T.E. (1986). Assessment of cognitive factors in chronic pain: a worthwhile enterprise? *J Consult Clin Psychol, 54*(6), 760–8.

Turk, D.C., Meichenbaum, D. & Genest, M. (1983). *Pain and behavioral medicine: A cognitive-behavioral perspective*. New York: Guilford Press.

Turner, J.A. (1996). Educational and behavioral interventions for back pain in primary care. *Spine, 21*, 2851–9.

Van Damme, S., Legrain, V., Vogt, J. & Crombez, G. (2010). Keeping pain in mind: a motivational account of attention to pain. *Neurosci Biobehav Rev,* **34**, 204–13.

Van der Windt, D.A.W., Hay, E.M., Jellema, P., & Main, C.J. (2008). Psychosocial interventions for low back pain in primary care: Lessons learned from recent trials. *Spine,* **33**, 81–9.

Van Tulder, M.W., Ostelo, R., Vlaeyen, J.W.S., Linton, S.J., Morley, S.J. & Assendelft, W.J.J. (2001). Behavioral treatment for chronic low back pain: A systematic review within the framework of the Cochrane Back Review Group. *Spine,* **26**, 270–81.

Vlaeyen, J.W., de Jong, J., Geilen, M., Heuts, P.H. & Van Breukelen, G. (2001). Graded exposure in vivo in the treatment of pain-related fear: a replicated single-case experimental design in four patients with chronic low back pain. *Behav Res Ther,* **39**, 151–66.

Vlaeyen, J.W. & Linton, S.J. (2000). Fear-avoidance and its consequences in chronic musculoskeletal pain: a state of the art. *Pain,* **85**, 317–32.

Waddell, G. (2004). *The Back Pain Revolution* (2nd. edn.). Edinburgh: Churchill-Livingstone.

Whitfill, T., Haggard, R., Bierner, S.M., Pransky, G., Hassett, R.G. & Gatchel, R.J. (2010). Early intervention options for acute low back pain patients: a randomized clinical trial with one-year follow-up outcomes. *J Occup Rehabil,* **20**(2), 256–63.

# Part 9

# Clinical Approaches for Patients with Established Pain and Disability

## Chapter 28

# Physical Exercise Interventions and Low Back Pain

J. Bart Staal, Chris G. Maher, and William S. Shaw

## 28.1 Introduction

Although low back pain (LBP) is usually considered a benign disorder with a good prognosis, a spontaneous relapse of symptoms and disability is not uncommon (Henschke et al. 2008; Pengel et al. 2003). Besides the unpredictable course over time, it is generally assumed that the longer the pain and disability persists, the higher the chances are to develop a chronic stage of pain and disability with little prospect of a successful recovery (Frank et al. 1996; Pincus et al. 2002, 2006). Effective strategies are required to prevent such a deteriorated health condition from developing and to improve the coping skills and resources available to LBP sufferers.

In the literature, LBP is regularly classified according to the duration of symptoms: acute and subacute LBP constitutes an episode with a duration of less than 12 weeks, and chronic LBP describes an episode of pain with a duration longer than 12 weeks (Airaksinen et al. 2006; Koes et al. 2001; van Tulder et al. 2006). The subacute stage has been referred alternately to symptoms within 3–12 weeks from pain onset or 6–12 weeks from pain onset (Frank et al. 1996; Hayden et al. 2005a). Only in a minority of cases (approximately 15%) can the pathoanatomical source of LBP be identified. This leaves the majority of cases in the category of non-specific or uncomplicated LBP (Deyo et al. 1992). The type of LBP dealt with in this chapter is non-specific, unless stated otherwise.

Many treatment alternatives have been proposed for LBP throughout the last decades even though the evidence base for many treatments is still weak (Spitzer 1987; Airaksinen et al. 2006). One of the most promising intervention alternatives is physical exercise. In acute LBP, physical exercise is generally considered to have no beneficial value compared to no treatment or other conservative treatments (Hayden et al. 2005a). In cases of subacute or chronic LBP, however, physical exercises are viewed as a valuable treatment alternative for LBP and exercise has been recommended in a number of clinical guidelines for subacute and chronic LBP (Chou et al. 2007; Koes et al. 2001; Airaksinen et al. 2006). Nevertheless, there are still doubts with regard to the clinical importance of its effect size (van Tulder et al. 2007). Physical exercise treatments in clinical studies may, however, vary with regard to its underlying concepts, the types of exercises included, the frequency, intensity, and length of exercise sessions, and whether or not exercise is combined with other treatment components such as patient education or cognitive-behavioural approaches. This heterogeneity in the content of exercise treatments complicates our understanding of the real effects of physical exercise for LBP. Other aspects that might also influence these effects are the skills and experience of the caregiver and the exercise adherence and level of effort by the patient (Helmhout et al. 2008). The interpretation of studies on physical exercises, and LBP treatment in general, may further be hampered by the variation in the type of chronic LBP patients who participate in such studies. These patients can vary from those who have episodic LBP that is merely an annoyance, to those whose LBP prevents work and social participation and is accompanied by psychological distress (Dufour et al. 2010; Mayer 2010). There is some evidence that the profile of the patient can influence their response to exercise-based treatment (Haldorsen et al. 2002). Clear characterization of study populations in intervention studies is therefore very important.

In this chapter, we review the effects of physical exercise in subacute and chronic LBP. Although the Cochrane systematic literature review by Hayden et al. (2005) has provided a reasonable summary of the effects of physical exercise interventions, the present chapter will place more emphasis on the context of daily clinical practice, and how that may influence exercise outcomes. To accomplish this, we explored the PubMed and Embase databases for publications in the last 5 years with particular interest in relevant systematic reviews and additional randomized controlled trials. Based on this literature search, the most common types of exercise therapy will be described according to concept and content of treatment. For the purpose, we subdivide physical exercise interventions into the following types of exercise interventions:

◆ Exercises aimed at improving aspects of physical fitness (e.g. strength, muscle endurance, movement coordination).

◆ Specific spinal stabilization exercises.

◆ McKenzie exercises.

◆ Physical exercises from a cognitive-behavioural perspective (aimed at reducing fear or altering cognitions).

◆ Physical exercise interventions for disabled workers with LBP (i.e. the occupational healthcare perspective).

Although it should be noted that there may be some overlap, we believe this classification corresponds with the current literature and with clinical practice as common in many countries around the world. In addition, the effects of these subgroups of exercise therapies as reported in the literature will be summarized and their clinical implications will be discussed.

## 28.2 **Treatment aimed at increasing physical fitness and/or activity**

Many exercise programmes are aimed at increasing aspects of physical fitness such as muscle strength, muscle cross-sectional area, muscle endurance, and coordination of movements. In general, it is believed that the improvement of physical fitness and, consequently, an increase in habitual physical activity is beneficial for the LBP patient. This may also imply that reduced physical fitness and physical activity levels play a role in the aetiology of LBP (i.e. the de-conditioning syndrome). The evidence for this relationship is, however, still weak. In a Norwegian case–control study, which compared groups of chronic and subacute LBP patients with a group of healthy controls, it was found that abdominal and back muscle endurance were reduced when comparing chronic LBP patients to subacute LBP patients, and to healthy controls (Brox et al. 2005). A more recent systematic review on the longitudinal relationship between physical capacity and the risk of musculoskeletal disorders concluded that due to inconsistency in multiple studies there is inconclusive evidence for a relationship between trunk muscle strength, or mobility of the lumbar spine and the occurrence of LBP (Hamberg-van Reenen et al. 2007). Another systematic review on the association between physical de-conditioning and chronic LBP concluded that there was conflicting and limited evidence for the presence of cardiovascular de-conditioning and multifidus disuse in chronic LBP patients (Smeets et al. 2006).

The Cochrane systematic review on the effects of exercise therapy identified five trials in subacute populations with data available to calculate pooled estimates for pain and four trials for self-reported functioning (Hayden et al. 2005a). All trials used non-exercise comparison groups. The content of the exercise treatments of the included trials varied from extension, flexion and/ or more general exercises (Davies et al. 1979; Moffett et al. 1999; Storheim et al. 2003) to McKenzie exercises (Cherkin et al. 1998) and to graded activity interventions (Lindstrom et al. 1992; Staal et al. 2004), which are exercise interventions that follow a cognitive-behavioural approach. The pooled effects estimates for pain (i.e. 1.9 points at a 100-point scale) and functional status (i.e. 1.1 point at a 100-point scale) at short- and intermediate-term follow-up were small and non-significant leading to the conclusion that there was insufficient evidence to support or refute the effectiveness of exercise therapy in subacute LBP (Hayden et al. 2005a). In a more recent large (n=259) randomized controlled trial (RCT) by Pengel et al. physiotherapy-directed exercise was compared with advice and placebo treatment in a population of subacute LBP patients. This study showed that exercises were significantly, but only slightly, more effective for pain and functioning at 6 weeks when compared to a placebo treatment (Pengel et al. 2007).

The results of exercise treatments in chronic LBP populations are more promising than the results in subacute populations. The meta-analysis by Hayden et al. found statistically significant effects of exercise therapy in chronic LBP at short-, intermediate-, and long-term follow-up periods based on 46 studies. The pooled mean differences in improvement was 7.3 points (of 100 points) for pain and 2.5 points (of 100 points) for function at the earliest follow-up point and similar effects were found for the intermediate and long-term follow-up (Hayden et al. 2005a). The studies included were mostly conducted in healthcare settings, commonly used individually designed and delivered exercise programmes, and often included strengthening or trunk-stabilizing exercises. Conservative care was frequently added to the exercise programme, including treatment components such as advice to stay active and education, manual therapy, or even behavioural therapy (Hayden et al. 2005a). The authors of this review study concluded that exercise therapy seemed to be slightly effective in decreasing pain and improving function in adults with chronic LBP, particularly in healthcare populations (Hayden et al. 2005a). Similar conclusions were reported in the evidence review which accompanied the European guidelines for chronic LBP (Airaksinen et al. 2006). The authors found, based on a best-evidence rating system applied to 45 studies, strong evidence that exercise is more effective than general practitioners' (GPs') care for pain and disability reduction, and return-to-work at 3 to 6 months. Moderate evidence was found when the comparison group included passive treatments. Besides the comparison between exercise and GPs' care or other treatments, the authors also compared different types of exercise therapies to each other (Airaksinen et al. 2006). In one of these comparisons muscle reconditioning and strengthening exercises were compared to other types of exercises. Based on the results of eight randomized studies it was concluded that there was strong evidence for muscle reconditioning and strengthening exercises being not superior to other types of exercises. In addition, one study provided limited evidence that there are no differences between aerobic and either reconditioning or conventional physiotherapy exercises (Mannion et al. 1999; Mannion et al. 2001; Airaksinen et al. 2006).

Based on studies with available data in roughly the same set of studies Hayden et al performed a meta-regression analysis alongside their meta-analysis to investigate which types of exercise therapies are most beneficial for chronic LBP patients (Hayden et al. 2005b). The conclusions of this literature study were slightly different when compared to the European guideline evidence review. Of the different types of exercise treatments, stretching exercises demonstrated the largest improvements in function outcomes and muscle strengthening exercises the largest improvement in pain outcomes (Hayden et al. 2005b). Further, the meta-regression model revealed that the effects of exercise on pain and function outcomes were greater if the exercise programme was individually designed and supervised (including home exercises), had a high dose or intensity

(≥20 hours), and encompassed an additional conservative care intervention component (Hayden et al. 2005b). Although these results are interesting and seem to provide tools for daily clinical practice it should be noted that the effects found for pain and function outcomes were still not considered large enough to represent a clinically important effect (i.e. 10 and 20 points for pain and function scores respectively on a 100-point scale) (Hayden et al. 2005a, 2005b).

If exercise programmes are aimed at improving aspects of physical fitness, changes in physical fitness or performance are expected to be associated with changes in clinical symptoms or disability (Airaksinen et al. 2006). Of the 46 studies included in the European evidence review only seven studies investigated the relationships between pain and disability on the one hand, and spinal mobility/range of motion, trunk strength or trunk endurance on the other hand (Airaksinen et al. 2006). Among those studies only two studies reported weak associations between pain/disability and spinal mobility (correlation coefficient r= 0.2–0.4) (Elnaggar et al. 1991; Mannion et al. 1999) and trunk strength (correlation coefficient r=0.48) (Martin et al. 1986). Although these and other results (Airaksinen et al. 2006; Smeets et al. 2006) point out there is hardly any relationship between changes in pain and disability and direct changes in aspects of physical fitness or performance after engaging in exercise treatments, the research literature suggests that physical fitness and activity programmes are to some extent effective in chronic LBP patients. There are, however, still many questions with regards to optimal content of treatment and mechanisms of action of physical fitness and activity programmes that remain to be answered in future studies.

## 28.3 **Specific spinal stabilization exercises**

Specific spinal stabilization exercises are aimed at improving coordination, strength, and endurance of muscles involved in the active stabilization of the spine and trunk. Other terms that are used for this specific type of exercise therapy are segmental stabilization or core stabilization. According to Panjabi, spinal stability can be provided by the articular, muscular, and neural systems which together control intervertebral movement (Panjabi, 1992a, 1992b). The muscles involved in spinal stability can be subdivided in global and local muscles (Bergmark, 1989; Richardson and Jull, 1995; Standaert et al. 2008). The global muscles are the large torque producing muscles which link the pelvis to the thoracic cage. They provide general trunk stabilization and balance external loads. The local muscles are directly linked to the vertebrae and are assumed to be responsible for spinal stability (Richardson and Jull 1995). The local muscles targeted in spinal stabilization programmes are primarily deep spinal muscles, such as the lumbar multifidi and the transversus abdominis (Richardson and Jull 1995). The recruitment of these muscles is assumed to be altered in LBP patients and this needs to be enhanced and restored in order to reach pain reduction and functional recovery (Ferreira et al. 2006; Standaert et al. 2008). According to an experimental study by Hodges and Richardson (1996) the contraction of the transversus abdominis was delayed in LBP patients compared to healthy controls when responding to disturbances of the spine produced by arm movements. In another study it was shown that lumbar multifidus wasting was present in patients with acute and subacute LBP (Hides et al. 1994). The recovery of the multifidus muscle after acute LBP, which did not occur spontaneously, could be improved by means of specific localized exercise therapy (Hides et al. 1996). The results of these studies together with the findings of other studies (MacDonald et al. 2006; Standaert et al. 2008) gave support to the hypothesis that inefficient muscular stabilization of the spine is associated with sustained LBP. Following this model it seems obvious that exercise therapy should promote coordination and stabilization training of the lumbar spine musculature.

During spinal stabilization programmes patients are taught to recruit their deep spinal muscles. They are for example asked to gently draw in their abdominal wall in order to achieve isometric co-contraction of the transversus abdominis and multifidus (Richardson and Jull 1995). Progression can be achieved by increasing the holding time and the number of repetitions, and by gradually increasing from low loads with minimal body weight to more functional body positions with higher external loads. Furthermore, the exercise should not only be performed with a static neutral lumbar spine but also in more extreme static body positions. Finally, co-contraction of the deep spinal muscles have to be held in dynamic functional movements of the trunk (Richardson and Jull 1995).

Two systematic reviews were published in 2006 on the effects of spinal stabilization exercises for LBP. Rackwitz et al. (2006) conducted a systematic review on the effects of so-called segmental spinal stabilization exercises for acute, subacute and chronic LBP and Ferreira et al. (2006) summarized the effects of spinal stabilization exercises for spinal and pelvic pain and followed, if possible, a meta-analytical approach. Both systematic reviews were more or less based on the same set of studies and, not surprisingly, similar conclusions were found. In chronic LBP spinal stabilization exercises were found to be superior when compared to GPs' care but the additional value to general physiotherapeutic management was not clear (Ferreira et al. 2006; Rackwitz et al. 2006).

The systematic review by Ferreira et al. has recently been updated and now provides the most up-to-date information regarding the effectiveness of spinal stabilization exercises (Macedo et al. 2009). In this systematic review only trials were included which included participants with persistent non-specific LBP. Persistent LBP was defined as non-acute LBP of at least 6 weeks duration or recurrent LBP. The follow-up time points were subdivided in short-term follow-up (less than 3 months after randomization), intermediate term follow-up (at least 3 months and less than 12 months after randomization) and long-term follow-up (12 months follow-up or more). Relevant subgroups were created and pooled analyses were performed with pain, disability, and quality of life scales converted to 0–100 scales. The authors of the review distinguished four comparisons: (1) spinal stabilization versus minimal intervention (i.e. no intervention, general practitioners' care or education) or versus another type of intervention with spinal stabilization exercises added as a supplement; (2) spinal stabilization versus spinal manipulative therapy; (3) spinal stabilization versus other types of exercise therapy; and (4) spinal stabilization versus surgery (Macedo et al. 2009).

Four trials were identified that compared spinal stabilization exercises with either general practitioners' care or no intervention (Moseley, 2002; Niemisto et al. 2003; O'Sullivan et al. 1997; Shaughnessy and Caulfield 2004), and three trials compared spinal stabilization exercises added as a supplement to another intervention to this intervention alone (Goldby et al. 2006; Koumantakis et al. 2005; Stuge et al. 2004). The pooled results of these seven trials together showed statistically significant effects in favour of the spinal stabilization exercises for pain at short-term follow-up (effect = −14.3 points, 95% confidence interval [CI]: −20.4 to −8.1), intermediate-term follow-up (effect = 13.6, 95% CI: −22.1 to −4.1), and long-term follow-up (effect = −14.4, 95% CI: −23.1 to −5.7). Significant effects were also found for disability at long-term follow-up (effect = −10.8, 95% CI: −18.7 to −2.8) but no effects for quality of life. In four trials, spinal stabilization exercises were compared with spinal manipulative therapy (Critchley et al. 2007; Ferreira et al. 2007; Goldby et al. 2006; Rasmussen-Barr et al. 2003). In most comparisons the pooled effects were in favour of spinal stabilization although the effects were small and only reached significance in a few estimates (Macedo et al. 2009). Significant effects at intermediate term follow-up were found for pain (effect = −5.7, 95% CI: −10.7 to −0.8), disability (effect = −4.0, 95% CI: −7.6 to −0.4) and quality of life (effect = −6.0, 95% CI: −11.2 to −0.8). Five trials were identified which compared spinal stabilization exercises with other kinds of exercises (Critchley et al. 2007; Ferreira et al. 2007; Kladny et al. 2003; Miller et al. 2005; Stevens et al. 2007). A significant pooled effect, based on the results of three trials, was only found for disability at short-term follow-up (effect =−5.1, 95% CI: −8.7 to 1.4). No significant differences were found for the other effect estimates. Finally, one trial compared spinal stabilization exercises with surgery and found no significant differences between these two treatments (Brox et al. 2003).

The results of the systematic reviews described above indicate that spinal stabilization exercises may be effective in comparison to standard GPs' care, no intervention, or as a supplement to a more general physiotherapeutic management. There is no convincing evidence that spinal stabilization exercises are more effective than other kinds of exercise interventions, spinal manipulative therapy, or surgery.

## 28.4 **McKenzie therapy**

The McKenzie method is a popular treatment for the management of LBP. It includes both an assessment and a management component (May and Donelson 2008). While commonly considered as an exercise approach, the method emphasizes education and self-management and for some patients a lumbar roll is provided. Manual therapy is a less frequently used part of the treatment package. The method was developed by a New Zealand physiotherapist, Robin McKenzie, based upon his clinical observations of patients with LBP. The method has evolved over time and in this chapter we will briefly describe the method as described in McKenzie and May's 2003 texts (McKenzie and May, 2003a, 2003b).

In common with the approach advocated in clinical practice guidelines, the initial step in the McKenzie method is to exclude patients with confirmed or suspected serious pathology. Findings from the history-taking and physical examination are then used to determine the provisional classification of non-serious LBP into one of three syndromes: the derangement syndrome; the dysfunction syndrome; or the postural syndrome. LBP presentations that after five visits do not fit any of the above-mentioned syndromes are classified as 'other' or 'non-mechanical syndrome' and are considered not suitable for treatment with the method. Unlike most clinical practice guidelines the method does not distinguish between patients with non-specific LBP and radiculopathy; or advocate a different approach based upon the duration of the episode.

Most patients fit the derangement syndrome and for these patients the guiding treatment principle is to encourage directions of movement and postures that produced a proximal shift in pain (centralization) and that prevented distal migration of pain (peripheralization). It is important to note that this is not equivalent to generic prescription of extension exercises for all patients. In the dysfunction syndrome symptoms are thought due to adhesions, contracture, and adaptive shortening of soft tissues. Treatment of the dysfunction syndrome therefore emphasizes movements that encourage the process of remodelling of these tissues. A small percentage of patients seeking care for LBP fit the postural syndrome and these patients receive advice on the link between posture and pain, and posture correction. As mentioned previously, self-management is a major element in all three syndromes.

Most clinical practice guidelines do not provide separate recommendations for various types of exercise such as the McKenzie method. There are, however, two systematic reviews that have aimed to determine the effectiveness of McKenzie therapy. The 2004 Clare review (Clare et al. 2004) concluded that McKenzie therapy does result in a greater decrease in pain and disability in the short term than do other standard therapies. The effect of treatment was, however, quite small with the weighted mean difference and 95% CI being −8.6 (−13.7 to −3.5) for pain and −5.4 (−8.4 to −2.4) for disability where both outcomes were measured on a 0-100 scale. At intermediate follow-up the effect for disability was smaller still and not significant and there was no pooled estimate for pain.

The 2006 Machado review (Machado et al. 2005), similarly to the earlier review, noted that the effects observed for McKenzie method exercises in trials seemed quite small. A key finding of the Machado review was that five of the 11 located trials applied treatment in a generic fashion, with patients not receiving treatment matched to their clinical classification. These authors noted that this approach potentially underestimates the effect of treatment with the McKenzie method. Accordingly at the present point the efficacy of McKenzie therapy is unclear.

## 28.5 Physical exercises from a cognitive-behavioural perspective

In addition to physical exercise, cognitive-behavioural interventions have been highlighted as a possible treatment alternative for chronic LBP. Recommendations for cognitive-behavioural treatment are not uncommon (Airaksinen et al. 2006; Chou and Huffman, 2007), and there is evidence in support of such treatment programmes (Ostelo et al. 2005). Cognitive-behavioural treatment can be defined as a treatment that focuses on reducing disability through the modification of environmental contingencies and cognitive processes (Ostelo et al. 2005). Three behavioural approaches can be distinguished. Operant treatments aim at the modification of behaviour by positive reinforcement of healthy behaviours and withdrawal of attention towards pain behaviours, and time-contingent instead of pain-contingent management of pain patients (Fordyce 1976). Cognitive treatments aim to modify maladaptive cognitions, beliefs and expectations with regards to pain and disability, and respondent treatment aims to modify physiological responses (e.g. reducing muscle tension by means of relaxation exercises) (Ostelo et al. 2005).

Although cognitive-behavioural treatment seems, at least conceptually, very different in comparison to physical exercise interventions an overlap exists between these two approaches. First, in many multimodal treatment packages, elements of cognitive-behavioural treatments are combined with physical exercises and sometimes other elements to obtain an optimal content of intervention (Guzman et al. 2001; Karjalainen et al. 2001). Second, physical exercises are sometimes used as a mean to modify behaviour, cognitions or physiological response and can therefore be considered in these cases as a form of cognitive-behavioural treatment. For the purpose of this chapter we will limit the discussion to this combined form of treatment; in particular, operant and graded exposure treatment that incorporates physical exercise. Graded activity interventions are examples of operant treatments. According to the operant conditioning theory, as applied to LBP, the future occurrence of healthy behaviour tends to increase as a result of graded activity (i.e. gradually increased exercise intensity) and positive reinforcement, in contrast to inactive pain behaviour (Fordyce 1976; Lindstrom et al. 1992). The graded activity intervention can be described as an intervention that consists of individual counselling, education, and physical exercises, applied according to operant conditioning principles. Following this approach, Swedish investigators conducted a RCT, which compared a graded activity intervention to usual care in Swedish automobile industry (Lindström et al. 1992). The results of the study by Lindström and colleagues showed that the participants of the graded activity intervention returned to work significantly earlier than the control group (Lindström et al. 1992).

A similar RCT to Lindström et al (1992) was conducted by Staal et al in a population of Dutch airline workers (Hlobil et al. 2005; Staal et al. 2004). In this study the graded activity intervention consisted of two sessions of physical exercises a week, which were supervised by skilled physiotherapists. The exercises were based on the functional demands of specific work tasks and on individual functional capacity. Functional capacity was determined for each exercise by a number of baseline assessments in which the worker exercised to the limit of tolerance. The worker then set a quota of exercises to be performed at each exercise session. During the course of the intervention the load of the exercises was gradually increased towards a preset exercise goal, following a time-contingent exercise scheme. This means that the exercise quota were preset and independent of variation in the severity of pain. The exercise goals were further connected with return-to-work (RTW) goals, which were also set by the worker eventually after consulting the physiotherapist, and the intervention stopped when full return to regular work was achieved (Hlobil et al. 2005; Staal et al. 2004). The results of the study by Staal et al. were similar to those reported in the Swedish trial: graded activity resulted in significantly earlier return-to-work compared to the control group. No effects were found for pain and self-reported disability (Hlobil et al. 2005; Lindstrom et al. 1992; Staal et al. 2004). The study with Dutch airline workers was followed by a more or less similar study which compared graded activity to a participatory ergonomics intervention and to usual care. In this study, carried out in a heterogeneous group of workers from different companies, no effects were found for graded activity (Anema et al. 2007; Steenstra et al. 2006). The study authors attributed differences to the level of implementation and the large number of participating physiotherapy clinics. A total number of 47 physiotherapists had been involved in their study who all received additional training on treating pain patients according to an operant conditioning behavioural approach (Steenstra et al. 2006). However, it had not been checked to what extent the physiotherapists had the appropriate skills to follow this approach. In the study by Staal et al. this was regularly done which was in fact also easier due to the limited number of physiotherapist involved in this trial (Staal et al. 2004).

Two out of the three trials described above found favourable effects on return-to-work caused by a graded activity intervention. When we look at the evidence in a non-occupational healthcare setting the picture becomes less promising. Some RCTs, conducted in patients with chronic LBP, have compared graded activity-like interventions to active physical therapy (Smeets et al. 2008) and to guideline-based physiotherapy in primary care (van der Roer et al. 2008). Another RCT in acute and subacute patients found that augmenting physical therapy with either graded activity or graded exposure did not result in different effects at 6-month follow-up (George et al. 2008). The effects of graded activity versus usual care have also been investigated in patients recovering from first-time lumbar disc surgery but no effects were found in this study either (Ostelo et al. 2003).

Graded exposure *in vivo* is a cognitive-behavioural treatment approach that aims at restoring function by means of systematically reducing pain-related fear. Patients with LBP have to establish a personal graded hierarchy of fear-eliciting activities by using a series of photographs of daily activities (Leeuw et al. 2008). After that, they are gradually and systematically exposed to personally tailored and fear-provoking activities which are derived from the individual fear hierarchy based on the series of photographs (Leeuw et al. 2008). In an RCT, Woods and Asmundson compared graded exposure to graded activity and to a waiting-list group in a population of chronic LBP patients (Woods and Asmundson 2008). Significant effects were found in favour of the graded exposure group for several measures of pain-related fear compared to the other treatment conditions although not for pain-related disability (Woods and Asmundson 2008). More or less similar results were found in another RCT which compared graded exposure to graded activity over 6 months follow-up (Leeuw et al. 2008). No effects were found for symptoms and self-reported disability but graded exposure appeared to be superior in decreasing pain catastrophizing and perceived harmfulness (Leeuw et al. 2008).

Although some beneficial effects have been found in occupational settings, the overall evidence base for graded activity interventions is still not very strong. The same holds for graded exposure when compared with waiting-list controls and graded activity. Maybe these types of interventions are especially effective in particular subgroups of patients which need to be selected prior to the start of the intervention. Though this might seem an attractive hypothesis, it still needs to be confirmed in future studies.

## 28.6 **Exercise interventions to improve work endurance**

A number of exercise intervention trials for LBP have been specifically targeted to affected workers with the goal of facilitating a return to usual work or improving work endurance. These exercise programmes have been variously described as work conditioning, work hardening, functional restoration, physical conditioning, or function-centred rehabilitation. Although the content of work conditioning programmes has a substantial overlap with other types of exercise programmes, work conditioning programmes are usually tailored to meet the physical work demands of a specific job, and the primary goal of intervention is to reduce or prevent occupational disability. This can be accomplished by analysing job tasks, simulating physical job demands in exercise sessions, conducting exercise sessions in the workplace environment, advising to reduce awkward postures, and coaching to deal effectively with lingering or recurrent job discomfort. The impetus for work conditioning programmes has been to reduce the cost to the employer of sickness absence and disability associated with LBP, especially when pain is the result of a work injury. In recent years, however, the line between work conditioning and other exercise programmes has begun to blur as RTW has become a more prominent outcome in LBP treatment.

An extensive literature review of RCTs for work conditioning programmes among injured workers was conducted and published by the Cochrane Collaboration Group in 2003 (Schonstein et al. 2003), and this review captured most of the available trial results published before 2001. Eighteen RCTs involving work conditioning programmes were identified, and the authors concluded that work conditioning programmes were effective to reduce sick days for workers with chronic LBP (but not acute LBP) compared with usual care. However, this conclusion only applied to exercise programmes that: (1) integrated cognitive-behavioural approaches with intensive physical training (aerobic capacity, muscle strength and endurance, coordination); (2) were in some way work-related; and (3) were given and supervised by either a physiotherapist or a multidisciplinary team. Thus, there is a reasonable evidence base supporting the use of work conditioning programmes for working adults with chronic LBP, provided that the programme includes these characteristics. Other reviews published prior to 2003 (Guzman et al. 2001; Karjalainen et al. 2001; Teasell and Harth, 1996), presented more mixed conclusions, but a meta-analysis published in 2004 (Kool et al. 2004) also concluded that exercise programmes reduced sick leave in patients with non-acute, non-specific LBP.

One important result of the 2003 Cochrane Review (Schonstein et al. 2003) was to highlight differences and similarities among work conditioning programmes described in intervention trials. Some of the more significant contrasts between exercise programmes included: inpatient versus outpatient delivery, differences in programme duration (from 1 to 18 months), and differences in duration of follow-up (from 12 weeks to 12 months). Nearly all work conditioning programmes included a cognitive-behavioural component (to redirect patient goals toward functional improvement and away from pain relief), and most programmes involved direct patient supervision by a physiotherapist.

A number of RCTs of work conditioning programmes have been conducted since 2000, and many of these studies have sought to determine whether such programmes are cost-effective (Steenstra et al. 2003), how work conditioning programmes compare with other treatments (Jousset et al. 2004), and which patients are most likely to benefit (Hebert et al. 2008). These types of research questions have been driven by rapidly rising healthcare costs in many countries, which has led to an interest in making work conditioning programmes more streamlined or cost-effective. Other questions raised by researchers are whether benefits of work conditioning programmes might vary by the timing of intervention, by treatment confidence or other patient expectations, and by local contextual factors that relate to treatment settings and disability compensation systems (Staal et al. 2005).

One conclusion that can be drawn from studies of work conditioning programmes is that sickness absence can be further reduced if exercise is paired with a worksite visit, job modification, or other employer-based intervention (Karjalainen et al. 2001). For example, Loisel and colleagues (Loisel et al. 1997) found that a multidisciplinary work rehabilitation programme for workers with chronic LBP was more effective when combined with a workplace intervention employing participatory ergonomic approaches. This study was conducted with workers from participating employers who had expressed interest in improving disability outcomes. In a graded activity exercise trial that reduced lost days among airline workers, Staal and colleagues (Staal et al. 2004) also incorporated a number of workplace elements (return-to- work goal-setting, therapeutic modified duty, overcoming work avoidant beliefs) to improve outcomes. However, when workers are randomized from the general population, where employers may vary in their level of involvement and cooperation, an exercise programme may actually delay recovery. In a trial for subacute LBP (4–6 weeks absent from work), one study found that randomization to a graded activity exercise programme actually delayed RTW, while those randomized to a comparison workplace intervention had improved RTW outcomes (Anema et al. 2007). In summary, there is emerging evidence that a worksite visit and the cooperation of a supportive employer might be necessary to provide an effective bridge between supervised exercise and the realities of physical job requirements.

Recent studies have also highlighted the need for physiotherapists and other providers to consider psychological and workplace factors that might hinder recovery and the importance of incorporating appropriate counselling and advice as part of a restorative exercise protocol. Key workplace factors include heavy physical demands, the inability to modify work, job stress, an unsupportive workplace, job dissatisfaction, poor expectation of RTW, and fear of re-injury (Shaw et al. 2009). Key psychological factors include depressed mood, social isolation, pain catastrophizing, fear avoidant beliefs, and low self-efficacy for managing pain (Kendall and Burton 2009). While a work conditioning programme may not be sufficient to overcome all of these potential barriers to RTW, this information may be helpful for physiotherapists to set appropriate goals and expectations for an individualized work conditioning programme. Research is needed to improve screening methods of prognostic factors and relate these to specific strategies that might be employed in a work conditioning programme.

Efforts to identify subsets of patients most likely to benefit from work conditioning programmes have not been conclusive (van der Hulst et al. 2005). However, there is some evidence that a worker who believes work will inevitably lead to a more serious re-injury may be a good candidate for a work conditioning programme (George et al. 2008). This approach allows workers to experience gradual success in improved functional capacity, and this counters a pre-existing belief that increased activity will inevitably lead to increased pain. This has been offered as the explanation for work conditioning programmes to show greater improvements in self-reported work ability and lost days compared with conventional physiotherapy (Kool et al. 2005, 2007; Roche et al. 2007).

In summary, randomized trials have provided evidence that work conditioning programmes are effective to reduce sickness absences related to LBP, but it is unclear whether these benefits are mediated by increases in muscle strength or endurance, by improved coping strategies, or by global improvements in perceived health and self-efficacy. Work conditioning programmes may be more effective when they incorporate customized patient education and counselling and worksite visits.

## 28.7 **Conclusion**

Exercise is generally considered a valuable treatment strategy for subacute and chronic LBP. The study results summarized in this chapter confirm this common thought. Nevertheless, the presented results need to be interpreted with caution. In general, the effects which have been found and reported for physical exercises are rather small. The pooled effect estimates as described in the Cochrane review by Hayden and colleagues for subacute LBP were very small and not significant (i.e. 1.9 points at a 100-point scale for pain and 1.1 points at a 100-point scale for function) and somewhat larger (i.e. 7.3 points at a 100-point scale for pain and 2.5 points at a 100-point scale for function) but significant for chronic LBP (Hayden et al. 2005a). Although reaching statistical significance is important, the clinical importance of effect sizes should not be disregarded: are the effects important from the perspective of the back pain sufferer? Research has been done, also in the field of LBP, to determine which effect size could be considered clinically important (van Tulder et al. 2007). Based on earlier clinimetric studies between-group differences were considered clinically important if the magnitude was 20% or more for pain and 10% or more for functioning (van Tulder et al. 2007). Van Tulder and colleagues investigated to what extent the significant effects as reported in the Cochrane review on exercise therapy and LBP reached an appropriate level of clinical importance. Of the 18 trials in the Cochrane review which reported significant effects in favour of the exercise group only six reported effect sizes that met these standards of clinical importance (van Tulder et al. 2007). This implies that it is questionable whether the effects reported in at least two-third of the trials affect the pain and disability as perceived by the patient.

We can not conclude that one type of exercise is clearly more beneficial than other types of exercise since the differences between exercise therapies are either small or non-significant. If this is true, less intense exercise therapies are to be preferred especially when viewed from a cost-effectiveness perspective (Heymans et al. 2006). In clinical practice, patient preferences regarding exercise treatments should not be ignored since expectations, confidence, and satisfaction regarding the chosen treatment strategy can influence treatment success (Helmhout et al. 2008). Another challenge for back pain researchers is to find out if particular patient groups are more or less likely to respond to specific exercise programmes (Helmhout et al. 2008; Staal et al. 2008). Subgroup analyses in RCTs are therefore needed as well as clear characterization of study populations and exercise treatments which are matched to individual patient characteristics. It has been reported that a classification approach in order to match treatments to patients resulted in improved disability when compared with treatment unmatched to this classification (Brennan et al. 2006). Other studies indicated that patients with a directional preference to movement, had better results when they exercised in the preferred direction compared to exercises in a random direction or opposite direction (Long et al. 2004) and that patients with high fear-avoidance beliefs improve more with exercise treatment addressing fear-avoidance than with standard care (George et al. 2003). It has also been suggested that patients with relatively low levels of disability and fear-avoidance beliefs have higher chances of RTW as a result of a graded activity programme (Staal et al. 2008). Research on clinical prediction rules to predict who is likely to respond to an exercise programme is however still scarce and inconclusive (Hicks et al. 2005; Teyhen et al. 2007).

Although the evidence is not very strong, physical exercise can still be considered a beneficial and also safe strategy for LBP (Staal et al. 2005). The exact working mechanisms are not clear yet and may be related to improved aspects of physical fitness, altered mood, fears and behaviour, decreased sensitization, or combinations of these different mechanisms. Physical exercise matches well with an active self-management approach in which patients become more and more responsible for their back health. For a large majority of patients this could be followed by a physically active lifestyle with little support of care providers despite eventual still existing pain.

# References

Airaksinen, O., Brox, J. I., Cedraschi, C., *et al.* (2006). Chapter 4. European guidelines for the management of chronic nonspecific low back pain. *Eur Spine J*, **15**(Suppl 2), S192–300.

Anema, J. R., Steenstra, I. A., Bongers, P. M. *et al.* (2007). Multidisciplinary rehabilitation for subacute low back pain: graded activity or workplace intervention or both? A randomized controlled trial. *Spine*, **32**, 291–8.

Bergmark, A. (1989). Stability of the lumbar spine. A study in mechanical engineering. *Acta Orthop Scand Suppl*, **230**, 1–54.

Brennan, G. P., Fritz, J. M., Hunter, S. J., Thackeray, A., Delitto, A. & Erhard, R. E. (2006). Identifying subgroups of patients with acute/subacute "non-specific" low back pain: results of a randomized clinical trial. *Spine*, **31**, 623–31.

Brox, J. I., Sorensen, R., Friis, A. *et al.* (2003). Randomized clinical trial of lumbar instrumented fusion and cognitive intervention and exercises in patients with chronic low back pain and disc degeneration. *Spine*, **28**, 1913–21.

Brox, J. I., Storheim, K., Holm, I., Friis, A. & Reikeras, O. (2005). Disability, pain, psychological factors and physical performance in healthy controls, patients with sub-acute and chronic low back pain: a case-control study. *J Rehabil Med*, **37**, 95–9.

Cherkin, D. C., Deyo, R. A., Battie, M., Street, J. & Barlow, W. (1998). A comparison of physical therapy, chiropractic manipulation, and provision of an educational booklet for the treatment of patients with low back pain. *N Engl J Med*, **339**, 1021–9.

Chou, R. & Huffman, L. H. (2007). Nonpharmacologic therapies for acute and chronic low back pain: a review of the evidence for an American Pain Society/American College of Physicians clinical practice guideline. *Ann Intern Med*, **147**, 492–504.

Chou, R., Qaseem, A., Snow, V., *et al.* (2007). Diagnosis and treatment of low back pain: a joint clinical practice guideline from the American College of Physicians and the American Pain Society. *Ann Intern Med*, **147**, 478–91.

Clare, H. A., Adams, R. & Maher, C. G. (2004). A systematic review of efficacy of McKenzie therapy for spinal pain. *Aust J Physiother*, **50**, 209–16.

Critchley, D. J., Ratcliffe, J., Noonan, S., Jones, R. H. & Hurley, M. V. (2007). Effectiveness and cost-effectiveness of three types of physiotherapy used to reduce chronic low back pain disability: a pragmatic randomized trial with economic evaluation. *Spine*, **32**, 1474–81.

Davies, J. E., Gibson, T. & Tester, L. (1979). The value of exercises in the treatment of low back pain. *Rheumatol Rehabil*, **18**, 243–7.

Deyo, R. A., Rainville, J. & Kent, D. L. (1992). What can the history and physical examination tell us about low back pain? *JAMA*, **268**, 760–5.

Dufour, N., Thamsborg, G., Oefeldt, A., Lundsgaard, C., Stender, S. (2010). Treatment of chronic low back pain: a randomized, clinical trial comparing group-based multidisciplinary biopsychosocial rehabilitation and intensive individual therapist-assisted back muscle strengthening exercise. *Spine*, **35**, 469–76.

Elnaggar, I. M., Nordin, M., Sheikhzadeh, A., Parnianpour, M. & Kahanovitz, N. (1991). Effects of spinal flexion and extension exercises on low-back pain and spinal mobility in chronic mechanical low-back pain patients. *Spine*, **16**, 967–72.

Ferreira, P. H., Ferreira, M. L., Maher, C. G., Herbert, R. D. & Refshauge, K. (2006). Specific stabilisation exercise for spinal and pelvic pain: a systematic review. *Aust J Physiother*, **52**, 79–88.

Ferreira, M. L., Ferreira, P. H., Latimer, J., *et al.* (2007). Comparison of general exercise, motor control exercise and spinal manipulative therapy for chronic low back pain: A randomized trial. *Pain*, **131**, 31–7.

Fordyce, W. (1976). *Behavioral methods for chronic pain and illness.* St. Louis, MO: CV Mosby.

Frank, J. W., Brooker, A. S., Demaio, S. E., *et al.* (1996). Disability resulting from occupational low back pain. Part II: What do we know about secondary prevention? A review of the scientific evidence on prevention after disability begins. *Spine,* **21,** 2918–29.

George, S. Z., Fritz, J. M., Bialosky, J. E. & Donald, D. A. (2003). The effect of a fear-avoidance-based physical therapy intervention for patients with acute low back pain: results of a randomized clinical trial. *Spine,* **28,** 2551–60.

George, S. Z., Fritz, J. M. & Childs, J. D. (2008). Investigation of elevated fear-avoidance beliefs for patients with low back pain: a secondary analysis involving patients enrolled in physical therapy clinical trials. *J Orthop Sports Phys Ther,* **38,** 50–8.

Goldby, L. J., Moore, A. P., Doust, J. & Trew, M. E. (2006). A randomized controlled trial investigating the efficiency of musculoskeletal physiotherapy on chronic low back disorder. *Spine,* **31,** 1083–93.

Guzman, J., Esmail, R., Karjalainen, K., *et al* (2001). Multidisciplinary rehabilitation for chronic low back pain: systematic review. *BMJ,* **322,** 1511–16.

Haldorsen, E. M., Grasdal, A. L., Skouen, J. S., Risa, A. E., Kronholm, K. & Ursin, H. (2002). Is there a right treatment for a particular patient group? Comparison of ordinary treatment, light multidisciplinary treatment, and extensive multidisciplinary treatment for long-term sick-listed employees with musculoskeletal pain. *Pain,* **95,** 49–63.

Hamberg-Van Reenen, H. H., Ariens, G. A., Blatter, B. M., Van Mechelen, W. & Bongers, P. M. (2007). A systematic review of the relation between physical capacity and future low back and neck/shoulder pain. *Pain,* **130,** 93–107.

Hayden, J. A., Van Tulder, M. W., Malmivaara, A. V. & Koes, B. W. (2005a). Meta-analysis: exercise therapy for nonspecific low back pain. *Ann Intern Med,* **142,** 765–75.

Hayden, J. A., Van Tulder, M. W. & Tomlinson, G. (2005b). Systematic review: strategies for using exercise therapy to improve outcomes in chronic low back pain. *Ann Intern Med,* **142,** 776–85.

Hebert, J., Koppenhaver, S., Fritz, J. & Parent, E. (2008). Clinical prediction for success of interventions for managing low back pain. *Clin Sports Med,* **27,** 463–79, ix–x.

Helmhout, P. H., Staal, J. B., Maher, C. G., Petersen, T., Rainville, J. & Shaw, W. S. (2008). Exercise therapy and low back pain: insights and proposals to improve the design, conduct, and reporting of clinical trials. *Spine,* **33,** 1782–8.

Henschke, N., Maher, C. G., Refshauge, K. M., *et al.* (2008). Prognosis in patients with recent onset low back pain in Australian primary care: inception cohort study. *BMJ,* **337,** a171.

Heymans, M. W., De Vet, H. C., Bongers, P. M., Knol, D. L., Koes, B. W. & Van Mechelen, W. (2006). The effectiveness of high-intensity versus low-intensity back schools in an occupational setting: a pragmatic randomized controlled trial. *Spine,* **31,** 1075–82.

Hicks, G. E., Fritz, J. M., Delitto, A. & McGill, S. M. (2005). Preliminary development of a clinical prediction rule for determining which patients with low back pain will respond to a stabilization exercise program. *Arch Phys Med Rehabil,* **86,** 1753–62.

Hides, J. A., Stokes, M. J., Saide, M., Jull, G. A. & Cooper, D. H. (1994). Evidence of lumbar multifidus muscle wasting ipsilateral to symptoms in patients with acute/subacute low back pain. *Spine,* **19,** 165–72.

Hides, J. A., Richardson, C. A. & Jull, G. A. (1996). Multifidus muscle recovery is not automatic after resolution of acute, first-episode low back pain. *Spine,* **21,** 2763–9.

Hlobil, H., Staal, J. B., Twisk, J., *et al.* (2005). The effects of a graded activity intervention for low back pain in occupational health on sick leave, functional status and pain: 12-month results of a randomized controlled trial. *J Occup Rehabil,* **15,** 569–80.

Jousset, N., Fanello, S., Bontoux, L., *et al.* (2004). Effects of functional restoration versus 3 hours per week physical therapy: a randomized controlled study. *Spine,* **29,** 487–93; discussion 494.

Karjalainen, K., Malmivaara, A., Van Tulder, M., *et al.* (2001). Multidisciplinary biopsychosocial rehabilitation for subacute low back pain in working-age adults: a systematic review within the framework of the Cochrane Collaboration Back Review Group. *Spine,* **26,** 262–9.

Kendall, N. A., Burton, A.K. (2009). Tackling musculoskeletal problems: a guide for clinic and workplace. Identifying obstacles using the psychosocial flags framework. Norwich: TSO Information and Publishing Solutions (The Stationery Office).

Kladny, B., Fischer, F. C. & Haase, I. (2003). [Evaluation of specific stabilizing exercise in the treatment of low back pain and lumbar disk disease in outpatient rehabilitation]. *Z Orthop Ihre Grenzgeb*, **141**, 401–5.

Koes, B. W., Van Tulder, M. W., Ostelo, R., Burton, A. & Waddell, G. (2001). Clinical guidelines for the management of low back pain in primary care: an international comparison. *Spine*, **26**, 2504–13; discussion 2513–14.

Kool, J., De Bie, R., Oesch, P., Knusel, O., Van den Brandt, P. & Bachmann, S. (2004). Exercise reduces sick leave in patients with non-acute non-specific low back pain: a meta-analysis. *J Rehabil Med*, **36**, 49–62.

Kool, J. P., Oesch, P. R., Bachmann, S., Knuesel, O., *et al.* (2005). Increasing days at work using function-centered rehabilitation in nonacute nonspecific low back pain: a randomized controlled trial. *Arch Phys Med Rehabil*, **86**, 857–64.

Kool, J., Bachmann, S., Oesch, P., *et al.* (2007). Function-centered rehabilitation increases work days in patients with nonacute nonspecific low back pain: 1-year results from a randomized controlled trial. *Arch Phys Med Rehabil*, **88**, 1089–94.

Koumantakis, G. A., Watson, P. J. & Oldham, J. A. (2005). Trunk muscle stabilization training plus general exercise versus general exercise only: randomized controlled trial of patients with recurrent low back pain. *Phys Ther*, **85**, 209–25.

Leeuw, M., Goossens, M. E., Van Breukelen, G. J., *et al.* (2008). Exposure in vivo versus operant graded activity in chronic low back pain patients: results of a randomized controlled trial. *Pain*, **138**, 192–207.

Lindström, I., Ohlund, C., Eek, C., Wallin, L., *et al.* (1992). The effect of graded activity on patients with subacute low back pain: a randomized prospective clinical study with an operant-conditioning behavioral approach. *Phys Ther*, **72**, 279–90.

Loisel, P., Abenhaim, L., Durand, P., *et al.* (1997). A population-based, randomized clinical trial on back pain management. *Spine*, **22**, 2911–18.

Long, A., Donelson, R. & Fung, T. (2004). Does it matter which exercise? A randomized control trial of exercise for low back pain. *Spine*, **29**, 2593–602.

Macdonald, D. A., Moseley, G. L. & Hodges, P. W. (2006). The lumbar multifidus: does the evidence support clinical beliefs? *Man Ther*, **11**, 254–63.

Machado, L. A., Maher, C. G., Herbert, R. D., Clare, H. & Mcauley, J. (2005). The McKenzie Method for the management of acute non-specific low back pain: design of a randomised controlled trial [ACTRN012605000032651]. *BMC Musculoskelet Disord*, **6**, 50.

Macedo, L. G., Maher, C. G., Latimer, J. & Mcauley, J. H. (2009). Motor control exercise for persistent, nonspecific low back pain: a systematic review. *Phys Ther*, **89**, 9–25.

Mannion, A. F., Muntener, M., Taimela, S. & Dvorak, J. (1999). A randomized clinical trial of three active therapies for chronic low back pain. *Spine*, **24**, 2435–48.

Mannion, A. F., Muntener, M., Taimela, S. & Dvorak, J. (2001). Comparison of three active therapies for chronic low back pain: results of a randomized clinical trial with one-year follow-up. *Rheumatology (Oxford)*, **40**, 772–8.

Martin, P. R., Rose, M. J., Nichols, P. J., Russell, P. L. & Hughes, I. G. (1986). Physiotherapy exercises for low back pain: process and clinical outcome. *Int Rehabil Med*, **8**, 34–8.

May, S. & Donelson, R. (2008). Evidence-informed management of chronic low back pain with the McKenzie method. *Spine J*, **8**, 134–41.

Mayer, T.G. (2010). Point of view. *Spine*, **35**, 477.

Mckenzie, R. & May, S. (2003a). *The lumbar spine: Mechanical Diagnosis & Therapy*, vol. 1. Waikanae: New Zealand Spinal Publications.

Mckenzie, R. & May, S. (2003b). *The lumbar spine: Mechanical Diagnosis & Therapy*, vol. 2. Waikanae: New Zealand, Spinal Publications.

Miller, E., Schenk, R., Karnes, J. & Rousselle, J. (2005). A comparison of the McKenzie approach to a specific spine stabilization program for chronic low back pain. *The Journal of Manipulative and Manual Therapy,* **13**, 103–12.

Moffett, J. K., Torgerson, D., Bell-Syer, *et al.* (1999). Randomised controlled trial of exercise for low back pain: clinical outcomes, costs, and preferences. *BMJ,* **319**, 279–83.

Moseley, L. (2002). Combined physiotherapy and education is efficacious for chronic low back pain. *Aust J Physiother,* **48**, 297–302.

Niemisto, L., Lahtinen-Suopanki, T., Rissanen, P., Lindgren, K. A., Sarna, S. & Hurri, H. (2003). A randomized trial of combined manipulation, stabilizing exercises, and physician consultation compared to physician consultation alone for chronic low back pain. *Spine,* **28**, 2185–91.

O'Sullivan, P. B., Phyty, G. D., Twomey, L. T. & Allison, G. T. (1997). Evaluation of specific stabilizing exercise in the treatment of chronic low back pain with radiologic diagnosis of spondylolysis or spondylolisthesis. *Spine,* **22**, 2959–67.

Ostelo, R. W., De Vet, H. C., Vlaeyen, J. W., *et al.* (2003). Behavioral graded activity following first-time lumbar disc surgery: 1-year results of a randomized clinical trial. *Spine,* **28**, 1757–65.

Ostelo, R. W., Van Tulder, M. W., Vlaeyen, J. W., Linton, S. J., Morley, S. J. & Assendelft, W. J. (2005). Behavioural treatment for chronic low-back pain. *Cochrane Database Syst Rev,* **1**, CD002014.

Panjabi, M. M. (1992a). The stabilizing system of the spine. Part I. Function, dysfunction, adaptation, and enhancement. *J Spinal Disord,* **5**, 383–9.

Panjabi, M. M. (1992b). The stabilizing system of the spine. Part II. Neutral zone and instability hypothesis. *J Spinal Disord,* **5**, 390–6.

Pengel, L. H., Herbert, R. D., Maher, C. G. & Refshauge, K. M. (2003). Acute low back pain: systematic review of its prognosis. *BMJ,* **327**, 323.

Pengel, L. H., Refshauge, K. M., Maher, C. G., Nicholas, M. K., Herbert, R. D. & McNair, P. (2007). Physiotherapist-directed exercise, advice, or both for subacute low back pain: a randomized trial. *Ann Intern Med,* **146**, 787–96.

Pincus, T., Burton, A. K., Vogel, S. & Field, A. P. (2002). A systematic review of psychological factors as predictors of chronicity/disability in prospective cohorts of low back pain. *Spine,* **27**, E109–20.

Pincus, T., Vogel, S., Burton, A. K., Santos, R. & Field, A. P. (2006). Fear avoidance and prognosis in back pain: a systematic review and synthesis of current evidence. *Arthritis Rheum,* **54**, 3999–4010.

Rackwitz, B., De Bie, R., Limm, H., Von Garnier, K., Ewert, T. & Stucki, G. (2006). Segmental stabilizing exercises and low back pain. What is the evidence? A systematic review of randomized controlled trials. *Clin Rehabil,* **20**, 553–67.

Rasmussen-Barr, E., Nilsson-Wikmar, L. & Arvidsson, I. (2003). Stabilizing training compared with manual treatment in sub-acute and chronic low-back pain. *Man Ther,* **8**, 233–41.

Richardson, C. A. & Jull, G. A. (1995). Muscle control-pain control. What exercises would you prescribe? *Man Ther,* **1**, 2–10.

Roche, G., Ponthieux, A., Parot-Shinkel, E., *et al.* (2007). Comparison of a functional restoration program with active individual physical therapy for patients with chronic low back pain: a randomized controlled trial. *Arch Phys Med Rehabil,* **88**, 1229–35.

Schonstein, E., Kenny, D. T., Keating, J. & Koes, B. W. (2003). Work conditioning, work hardening and functional restoration for workers with back and neck pain. *Cochrane Database Syst Rev,* **1**, CD001822.

Shaughnessy, M. & Caulfield, B. (2004). A pilot study to investigate the effect of lumbar stabilisation exercise training on functional ability and quality of life in patients with chronic low back pain. *Int J Rehabil Res,* **27**, 297–301.

Shaw, W., Van der Windt, D., Main, C., Loisel, P., Linton, S. & the "Decade of the Flags" Working Group. (2009). Early patient screening and intervention to address individual-level occupational factors ("blue flags") in back disability. *J Occup Rehabil,* **19**, 64–80.

Smeets, R. J., Wade, D., Hidding, A., Van Leeuwen, P. J., Vlaeyen, J. W. & Knottnerus, J. A. (2006). The association of physical deconditioning and chronic low back pain: a hypothesis-oriented systematic review. *Disabil Rehabil, 28*, 673–93.

Spitzer, W. O., Leblanc, F.E., Dupuis, M. (1987). Scientific approach to the assessment and management of activity-related spinal disorders. A monograph for clinicians. Report of the Quebec Task force on Spinal disorders. *Spine, 12*, 1–59.

Staal, J. B., Hlobil, H., Twisk, J. W., Smid, T., Koke, A. J. & Van Mechelen, W. (2004). Graded activity for low back pain in occupational health care: a randomized, controlled trial. *Ann Intern Med, 140*, 77–84.

Staal, J. B., Rainville, J., Fritz, J., Van Mechelen, W. & Pransky, G. (2005). Physical exercise interventions to improve disability and return to work in low back pain: current insights and opportunities for improvement. *J Occup Rehabil, 15*, 491–505.

Staal, J. B., Hlobil, H., Koke, A. J., Twisk, J. W., Smid, T. & Van Mechelen, W. (2008). Graded activity for workers with low back pain: who benefits most and how does it work? *Arthritis Rheum, 59*, 642–9.

Standaert, C. J., Weinstein, S. M. & Rumpeltes, J. (2008). Evidence-informed management of chronic low back pain with lumbar stabilization exercises. *Spine J, 8*, 114–20.

Steenstra, I. A., Anema, J. R., Bongers, P. M., De Vet, H. C. & Van Mechelen, W. (2003). Cost effectiveness of a multi-stage return to work program for workers on sick leave due to low back pain, design of a population based controlled trial [ISRCTN60233560]. *BMC Musculoskelet Disord, 4*, 26.

Steenstra, I. A., Anema, J. R., Bongers, P. M., De Vet, H. C., Knol, D. L. & Van Mechelen, W. (2006). The effectiveness of graded activity for low back pain in occupational healthcare. *Occup Environ Med, 63*, 718–25.

Stevens, V., Grombez, G. & Parleviet, T. (2007). The effectiveness of specific exercise therapy versus device exercise therapy in the treatment of chronic low back pain patients. 6th Interdisciplinary World Congress of Low Back and Pelvic Pain. Barcelona.

Storheim, K., Brox, J. I., Holm, I., Koller, A. K. & Bo, K. (2003). Intensive group training versus cognitive intervention in sub-acute low back pain: short-term results of a single-blind randomized controlled trial. *J Rehabil Med, 35*, 132–40.

Stuge, B., Laerum, E., Kirkesola, G. & Vollestad, N. (2004). The efficacy of a treatment program focusing on specific stabilizing exercises for pelvic girdle pain after pregnancy: a randomized controlled trial. *Spine, 29*, 351–9.

Teasell, R. W. & Harth, M. (1996). Functional restoration. Returning patients with chronic low back pain to work – revolution or fad? *Spine, 21*, 844–7.

Teyhen, D. S., Flynn, T. W., Childs, J. D. & Abraham, L. D. (2007). Arthrokinematics in a subgroup of patients likely to benefit from a lumbar stabilization exercise program. *Phys Ther, 87*, 313–25.

Van der Hulst, M., Vollenbroek-Hutten, M. M. & IJzerman, M. J. (2005). A systematic review of sociodemographic, physical, and psychological predictors of multidisciplinary rehabilitation-or, back school treatment outcome in patients with chronic low back pain. *Spine, 30*, 813–25.

Van der Roer, N., Van Tulder, M., Barendse, J., Knol, D., Van Mechelen, W. & De Vet, H. (2008). Intensive group training protocol versus guideline physiotherapy for patients with chronic low back pain: a randomised controlled trial. *Eur Spine J, 17*, 1193–200.

Van Tulder, M., Becker, A., Bekkering, T., *et al.* (2006). Chapter 3. European guidelines for the management of acute nonspecific low back pain in primary care. *Eur Spine J, 15*(Suppl 2), S169–91.

Van Tulder, M., Malmivaara, A., Hayden, J. & Koes, B. (2007). Statistical significance versus clinical importance: trials on exercise therapy for chronic low back pain as example. *Spine, 32*, 1785–90.

Woods, M. P. & Asmundson, G. J. (2008). Evaluating the efficacy of graded in vivo exposure for the treatment of fear in patients with chronic back pain: a randomized controlled clinical trial. *Pain, 136*, 271–80.

Chapter 29

# Contextual Cognitive-Behavioural Therapy for Chronic Pain (Including Back Pain)

Lance M. McCracken

## 29.1 Introduction

Although many of the distressing and unwanted experiences of chronic pain are controllable to some extent or other, this is in most cases incomplete, and some attempts to control these experiences can themselves directly cause problems. It is possibly a cruel irony that many ways to attempt to reduce pain, in conditions of chronic pain, do not improve daily living but curtail it. This problem is illustrated in effects of prolonged rest, withdrawal from activity, or pain-related retirement. It is also illustrated in expense, time, and hope spent in the search for new treatments, and in adverse effects from medications. The choice to try to avoid pain typically includes costs. These often include reduced participation in what would otherwise be important activities and experiences for people with pain. Recent theoretical developments help us to understand how behaviour patterns can become dominated by experiences that ostensibly 'need' to be avoided, modified, or controlled, rather than guided by experiences of personal goals or values, and these theoretical developments are yielding new directions for treatment.

## 29.2 The history of behavioural and cognitive-behavioural approaches to chronic pain

There has been a natural and healthy evolution within the cognitive and behavioural therapies both for chronic pain and outside of work on chronic pain. It is worth reviewing this evolution. If we better understand the course this is taking, the work we do may better align with what is progressive in this process.

More than 40 years ago it was suggested that we could do better than to look at chronic pain as either a physical problem or a psychogenic problem and that we could take a direct interest in patient functioning and behaviour. It was further suggested that we could do this without requiring that we understand specific sources of the pain inside the skin, in the structures or functions of tissues or organs. This approach specifically called for a focus on patient behaviour, learning principles, and social circumstances as a means for understanding and for reducing the suffering and disability of those with chronic pain. This was called the 'operant behavioural' approach (Fordyce 1976). In turn, roughly 25 years ago, an expansion of this focus was called for, an expansion including patients' interpretations, beliefs, other cognitive processes, and pain coping strategies. This approach was referred to as 'cognitive-behavioural' or as cognitive-behavioural therapy (CBT; Turk et al. 1983).

During the four decades of developments in treatment for chronic pain a series of other developments also have occurred. These either were simply little discussed in relation to chronic pain, perhaps because they did not register as relevant during earlier times, or had not occurred until very recently. CBT for chronic pain had considerable early success and there may have been little reason to look elsewhere to improve upon the results obtained (e.g. Flor et al. 1992). These developments that were happening but not intersecting with the mainstream of CBT for chronic pain include, for example, mindfulness (Kabat-Zinn 1990), functional analytic psychotherapy (Kohlenberg and Tsai 1991), dialectical behaviour therapy (Linehan 1993), acceptance and commitment therapy (ACT, Hayes et al. 1999a), and, more recently, updated versions of traditional methods such as behavioural activation (e.g. Martell et al. 2004; Dimidjian et al. 2006), and an application of ACT for chronic pain called contextual cognitive-behavioural therapy (CCBT; McCracken et al. 2005). The chapter focuses on some of these developments, their implications for treatment of chronic pain, and research results that have accumulated in their favour.

## 29.3 **What is CCBT?**

CCBT is a version of Acceptance and Commitment Therapy (ACT) that developed as an interdisciplinary, primarily group-based, treatment format for chronic pain. It is an approach that arises from within the wider family of CBT for chronic pain (McCracken 2005a). It includes a broad, deep, and theoretically integrated conceptual model and adds a number of distinctive therapeutic processes to those that are currently available within CBT. Its theoretical foundation is what is called *functional contextualism* (Hayes et al. 1999a), an approach that is pragmatic, non-mechanistic, behaviourally-focused, and cognitive. CCBT integrates the differing emphases from the operant and cognitive behavioural approaches so that its analyses wholly consider the environment, overt behaviour, cognition, and emotion. The 'environment' within CCBT, however, is defined not merely as the 'outside world' around behaviour. It is defined with two dimensions, historical and situational, and is referred to as 'context'. Behaviour arises in situations due to the influences exerted by events present in these situations by virtue of the individual's unique history. Another way to say this is that a situation cannot be understood in its influence over behaviour except in relation to the history that gives the situation that influence or, loosely, its 'meaning'. This context is also 'transdermal,' it crosses the barrier of the skin, as elements of context invariably involve sensations in the body or content of cognitive responses, such as thoughts or images.

From a functional contextual standpoint cognitive and emotional experiences are considered in a particular fashion, not based on whether they have a maladaptive form or structure, but based on how they are coordinated with individual responses and patterns of behaviour. Here it is the influence exerted by thoughts and feelings that is of primary concern and not whether these feel uncomfortable or specify frightening or unwanted experiences. Thus, behaviour is considered contextually determined through relations with events in the environment, both inside and outside the skin, relations determined by the individual's history, most particularly in the form or their learning history, but also including their cultural and genetic history. This functional contextual philosophy entails a certain model of truth, such as the truth of a model of cause and effect. Hypotheses are not considered true or false in an ultimate sense, as in the type of truth that might exist as a reality waiting to be uncovered in nature. The model of truth here considers 'workability' as the criteria. An analysis is true when it effectively meets the goals laid out for the analyses. This is called a 'pragmatic' approach to truth as distinguishable from an objectivist or rationalist approach. This may seem an esoteric or unnecessary distinction but the spirit of it infuses both contextual behavioural science and therapy methods that emerge from it.

Within the CCBT framework people suffer largely from normal processes of thinking and language, from how these interact with direct experience, and from the ways these interactions engender psychological inflexibility (Hayes et al. 1999a; McCracken 2005). The processes underlying psychological inflexibility include experiential avoidance, cognitive fusion, values-failures, loss of contact with present moment, preoccupation with self-as-content, and failures of committed action (Hayes et al. 2006). The parallel therapeutic processes in relation to these include acceptance, cognitive defusion, values clarification and values-based action, moment-to-moment awareness, contact with self-as-context, and committed action. These processes are not wholly independent from each other, and they substantially overlap in the qualities they add to behaviour patterns. The purpose of this chapter is to review these processes underlying CCBT and summarize data supporting their applicability to chronic pain management.

## 29.4 **Acceptance of chronic pain**

We provided a number of functionally similar definitions of acceptance of chronic pain in the past (e.g. McCracken 1998; McCracken et al. 2004). In essence it is a willingness to actively contact pain. It is a quality of behaviour that is realistic, flexible, practical, and free from unnecessary restrictions from pain. It is the engagement in activity with pain present plus an absence of attempts to control or avoid pain (McCracken et al. 2004). The most commonly used measure of acceptance of pain is the Chronic Pain Acceptance Questionnaire (CPAQ; Geiser 1992; McCracken et al. 2004; Volwes et al. 2008).

Currently there are more than 35 published studies of acceptance of pain including experiments (e.g. Hayes et al. 1999b; Gutierrez et al. 2004; Masedo and Esteve 2007), clinical studies (e.g. McCracken 1998; McCracken and Eccleston 2003; Viane et al. 2003; McCracken et al. 2004, McCracken and Eccleston 2005; Cheung et al. 2008; Mason et al. 2008), and treatment outcome studies (Dahl et al. 2004; McCracken et al. 2005, 2007b; Volwes and McCracken 2008; Wicksell et al. 2008). All of these studies support the role of acceptance as a process that appears to lessen the impact of pain on behaviour. In the clinical studies employing both retrospective and prospective designs, acceptance of chronic pain has been shown to significantly correlate with patient physical, social, and emotional functioning, work status, and medication use. These relations hold independent of pain and relevant patient background variables, such as gender, age, education, and pain duration. It has been demonstrated that, in relation to key aspects of patient functioning, such as anxiety, depression, and physical and psychosocial disability, a measure of acceptance of chronic pain is a significantly better predictor than a commonly used measure of coping with pain (McCracken and Eccleston 2003; McCracken and Eccleston 2006), a measure of attention and vigilance to pain (McCracken 2007), and about equal to a measure of catastrophizing (Vowles et al. 2007).

It is possible to summarize the magnitude of the relations between acceptance of pain as measured by the CPAQ and measures of patient functioning. This can be done, for example, by selecting a number of studies that used similar measure of patient functioning and combining their findings. Four studies based on entirely independent samples were readily identified meeting these criteria (McCracken and Eccleston 2003; Nicholas and Asghari 2006; McCracken et al. 2007; Cheung et al. 2008). Table 29.1 shows the results from combining the correlation analyses of these studies. The mean correlations from these analyses (combined N=811) between the CPAQ total score and measures of anxiety, depression, physical disability, and psychosocial disability, were $r=0.59$, $r=0.60$, $r=0.39$, and $r=0.52$, respectively.

The constituent parts of acceptance as measured by the CPAQ, activity engagement and pain willingness, have been questioned with the suggestion that the pain willingness component is

**Table 29.1** Summary of correlation studies of acceptance of pain as measured with the CPAQ in relation to measure of patient, emotional, physical, and psychosocial functioning

| Domain of Functioning | Range r | Mean r |
|---|---|---|
| Anxiety | −0.44 to −0.72 | −0.60 |
| Depression | −0.56 to −0.66 | −0.59 |
| Physical Disability | −0.26 to −0.47 | −0.39 |
| Psychosocial disability | −0.42 to −0.63 | −0.52 |

Note: these data based on four independent studies, total N=811.

possibly unnecessary (Nicholas and Asghari 2006). Nonetheless, there are conceptual, empirical, and clinical bases for continued inclusion of both components (McCracken et al. 2007). In a recent study the dual factor structure of the CPAQ was replicated in a large sample (N=333) and confirmed in a second independent sample (N=308; Vowles et al. 2008). It was also discovered based on cluster analyses that most patients seeking treatment for chronic pain have relatively similar scores on both subscales of the CPAQ. However, in these data there was a large group (45% of the study sample) who were relatively high on one scale, activity engagement, and low on the other, pain willingness. These patients represent a group who essentially report they are active but they also report they must eliminate their pain. This group is interesting because this presentation is somewhat discordant. One might speculate that they are presenting their life as intact even though it is not, such as to portray a positive appearance. Possibly their life is intact in many ways but their pain experience is weighing heavily upon them mentally and emotionally. This latter group may be important to identify as their treatment needs may be very specific. Perhaps they will not require behavioural activation strategies or physical rehabilitation but some of psychological work do address a different range of mental or emotional impacts of pain. Other scenarios are possible as well. Perhaps these patients are the proverbial 'activity cyclers' or those who chronically overdo activity (e.g. McCracken and Samuel 2007) (reviewed in this volume in Chapters 15 and 27).

Acceptance can be open to a number of varying definitions and can be overall a difficult process to understand. For example, it is easy to assume that acceptance is a form of belief or way of thinking, such as a belief that pain is not controllable or the belief that it will be a permanent experience. It also has been likened to a form of positive thinking or belief, such as the belief that one can function with pain (Nicholas and Asghari 2006). From the patient's perspective, acceptance may have a negative quality or may be equated with giving up or quitting. In our applications of the term, it is not intended to mean any of these things. According to a particularly functional contextual definition it is a process that includes thinking and believing but is not determined solely by the content of thinking and believing. It is not an exclusively mental process but a quality of whatever action is taken in relation to pain. It is the quality of not struggling with it, of allowing room in experience for it, and being willing to have it present. Whether the person experiencing pain thinks or believes in these processes is another matter. It is not a global act of quitting but selective actions of quitting responses to pain that take pain as a barrier to functioning or as an experience that must change for healthy functioning to proceed. When acceptance is present in behaviour contact with pain coordinates awareness, observing, or flexible responding; not avoiding, wrestling, bracing or restricted responding. Positive thinking or optimistic beliefs may achieve an ostensibly similar behaviour pattern, but this may be a more limited version of the behaviour pattern, one that depends on the content of thoughts and beliefs and is hostage to the capriciousness of these.

## 29.5 **Cognitive de-fusion**

As humans we have at least one ability that other animals do not have: we can experience events located in other places and times as if they are present. When we do this we then respond accordingly, with the emotional experiences and actions occasioned by the influences these events hold, again, even though the events themselves are not present. It is our ability to speak and think and 'listen' to the content of speaking and thinking that makes this so. As a result much of the time we do not have direct contact with experiences around us in life but only with verbally constructed or modified versions of these experiences. Our day-to-day contact with the world around us is constantly filtered and our psychological experiences altered through our interpretations, evaluations, thoughts, and beliefs. 'Cognitive fusion' is the description of this process by which our thoughts become merged and undifferentiated from the events they describe or the person who has them (Hayes et al. 1999a).

Most versions of CBT include work with thoughts and beliefs in some way, whether that be, for example, a focus on identifying and restructuring irrational beliefs (Ellis 1994), or on disputing or altering automatic thoughts and schemas (Beck 1976). There are, however, many forms of CBT, and these focus on differing levels, forms, or processes of cognition and can apply differing methods for addressing these. This has led to the criticism that CBT lacks a unifying theory of change (David and Szentagotai 2006). In fact, studies of CBT in patients with anxiety and depression have questioned whether changes in dysfunctional attitudes are primarily responsible for benefits of CBT (Burns and Spangler 2001) and whether methods directed at change in automatic thoughts or core schemas are necessary for positive treatment outcomes (Jacobson et al. 1996; Dimidjian et al. 2006). A comprehensive review of component analysis and mediation studies of CBT found little evidence for the role of cognitive change as causal in the symptom improvements achieved in CBT (Longmore and Worrell 2007).

The model of cognition and cognitive processes underlying CCBT is based directly on the approach from ACT (Hayes et al. 1999a). Within this approach cognitive processes are considered at two levels, the level of content, including the form or frequency of thoughts, and the level of function or context, including the situation that determines the impact thoughts exert on other responses. While treatment methods may include a focus on either level, a relative emphasis in CCBT and ACT is placed on contextual change. Notice, however, that when treatment methods imply that cognitive content determines behaviour and that cognitive change is necessary for behaviour change, this increases the behaviour regulatory influences of thoughts, which, ironically, holds the potential to create greater difficulties.

A core therapeutic process in ACT is what is called 'cognitive defusion'. This process entails a loosening of the influence of thought content on behaviour and increasing contact between behaviour and potential influences beyond thought content. Through methods that promote cognitive defusion, the chronic pain sufferer becomes more aware of the *process* of thinking, and less entangled in the *content* of thinking. From this process they can respond more flexibly while in contact with otherwise distressing, discouraging, or restricting thoughts. Cognitive defusion means a weakening of the role of thoughts as the sole or overwhelming basis for action without necessarily reformulating the content of thoughts. This does not mean blocking thoughts or even reducing 'attention' to thoughts, but does include contacting thoughts in a particular way. By bringing behaviour in contact with thoughts in a defused and less exclusive fashion, and altering the way they are experienced, in a broader context, cognitive defusion allows free and healthy action without the necessity of positive thoughts and beliefs. This is particularly helpful when positive thoughts or beliefs can be impossible to achieve or to maintain.

Cognitive defusion methods generally approach thought content indirectly. These methods include the use of metaphor, paradox, humour, confusion, and experiential exercises

(Hayes et al. 1999a). They typically do not include logical confrontation, direct verbal persuasion, or empirical verification (Hayes et al. 1999a). Again, methods that seek to directly reformulate the content of thoughts tend to emphasize the importance of this content and of changing it and therefore tend to solidify the controlling role of thoughts over behaviour rather than dismantle it. Responses that attempt to change thought content are themselves responses controlled by that thought content.

Confrontation of dysfunctional beliefs and cognitions, as is done in cognitive therapy can achieve a degree of cognitive defusion. These methods typically include methods to identify thoughts *as thoughts* and then include recording this on paper and looking at the reality around these thoughts. Each of these methods, which on the surface form part of a process of changing thoughts, can as a side effect alter the influence of the thought even before the stage at which a more rational or accurate thought is concocted. Again, the potential drawback of methods that direct themselves at change in content is that they can emphasize the necessity of rational thinking and reinforce the behavioural imperative of doing, or feeling emotionally, what the literal content of thought demands one to do or feel.

Methods for targeting cognitive fusion include exercises that raise awareness of: (1) the experience of having a thought rather than being stuck in the content of the thought; (2) the experience of difficulties presented by trying to control thoughts; (3) the un-workability of following some thought content; and (4) the ability to act according to what the person feels is important while in contact with thoughts that 'say' otherwise. These forms of 'awareness' so to speak add certain qualities to subsequent behaviour creating flexibility in the relationship between thoughts and action.

## 29.6 Values clarification and values-based action

'Values' can be defined as chosen life directions. They are qualities of behaviour that reflect what the individual cares most about in their life. Values are an individual's answers to the question, 'What do you want your life to stand for?' (Hayes et al. 1999a). Values-based processes are particularly useful in chronic pain when the pain sufferer's behaviour has become stuck in a focus on pain, and other unwanted experiences, and has lost contact with what they would otherwise hold as most important. For many chronic pain sufferers daily life can be about struggling with pain, trying to control it, and seeking relief from, it. As this dominates their daily activity, their interests in family, friends, intimate relations, work, and health, or other concerns become subordinated. A focus on clarifying values, on making them present when choices appear, and on enhancing values-based action, can counter a nearly exclusive focus on pain as the primary guide for action.

Values-related processes have been discussed in relation to a number of differing psychological treatment approaches in the past, including client-centred therapy (Rogers 1964) and motivational interviewing (Wagner and Sanchez 2002). However, values do not appear to have been explicitly emphasized in CBT in the past as they have been in ACT and CCBT. Notice, values are not the same as goals. Goals have a primarily practical, concrete, and achievable quality and values do not. Values are chosen ongoing directions. Goals tend to be future-focused and outcome oriented. Values are present focused and process oriented. A number of recent attempts to measure values-related processes have arisen from this new emphasis, both in general samples (Wilson and Murrell 2004) and in individuals with chronic pain (McCracken and Yang 2006; McCracken and Vowles 2008).

We developed a brief measure of values and values-based action in a study of 140 consecutive patients with chronic pain seen for an assessment in a specialty pain centre in the UK. This measure is called the Chronic Pain Values Inventory (CPVI; McCracken and Yang 2006). The CPVI asks patients to consider the values they hold in domains of family, intimate relations, friends, work, health, and growth or learning. They are first asked to rate the importance with which they hold their values and then the success they have had in living according to them, both on a 0–5 scale. Results from this study demonstrated that patients' importance ratings in each domain are significantly higher than their success ratings. As predicted, average success ratings positively correlated with acceptance of pain and negatively correlated with a self-report measure of pain-related avoidance. These average success ratings also significantly correlated with measures of disability, depression, and pain-related anxiety. In regression analyses, these ratings accounted for significant variance in these same variables independent of acceptance of pain, suggesting that these two processes combined can account for significant unique variance in patient functioning (McCracken and Yang 2006). A later study of chronic pain sufferers conducted prospectively, over an 18.5-week interval, showed similar results, that acceptance of pain and values-based action in combination measured at one time account for significant variance (6.5% to 27.0%) in pain-related distress, depression, and disability at the later point in time (McCracken and Vowles 2008).

Values clarification is often a challenging process, sometimes fraught with emotional or practical barriers (Hayes et al. 1999a). It requires in most cases that patients consider circumstances that may be very distressing. When people honestly identify what they care most about and at the same time realize they are not acting in accord with that, they may experience painful feelings of loss, embarrassment, shame, or guilt. This distress from clarifying values may lead patients to avoid doing so, such as during treatment. Further, many people find it difficult to identify what is important to them in a way that is not significantly influenced, or even completely obscured, by what significant others or society in general regard as important. This can produce actions that are superficial or lack deep meaning for a person. Taking a course of action to avoid disapproval from others is negatively controlled and is not the same behaviour pattern as taking it under positive influences, in the service of what one about cares most. Finally, patients may immediately dismiss particular directions their lives may take and label them as 'impossible.' This dismissal and automatic judgement, however, may be misleading and may unnecessarily exclude a real possibility, even if the possible movements in the direction of the value in question are small or slow (Hayes et al. 1999a; McCracken 2005a).

## 29.7 **Mindfulness**

Chronic pain sufferers, like any one of us, can find themselves excessively 'caught up' with their thoughts and their own reactions to sensations in their body, and their emotional experiences. This entanglement can lead to disorganized, impulsive, or ineffective behaviour. They can have the natural pain, stress, and unwanted experiences in life magnified in their effects on their behaviour by the ways they struggle, defend against, and harden their stance toward these things. They may multiply their distress by feeling and acting distressed about their distress, and so on (e.g. McCracken and Keogh, 2009). These processes entail a loss of contact with the present moment and a tendency to react to experiences automatically in ways that hinder healthy functioning. A therapeutic response to counteract these processes of suffering is training in a skill set including direct, present-focused, and accepting awareness, or what is called mindfulness (Kabat-Zinn 1990). Said in a more technical fashion, mindfulness is a process of contact with experiences, such as thoughts, mental images, urges, and emotional feelings that alters some of the otherwise automatic and misleading functions of these experiences. The predominant attitudes of mindfulness include openness, curiosity, and compassion.

Mindfulness differs from better-known methods such as relaxation, for example. Relaxation is often done for the specific purpose of controlling what is experienced, usually to reduce distressing sensations or emotions. Mindfulness, on the other hand, is done for the purpose of simply being aware of sensations and emotions without doing anything else about them. Guided imagery exercises are another example. Imagery exercises are often done to change the content of what is being experienced in order to gain the emotional, physical, or behavioural effects that come with that. Mindfulness is done to observe and learn about whatever content spontaneously occurs in experience while also maintaining a connection with the present moment, an attitude of interest, but a neutral attitude with respect to needing to take any action. There are many types of mindfulness exercises. Some of these include a focus on the body, on sensations of breathing, or on sensations during movement (Kabat-Zinn 1990), and some include the use of an imagined scene as a framework for contacting one's experiences mindfully (Hayes et al. 1999a).

Although mindfulness has been of formal interest within pain management for more than 20 years, there is still a relative lack of evidence regarding its usefulness. There are uncontrolled trials supporting the role of mindfulness-based methods in treatment for chronic pain (Kabat-Zinn et al. 1985; Kaplan et al. 1993). Meta-analyses of mindfulness-based treatments for a range of conditions including pain also conclude that these treatments are of potential benefit for those with chronic pain (Baer 2003; Grossman et al. 2004). There are three recent randomized trials of mindfulness that have produced significant results in relation to symptoms of depression in women with fibromyalgia (Sephton et al. 2007), in relation to acceptance of pain and for physical functioning in older adults (Morone et al. 2008), and in relation to coping, emotional functioning, and joint tenderness in patients with rheumatoid arthritis, particularly those with a history of depression (Zautra et al. 2008).

Relatively few studies of mindfulness have attempted to measure the process or processes involved and examine them in relation to measures of patient functioning. We completed a study of mindfulness in patients with chronic pain (McCracken et al. 2007) in which we administered the Mindful Attention Awareness Scale (MAAS; Brown and Ryan 2003) to a sample of 105 consecutive patients seeking specialty treatment in the UK. The MAAS is a 15-item measure of mindfulness in which all of the item content is negatively-keyed (i.e. 'I could be experiencing some emotion and not be conscious of it until some time later,' 'I find it difficult to stay focused on what's happening in the present,' 'I find myself preoccupied with the future or the past'). Items are rated from 1 ('almost always') to 6 ('almost never') and are summed to produce a single summary score. Correlation analyses of the MAAS showed that mindfulness was positively correlated with acceptance of pain (r=0.28), as predicted. It was also negatively correlated with measures of pain-related distress, anxiety, depression, interference with cognitive functioning, and pain medication use. In multiple regression analyses in which age, gender, education, duration of pain, pain intensity, and acceptance of pain, were entered first, mindfulness accounted for significant increments in explained variance for five of eight measures of patient functioning, including depression, pain-related anxiety, as well as physical, psychosocial, and 'other' disability. The strength of these results with regard to mindfulness is highlighted by the fact that acceptance of pain, entered before mindfulness in each equation, is a reliably strong predictor of patient functioning. Mindfulness was a particularly good predictor of depression where it accounted for 11.0% of the variance after the series of other potential predictors were taken into account. The variance in these equations accounted for by acceptance of pain and mindfulness combined averaged 28.0% across the eight equations (McCracken et al. 2007).

Acceptance, ACT, and mindfulness are often discussed together, particularly in relation to 'expanding the cognitive-behavioural tradition' (e.g. Hayes et al. 2004). There is clearly a shared sensibility between ACT and mindfulness but these approaches come from different traditions: ACT from the behaviour analytic side of the cognitive and behavioural therapies, a family of therapy approaches that are no more than 50 years old; and mindfulness from eastern spiritual practices, practices that are about 3000 years old. ACT includes six partly overlapping therapeutic processes: acceptance, contact with the present, values-based action, committed action, self-as-context, and cognitive defusion (Hayes et al. 2006). Although this does not appear in formal technical analyses or in popular definitions of mindfulness, mindfulness appears to include four of these ACT processes: acceptance, contact with the present, self-as-context, and cognitive defusion.

There is only one study we have identified in which processes underlying mindfulness were investigated in a sample of people with chronic pain. This is a study that again used the MAAS (McCracken and Thompson 2009). This study of mindfulness included 150 persons seeking treatment for chronic pain. There data from the MAAS were factor analysed and yielded four factors: Acting with Awareness (e.g. 'I could be experiencing some emotion and not be conscious of it until some time later'), Present Focus (e.g. I find myself preoccupied with the future or the past'), Responsiveness (e.g. 'I tend not to notice feelings of physical tension or discomfort until they really grab my attention'), and Social Awareness (e.g. 'I forget a person's name almost as soon as I've been told it for the first time'). Subsequent correlation analyses showed that just two of these factors: Acting with Awareness and Present Focus appeared to account for the relations of the overall mindfulness process with measures of emotional, physical, and social functioning in these patients. In fact, the Present Focus factor emerged as the strongest predictor of patient functioning, achieving particularly strong correlations with psychosocial disability, r = −0.60, and depression, r = −0.60, both p < 0.001 (See Figure 29.1).

## 29.8 **Chronic pain in a social context**

While social influence is widely acknowledged in chronic pain, current models of social influence appear limited. These models are often univariate, mechanistic, static, or unidirectional

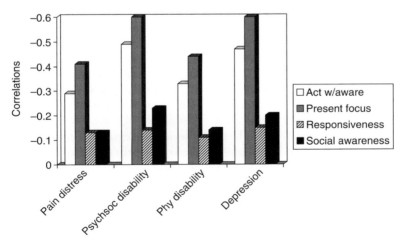

**Fig. 29.1** Correlations of mindfulness factors from the Mindful Attention Awareness Scale with measures of patient functioning (N=150). Note: correlations marked by bars above the dashed line significant at p <0.05. Pain distress measured with a 0–10 rating from 'not at all distressing' to 'extremely distress;' psychosocial and physical disability measures with the Sickness Impact Profile (Bergner et al. 1981); and depression measured with the British Columbia Major Depression Inventory (Iverson and Remick 2004). Data from McCracken and Thompson (2009).

(e.g. Peat et al. 2004; Schwartz et al. 2005). A functional contextual approach to chronic pain has several implications for the role of social influence in chronic pain and suffering. These include a potentially more incisive and complex analysis of the role of significant others in chronic pain (McCracken, 2005b), models of 'self' and identity (Crombez et al. 2003) and the role of social influences in the context of treatment (McCracken 2005a).

Social influence on chronic pain has been of interest to researcher and clinicians for at least 40 years. For most of that time, however, the role of social responses in chronic pain has been considered in relation to processes of reinforcement or punishment for overt displays of pain and disability, so-called 'pain behaviour' (Fordyce 1976). Alternately, social influence has also been considered in relation to buffering or stressing effects on emotional experience of chronic pain (Cano et al. 2004; reviewed in this volume in Chapter 17). A complete social analysis of chronic pain from a functional contextual approach is well beyond the scope of this chapter. However, a few illustrative examples of how social influence might be analysable from a more contextual approach are possible (McCracken 2005b).

One important point is to observe that people engage in behaviour strongly determined by social experience everyday of their life, even when there are no other people present, and obviously this will be true for chronic pain sufferers. This is a key distinction, from a contextual standpoint, what makes behaviour socially determined is not the immediate presence of others but a history of social influence that coordinates the current behaviour. When patients have experiences of guilt, shame, humiliation, self-criticism, and even anger, these experiences, the behaviour that attends them, and the relationship between the two is certainly social in origin.

Surely social and non-social influences will be woven together in complex ways and social influence may be present where it is not expected. For example, a person with pain who responds to experiences of that pain with activity avoidance may have that pattern so tightly controlled by present experiences of thoughts and emotions that other immediate social influences play little role. In contrast, consider social aspects of learning by instruction or observing the behaviour of others, or consider the social roots of guilt and how strong an influence guilt can play over behaviour patterns.

The apparent solicitousness or aversiveness of a social response may have little to do with its effect on behaviour and again there may be unexpected results. For example, a patient who acts with increasing avoidance and passivity may have this behaviour pattern strengthened (not weakened) if it meets angry or frustrated reactions from their environment, particularly if they feel invalidated or like their pain experience is not being treated as legitimate. Most of us will rigidly defend against being disbelieved. On the other hand a patient whose difficulties in functioning meet offers of help may respond by hiding these difficulties in the future or by struggling to carry on without help, such as when receiving help includes feeling dependent on others, like a burden, or like an 'invalid.' Either of these ostensibly different patterns could strengthen a pattern of behaviour that limits functioning in the longer term (McCracken 2005a, 2005b). From the perspective presented here it is not the appearance of the response as either 'solicitous' or 'punishing' that is critical but it is the psychological context in which it occurs, including the pain sufferer's history, that gives those responses their meaning and function.

There are many different conceptualizations of 'self.' For example, the self can be understood as an object or subject, 'self-as known' or 'self-as-knower' (James 1950). There is general agreement that our sense of self is essentially social in origin (James 1950; Skinner 1953). We increasingly learn who we are, in a sense, as this becomes important for others. In turn, we experience an inclination to act consistently with this sense of our self (Hayes et al. 1999a). To act unpredictably or 'not like our self' is often experienced as aversive by other and is discouraged in their responses. From another viewpoint, however, this sense of self of social origin is basically a story, a constructed or conceptualized sense of self that is not the same as the actual person as a human being or biological organism.

A number of different problems can arise from this situation of the conceptualized self for those with chronic pain. Social pressure for behavioural consistency will inevitably come to bear on chronic pain sufferers. This is particularly pertinent in situations where such consistency is either impossible or unworkable. Chronic pain is associated with changes in roles and behaviour, changes that occur in relation to private experiences that cannot be observed and are not fully understood by others. This can be distressing, such as when expectations from others are not met, and this lead them to criticize or express disappointment. It can also be restricting on functioning, such as when essentially arbitrary social influences press for behaviour patterns that are consistent to the outside observer but essentially ineffective.

It is a natural process of thinking and speaking in a social context that we can come to hold too tightly onto a certain sense or our self, a self made up of our thoughts and beliefs about who we are. This self we can refer to as 'self-as-content' (Hayes et al. 1999a). For chronic pain sufferers strongly held beliefs such as 'I never need help from others,' 'I never quit,' 'I am always happy,' 'I never talk about my feelings,' or 'I am always the victim,' can rigidly determine behaviour patterns and prevent change in behaviour that would otherwise entail better functioning. If the belief 'I never need help from others' is defended in action as a matter of personal identity, seeking help, even when this is the most effective available action, may not occur. Likewise, if the belief 'I never quit' is followed in the face of a behaviour pattern that consistently meets unwanted consequences, whether this be in seeking medical treatments that consistently fail, staying in an unhealthy relationship, or following an unrealistic program of physical exercise, then this behaviour pattern is unworkable. From this type of analysis treatment approaches for chronic pain can advocate the development in treatment of a different sense of self, a self that is not determined in the content of thought and belief, but emerges as an awareness of this content, a sense of self as the location where this content occurs, a sense of 'self as context' (Hayes et al. 1999a; McCracken 2005a).

Many individuals with complex problems of chronic pain will have experienced the feeling of being disbelieved, may be highly attuned to this possibility in subsequent healthcare visits, and may want to avoid it. This is understandable. To suffer and to have the legitimacy of that suffering doubted can be to feel accused of lying, or that one will be abandoned with uncontrollable pain. This is a situation any person would fight to avoid. And perhaps the most natural response to this situation is to try to 'prove' there is something wrong. When the pain sufferer's behaviour is under this kind of influence it is a serious dilemma for treatment. It might be difficult or impossible for a person to prove they are suffering and to recover lost functioning at the same time. As the consequences associated with being disbelieved are often painful or frightening, even actions that hint at disbelief may be experienced as such. For example, to imply that certain activities may be done without pain relief may be to send a message that sounds illogical or expresses disbelief. Requests for actions that appear 'impossible' can feel de-legitimizing, and can be experienced as discounting a person's pain, even if these are expressed with the best of intentions.

Treatments like CCBT are intensive and highly emotionally evocative. They require great care in the development of the relationships between treatment participants and treatment providers. A primary focus of treatment includes creating occasions when patients will contact painful experiences, specifically as these are a necessary part of making the changes they desire. It is typically on these occasions in daily life that the patient's behaviour is failing to serve their goals and values. These occasions provide the opportunity for developing different and more effective actions, actions that engender flexibility rather than struggling or avoidance. In order to effectively deliver treatment of this type, treatment providers will need a well developed analysis or conceptualization of the behaviour problems being targeted. They will also require repeated patient consent, and adequate rapport to create occasions that are clinically relevant and unlikely to punish the very behaviour patterns that are trying to be developed (Kohlenberg and Tsai 1991).

It is presumed that effective therapeutic behaviour will require psychological flexibility on the part of the treatment provider, including acceptance of painful psychological experiences, contact with the present moment, values-based action, and cognitive defusion. In our work we have shown that these qualities in healthcare worker behaviour are correlated with greater health and well-being in healthcare provider themselves and in less hindrance from patients' pain in the performance of work-related activities (McCracken and Yang 2008), however, we have not yet demonstrated fully that these qualities produce better treatment results, again, as we presume they will. This will require further study.

## 29.9 **Treatment outcome from contextual approaches to chronic pain**

Despite the relatively recent development of contextual approaches, there are now many published randomized controlled trials of these approaches for a range of behaviour problems. This includes at least 20 published trials of ACT in a wide range of clinical areas (Hayes et al. 2006) and more than six trials of mindfulness-based methods in relation to chronic pain alone (Baer et al. 2003). There are two published, small-scale, randomized trials of ACT related to chronic pain (Dahl et al. 2004; Wicksell et al. 2008) and at least three other effectiveness trails of ACT-based treatment that did not include randomization to separate treatment conditions (McCracken et al. 2005, 2007; Vowles and McCracken 2008).

Of the two randomized trials of ACT related to chronic pain one applied this approach to persons at risk for long-term disability due to pain and stress in a work setting (Dahl et al. 2004). This trial showed dramatically reduced missed workdays and healthcare use from four hours of treatment. The other ACT trial in this area included persons with chronic pain associated with whiplash in a specialty pain centre (Wicksell et al. 2008). This trial showed significant improvements in disability, life satisfaction, fear, and depression from 10 sessions. Both of these studies were conducted in Sweden. Both included 'treatment as usual' as the control condition.

All three of our treatment trials were conducted as analyses of an actual ongoing tertiary care treatment service operating within the National Health Service in the UK. This service is designed for people with highly complex cases of chronic pain that have repeatedly failed to benefit from other primary and secondary care services. As mentioned, in this respect our analyses of treatment outcome results are a test of the application of a treatment model to actual clinical practice and are therefore more akin to effectiveness studies than efficacy trials. Further, as a publicly funded national specialty service, providing services to pain sufferers who have few other options, our patient selection criteria for services are particularly inclusive.

Our first study of treatment outcome included 108 chronic pain sufferers, about half of whom reported back pain as their primary problem (McCracken et al. 2005). They participated in 3- or 4-week, group-based, treatment delivered by an interdisciplinary team of physiotherapists, occupational therapists, nurses, physicians, and clinical psychologists. This treatment included graded physical conditioning, exposure-based methods, skills training, education, mindfulness training, and experiential psychological methods based on the ACT and CCBT model (McCracken 2005a). The comparison condition for this study consisted of data from a waiting interval priory to treatment that was an average of 3.9 months in duration. Hence there was no randomization to conditions.

The analyses in our first treatment study were based on outcome measures collected at initial assessment, the start of treatment, immediately post treatment, and at a three-month follow-up visit for a consecutive sample. Results showed that patient functioning remained unchanged during the waiting phase prior to treatment but significantly improved in nine key domains following treatment and remained significantly improved on all measured domains at follow-up. These domains included pain, depression, pain-related anxiety, physical disability, psychosocial disability, daily rest, walking speed, activity tolerance, and medication use (all p <0.001). Other results showed that acceptance of pain significantly increased during treatment and changes in acceptance were significantly correlated with changes in other key outcome variables (McCracken et al. 2005).

In our second outcome study we examined clinically significant change in a subset of highly disabled patients (n=53), about 60% of whom reported back or whole body pain (McCracken et al. 2007). These are patients we treat in a hospital-based course because they have extremely limited mobility and self-care and thus are unable to participate in any pain management course without nursing support for transfers, mobility, bathing, or dressing. These patients significantly improved at post treatment in pain-related distress, physical and psychosocial disability, depression, anxiety, directly assessed activity tolerance, and hours spent resting during the day due to pain. The average effect size across outcome variables was $d = 0.75$. Based on analyses that take into account degree of temporal stability in outcome measures (Jacobson et al. 1999), 47.6% of patients demonstrated reliable improvement in total disability and 61.9% demonstrated reliable improvement in depression scores. Applying criteria for 'recovery' based on level of post treatment functioning of successfully treated standard cases from our service, 52.8% of the highly disabled patients met criteria for clinical recovery in a least one primary outcome domain, including physical or psychosocial disability, or depression (McCracken et al. 2007). This is equivalent to saying that for every 1.9 highly disabled patients treated with this approach one achieves recovery in at least one key domain of functioning. It will be noticed that once again there was no randomization to an active or control condition. All patients were assigned to active treatment. The design allowed for pre to post comparisons and comparison between two groups who differed in their initial level of disability.

In our most recent investigation we examined treatment outcome and process in 171 consecutive patients that were an entirely independent sample from the previous trials (Vowles and McCracken 2008). As with the previous trials the effects of treatment were broad, as reflected in multiple measures of pain, emotional, physical, and social functioning, healthcare use, and directly assessed physical performances. Effect sizes at post treatment averaged $d = 1.07$ and at three month follow-up averaged $d = 0.89$. Based on reliable change analyses 75.4% of patients were reliably improved in at least one domain, including anxiety, depression, or disability. Change in the combined processes of acceptance of pain and values-based action accounted for significant variance in improvements during treatment or at follow-up in each of seven key measures of functioning. Average variance accounted for at post treatment was 15% and at follow-up was 17%.

## 29.10 **Summary**

In many ways our main cognitive-behavioural treatment methods for chronic pain have stayed very much the same for the past 25 years. Perhaps this is a product of early success (Flor et al. 1992). There could be other factors: a lack of a truly well-integrated and progressive theory of human behaviour and suffering. Maybe there were other battles, such as to hold onto some piece of territory in a field where psychological methods are clearly the underdog. Psychological methods for pain are set in a culture where solutions for pain that look like a fix, including medications or even high technology devices, have much greater immediate appeal. These apparent solutions it seems are much more enticing than approaches that require learning, facing discomfort and uncertainty, approaches that say the answer to your pain requires change in your behaviour.

At the same time that CBT for pain was enjoying its successes clinical psychology outside of pain management has been growing and changing faster than inside pain management. This is an impression, said with no data. If it is true, what does it mean?

Increasing research findings outside of pain management and, increasingly, inside of pain management, demonstrate that there is more than one way to live a full life when one has been suffering with chronic pain. Methods available from CBT as it has been practised for 25 years are one way (Morley et al. 1999). These methods are varied but tend to include training in coping and methods designed predominantly to change, control, or decrease unwanted physical and emotional feelings, or dysfunctional or misleading thoughts and beliefs (e.g. Williams et al. 1996; DeJong et al. 2005). Another way, rather than coping with or attempting to control feelings, thoughts, or beliefs, is to a focus on contextual change around all of the painful and discouraging experiences that arise with chronic pain.

Contextually-based therapies, like ACT and CCBT or mindfulness-based approaches, aim to manipulate the contextual elements that afford psychological experiences their influence over behaviour patterns. They do not primarily aim to manipulate the content of psychological experiences themselves. They aim not to decrease sensations, emotions and thoughts but to modify how they are experienced. Contextual change is not superficial. It attempts to get to the roots from which suffering and behaviour disruption emerge, largely in the interaction of processes of language and cognition with direct experience. Contextual processes are perhaps less naturally apparent in our everyday experience. Contextual methods are perhaps subtle, sometimes illogical, metaphorical or paradoxical, not dominantly change-oriented, and typically flexible in their balance between change and acceptance.

There are now more than ten recent trials investigating contextual approaches for chronic pain, including acceptance or mindfulness-based methods. Six of these are fully randomized and controlled and some of the remaining ones are non-randomized or partially controlled effectiveness studies. Most of controlled studies are small in scale. Findings from these studies are encouraging. They are encouraging because they show impacts on variables of high importance, such as work status and healthcare use. They are also encouraging because they include process analyses. There is additional work to do: larger randomized trials, and development work to produce versions of treatment that allow greater access, outside of specialty care, and versions that deliver greater impact more efficiently.

## References

Bach, P. and Hayes, S.C. (2002). The use of Acceptance and Commitment Therapy to prevent the rehospitalization of psychotic patients: a randomized controlled trial. *Journal of Consulting and Clinical Psychology*, **70**, 1129–39.

Baer, R.A. (2003). Mindfulness training as a clinical intervention: a conceptual and empirical review. *Clinical Psychology Research and Practice*, **10**, 125–43.

Beck, A.T. (1976). *Cognitive therapy and the emotional disorders*. New York: Meridian.

Bond, F.W. and Bunce, D. (2000). Mediators of change in emotion-focused and problem-focused worksite stress management interventions. *Journal of Occupational Health Psychology*, **5**, 156–63.

Brown, K.W. and Ryan, R.M. (2003). The benefits of being present: mindfulness and its role in psychological well-being. *Journal of Personality and Social Psychology*, **84**, 822–48.

Burns, D.D. and Spangler, D.L. (2001). Do changes in dysfunctional attitudes mediate changes in depression and anxiety in cognitive behavioral therapy? *Behavior Therapy*, **32**, 337–69.

Cano, A., Gillis, M., Heinz, W., Geisser, M., and Foran, H. (2004). Marital functioning, chronic pain, and psychological distress. *Pain,* **107,** 99–106.

Cheung, N.M., Wong, T.C.M., Yap, J.C.M., and Chen, P.P. (2008). Validation of the Chronic Pain Acceptance Questionnaire (CPAQ) in Cantonese-speaking Chinese patients. *Journal of Pain,* **9,** 823–832.

Crombez, G., Morley, S., McCracken, L.M., Sensky. T., and Pincus, T. (2003). Self, identity and acceptance in chronic pain. In J.O. Dostrovsky, D.B. Carr, M. Koltzenburg (Eds.) *Proc. 10th World Congress on Pain,* Vol. 24, pp. 651–9. Seattle: IASP Press.

Dahl, J., Wilson, K.G. and Nilsson, A. (2004). Acceptance and Commitment Therapy and the treatment of persons at risk for long-term disability resulting from stress and pain symptoms: a preliminary randomized trial. *Behavior Therapy,* **35,** 785–801.

David, D. and Szentagotai, A. (2006). Cognitions in cognitive-behavioral psychotherapies: toward an integrative model. *Clinical Psychology Review,* **26,** 284–98.

De Jong, J.R., Vlaeyen, J.W.S., Onghena, P., Cuypers, C., den Hollander, M. and Ruijgrok, J. (2005). Reduction of pain-related fear in complex regional pain syndrome type I: the application of graded exposure in vivo. *Pain,* **116,** 264–275.

Dimidjian, A., Hollon, S.D., Dobson, K.S., *et al.* (2006). Randomized trial of behavioral activation, cognitive therapy, and antidepressant medication in the acute treatment of adults with major depression. *Journal of Consulting and Clinical Psychology,* **74:** 658–70.

Ellis, A. (1994). *Reason and emotion in psychotherapy* (Rev. edn.). Secaucus, NJ: Birch Lane.

Flor, H., Frydrich, T., Turk, D.C. (1992). Efficacy of multidisciplinary pain treatment centers: a meta-analytic review. *Pain,* **49,** 221–230.

Fordyce, W.E. (1976). *Behavioral methods for chronic pain and illness.* Saint Louis, MO: Mosby.

Geiser, D.S. (1992). A Comparison of acceptance-focused and control-focused psychological treatments in a chronic pain treatment center. Unpublished Doctoral Dissertation, Reno: University of Nevada.

Grossman, P., Niemann, L., Schmidt, S. and Walach, H. (2004). Mindfulness-based stress reduction and health benefits: a meta-analysis. *Journal of Psychosomatic Research,* **57,** 35–43.

Gutierrez, O., Luciano, C., Rodriguez, M. and Fink, B.C. (2004). Comparison between an acceptance-based and a cognitive-control-based protocol for coping with pain. *Behavior Therapy,* **35,** 767–83.

Hayes, S.C., Strosahl, K. and Wilson, K.G. (1999a). *Acceptance and Commitment Therapy: An experiential approach to behavior change.* New York: Guildford Press.

Hayes, S.C., Bissett, R.T., Korn, A., *et al.* (1999b).The impact of acceptance versus control rationales on pain tolerance. *Psychological Record,* **49,** 33–47.

Hayes, S.C., Follette, V.M. and Linehan, M.M. (2004). *Mindfulness and acceptance: expanding the cognitive-behavioral tradition.* New York: The Guilford Press.

Hayes, S.C., Luoma, J.B., Bond, F.W., Masuda, A. and Lillis, J. (2006). Acceptance and Commitment Therapy; model, processes and outcomes. *Behaviour Research and Therapy,* **44,** 1–25.

Iverson, G.L. and Remick, R. (2004). Diagnostic accuracy of the British Columbia Major Depression Inventory. *Psychological Reports,* **95,** 1241–1247.

Jacobson, N.S., Dobson, K.S., Truax, P.A., *et al.* (1996). A component analysis of cognitive-behavioral treatment for depression. *Journal of Consulting and Clinical Psychology,* **64,** 295–304.

Jacobson, N.S., Roberts, L.J., Berns, S.B. and McGlinchey, J.B. (1999). Methods from defining and determining the clinical significance of treatment effects: description, application, and alternatives. *Journal of Consulting and Clinical Psychology,* **67,** 300–7.

Jacobson, N.S., Christensen, A., Prince, S.E., Codova, J. and Eldridge, K. (2000). Integrative behavioral couple therapy: an acceptance-based, promising new treatment for couple discord. *Journal of Consulting and Clinical Psychology,* **68,** 351–5.

James, W. (1950). *Principles of psychology* (reprint edition). New York: Dover Publications.

Kabat-Zinn, J. (1990). *Full catastrophe living: using the wisdom of your body and mind to face stress, pain, and illness.* New York: Dell Publishing.

Kabat-Zinn, J., Lipworth, L. and Burney, R. (1985). The clinical use of mindfulness meditation for self-regulation of chronic pain. *Journal of Behavioral Medicine*, **8**, 163–90.

Kaplan, K.H., Goldenberg, D.L. and Galvin-Nadeau, M. (1993). Impact of a meditation-based stress reduction program on fibromyalgia. *General Hospital Psychiatry*, **15**, 284–9.

Kohlenberg, R.J. and Tsai, M. (1991). Functional analytic psychotherapy: creating intense and curative therapeutic relationships. New York: Springer.

Longmore, R.J. and Worrell, M. (2007). Do we need to challenge thoughts in cognitive behavior therapy. *Clinical Psychology Review*, **27**, 173–87.

Ma, S.H. and Teasdale, J.D. (2004). Mindfulness-based cognitive therapy for depression: replication and exploration of differential relapse prevention effects. *Journal of Consulting and Clinical Psychology*, **72**, 31–40.

Martell, C., Addis, M. and Dimidgian, S. (2004). Finding the action in behavioral activation, in S.C. Hayes, V.M. Follette, M.M. Linehan (ed), *Mindfulness and acceptance: expanding the cognitive-behavioral tradition*, pp. 152–67. New York: The Guilford Press.

Masedo, A.I. and Esteve, M.R. (2007). Effects of suppression, acceptance and spontaneous coping on pain tolerance, pain intensity and distress. *Behaviour Research and Therapy*, **45**, 199–209.

Mason, V.L., Mathias, B. and Skevington, S.M. (2007). Accepting low back pain: is it related to good quality of life? *Clinical Journal of Pain*, **24**, 22–9.

McCracken, L.M. (1998). Learning to live with the pain: acceptance of pain predicts adjustment in persons with chronic pain. *Pain*, **74**, 21–7.

McCracken, L.M. (2005a). *Contextual Cognitive-Behavioral Therapy for chronic pain, Progress in pain research and management, vol 33*. Seattle, WA: IASP Press.

McCracken, L.M. (2005b). Social context and acceptance of chronic pain: the role of solicitous and punishing responses. *Pain*, **113**, 155–9.

McCracken, L.M. (2007). A contextual analysis of attention to chronic pain: what the patient does with their pain may be more important than their awareness or vigilance alone. *The Journal of Pain*, **8**, 230–6.

McCracken, L.M. and Eccleston, C. (2003). Coping or acceptance: what to do with chronic pain? *Pain*, **105**, 197–204.

McCracken, L.M. and Eccleston, C. (2005). A prospective study of acceptance of pain and patient functioning with chronic pain. *Pain*, **118**, 164–9.

McCracken, L.M. and Eccleston, C. (2006). A comparison of the relative utility of coping and acceptance-based measures in a sample of chronic pain sufferers. *European Journal of Pain*, **10**, 23–9.

McCracken, L.M. and Keogh, E. (2009). Acceptance, mindfulness, and values-based action may counteract fear and avoidance of emotions in chronic pain: An analysis of anxiety sensitivity. *The Journal of Pain*, **10**, 408–15.

McCracken, L.M. and Samuel, V.M. (2007). The role of avoidance, pacing, and other activity patterns in chronic pain. *Pain*, **130**, 119–125.

McCracken, L.M. and Thompson, M. (2009). Components of mindfulness in patients with chronic pain. *Journal of Psychopathology and Behavioral Assessment*, **31**, 75–82.

McCracken, L.M. and Vowles, K.E. (2008). A prospective analysis of acceptance of pain and values-based action in patients with chronic pain. *Health Psychology*, **27**, 215–20.

McCracken, L.M. and Yang, S-Y. (2006). The role of values in a contextual cognitive-behavioral analysis of chronic pain. *Pain*, **123**, 137–45.

McCracken, L.M. and Yang, S-Y. (2008). A contextual cognitive-behavioral analysis of rehabilitation workers' health and well-being: influences of acceptance, mindfulness, and values-based action. *Rehabilitation Psychology*, **53**, 479–85.

McCracken, L.M., Vowles, K.E. and Eccleston, C. (2004). Acceptance of chronic pain: component analysis and a revised assessment method. *Pain*, **107**, 159–66.

McCracken, L.M., Vowles, K.E. and Eccleston, C. (2005). Acceptance-based treatment for persons with complex, longstanding chronic pain: a preliminary analysis of treatment outcome in comparison to a waiting phase. *Behaviour Research and Therapy*, **43**, 1335–46.

McCracken, L.M., Vowles, K. and Thompson, M. (2007a). Comment on Nicholas and Asghari. *Pain,* **128**, 283–4.

McCracken, L.M., MacKichan, F. and Eccleston, C. (2007b). Contextual Cognitive-Behavioral Therapy for severely disabled chronic pain sufferers: effectiveness and clinically significant change. *European Journal of Pain,* **11**, 341–322.

McCracken, L.M., Gauntlett-Gilbert, J. and Vowles K. (2007c). The role of mindfulness in a contextual cognitive-behavioral analysis of chronic pain-related suffering and disability. *Pain,* **131**, 63–69.

Morley, S., Eccleston, C. and Williams, A.C. (1999). Systematic review and meta-analysis of randomized controlled trials of cognitive behaviour therapy and behaviour therapy for chronic pain in adults, excluding headache. *Pain,* **80**, 1–13.

Morone, N.E., Greco, C.M. and Weiner, D.K. (2008). Mindfulness meditation for treatment of chronic low back pain in older adults: a randomized controlled pilot study. *Pain,* **134**, 310–19.

Nicholas, M.K. and Asghari, A. (2006). Investigating acceptance in adjustment to chronic pain: is acceptance broader than we thought? *Pain,* **124**, 269–79.

Peat, G., Thomas, E., Handy, J. and Croft, P. (2004). Social networks and pain interference with daily activities in middle and old age. *Pain,* **112**, 397–405.

Rogers, C.R. (1964). Toward a modern approach to values: the valuing process in the mature person. *Journal of Abnormal and Social Psychology,* **68**, 160–7.

Sephton, S.E., Salmon, P., Weissbecker, I., *et al.* (2007). Mindfulness meditation alleviates depressive symptoms in women with fibromyalgia: results of a randomized clinical trial. *Arthritis & Rheumatism (Arthritis Care and Research),* **57**, 77–85.

Skinner, B.F. (1953). *Science and human behavior.* New York: The Free Press.

Schwartz, L., Jensen, M.P., Romano, J.M. (2005). The development and psychometric evaluation of an instrument to assess spouse responses to pain and well behavior in patients with chronic pain: the Spouse Response Inventory. *Journal of Pain,* **6**, 243–52.

Turk, D.C., Meichenbaum, D. and Genest, M. (1983). *Pain and behavioral medicine: a cognitive-behavioral perspective.* New York: The Guilford Press.

Viane, I., Crombez, G., Eccleston, C., *et al.* (2003). Acceptance of pain is an independent predictor of mental well-being in patients with chronic pain: empirical evidence and reappraisal. *Pain,* **106**, 65–72.

Vowles, K.E. and McCracken, L.M. (2008). Acceptance and values-based action in chronic pain: a study of treatment effectiveness and process. *Journal of Consulting and Clinical Psychology,* **76**, 397–407.

Vowles, K.E., McCracken, L.M., McLeod, C. and Eccleston, C. (2008). The Chronic Pain Acceptance Questionnaire: confirmatory factor analysis and identification of patient subgroups. *Pain,* **140**, 284–91.

Wagner, C.C. and Sanchez F.P. (2002). The role of values in motivational interviewing. In W.R. Miller, S. Rollnick (Eds.) *Motivational interviewing: preparing people for change* (2nd edn.), pp. 284–98. New York: Guilford Press.

Wicksell, R.K., Ahlqvist, J., Bring, A., Melin, L. and Olson, G.L. (2008). Can exposure and acceptance strategies improve functioning and life satisfaction in people with chronic pain and whiplash-associated disorders (WAD)? A randomized controlled trial. *Cognitive Behavior Therapy,* **37**, 169–82.

Williams, A.C. de C., Richardson, P.H., Nicholas, M.K., *et al.* (1996). Inpatient vs. outpatient pain management: results of a randomized controlled trial. *Pain,* **66**, 13–22.

Wilson, K.G. and Murrell, A.R. (2004). Values work in Acceptance and Commitment Therapy. In S.C. Hayes, V.M. Follette, and M.M. Linehan (Eds.) *Mindfulness and acceptance: expanding the cognitive-behavioral tradition,* pp. 121–51. New York: Guilford Press.

Zautra, A.J., Davis, M.C., Reich, J.W., *et al.* (2008). Comparison of cognitive behavioral and mindfulness meditation interventions on adaptation to rheumatoid arthritis for patients with and without history or recurrent depression. *Journal of Consulting and Clinical Psychology,* **76**, 408–21.

Zettle, R.D., Rains, J.C. (1989). Group cognitive and contextual therapies in treatment of depression. *Journal of Clinical Psychology,* **45**, 436–45.

Chapter 30

# Rehabilitation Programmes to Prevent Severely Disabling Chronic Back Pain

Michael K. Nicholas and Rob J.E.M. Smeets

## 30.1 Introduction

Once pain has persisted for several months and is associated with marked interference in daily activities and depressed mood, low self-efficacy, catastrophizing thoughts, and fear-avoidance beliefs, the risk is very high for continuing deterioration and reduced chances of returning to work and pre-injury lifestyles. Previous chapters in this book have clearly described the importance of identifying and helping those considered to be at risk of this secondary disability as soon as possible. But despite the best efforts of primary healthcare providers, a proportion of cases will still end up with chronic pain and many will continue to seek help. In their pursuit of help they often run the added risk of iatrogenic complications—complications caused by the treatments and attention they receive rather than the original injury. In many countries injured workers will be at increasing risk of losing their jobs the longer they are away from the workplace. They may have to deal not just with their pain and the associated activity limitations, but also with financial pressures, relationship difficulties, and the unwanted effects of multiple treatments. This chapter is directed at this group of people and their management and rehabilitation options.

Typically, the aims of rehabilitation at this stage are multiple. While pain relief is often the immediate focus of the patient, it is often unlikely to be achieved and some accommodation will have to be made to that. But other goals may well be feasible. These may be described broadly as quality of life goals, and may include return to desired work, home or social activities, as well as improved sleep, mood, and health. Some of these may initially be quite basic activities of daily living or independent functioning, like sitting long enough to achieve a task on a computer or drive to the shops. Others may be more complex, but whatever the task, the fundamental principle in all rehabilitation is that success will require the active participation of the patient suffering from pain. Rehabilitation cannot be done to someone; it can only be done with him or her. This has important implications for healthcare providers and agencies responsible for facilitating rehabilitation. It means we need to consider not just the nature of the pain but also the person in pain and his perspectives, abilities and goals (or desires), as well as the context in which he lives—the workplace, the home, even the broader social environment via the available social support systems.

In previous chapters the early identification of those at risk as well as potential contributing personal and environmental factors were described, so they will not be repeated here. Instead, we will explore the tasks likely to be involved in helping those who have slipped through the early management 'net' and the evidence for the interventions employed as pain persists beyond the first few months.

## 30.2 **A conceptual framework for assessment and multidisciplinary rehabilitation**

Biopsychosocial models of pain have provided the most widely-accepted conceptual framework for pain rehabilitation for over 40 years and different versions of this model have been extensively described throughout this book. A version of a biopsychosocial approach has also been described for general use in the World Health Organization (WHO) International Classification of Functioning, Disability, and Health (2001). This classification has attempted to capture the key features of the biopsychosocial models and to provide a basis for operational definitions of these key elements. Specifically, it identifies three core elements: body systems (body functions and structures), the individual (activity) and society (participation), all of which are expected to interact (see Figure 30.1).

As can be seen in Figure 30.1, bodily functions and structures are defined as physiological functions of body systems or anatomical structures. Activity is defined as the capacity of the person to execute a task or action. This action is an inherent or intrinsic feature of the person himself, without the influence of varying environmental factors (e.g. bending forward). Participation is the actual performance of activities in the person's current environment aimed at engaging in a life situation (e.g. work, preparing a meal, picking up a child from school, driving the car to the supermarket, despite limited ability to bend forward, sit, stand, or walk). This account of a biopsychosocial model encourages the eliciting of information about the effects the environment (physical and social) as well as personal factors (such as age, education, fear of injury, motivation) may have on the person's actions. As such, it is expected to set the scene for possible interventions. Depending upon the assessed features of a particular individual patient, these interventions may vary from one person to another. Thus, if environmental factors (e.g. excessively rigid and unrealistic expectations for recovery by the workplace supervisor) appear to be acting as a barrier to an injured worker's rehabilitation then that would need to be addressed by the rehabilitation team as part of their intervention, possibly even through specific training for the workplace supervisor (e.g. Shaw et al. 2006, 2008). Equally, if the injured worker displayed strong

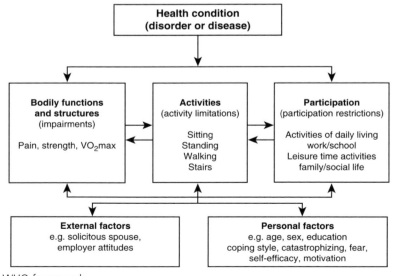

**Fig. 30.1** WHO framework.

catastrophic responses to his or her pain then they too would need to be targeted as part of the intervention plan (e.g. Sullivan et al. 2006).

An important feature of the WHO model is that it indicates specific types of data that might be collected and that, in turn, suggests the involvement of different disciplines in the assessment process, as few individuals would be expected to have the skills required to assess all elements. This provides overt encouragement for a multidisciplinary approach which would be expected to include a formulation of the individual case, ideally at a team meeting, followed by preparation of a treatment plan. This case formulation approach has a long history in behavioural therapies and was recently outlined for application to pain patients by Linton and Nicholas (2008).

## 30.3 **Importance of treatment settings and contexts**

The studies describing early interventions for low back pain (LBP) are usually conducted in primary care settings, such as general medical practitioner or private physiotherapy clinics, as well as hospital outpatient physiotherapy departments (e.g. Hay et al. 2005; Jellema et al. 2005; Pengel et al. 2007; Underwood et al. 2007). Typically, the focus of treatments in these settings is symptom relief and return to normal functioning at work or home as soon as possible. But as the pain becomes identified as more chronic and early interventions are not succeeding patients tend to be seen in a wider range of settings and by a wider range of healthcare providers, with some variation between countries and healthcare systems. Thus, different hospital departments, different specialists, and rehabilitation services staffed by a range of healthcare disciplines and even commercial healthcare institutes specialized in early return to work are often introduced. These might include orthopaedic surgeons, neurologists, anaesthesiologists, occupational or rehabilitation medicine specialists, clinical psychologists, social workers, occupational therapists, nurses specialized in pain management, as well as physiotherapists and providers of numerous complementary therapies (eg. Blyth et al. 2005; Loisel et al. 2002; Skouen et al. 2006; Smeets et al. 2006).

The focus of interventions can also start to shift. Instead of symptom relief and rapid return to normal lifestyle, the focus often moves towards symptom management and gradual return to normal lifestyle and in very severe cases adapting another lifestyle with new activities and roles. In many countries, not only may the treatment providers and the focus of treatment start to change as pain becomes more chronic, but other interested parties, such as third-party (e.g. workers compensation) insurers and the workers' employer, may begin to enter the picture. As pain becomes more chronic, while immediate return to work may become less of an expectation for both the healthcare providers and the patients, the third-party funder and the employer may well have quite different expectations. Franche et al. (2005a) tried to tease out a number of possible expectations, or paradigms, which might be held by the key stakeholders (the patient, the healthcare providers, the employer, the insurance company, the union, etc.) and to explore how these might influence outcomes. Potentially, where these paradigms differed or were in conflict, the effectiveness of even treatments with good supporting evidence might be reduced.

The presence of a compensation claim, for instance, has been widely recognized as a potential inhibitor of good treatment outcomes. This isn't just in rehabilitation settings. A meta-analysis by Harris (2005) found that the outcomes of surgery differed according to whether or not the patients had a compensation claim, regardless of country or type of surgery. Where the intervention takes place might also influence the outcomes achieved even when seemingly similar approaches are being taken. For example, Loisel et al. (2002) found that treatment that included being at work for workers with persisting back pain achieved fewer lost work days at long-term follow-up than treatments that did not include the workplace. A systematic review by Franche et al. (2005b) also found that when the treatment provider actively engaged with the workplace as part of the treatment process, better return to work outcomes and reduced costs were achieved (see Chapter 19 by Shaw et al. for further discussion of this topic).

The cultural and societal contexts can also play an important role in the way people with LBP behave. The results of a large population-based intervention (via advertisements on television and on bill boards by major roads) showed that changing the societal beliefs and expectations regarding the management of LBP, especially the activity restrictions due to pain, reduced the overall reporting of LBP, associated healthcare consumption and economic costs due to LBP (Buchbinder and Jolley 2004). Nevertheless, as the positive results tended to decline in the space of a few years once the advertising campaign ceased, reinforcement of the newly acquired beliefs seems to be important.

In sum, when considering the management of patients who do not respond to early intervention methods the tasks facing the treatment provider are likely to become more complex and to involve more stakeholders. In fact, if this is not recognized by the treatment provider who continues to treat the pain as if it were acute it is quite possible they run the risk of unintentionally making things worse and prolonging their patient's disability. These iatrogenic risks have been well described by others (e.g. Loeser 1996), but the point when the pursuit of pain relief should cease to be the focus and rehabilitation goals should become dominant will remain hotly debated.

## 30.4 **Timing of rehabilitation and decision rules**

To date, while there is general agreement that rehabilitation approaches should be commenced as early as possible, consensus is lacking on when that should be. In many countries there may be systemic obstacles to early intervention that may effectively restrict access to early rehabilitation. Nevertheless, even in the acute phase, it is argued that the aim of treatment providers should not only be to reduce the pain but also check for potential risk factors for the development of chronicity and associated disability (van der Windt et al. 2008). However, recent research has found that when primary healthcare providers (general practitioners or physiotherapists) are specifically trained to identify and address psychosocial risk factors for chronic disability, the results have been rather disappointing (Hay et al. 2005; Jellema et al 2005). In part, this has been attributed to the general practitioners having difficulty in identifying the psychosocial risk factors (Jellema et al. 2005). In the study by Hay and colleagues (2005) no treatment integrity was reported, but the therapists were provided training for only 2 days which might indicate that these rather inexperienced care-providers were not sufficiently trained to diagnose and treat psychosocial risk factors. In these two studies also, the number of patients with psychosocial risk factors in patients with (sub)acute complaints seemed rather low, diluting the potential effects of this intervention.

Timing is also strongly dependent on the financial resources available to the healthcare system as well as the accessibility and availability of well equipped and experienced healthcare providers. For example, in the Netherlands the access to a clinical psychologist in the primary care setting has recently been improved due to a change in the healthcare system. Nevertheless, the number of permitted sessions is limited and most patients have to pay additional fees and last but not least, the number of psychologists sufficiently trained in secondary prevention of chronic pain syndromes is too low to meet the demand. As a result many of these patients are being treated longer than necessary by other primary healthcare providers, mostly using a pain-focussed rather than a rehabilitation-focussed approach.

Given the evidence that untreated psychosocial factors are likely to lead to more patients with chronic pain and associated disability, the net result is that pain management and rehabilitation facilities become the last resort for an increasing number of people. But as there are relatively few of these facilities, their capacity to meet the demand is rapidly overtaken and long waiting times for assessment and treatment are commonplace. The delays involved can also pose a serious risk for further deterioration in the well-being of these patients. As most compensation systems for injured workers have built in time limits for return to work, so that those not back at work within a set time (e.g. 6 months) may lose their jobs, the additional risk posed by long waiting times is that these patients may lose their jobs while waiting for help. Once an injured worker loses his/her job, the chances of return to work following treatment decline rapidly. Thus, outcomes for rehabilitation are usually much worse when dealing with unemployed workers. Ideally, timing for rehabilitation in these systems should intervening before the worker has lost his/her job.

Identifying and targeting specific contributors to disability has long been argued as a logical development in pain rehabilitation. Turk (1990), and more recently Vlaeyen and Morley (2005), have argued that if we could select the right treatment for the right patient it would be both more effective and potentially more cost-effective. This approach requires assessing patients with specific features, such as depression or fear-avoidance responses and offering them interventions targeted more specifically at these features.

The use of decision rules that might guide the selection of suitable individuals for specific interventions has recently gained some momentum with the publication of a number of studies that have tested different selection methods. This topic has been well-covered already in an earlier chapter (Chapter 11), but some examples of applications are relevant here. These have ranged from workplace characteristics (e.g. Shaw et al. 2006) to specific psychological risk factors, especially heightened catastrophizing (see Chapter 13). Some studies have also described successful interventions in cases identified according to their overall psychosocial risk profile rather than any particular characteristic. For example, Gatchel et al. (2003 used a statistical algorithm to select acute LBP patients as high risk for developing chronic disability. These patients were randomly assigned to either a cognitive-behavioural functional restoration group or a treatment-as-usual group. At follow-up the functional restoration group displayed significantly fewer indices of chronic pain disability on a wide range of work, healthcare utilization, medication use, and self-reported pain variables. A recent Canadian study (Schultz et al. 2008) with subacute LBP workers also found that selection of patients based on their overall risk profile was more effective than usual care. Specifically, Schultz et al. showed that only those at high risk of protracted disability required a more comprehensive biopsychosocial intervention. A similar finding with more chronic cases was reported from a large Norwegian study by Haldorsen et al. (2002); in that study it was only the cases with the poorest prognosis (identified by operational criteria) who required more comprehensive pain rehabilitation.

Sullivan and Stanish (2003) also reported encouraging results with their community-based programme (the Pain-Disability Prevention [PDP] Programme) with patients who had a mean time off work of 7 months due to back pain. In that study the treatment by psychologists targeted identified risk factors, such as catastrophizing responses to pain, heightened fear of movement or re-injury, and depressed mood. Although not a randomized trial, a majority (60%) of PDP-treated clients returned to work, compared to an 18% base rate of return (achieved previously). Sullivan et al. (2005) showed that, of 215 injured workers who completed the PDP Programme, treatment-related reductions in pain catastrophizing significantly predicted return-to-work (RTW). A similar programme (the Progressive Goal Attainment Programme, PGAP) for primary care professionals (mainly physiotherapists and occupational therapists) with individuals who had been work disabled (on average just over 7 months) due to whiplash symptoms, and were selected on the basis of the same heightened psychological risk factors as those employed in the PDP Programme, achieved a 75% return to work rate compared to 50% in an earlier cohort with usual treatment (Sullivan et al. 2006).

A number of controlled studies have reported similar positive findings for various psychosocial interventions for selected patients with subacute LBP (Anema et al. 2007; Damush et al. 2003; Hagen et al. 2000; Hasenbring et al. 1999; Hlobil et al. 2005; Karjalainen et al. 2005; Linton et al. 2005; Schiltenwolf et al. 2006; Staal et al. 2002; van den Hout et al. 2003) and while these are not specifically trials of matching patients' characteristics to interventions, they are consistent with this idea.

In relation to persisting or chronic pain conditions, a number of reviews and meta-analyses of randomized controlled trials (RCTs) have reported consistent findings that for patients with disabling chronic pain conditions coordinated, multidisciplinary interventions based on cognitive-behavioural methods provide a generally effective option for rehabilitation (Airaksinen et al. 2006; Guzman et al. 2001; McCracken and Turk 2002; Morley et al. 1999; Nielsen and Weir 2001). In the main, these studies have demonstrated that quality of life indicators tend to improve, and be maintained for up to a year following these interventions. However, the achievement of goals like RTW were rarely addressed by many of these programmes (e.g. Williams et al. 1999). This prompted one reviewer to write that the results in this domain were inconsistent (Guzman et al. 2001). Even so, some studies have demonstrated that reasonable RTW outcomes can be achieved, but there are caveats.

One of the largest and best-designed RTW studies with a more chronic pain population was described by Haldorsen et al. (2002). Importantly, the Haldorsen et al. study pointed to one of the emerging trends in this area: the role of selection of suitable patients and targeting of identified risk factors for disability. In that study, the patients (with LBP duration at least 2 months and up to 2 years) were divided into three subgroups according to an operationally-defined algorithm for prognosis (good, medium and poor prognoses). The individuals in these groups were then randomly assigned to one of three levels of intervention: a light, advice-based approach by the general practitioner, a brief, structured advice and activity programme, and a comprehensive, multidisciplinary, cognitive-behavioural pain rehabilitation programme. The RTW results over the following year clearly demonstrated a dose-problem interaction, with the poor prognostic group having much stronger RTW outcomes after the comprehensive intervention relative to the two lighter 'doses'. On the other hand, the medium prognostic group did just as well with the medium-level intervention as in the comprehensive intervention, and the good prognostic group did just as well in the light, advice intervention. This indicated that it would be false economy to direct all patients to the comprehensive programme, but if selected well enough good results could be obtained from all three groups if they were assigned interventions according to assessed need.

Close examination of several other randomized controlled studies reveals a similar picture and reinforces the idea of selecting the right dose for the right patient. For example, Williams et al. (1999) showed that moderately disabled patients with mixed chronic pain conditions responded better to a 4-week comprehensive inpatient programme and maintained these gains at 1-year follow-up over a similarly disabled group who received a lighter dose in the form of $8 \times 3$-hour weekly sessions as outpatients, who still improved relative to baseline and a group receiving standard care from their general practitioner. Also, Marhold and Linton (2001) found that more disabled chronic back pain patients responded less well to a brief ($12 \times 2$ hour) outpatient cognitive-behavioural programme compared to a group of less chronic and less disabled back pain patients.

Although the contingencies and philosophies operating in many clinical settings will tend to mean that clinicians will try to do what they can with what they have available, the evidence is building to suggest that some patients will have a much better chance of successful rehabilitation if they receive a dose of treatment proportionate to their need. This means that vigorous representations may need to be made to ensure this happens. Recent experiences in the US health maintenance environment provides testimony to this imperative (Robbins et al. 2003).

There is certainly growing evidence that patients can be clustered according to various dimensions and that these can have different implications for outcomes (e.g. Boersma and Linton 2005), but studies in which patients are assigned to interventions according to their sub-group characteristics remain limited. Perhaps the closest example is provided by the Haldorsen et al. (2002) study. Clearly there is an urgent need to replicate and extend these findings in other countries.

Overall, it is still the case that while the logic of matching patients to treatments seems compelling and the available evidence is supportive, the lack of RCTs evaluating the approach is a handicap and must be a priority in the next few years. Fortunately, some studies of this type are underway and some answers should be available shortly. But more will be needed.

## 30.5 **Integrating/combining with other treatment modalities**

As noted in the earlier section on the implications of a biopsychosocial perspective for managing persisting pain, a multidimensional assessment will often indicate that multiple interventions might be appropriate in individual cases. While much of the research literature on interventions seems to focus on the delivery of single modality interventions (e.g. a trial of an analgesic or an exercise programme), the reality in clinical practice is that multiple interventions will be considered and a key question is whether they should be delivered in series (with the following interventions depending upon the outcome of the earlier ones) or in parallel (i.e. simultaneous delivery). Typically, these would be directed against different targets, but before commencing such a multidimensional intervention process adequate preparation of the patient, in addition to the development of a coordinated plan, would seem appropriate. This is especially since different interventions can easily appear at cross purposes. For example, a patient could be offered a drug to relieve pain while also being encouraged to accept the presence of the pain and to exercise despite the pain.

Traditionally, many have taken the approach of waiting for adequate analgesia to be established before commencing rehabilitation. Collett (2001) described this as 'capitalising on improved analgesia' (p. 140). Although this expectation may hold with acute pain, like postsurgical cases (Stein 2000) and with cancer pain (Bruera et al. 1999), the evidence for patients with chronic non-cancer pain still seeking help for their pain despite repeated trials of medication is not so supportive of this position (Nicholas et al. 2006).

Unfortunately, there are relatively few good examples of combined interventions in the pain literature and the vast majority of treatment studies report outcomes from one intervention performed in isolation (Turk 2001). In some of these cases the researchers report significant improvements across a range of outcome domains, but generalizing from these examples requires caution. For example, Dreyfuss et al. (2000) reported improvements in disability with radiofrequency neurotomy for patients with chronic lumbar zygapophysial joint pain (a procedure aimed at pain relief), but examination of the disability level of their sample on the Roland and Morris Disability Questionnaire (Roland and Morris 1983), revealed that the mean score at pretreatment was 7. This reflects only mild disability and is well below the levels typically reported in those attending multidisciplinary pain rehabilitation settings (Nicholas et al. 2008). De Jong et al. (2005), for example, reported a mean score of 15 on the Roland and Morris Questionnaire at pretreatment. This means we should be cautious about generalizing from the Dreyfuss study as the radiofrequency procedure has not been demonstrated in more disabled chronic pain populations. Nevertheless, it would be interesting to see if a combination of radiofrequency neurotomy and a pain management programme would yield better results than either alone in the more disabled populations. To date, this has not been reported.

Despite the inherent difficulties in providing combined treatment modalities, there is emerging evidence that a strategy of combining treatments aimed at different targets in chronic pain patients can lead to better results than a single treatment on its own. In an uncontrolled trial Molloy et al. (2004) reported significant gains in mood and disability for patients diagnosed with failed back surgery syndrome when they were treated with a combination of an implanted spinal cord stimulator or a morphine pump plus a comprehensive 3-week, multidisciplinary cognitive-behavioural pain management programme rather than either an implant or a programme alone. This suggests that such combined approaches are possible, but no RCTs have yet been reported.

There are studies that have combined pharmacotherapy and rehabilitation interventions. For example, Holroyd et al. (1995, 2001) found that the combination of propranolol hydrochloride with relaxation plus biofeedback, as well as tricyclic antidepressants plus stress management training was more effective for reducing migraine headache activity than either of these interventions when used alone. Similarly, Kishino et al. (2000) reported that a combination of a psychological intervention that targeted patient motivation and exercise was superior to a graded exercise programme in patients with chronic back pain seen following spinal surgery. In patients with rheumatoid arthritis, Leibing et al. (1999) found that the combination of pharmacological and cognitive-behavioural treatment (CBT) achieved greater improvements on measures of depression, helplessness, affective pain scores and improved coping or adjustment compared to standard rheumatological (pharmacological) treatment. As a result the authors recommended the use of CBT as an effective adjunct to standard (rheumatological) treatment of rheumatoid arthritis outpatients. Similar findings were reported by Sharpe et al. (2001) following a randomized controlled trial with patients who had recent onset (less than 2 years) seropositive rheumatoid arthritis. To date, however, despite repeated calls (e.g. Haythornthwaite 2005; Turk 2001) there is a lack of trials of combined pharmacotherapy and multidisciplinary pain management in patients with chronic LBP.

It can be argued that many multidisciplinary CBT programmes are a form of combined intervention (e.g. van Tulder et al. 2000), but while they combine members of different disciplines in a coordinated way, typically they are driven by a self-management and rehabilitation philosophy and all elements are focused on equipping the participants to function as independently as possible of healthcare providers. This usually means medication is withdrawn (e.g. Nicholas 2008) rather than introduced, and that physical therapy involvement is more like that of a trainer than a 'hands-on' therapist (like manipulation). In this section we have defined combined interventions as those that target different aspects of a case simultaneously, based on a biopsychosocial assessment and case-formulation. These may include pharmacological or surgical interventions (i.e. dependent upon the healthcare provider) being provided alongside self-management approaches. While there is broad evidence in support of this approach, some of which was described earlier, there is clearly a need for more applied studies. In a review of outcomes from multidisciplinary pain clinics Clark (2000) found that multidimensional interventions were more effective across a range of dimensions compared to single modality (mostly medical) treatments alone. These findings should not be that surprising, but they do not overcome the need for more studies designed to test the combined hypothesis specifically. Of course, at a practical level the obstacles facing those trying to integrate different treatment modalities should not be underestimated. In addition to the challenges of grappling with the content of treatment packages, the treatment providers still face the task of integrating the treatment processes with the patient's social environment. This will be addressed in the next section.

## 30.6 **Integrating with the social environment**

Although most pain rehabilitation is conducted under the banner of a biopsychosocial model, recent reviews have questioned the degree to which the social (or environmental component) is included in intervention studies (Blyth et al. 2007). However, there is growing evidence for the value of including this often neglected dimension in pain rehabilitation. Much of the stimulus for this seems to have come from occupational rehabilitation, but some have been exploring the utility of including patients' families in the treatment process as well (Newton-John, 2002). The same applies for healthcare professionals involved in the care of patients with chronic pain related disability, especially since it is evident that their attitudes and beliefs influence treatment content and outcome. For example, clinicians with more biomedical orientations tend to give advice which results in a less active lifestyle (Bishop et al. 2008; Houben et al. 2005).

One of the early studies of occupational rehabilitation noted that better RTW outcomes were achieved when employers had what they termed 'proactive RTW policies' (Hunt and Harbeck 1993). That is, they had policies that tried to accommodate to the needs of injured workers and to facilitate their return to work rather than waiting for a medical interventions to do it for them. More recently, in a systematic review of this literature Franche et al. (2005a) concluded that there was moderately strong evidence from seven studies to support the value of liaison between healthcare providers and their patients' workplaces in facilitating RTW. The importance of including the workplace in rehabilitation for injured workers was further reinforced by the experience of McCluskey et al. (2006) who found their guideline-based return to work programme for injured workers was effectively undermined by the workplace's policies. Similarly, Shaw et al. (2006) have demonstrated that providing specific training for workplace supervisors was very effective in reducing workplace disability with injured workers.

Despite this evidence there is surprisingly little information in the pain rehabilitation literature of efforts to incorporate linkages to the workplace as an element of this work. In part, this may be due to health system limitations within many countries, especially those where return to work is not seen as a goal of healthcare (e.g. Waddell et al. 2002). To the extent that this means direct efforts to help injured workers return to work may be discouraged then it should not be surprising that links to workplaces are rarely included in many public hospital pain rehabilitation services (e.g. McCracken et al. 2007; Williams et al. 1996). However, given the known benefits of work on health and wellbeing it would seem an important area for expansion in these types of programmes in the future (Waddell et al. 2003). In some countries the public authority responsible for injured workers has directly funded pain rehabilitation services. In Canada, for example Tschernetzki-Neilson et al. (2007) described improved RTW outcomes achieved by the services in one state when the focus of rehabilitation was shifted from processes and functional capacity to RTW. This study underscored the point that system-level changes may be needed to bring about some changes in rehabilitation outcomes (see Chapter 19 for a fuller discussion).

While the logic of this extension of pain rehabilitation from the clinic to the workplace (and home) is not difficult to grasp, reliably delivering it in practice is a major problem in many health systems. This is especially the case where health has traditionally been closely defined within a biomedical perspective or paradigm. As Franche et al. (2005b) pointed out, the paradigm for healthcare providers has typically focussed on the individual patient, his or her medical status, and treatments accepted under local funding arrangements. RTW in this paradigm is left to the patient to undertake once they are medically 'better'. There is usually no direct benefit for the healthcare funders if the patient returns to work. In the UK, for example, the National Health Service is responsible for funding health services, but whether a patient returns to work or not makes no difference to the health service funding, though it may to the Department of Work and Pensions which is responsible for pensions if the person does not RTW (Waddell et al. 2002). However, the Department of Work and Pensions makes no contribution to the funding of health services, so they cannot differentially support treatments that might help someone RTW.

There is clearly an imperative for considering major social outcomes, such as RTW by injured workers, beyond the specific biomedical, diagnostic framework, regardless of the site of pain. This calls for approaches that can accommodate a real biopsychosocial perspective, not just a bio-psycho version that is so often presented (e.g. Blyth et al. 2007). To date, there are no examples in the pain literature of outcomes from comprehensive initiatives that target the full range of factors that may contribute to ongoing pain-related disability. However, there are examples of national and state-based rehabilitation or injury management systems that have reported attempts to engage in these processes (e.g. Kendall et al. 2004; Tschernetzki-Neilson et al. 2007; WorkCoverNSW 2008).

## 30.7 **Research agenda: the future**

Multidisciplinary pain management programmes have been proven effective, but effect sizes are typically only moderate. Possible reasons for this have been advanced but definitive evidence for interventions that reliably achieve better outcomes remains scarce. The case for more comprehensive interventions that might include multidisciplinary programmes, but other facets as well, has been argued here as a logical response to the shortcomings of the current literature. However, good evidence for the superiority of more comprehensive approaches over more narrowly focussed approaches is still limited. Despite the inherent difficulties of large scale research on comprehensive approaches it is hard to see how this field can make further real progress without such projects. This calls for researchers in this area to move out of the clinic and to negotiate with those responsible for broader aspects of the injury management and rehabilitation systems. Fortunately, there are precedents upon which we can draw at least inspiration (e.g. Loisel et al. 2002), but the difficulties should not be underestimated—as some have found to their cost (e.g. McClusky et al. 2006).

Despite the clear need for evaluation of more comprehensive interventions over single modality approaches, at the individual level, results vary greatly and for a proportion of individuals this treatment is not successful at all. The question of 'What works for whom?' remains only partially answered. Some individually targeted interventions for certain risk factors have been described and these do seem promising but more of these studies are urgently needed. Many studies have suffered from insufficient power to explore these questions, but it is also likely that interventions that are too narrowly focussed may miss important individual targets (e.g. just focussing on fear of movement through graded activity when over-reliance of medication may also need attention). In the 9 years since Haldorsen et al. (2002) published their study comparing level of intervention with level of prognostic signs, no other study has come near the degree of 'real world' testing of multidisciplinary interventions that group achieved. More of these sorts of studies must be a high priority. This review has also found remarkably few studies that investigate the integration of multiple, simultaneous interventions, particularly combining psychological-behavioural and medical-surgical regimes, still appear rarely in the research literature even though they are common in clinical practice. There are good examples in the literature which ought to be amenable to replication or adaptation (e.g. Leibing et al. 1999; also see Haythornthwaite et al. 2005). Innovative designs, such as N = 1 methods, might represent a means for further exploration of this topic in clinically meaningful ways (e.g. Linton and Nicholas 2008).

This review also raises the question of should we expect there to be a treatment to help everyone? As pointed out earlier (and in Chapters 19 and 24), work-related issues and motivational issues are likely to remain significant barriers to successful rehabilitation programmes, largely because they cannot be reliably controlled by the providers of these interventions. At a pragmatic level, if providers cannot change the system in which they work then identifying those individuals who are likely to respond to current interventions, given their limitations, remains a worthwhile focus for research, despite limited results to date (Underwood et al. 2007). The corollary in this regard is to explore ways of helping those who are unlikely to benefit from available options. This might mean shifting the focus from pain management or pain rehabilitation per se, to dealing with interpersonal or family issues, as exemplified in work on communications and anger management with pain populations (e.g. Greenwood et al. 2003).

While consensus on the content, intensity and duration of treatment modalities necessary for successfully preventing disability remains elusive, there is growing evidence for specific features of these interventions for particular patient subgroups (Guzman et al. 2001; Haldorsen et al. 2002; Smeets et al. 2006). Long-term effectiveness and adherence to behavioural change remains a challenge that is likely to be beyond the resources of most pain rehabilitation programmes in isolation. The analysis presented here (and elsewhere in this book) suggests that answers to these questions are likely to come from work on patient selection for programmes, tailored interventions, and the peri-programme environment, such as the workplace, other treatment providers, and the broader context of the rehabilitation system, rather than a healthcare facility alone.

# References

Airaksinen, O., Brox, J.I., Cedraschi, C. et al. (2006). European guidelines for the management of chronic nonspecific low back pain. *European Spine Journal*, **15** (Suppl. 2), S192–S300.

Anema, J.R., Steenstra, I.A., and Bongers, P.M. (2007). Multidisciplinary rehabilitation for subacute low back pain: graded activity or workplace intervention or both? A randomized controlled trial. *Spine*, **32**, 291–8.

Bishop, A., Foster, N., Thomas, E. et al. (2008). How does the self-reported clinical management of patients with low back pain relate to the attitudes and beliefs of health care practitioners? A survey of UK general practitioners and physiotherapists. *Pain* **135**, 187–95.

Blyth, F.M., March, L., Nicholas, M.K. and Cousins, M.J. (2005). Self-management of chronic pain: a population-based study. *Pain*, **113**, 285–92.

Blyth, F.M., Macfarlane, G.J., and Nicholas, M.K. (2007). Understanding the role of psychosocial factors in the development of chronic pain: the key to better outcomes for patients? *Pain*, **129**, 8–11.

Boersma, K., and Linton, S.J. (2005). Screening to identify patients at risk profiles of psychological risk factors for early intervention. *Clinical Journal of Pain*, **21**, 38–43.

Boersma, K. and Linton, S.J. (2006) Psychological processes underlying the development of a chronic pain problem: a prospective study of the relationship between profiles in the fear-avoidance model and disability. *Clinical Journal of Pain* **22**, 160–6.

Bruera, E., Walker, P., and Lawlor, P. (1999). Opioids in cancer pain. In Stein, C. (Ed.). *Opioids in Pain Control: Basic and Clinical Aspects*, pp. 309–24. Cambridge University Press, Cambridge.

Buchbinder. R., and Jolley, D. (2004). Population based intervention to change back pain beliefs: three year follow up study. *British Medical Journal*, **328**, 321.

Clark, T.S. (2000). Interdisciplinary treatment for chronic pain: is it worth the money? *Baylor University Medical Center Procedings*, **13**, 240–3.

Collett, B.J. (2001). Chronic opioid therapy for noncancer pain. *British Journal of Anaesthesia*, **87**, 133–44.

Damush, T.M., Weinberger, W., Perkins, S.M. et al. (2003). The long term effects of a self-management program for inner city primary care patients with acute low back pain. *Archives of Internal Medicine*, **163**, 2632–8.

de Jong, J.R., Vlaeyen, J.W.S., Onghena, P., Goosens, M.E.J.B., Geilen, M. and Mulder, H. (2005). H. Fear of movement/reinjury in chronic low back pain. Education or exposure in vivo as mediator to fear reduction. *Clinical Journal of Pain*, **21**, 9–17.

Dreyfuss, P., Halbrook, B., Pauze, K., Joshi, A., McLarty, J. and Bogduk, N. (2000). Efficacy and validity of radiofrequency neurotomy for chronic lumbar zygapophysial joint pain. *Spine*, **25**, 1270–7.

Franche, R.-L., Cullen,K., Clarke, J., Irvin, E., Sinclair, S. and Frank, J. (2005a). Workplace-based return to work interventions: A systematic review of the quantitative literature. *Journal of Occupational Rehabilitation,* **15**(4), 607–32.

Franche, R-L., Baril, R., Shaw, W., Nicholas, M.K. and Loisel, P. (2005b). Workplace-based return-to-work interventions: Optimizing the role of stakeholders in implementation and research. *Journal of Occupational Rehabilitation* **15**(4), 525–42.

Gatchel, R.J., Polatin, B.P., Noe, C. et al. (2003). Treatment- and cost-effectiveness of early intervention for acute low-back pain patients: A one-year prospective study. *Journal of Occupational Rehabilitation,* **13**, 1–9.

Greenwood, K.A., Thurston, R., Rumble, M.,Waters, S.J. and Keefe, F.J.(2003). Anger and persistent pain: current status and future directions. *Pain,* **103**, 1–5

Guzman, J., Esmail, R., Karjalainen, K., et al. (2001). Multidisciplinary rehabilitation for chronic low back pain: systematic review. *British Medical Journal,* **322**, 1511–16.

Hagen, E.M., Eriksen, H.R., and Ursin, H. (2000). Does early intervention with a light mobilization program reduce long-term sick leave for low back pain? *Spine,* **25**, 1973–76.

Haldorsen, E.M.H., Grasdal, A.L., Skouen, J.S. et al.(2002). Is there a right treatment for a particular patient group? Comparison of ordinary treatment, light multidisciplinary treatment, and extensive multidisciplinary treatment for long-term sick-listed employees with musculoskeletal pain. *Pain,* **95**, 49–63.

Harris, I.A. (2005). Association between compensation status and outcome after surgery: a meta-analysis. *Journal of the American Medical Association,* **293**, 1644–52.

Hasenbring, M., Ulrich, H.W., Hartmann, M. et al. (1999). The efficacy of a risk factor based cognitive behavioral intervention and EMG-biofeedback in patients with acute sciatic pain: an attempt to prevent chronicity. *Spine* **24 (23)**, 2525–35.

Hay, E.M., Mullis, R., Lewis, M. et al. (2005). Comparison of physical treatments versus a brief pain management programme for back pain in primary care: a randomised clinical trial in physiotherapy practice. *Lancet,* **365**, 2024–30.

Haythornthwaite, J.A. (2005). Clinical trials studying pharmacotherapy and psychological treatments and together. *Neurology,* **65**(suppl 4), S20–S31.

Hlobil, H., Staal, B.J., Twisk, J. et al. (2005). The effects of a graded activity intervention for low back pain in occupational health on sick leave, functional status and pain: 12-month results of a randomized controlled trial. *Journal of Occupational Rehabilitation,* **15**, 569–80.

Holroyd, K.A., O'Donnell, F.J., Stenland, M. et al. (2001). Management of chronic tension-type headache with tricyclic antidepressant medication, stress management therapy, and their combination - a randomized controlled trial. *Journal of the American Medical Association,* **285**, 2208–17.

Holroyd, K.A., France, J.L., Cordingley, G.E., et al. (1995). Enhancing the effectiveness of relaxation-thermal biofeedback with propranolol hydrochloride. *Journal of Consulting and Clinical Psychology,* **63**, 327–36.

Houben, R.M.A., Ostelo, R.W.J.G., Vlaeyen, J.W.S. et al. (2005) Health care providers' orientations towards common low back pain predict perceived harmfulness of physical activities and recommendations regarding return to normal activity. *European Journal of Pain,* **9**, 173–83.

Hunt, A. and Harbeck, R. (1993). *The Michigan Disability Prevention Study.* WE Upjohn Institute for Employment Research, Kalamazoo, MI.

Jellema, P., van der Windt, D.A.M.W., van der Horst, H.E., Twisk, J.W.R., Stalman, W.A.B. and Bouter, L.M. (2005). Should treatment of (sub)acute low back pain be aimed at psychosocial prognostic factors? Results of a cluster-randomised clinical trial in general practice. *British Medical Journal,* **331**, 84–90.

Karjalainen, K., Malmivaara, A., Mutanen, P., Roine, R., Hurri, H. and Pohjolainen, T. (2004). Mini-intervention for subacute low back pain two-year follow-up and modifiers of effectiveness. *Spine,* **29**, 1069–76.

Kendall, N.A.S., Linton, S.J., and Main, C.J. (2004). *Guide to Assessing Psych-social Yellow Glagsin Acute Low Back Pain: Risk Factors for Long-Term Disability and Work Loss*. Accident Compensation Corporation and the New Zealand Guidelines Group, Wellington, New Zealand

Kishino, N.D., Polatin, P.B., Brewer, S. and Hoffman, K. (2000). Long-term effectiveness of combined spinal surgery and functional restoration: a prospective study. *Journal of Occupational Rehabilitation*, **10**, 235–9.

Leibing, E., Pfingsten, M., Bartman, U., Leibing, U.R. and Gerhard, S. (1999). Cognitive-behavioral treatment in unselected rheumatoid arthritis outpatients. *Clinical Journal of Pain*, **15**, 58–66.

Linton, S.J., Boersma, K., Jansson, M., Svärd, L., and Botvalde, M. (2005). The Effects of Cognitive-Behavioral and Physical Therapy Preventive Interventions on Pain-Related Sick Leave: A Randomized Controlled Trial. *Clinical Journal of Pain*, **21**, 109–19.

Linton, S.J. and Nicholas, M.K. (2008). After assessment, then what? Integrating findings for successful case formulation and treatment tailoring. In Breivik, H., Campbell, W.J., Nicholas, M.K. (Eds.) *Practice and Procedures, Textbook of Clinical Pain Management* 2nd edition, Hodder Arnold, New York, pp. 95–106.

Loeser, J.D. (1996). Mitigating the dangers of pursuing cure. In: Cohen, M.J.M., Campbell, J.N. (eds.) *Pain Treatment Centers at a Crossroads: A Practical and Conceptual Reappraisal*. IASP Press, Seattle, WA, pp. 101–8.

Loisel, P., Lemaire, J., Poitras, S. et al. (2002). Cost-benefit and cost-effectiveness analysis of a disability prevention model for back pain management: a six year follow up study. *Occupational and Environmental Medicine*, **59**, 807–15.

Marhold, C., Linton, S.J. and Melin, L. (2001).A cognitive-behavioral return-to-work program: effects on pain patients with a history of long-term versus short-term sick leave. *Pain*, **91**, 155–63

McCluskey, S., Burton, A.K. and Main, C.J. (2006). The implementation of occupational health guidelines principles for reducing sickness absence due to musculoskeletal disorders. *Occupational Medicine*, **56**, 237–42.

McCracken, L.M. and Turk, D.C. (2002). Behavioral and cognitive-behavioral treatment for chronic pain: outcome, predictors of outcome, and treatment process. *Spine*, **27**(22), 2564–73.

McCracken, L. M., MacKichan, F. and Eccleston, C. (2007). Contextual cognitive-behavioral therapy for severely disabled chronic pain sufferers: Effectiveness and clinically significant change. *European Journal of Pain*, **11**, 314–22.

Molloy, A.R., Nicholas, M.K., Asghari, A. et al. (2006). Does a combination of intensive cognitive-behavioural pain management and a spinal implantable device confer any advantage? A preliminary examination. *Pain Practice*, **6**, 96–103.

Morley, S., Eccleston, C. and Williams, A. (1999). Systematic review and meta-analysis of randomized controlled trials of cognitive behaviour therapy and behaviour therapy for chronic pain in adults, excluding headache. *Pain*, **80**(1–2), 1–13.

Newton-John, T.R.O. (2002) Solicitousness and chronic pain: a critical review. *Pain Rev*, 9(1), 7–27.

Nicholas, M.K. (2008). Pain management in musculoskeletal conditions. *Best Practice in Research and Clininical Rheumatology*, **22**(3), 451–70.

Nicholas, M.K., Molloy, A.R. and Brooker, C. (2006). Using opioids with persisting, noncancer pain: A biopsychosocial perspective. *Clinical Journal of Pain*, **22**(2), 137–46.

Nicholas, M.K., Asghari, A. and Blyth, F.M. (2008). What do the numbers mean? Normative data in chronic pain measures. *Pain*, **134**, 158–73.

Nielson, W. and Weir, R. (2001). Biopsychosocial approaches to the treatment of chronic pain. *Clinical Journal of Pain*, **17**, S114–127.

Pengel, L.H.M., Refshauge, K.M., Maher, C.G., Nicholas, M., Herbert, R.D. and McNair, P. (2007). Physiotherapist-directed exercise, advice, or both for sub-acute low back pain: a randomized controlled trial. *Annals of Internal Medicine*, **146**(11), 787–96.

Robbins, H., Gatchel, R.J., Noe, C. et al. (2003). A prospective one-year outcome study of interdisciplinary chronic pain management: Compromising its efficacy by managed care policies. *Anesthesia and Analgesia*, **97**, 156–62.

Roland, M. and Morris, R. (1983). A study of the natural history of back pain. Part 1.Development of a reliable and sensitive measure of disability in low-back pain. *Spine*, **8**, 141–4.

Schiltenwolf, M., Buchner, M., Heindl, B., von Reumont, J., Müller, A., and Eich, W. (2006). Comparison of a biopsychosocial therapy (BT) with a conventional biomedical therapy (MT) of subacute low back pain in the first episode of sick leave: a randomized controlled trial. *European Spine Journal*, **15**, 1083–92.

Schultz, I.Z., Crook, J., Berkowitz, J., Milner, R., Meloche, G.R. and Lewis, M.L. (2008). A prospective study of the effectiveness of early intervention with high-risk back-injured workers – a pilot study. *Journal of Occupational Rehabilitation*, **18**, 140–51.

Sharpe, L., Sensky, T., Timberlake, N., et al. (2001). A blind, randomized, controlled trial of cognitive-behavioural intervention for patients with recent onset rheumatoid arthritis: preventing psychological and physical morbidity. *Pain*, **89**, 275–83.

Shaw, W.S., Robertson, M.M., McLellan, R.K., Verma, S. and Pransky, G. (2006). A controlled case study of supervisor training to optimize response to injury in the food processing industry. *Work*, **26**,107–14.

Shaw, W.S., Quan-nha Hong, Q., Pransky, G. and Loisel, P. (2008). A Literature Review Describing the Role of Return-to-Work Coordinators in Trial Programs and Interventions Designed to Prevent Workplace Disability. *Journal of Occupational Rehabilitation*, **18**, 2–15

Skouen, J.S., Grasdal, A. and Haldorsen, E.M.H. (2006). Return to work after comparing outpatient multidisciplinary treatment programs versus treatment in general practice for patients with chronic widespread pain. *European Journal of Pain*, **10**, 145–52.

Smeets, R.J.E.M., Vlaeyen, J.W.S., Kester, A.D.M. and Knottnerus, J.A. (2006). Reduction of Pain Catastrophizing Mediates the Outcome of Both Physical and Cognitive-Behavioral Treatment in Chronic Low Back Pain. *Journal of Pain*, **7**(4), 261–71.

Staal, J.B., Hlobil, H., van Tulder, M.W., Koke, A.J.A., Smid, T., and van Mechelen, W. (2002). Return-to-work interventions for low back pain. A descriptive review of contents and concepts of working mechanisms. *Sports Medicine*, **32**, 251–67.

Stein, C. (2000). What's wrong with opioids in chronic pain? *Current Opinion in Anesthesiology*, **13**, 557–9.

Sullivan, M.J. and Stanish, W.D. (2003). Psychologically based occupational rehabilitation: The Pain-Disability Prevention Program. *Clinical Journal of Pain*, **19**, 97–104.

Sullivan, M.J., Ward, L.C., Tripp, D., Adams, H. and Stanish, W.D. (2005). Secondary prevention of work disability: Community-based psychosocial intervention for musculoskeletal disorders. *Journal of Occupational Rehabilitation*, **15**(3), 377–92.

Sullivan, M.J., Adams, H., Rhodenizer, T. and Stanish, W.D. (2006). A psychosocial risk factor-targeted intervention for the prevention of chronic pain and disability following whiplash injury. *Physical Therapy*, **86**(1), 8–18.

Tschernetzki-Neilson, P.J., Brintnell, S., Haws, C. and Graham, K. (2007). Changing to an outcome-focused program improves return to work outcomes. *Journal of Occupational Rehabilitation*, **17**, 473–86.

Turk, D.C. (1990). Customizing treatment for chronic pain patients: who, what, and why. *Clinical Journal of Pain*, **6**(4), 255–70.

Turk, D.C. (2001). Combining somatic and psychosocial treatment for chronic pain patients: perhaps 1 + 1 does = 3. *Clinical Journal of Pain*, **17**(4), 281–3.

Turk, D.C. and Okifuji, A. (1998). Treatment of chronic pain patients: clinical outcomes, cost-effectiveness, and cost-benefits of multidisciplinary pain centers. *Critical Reviews in Physical Rehabilitation Medicine*, **10**, 181–208.

Underwood, M.R., Morton, V. and Farrin, A. (2007). Do baseline characteristics predict response to treatment for low back pain? Secondary analysis of the UK BEAM dataset. *Rheumatology*, **46**(8), 1297–302.

van den Hout, J.H., Vlaeyen, J.W., Heuts, P.H., Zijlema, J.H. and Wijnen, J.A.(2003). Secondary prevention of work-related disability in nonspecific low back pain: Does problem-solving therapy help? A randomized clinical trial. *Clinical Journal of Pain*, **19**, 87–96.

van der Windt, D., Hay, E., Jellema, P. and Main, C.J.(2008). Psychosocial interventions for low back pain in primary care: Lessons learned from recent trials. *Spine*, **33**, 81–89.

van Tulder, M.W., Ostelo, R.W.J.G., Vlaeyen, J.W.S., et al. (2000). Behavioural treatment for chronic low-back pain. *The Cochrane Database of Systematic Reviews*, **2**, CD002014.

Vlaeyen, J.W.S., de Jong, J., Geilen, M., Heuts, P.H.T.G. and van Breukelen, G. (2002). The treatment of fear of movement/(re)injury in chronic low back pain: further evidence on the effectiveness of exposure in vivo. *Clinical Journal of Pain*, **18**, 251–61.

Vlaeyen, J.W.S. and Morley, S. (2005). Cognitive-Behavioral Treatments for Chronic Pain: What Works for Whom? *Clinical Journal of Pain*, **21**, 1–8.

Waddell, G., Aylward, M. and Sawney, P. (2002). *Back pain, incapacity for work and social security benefits: An international literature review and analysis.* The Royal Society of Medicine Press, London.

Waddell, G., Burton, A. K. and Main, C. J. (2003). *Screening of DWP clients for risk of long-term incapacity: a conceptual and scientific review.* Royal Society of Medicine Monograph; Royal Society of Medicine Press, London.

WHO. (2001). *The International Classification of Functioning, Disability and Health (ICF).* 2nd ed. WHO, Geneva.

Williams, A.C. Nicholas, M.K., Richardson, P.H., Pither, C.E. and Fernandes, J. (1999). Generalizing from a controlled trial: the effects of patient preference versus randomization on the outcome of inpatient versus outpatient chronic pain management. *Pain*, **83**(1), 57–65.

Williams, A.C., Richardson, P.H., Nicholas, M.K. et al. (1996). Inpatient versus outpatient pain management: results of a randomised controlled trial. *Pain*, **66**, 13–22.

WorkCover NSW. (2006).*Management of Soft Tissue Injuries (General Guide, Insurer Guide and version for Treatment Providers)*, Locked Bag 2906, Lisarow, NSW 2252, Australia.

# Index